Mental Health Care for Elite Athletes

Claudia L. Reardon

Editor

Mental Health Care for Elite Athletes

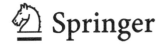 Springer

Editor
Claudia L. Reardon
Department of Psychiatry
University of Wisconsin School of Medicine and Public Health
Madison, WI, USA

ISBN 978-3-031-08363-1   ISBN 978-3-031-08364-8   (eBook)
https://doi.org/10.1007/978-3-031-08364-8

This Springer imprint is published by the registered company Springer Nature Switzerland AG
The registered company address is: Gewerbestrasse 11, 6330 Cham, Switzerland

For elite athletes everywhere. We know that any perception of your life being easy, your performance effortless, is a fallacy. You are worthy human beings—more than the number on the scoreboard or the time on the jumbotron.

Preface

Those of us working with elite athletes—collegiate, professional Olympic, and Paralympic—know the real deal. We see the pain every day. It is far from the life of luxury and ease that some seem to perceive. When I see athletes being ridiculed in television media, or blasted on social media, it all but brings me to tears. When I see them being discussed with venom and judgment, as if they are immune to criticism, I cannot help but think of the friend, the family member, the PERSON they are. Tomorrow I might see that athlete in my psychiatry practice. And what I see is their humanity, their suffering, their fallibility.

When you watch a top-level athlete perform at the Olympics or the national championships or the fill-in-the-blank other major competition, it looks easy, effortless, and glamorous. They are strong, confident, poised, and beautiful. Right? And also maybe they have major depressive disorder. Perhaps they are suicidal. They might have a crushing panic attack later tonight. An eating disorder may plaque their every waking thought.

Sometimes such mental health symptoms and disorders might be completely coincidental to their role as athlete. All too often, though, the system of high-level sport that the world and its institutions have set up for them is a prime driver of their symptoms.

How does it feel to be made into a commodity? It gnaws at you—even if you can't exactly pinpoint the source of angst—when your coaches, sponsors, agents, and even maybe your loved ones and medical treatment team give you differential attention depending on your most recent sports performance.

How does it feel to not have an exit option from sport, even if it is driving you to the breaking point? What if the only thing your friends and family ask about when you go "back home" is how your sport is going? There would be nothing for them to discuss otherwise. You'd be nothing otherwise. What if your sport is the only avenue through which you can attend college, or support your family, because there otherwise aren't funds or other options?

Sport promotes a sense of competence, higher academic and occupational functioning, and social and emotional growth. It is a driver of many good things. Except when it isn't. Except when it is the perfect recipe for disaster. Disaster of the mind.

This book is borne of many years of international collaborations. The contributors were carefully, thoughtfully hand-chosen as genuinely "getting it." They care about the athletes. They see the pain and work tirelessly to improve it. I hope you will be inspired to do the same.

Madison, WI, USA   Claudia L. Reardon

Contents

Scope of the Problem of Mental Health Symptoms and Disorders in Elite Athletes

Simon M. Rice, Courtney C. Walton, Lisa Olive, Claudia L. Reardon, and Rosemary Purcell

Mental health is identified as an integral dimension of elite athlete well-being. Entwined with other aspects of physical health and athletic performance, attention to mental health will reduce suffering and bolster quality of life in elite athletes [1], and assist in simultaneously normalising and de-stigmatising mental health concerns for broader society [2]. Up until recently, mental health has not been a major area of focus or training for sports medicine practitioners [3], with other health professionals (e.g. psychologists, mental health nurses) or sub-specialities of medicine (e.g. primary care physicians, psychiatrists) usually providing care for affected athletes. Consequently, as a broad population, elite athletes have been largely ignored in relation to mental health programming [3]. This has occurred in spite of the unique stressors associated with high-performing athletic careers [4]. Increasingly, the emergent fields of sports psychiatry and clinical sports psychology have catalysed greater attention to the identification and management of mental health symptoms and disorders among elite athletes [5, 6]. Together, with insights from the disciplines of sports and performance psychology, athlete mental health is now seen as an important field of multidisciplinary research and practice.

This chapter provides a foundational perspective on the scope of the problem of elite athlete mental health symptoms and disorders, providing context and background information for the proceeding chapters. The chapter commences with an outline of why the developmental phase of emerging adulthood is a period of unique risk for mental health symptom incidence, and how this stage is relevant for elite athletes. The chapter then progresses to a summary of current elite athlete epidemiological data, highlights key risk and protective factors, and concludes with a rationale for why a focus on athlete mental health is essential in supporting integrated care for the well-being and performance of athletes.

Emerging Adulthood and Mental Health

The years of emerging adulthood span the age range of 18–25 years [7]. Emerging adulthood reflects five theorised developmental features that are most prominently experienced during these years. The five developmental features are characterised by: *identity exploration* leading to subsequent enduring identity choices, *instability* due to identity explorations and associated experiences, *self-focus* where knowledge, skills, and self-understanding are developed for later adult life, *feeling in-between* with neither fixed adolescent or proper adulthood identities and *possibilities/optimism* about entering adult life and a sense of positivity about what lies ahead [8].

The emerging adulthood concept is particularly relevant for elite athletes for two key reasons. Firstly, the years of 18–25 overlap with the peak competitive years for athletic achievement [9]. While there are of course exceptions to this—especially among endurance sports (where athletes are often older) and gymnastics (where athletes are often younger)—the vast majority of peak athletic achievement occurs in the 20s. Illustrating this, the mean age of world class swimmers is 22.7 and 23.2 years for females and males, respectively [10]. Secondly, the years of emerging adulthood and peak athletic competition also overlap with the peak

S. M. Rice (✉) · C. C. Walton · R. Purcell
Elite Sport and Mental Health, Orygen, Melbourne, VIC, Australia

Centre for Youth Mental Health, The University of Melbourne, Melbourne, VIC, Australia
e-mail: simon.rice@orygen.org.au; courtney.walton@orygen.org.au; rosie.purcell@orygen.org.au

L. Olive
Elite Sport and Mental Health, Orygen, Melbourne, VIC, Australia

Centre for Youth Mental Health, The University of Melbourne, Melbourne, VIC, Australia

School of Psychology, Deakin University, Geelong, VIC, Australia
e-mail: lisa.olive@deakin.edu.au

C. L. Reardon
Department of Psychiatry, University of Wisconsin School of Medicine and Public Health, Madison, WI, USA
e-mail: clreardon@wisc.edu

incidence age range for the emergence of mental health problems. [11] Research demonstrates that over 50% of mental health disorders onset prior to age 15, with 63–75% presenting by 25 years [11, 12]. Mental health ranks among the most important concerns voiced by young people, across high-, middle-, and low-income countries [13]. Consequently, specific youth mental health models have been developed to address the specific psychosocial needs of emerging adults, with a focus on accessible, low-stigma, and timely early intervention [13, 14]. Drawing these lines of research together, recent empirical work indicates that relative to older cohorts, those aged 18–25 years do indeed report significantly higher ratings for features of emerging adulthood (e.g. identity exploration, self-focus, instability, possibilities/optimism), in addition to higher endorsement of symptoms of mental health disorders [8]. This age range also overlaps with key developmental considerations related to mental health including seeking of autonomy, enhanced awareness of pressure to conform with peers (and/or perceived gender or other cultural norms), exploration of sexual identity, increased access to information and technology, hormonal changes, increasing salience of emotional responses to social stimuli, and changes to motivation [15]. The following section defines key constructs within mental health and examines the prevalence and experiences of mental health symptoms and disorders among elite athletes.

High and Low Prevalence Disorders

The World Health Organisation (WHO) defines health as a state of physical, mental, and social well-being rather than merely the absence of disease [16]. More specifically, mental health is conceptualised as a state where individuals are able to realise their own abilities, cope, and respond to the expected stressors of life, productively work and achieve, and contribute meaningfully to their community [17]. As mental health disorders account for close to one-in-six deaths globally [18], they rank among the most substantial causes of death worldwide; however, there is inequitable access to treatment across the globe. The WHO estimates that 76–85% of people with severe mental health disorders who reside in low- and middle-income countries receive no treatment [19]. Resourcing and the level of access elite athletes have to evidence-based intervention are therefore important considerations outside of high-income countries or settings.

Mental health disorders are often delineated into high prevalence (or common) disorders and low prevalence disorders according to their occurrence in the general population. High prevalence disorders include mood, anxiety, somatoform, and substance use disorders, as these are relatively frequently observed in general primary care settings [20]. High prevalence disorders are usually responsive to psychothera-

peutic intervention (e.g. talk-based therapy), although combination therapy (e.g. antidepressant or anxiolytic medication together with talk-based therapy) may be needed in some instances. A small proportion of the general population will experience severe or complex presentations necessitating multidisciplinary team-based care (e.g. medical/psychiatry, psychological/case management, psychosocial recovery support) [21].

Low prevalence disorders are less likely to be experienced in the general population, comprising psychotic disorders (including schizophrenia), bipolar disorder, and eating disorders [22]. In general, low prevalence disorders tend to be associated with higher levels of functional impairment and treatment/service usage [23]. While the prevalence of psychotic, bipolar, and eating disorders in elite athlete populations is unclear, symptoms of these disorders are not necessarily incompatible with athletic achievement [24], especially when these conditions are well managed, in remission, or if the athlete is in a euthymic state. Consequently, it is important for medical and other mental health practitioners working in the elite sport context to be familiar with high and low prevalence disorders and key management considerations. Practitioners are directed to subsequent chapters of this text, in addition to the International Olympic Committee (IOC) expert consensus statement on mental health in elite athletes [1] and the associated papers on specific disorders for further information.

While prevalence data for mental health symptoms and disorders among elite athletes continues to emerge, high-quality studies using structured clinical interviews are lacking. Current best estimates of prevalence are reported in the 2019 meta-analysis from Gouttebarge and colleagues [25] pooling athlete self-report data. This meta-analytic review concluded that approximately 19.6% of elite athletes experience symptoms of psychological distress, 26.4% experience sleep disturbance symptoms, 33.6% experience symptoms of anxiety and/or depression, and 18.8% of athletes report symptoms of alcohol misuse, with broadly comparable rates experienced among retired athletes. A subsequent meta-analysis by Rice and colleagues [26] examined predictors of symptomatic anxiety (excluding competitive anxiety) and found that career dissatisfaction, female gender, younger age, musculoskeletal injury, and recent adverse life events were all associated with higher athlete anxiety. While the epidemiology of athlete mental health problems is becoming stronger, important questions related to mental health symptom prevalence remain, including specific understandings of pathways of impairment and recovery among athletes experiencing threshold disorder and/or mental health crisis (e.g. suicide risk or attempt [27, 28]), although guidelines for managing acute mental health symptoms among athletes are available [29].

General and Athlete-Specific Risk Factors

Development of positive mental health among elite athletes requires attention to key risk and protective factors that may increase (or decrease) the likelihood of symptom onset, maintenance or recurrence. It is important to consider the multidimensional nature of contributors to mental health problems, commonly referred to within the biopsychosocial framework [30]. Biopsychosocial approaches are increasingly being applied to athletic settings [31–33] and conceptualise the multiple social, psychological, and biological determinants of an athlete's mental health functioning.

General biopsychosocial risk factors for the development of mental health problems during late adolescence and emerging adulthood range from biological and genetic factors including family history of mental health problems and problematic substance use, through to psychological and social factors including exposure to traumatic events (e.g. physical abuse, sexual abuse, family violence, bereavement), experiences of discrimination, on-going life stressors, relationship difficulties, and financial problems [34, 35]. Among elite athletes specifically, identified risk factors for experiencing mental health symptoms include current injury status, prior history of a mental health problem, experiences of adverse life events, forced or unplanned retirement, sport-specific stressors including travel and (social) media pressures, help-seeking stigma, ineffective coping, maladaptive personality traits (e.g. perfectionism), and lack of social support from family, teammates, and/or coaches [36, 37]. Some evidence also suggests gender differences in mental health problems for elite athletes, whereby women athletes report higher rates of mental health symptoms, lower rates of well-being, and more frequent exposures to interpersonal conflict, financial hardship, and discrimination relative to men athletes [38]. Recent evidence suggests little difference in mental health outcomes between athletes competing in para sports and non-para sport athletes [39]. Finally, managing performance disappointment is an essential aspect of elite athlete mental health, and there is a growing literature on acceptance, compassion-based, and cognitive treatments that may assist in supporting athletes in instances of perceived failure (as well as managing other mental health risks) [40–42].

Sports administrators, coaches, and support staff should be aware of mental health protective factors among elite athletes, creating opportunities to integrate and maximise these wherever possible. General mental health protective factors include protective and supportive peer and familial relationships, positive lifestyle factors (diet, exercise), perceived mastery and autonomy, and vocational and educational engagement [34, 43]. Among elite athletes, sports-specific factors include positive relationships and supports in the sporting environment, organisation-wide mental health literacy, an athletic environment characterised as mastery-oriented, use of active behavioural coping strategies, and where appropriate, successful adjustment to competitive retirement—which requires sufficient attention and planning during competitive years [36, 37]. In addition, athletes who hold positive attitudes towards mental health help seeking (often as a result of efforts to promote mental health literacy) are more likely to engage with effective supports and interventions relative to athletes experiencing mental health stigma. Understanding athlete help seeking barriers can ensure these obstacles are addressed.

Help Seeking and Help Seeking Barriers

Athletes have been shown to hold less positive attitudes towards mental health help seeking than the general community [44]. A recent systematic review examining cultural influences and barriers to athletes seeking treatment identified four major contributors preventing athlete mental health help seeking: stigma, low mental health literacy, negative past experience with mental health treatment-seeking, and busy schedules [45]. Additionally, hypermasculinity was identified as a barrier specific to males. As mentioned above, mental health literacy programmes are able to improve mental health literacy and shift attitudes in relation to stigma. Mental health literacy programmes have been discussed in the various position statements on athlete mental health that have been published in recent years [46], underscoring the importance of these initiatives. In addition, the dissemination of mental health awareness messaging should be provided to key support people linked to the athlete, including partners, friends, family, coaching and administration staff, as these people are often the first point of contact for athletes experiencing emerging mental health symptoms rather than mental health professionals. However, for this to occur successfully, collaborative efforts are required between sports medicine practitioners, psychiatrists, psychologists, and other mental health professionals who are mindful of the athletic context and associated opportunities and limitations for messaging. Organisational factors should be considered, and a growing area of research inquiry and practice relates to psychological safety.

Psychological Safety in Elite Sport Settings

In its broadest sense, psychological safety refers to an individual experiencing feelings of safety to take interpersonal risks or make mistakes without fear of negative consequences [47]. A recent systematic review of 67 sport-based studies found that psychological safety in sport contexts was conceptualised as a group level construct that is perceived (and reported) at an individual level, defined as the perception that one is protected from, or unlikely to be at risk of, psychological harm in sport [48]. Since its original application in organisational settings, the concept of psychological safety has been applied to numerous contexts, including healthcare, education, manufacturing, and technology settings [49]. Evidence supports a range of positive outcomes associated with psychologically safe teams, including facilitated learning, task and team performance, engagement, and creativity [50]. These benefits are thought to occur because psychological safety allows teams to provide open feedback, discuss errors, collaborate, and experiment with new ideas [49]. Psychological safety may also act as an environmental protective factor against mental health symptoms or disorders [51, 52], possibly given the increased openness and vulnerability that the concept enables between team members.

The IOC Mental Health in Elite Athletes Toolkit, published in 2021, assists stakeholders to develop and implement initiatives that protect and promote the mental health and well-being of elite athletes [53]. A core component involved in the protection and promotion of elite athlete mental health outlined by the IOC Toolkit is the concept of psychological safety—defined in the Toolkit as the creation of athletic environments enabling athletes to be comfortable being themselves, feeling able to take necessary interpersonal risks, having the sufficient knowledge and understanding about mental health symptoms and disorders, and experiencing a sense of comfort in being able to seek mental health help if needed. The concept of psychological safety intuitively lends itself to safeguarding athlete mental health; however, the operationalisation of psychological safety occurs at the organisational level, influenced by organisational culture including policies, procedures, and behaviours that communicate a sense of safety (or otherwise) to the athlete. There are efforts underway to assess psychological safety in elite sport contexts using valid and reliable approaches, with promising early findings. Preliminary data from our research group has identified that domains of sport psychological safety, as assessed by a novel scale, were inversely related to general and athlete-specific psychological distress, and positively associated with psychological well-being among elite athletes [54].

While the concept of psychological safety is well established as foundational to underpinning the culture of high-performing teams across corporate and medical sectors [55], there has been comparatively less integration of the concept within the elite sports setting. It is likely that the IOC Toolkit and other efforts will help catalyse attention to the ways in which the sports sector can focus on enhancing psychological safety. Emerging evidence suggests that sport environments that are psychologically safe have the capacity to enhance teamwork and satisfaction with team performance and act as a buffer against athlete burnout [56]. Importantly, mental health literacy programmes have been shown to impact factors that contribute to creating and maintaining psychologically safe climates, including reducing stigma, normalising mental health symptoms, and increasing confidence and intentions to help others [57]. In summary, organisational-level variables such as psychological safety should be considered important in the broader ecology of athlete mental health and appreciated as an important cultural influence on athlete well-being outcomes [58].

Cultures of Care for Elite Athlete Mental Health

The established field of youth mental health is underpinned by an early intervention framework focussing on accessible and youth-friendly cultures of care. Box 1.1 outlines important concepts from the youth mental health field that can be applied to the elite athlete context to ensure best practice. While it is acknowledged that limited resourcing for mental health programmes in many elite sports settings will prohibit the development of specialised or bespoke services, similar to the developing cultures of psychological safety (which can be achieved through low-cost policy and practice changes), many aspects of youth-focussed practice can be provided within modifications or augmentation to existing service models for youth and young adults alike.

Box 1.1 Key Considerations for Sports Settings Regarding Youth and Young Adult Mental Health Interventions [59]

- Stakeholder (youth) consultation in service design and delivery
- Development of youth-friendly, stigma-free cultures of care
- Sensitivity to developmental factors and challenges experienced by emerging adults including integrating shared decision-making
- Provision of psychoeducation and mental health literacy support for caregivers (e.g. partners, families)
- Use of preventive and optimistic frameworks that emphasise evidence-based and evidence-informed early intervention
- Person-centred care, organised around the needs of the young person including flexibility with appointment hours as needed
- Flexible points of re-entry to care as needed, particularly around periods of transition, which may heighten mental health risks

There is a need for new, athlete-specific models of mental health care to capitalise on an early intervention framework for youth mental health [58]. Wherever possible, this should ensure early detection and prompt access to high-quality, evidence-based interventions. Growing momentum is developing around the implementation of mental health screening programmes alongside physical health checks for elite athletes [60], especially given athlete-specific screening tools and assessment procedures are now recommended [61, 62]. In a number of countries, specialised models of care have been developed and evaluated to support elite athlete mental health, with a focus on acceptability and engagement [63]. For example, the national Mental Health Referral Network developed by the Australian Institute of Sport (AIS) provides an example of a decentralised model of care where mental health clinicians experienced in evidence-based intervention and the elite sport environment provide confidential treatment to elite athletes, coordinated centrally and funded by the AIS [3, 64]. While similar models of care are provided in other sport settings internationally, high-quality athlete-specific mental health intervention is not universally available, especially in many low- and middle-income settings. Nonetheless, lower resource interventions and initiatives are becoming increasingly available globally, and impactful organisational approaches (e.g. psychological safety [65]) can be instituted at relatively low cost.

Conclusion

Athletes are susceptible to mental health problems by virtue of both being human and the additional risk factors experienced in sport. The broad range of health and sporting professionals working in elite sport will encounter athletes experiencing metal health symptoms and disorders. There is opportunity for practitioners to view interactions with athletes experiencing mental health symptoms as a standard part of their role, referring on to specialists as they would for the management of other physical health concerns. Important progress has been achieved in improving athlete mental health across the last decade. This momentum will continue to catalyse on-going efforts in stigma reduction and mental health-related attitudes, positively impacting broader tiers of competition (e.g. junior and community sport), and population health more generally.

References

1. Reardon CL, Hainline B, Aron CM, et al. Mental health in elite athletes: International Olympic Committee consensus statement. Br J Sports Med. 2019;53(11):667–99.
2. Walton CC, Purcell R, Rice S. Addressing mental health in elite athletes as a vehicle for early detection and intervention in the general community. Early Interv Psychiatry. 2019;13(6):1530–2.
3. Rice S, Butterworth M, Clements M, et al. Development and implementation of the national mental health referral network for elite athletes: a case study of the Australian Institute of Sport. Psychology. 2020;4(S1):27–35.
4. Rice S, Walton CC, Gwyther K, Purcell R. Mental health. In: Arnold R, Fletcher D, editors. Stress, well-being, and performance in sport. New York: Routledge; 2021.
5. Donohue B, Murphy S, Rice S, Carr C. Clinical sport psychology in practice: sport-specific roles, settings, strategies, and recommendations for its advancement. In: The Routledge handbook of clinical sport psychology. New York: Routledge; 2021. p. 11–24.
6. Reardon CL, Factor RM. Sport psychiatry. Sports Med. 2010;40(11):961–80.
7. Arnett JJ. Emerging adulthood: what is it, and what is it good for? Child Dev Perspect. 2007;1(2):68–73.
8. Arnett JJ, Mitra D. Are the features of emerging adulthood developmentally distinctive? A comparison of ages 18–60 in the United States. Emerg Adulthood. 2020;8(5):412–9.
9. Allen SV, Hopkins WG. Age of peak competitive performance of elite athletes: a systematic review. J Sports Med. 2015;45(10):1431–41.
10. Mallett A, Bellinger P, Derave W, Osborne M, Minahan C, Coaching. The age, height, and body mass of olympic swimmers: a 50-year review and update. Science. 2021;16(1):210–23.
11. Kessler RC, Berglund P, Demler O, Jin R, Merikangas KR, Walters EE. Lifetime prevalence and age-of-onset distributions of DSM-IV disorders in the National Comorbidity Survey Replication. Arch Gen Psychiatry. 2005;62(6):593–602.
12. Solmi M, Radua J, Olivola M, et al. Age at onset of mental disorders worldwide: large-scale meta-analysis of 192 epidemiological studies. Mol Psychiatry. 2021;2021:1–15.
13. Patel V, Flisher AJ, Hetrick S, McGorry P. Mental health of young people: a global public-health challenge. Lancet. 2007;369(9569):1302–13.
14. McGorry P, Trethowan J, Rickwood D. Creating headspace for integrated youth mental health care. World Psychiatry. 2019;18(2):140.
15. WHO. Adolescent mental health 2020. https://www.who.int/news-room/fact-sheets/detail/adolescent-mental-health2021.
16. WHO. Constitution of the world health organisation. Geneva: WHO; 2006.
17. WHO. Mental health: a state of well-being. 2014. https://www.who.int/features/factfiles/mental_health/en/2021.
18. Walker ER, McGee RE, Druss BG. Mortality in mental disorders and global disease burden implications: a systematic review and meta-analysis. JAMA Psychiat. 2015;72(4):334–41.
19. WHO. Mental health action plan 2013-2020. Geneva: WHO; 2013.
20. Ansseau M, Dierick M, Buntinkx F, et al. High prevalence of mental disorders in primary care. J Affect Disord. 2004;78(1):49–55.
21. Rice SM, McKechnie B, Cotton S, et al. Severe and complex youth depression: Clinical and historical features of young people attending a tertiary mood disorders clinic. Early Interv Psychiatry. 2021;16(3):316–22.
22. Baxter AJ, Patton G, Scott KM, Degenhardt L, Whiteford HA. Global epidemiology of mental disorders: what are we missing? PLoS One. 2013;8(6):e65514.
23. McGrath JJ, Charlson F, Whiteford HA. Challenges and options for estimating the prevalence of schizophrenia, psychotic disorders, and bipolar disorders in population surveys. 2016. http://sites.nationalacademies.org/cs/groups/dbassesite/documents/webpage/dbasse_173004.pdf
24. Currie A, Gorczynski P, Rice SM, et al. Bipolar and psychotic disorders in elite athletes: a narrative review. Br J Sports Med. 2019;53(12):746–53.
25. Gouttebarge V, Castaldelli-Maia JM, Gorczynski P, et al. Occurrence of mental health symptoms and disorders in current and former elite athletes: a systematic review and meta-analysis. Br J Sports Med. 2019;53(11):700–6.

26. Rice SM, Gwyther K, Santesteban-Echarri O, et al. Determinants of anxiety in elite athletes: a systematic review and meta-analysis. Br J Sports Med. 2019;53(11):722–30.

27. Newman HJ, Howells KL, Fletcher D. The dark side of top level sport: an autobiographic study of depressive experiences in elite sport performers. Front Psychol. 2016;7:868.

28. Doherty S, Hannigan B, Campbell MJ. The experience of depression during the careers of elite male athletes. Front Psychol. 2016;7:1069.

29. Currie A, McDuff D, Johnston A, et al. Management of mental health emergencies in elite athletes: a narrative review. Br J Sports Med. 2019;53(12):772–8.

30. Engel GL. The clinical application of the biopsychosocial model. In: The Journal of Medicine and Philosophy, vol. 1981; 1981. p. 101–24.

31. DeFreese J. Athlete mental health care within the biopsychosocial model. West Deptford: SLACK Incorporated Thorofare; 2017.

32. von Rosen P, Frohm A, Kottorp A, Fridén C, Heijne A. Multiple factors explain injury risk in adolescent elite athletes: applying a biopsychosocial perspective. Scand J Med Sci Sports. 2017;27(12):2059–69.

33. Solomon GS, Haase RF. Biopsychosocial characteristics and neurocognitive test performance in National Football League players: an initial assessment. Arch Clin Neuropsychol. 2008;23(5):563–77.

34. Barnes GE, Mitic W, Leadbeater B, Dhami MK. Risk and protective factors for adolescent substance use and mental health symptoms. Can J Commun Ment Health. 2009;28(1):1–15.

35. Dooley B, Fitzgerald A, Giollabhui N. The risk and protective factors associated with depression and anxiety in a national sample of Irish adolescents. Ir J Psychol Med. 2015;32(1):93–105.

36. Küttel A, Larsen CH. Risk and protective factors for mental health in elite athletes: a scoping review. Int Rev Sport Exerc Psychol. 2020;13(1):231–65.

37. Purcell R, Rice S, Butterworth M, Clements M. Rates and correlates of mental health symptoms in currently competing elite athletes from the Australian National high-performance sports system. Sports Med. 2020;50(9):1683–94.

38. Walton CC, Rice S, Gao CX, Butterworth M, Clements M, Purcell R. Gender differences in mental health symptoms and risk factors in Australian elite athletes. BMJ Open Sport Exerc Med. 2021;7(1):e000984.

39. Olive LS, Rice S, Butterworth M, Clements M, Purcell R. Do rates of mental health symptoms in currently competing elite athletes in paralympic sports differ from non-para-athletes? Sports Med. 2021;7(1):1–9.

40. Henriksen K, Hansen J, Larsen CH. Mindfulness and acceptance in sport: How to help athletes perform and thrive under pressure. New York: Routledge; 2019.

41. Mosewich AD. Self-compassion in sport and exercise. In: Handbook of sport psychology. Hoboken: Wiley; 2020. p. 158–76.

42. Jordana A, Turner MJ, Ramis Y, Torregrossa M. A systematic mapping review on the use of rational emotive behavior therapy (REBT) with athletes. Int Rev Sport Exerc Psychol. 2020;2020:1–26.

43. Piechaczek CE, Pehl V, Feldmann L, et al. Psychosocial stressors and protective factors for major depression in youth: evidence from a case–control study. Child Adolesc Psychiatry Ment Health. 2020;14(1):1–11.

44. Watson JC. College student-athletes' attitudes toward help-seeking behavior and expectations of counseling services. J Coll Stud Dev. 2005;46(4):442–9.

45. Castaldelli-Maia JM, Gallinaro JG, Falcão RS, et al. Mental health symptoms and disorders in elite athletes: a systematic review on cultural influencers and barriers to athletes seeking treatment. Br J Sports Med. 2019;53(11):707–21.

46. Gorczynski P, Currie A, Gibson K, et al. Developing mental health literacy and cultural competence in elite sport. J Appl Sport Psychol. 2020;2020:1–15.

47. Edmondson A. Psychological safety and learning behavior in work teams. Adm Sci Q. 1999;44(2):350–83.

48. Sutcliffe J, Mayland, E., Schweickle, M., McEwan, D., Swann, C., Vella, S. Psychological safety in sport: a systematic review and concept analysis. Canadian Society for Psychomotor Learning and Sport Psychology Conference. 2021.

49. Newman A, Donohue R, Eva N. Psychological safety: a systematic review of the literature. Hum Resour Manag Rev. 2017;27(3):521–35.

50. Frazier ML, Fainshmidt S, Klinger RL, Pezeshkan A, Vracheva V. Psychological safety: a meta-analytic review and extension. Pers Psychol. 2017;70(1):113–65.

51. Vévoda J, Vévodová Š, Nakládalová M, et al. The relationship between psychological safety and burnout among nurses. Occup Med. 2016;2:68.

52. Zhao F, Ahmed F, Faraz NA. Caring for the caregiver during COVID-19 outbreak: does inclusive leadership improve psychological safety and curb psychological distress? A cross-sectional study. Int J Nurs Stud. 2020;110:103725.

53. Committe IO. Mental health in elite athletes toolkit. 2021.

54. Rice S, Walton C, Pilkington V, Gwyther K, Olive L, Lloyd M, Kountouris A, Butterworth M, Clements M, Purcell R. Psychological safety in elite sport settings: development and validation of the sport psychological safety inventory. 2021.

55. Edmondson AC, Lei Z. Psychological safety: the history, renaissance, and future of an interpersonal construct. Annu Rev Organ Psych Organ Behav. 2014;1(1):23–43.

56. Fransen K, McEwan D, Sarkar M. The impact of identity leadership on team functioning and well-being in team sport: is psychological safety the missing link? Psychol Sport Exerc. 2020;51:101763.

57. Breslin G, Shannon S, Haughey T, Donnelly P, Leavey G. A systematic review of interventions to increase awareness of mental health and well-being in athletes, coaches and officials. Syst Rev. 2017;6(1):1–15.

58. Purcell R, Gwyther K, Rice SM. Mental health in elite athletes: increased awareness requires an early intervention framework to respond to athlete needs. J Sports Med. 2019;5(1):1–8.

59. McGorry PD, Goldstone SD, Parker AG, Rickwood DJ, Hickie IB. Cultures for mental health care of young people: an Australian blueprint for reform. Lancet Psychiatry. 2014;1(7):559–68.

60. Drew M, Petrie TA, Palmateer T. National Collegiate Athletic Association Athletic Departments' mental health screening practices: who, what, when, and how. J Clin Sport Psychol. 2021;1:1–17.

61. Rice S, Olive L, Gouttebarge V, et al. Mental health screening: severity and cut-off point sensitivity of the athlete psychological strain questionnaire in male and female elite athletes. BMJ Open Sport Exerc Med. 2020;6(1):e000712.

62. Gouttebarge V, Bindra A, Blauwet C, et al. International olympic committee (IOC) sport mental health assessment tool 1 (SMHAT-1) and sport mental health recognition tool 1 (SMHRT-1): towards better support of athletes' mental health. Br J Sports Med. 2021;55(1):30–7.

63. Donohue B, Gavrilova Y, Galante M, et al. Controlled evaluation of an optimization approach to mental health and sport performance. J Clin Sport Psychol. 2018;12(2):234–67.

64. Olive L, Rice S, Butterworth M, Spillane M, Clements M, Purcell R. Creating a national system to support mental health and enhance well-being across high performance sport. Ment Health Elite Sport. 2021;2021:68–79.

65. Rice S, Walton CC, Pilkington V, et al. Psychological safety in elite sport settings: a psychometric study of the Sport Psychological Safety Inventory. BMJ Open Sport & Exercise Medicine. 2022;8(2):e001251.

General Approaches to Management of Mental Health in Elite Athletes: Psychotherapy

Tim Herzog, Kristine M. Eiring, and Jessica D. Bartley

Elite Athlete Mental Health

Elite athletes are those performing at the national and international level; they are among the best in their country at their sport [1]. Similarly, the International Olympic Committee (IOC) Mental Health Working Group defines elite athletes as Olympic, Paralympic, professional, or collegiate athletes, though the IOC acknowledges that this categorization is abstract and risks overlooking other individuals who have devoted significant time and effort to the pursuit of athletic excellence [2]. Much of what is discussed in this chapter may also apply to this larger pool of athletes. For athletes, performance can impact mental health, and mental health can impact performance. Athletes have a unique set of pressures, in addition to dealing with the same stressors as everyone else, whether interpersonal, financial, and otherwise. As Reardon et al. [2] noted, mental health symptoms and disorders are common in elite athletes and can interfere with performance. Therefore, mental and physical health cannot be separated, and it is imperative to care for athletes holistically.

According to the Global Burden of Diseases, Injuries, and Risk Factors Study [3], around 13% of the global population is currently struggling with a mental health disorder. Elite athletes are not immune to mental health issues, and in some instances, they may be at greater risk. The International Classification of Diseases (ICD-11) describes mental, behav-

ioral, and neurodevelopmental disorders as "syndromes characterised by clinically significant disturbance in an individual's cognition, emotional regulation, or behaviour that reflects a dysfunction in the psychological, biological, or developmental processes that underlie mental and behavioural functioning. These disturbances are usually associated with distress or impairment in personal, family, social, educational, occupational, or other important areas of functioning [4]. Mental health can be amorphous, and the ICD-11 provides a language for communication between professionals but often does not present the whole picture. For athletes, labels sometimes have utility but sometimes contribute to stigma [5, 6]. Further, practitioners must be mindful of diagnostic challenges that may be more prevalent when working with athletes (e.g., overtraining syndrome versus major depression; aggression; narcissism; and entitlement [7].

Anxiety disorders are the most common mental health disorders worldwide, and prevalence among the general population and elite athletes is comparable at around 10.6–12.0% [8]. Major depression is the second leading cause of disability worldwide [9]. While prevalence of mental health disorders is often unclear with elite athletes, a systematic review of mental health studies of elite athletes noted the prevalence rate for depression among elite athletes is relatively comparable to the general population [10]. Sleep is often closely tied to mental health and is paramount for optimal performance in athletics (e.g., via effects on reaction time), and sleep deprivation is destructive for performance, recovery, and mental health [11, 12]. Studies consistently show that athletes tend to fall short of total sleep time and sleep efficiency recommendations [13]. Treating insomnia may be helpful to athletes even if sleep disruptions do not reach the level of chronic insomnia, and treatment of major depressive disorder is twice as likely to be successful when insomnia is treated directly [14, 15]. In discussing depression, and mental health in general, potential for suicide is always concerning. Suicide rates for elite athletes are lower compared to the general population, but elite athletes are nonetheless at risk

T. Herzog (✉)
Reaching Ahead LLC, Annapolis, MD, USA
e-mail: tim@reachingahead.com

K. M. Eiring
Kristine M. Eiring, PhD LLC, Madison, WI, USA
e-mail: dreiring@dreiring.us

J. D. Bartley
Mental Health Services, United States Olympic and Paralympic Committee, Colorado Springs, CO, USA

Graduate School of Professional Psychology, University of Denver, Denver, CO, USA
e-mail: Jessica.Bartley@usopc.org; Jessica.Bartley@du.edu

© The Author(s), under exclusive license to Springer Nature Switzerland AG 2022
C. L. Reardon (ed.), *Mental Health Care for Elite Athletes*, https://doi.org/10.1007/978-3-031-08364-8_2

for suicide and should be properly treated and mitigating circumstances decreased [2].

Depending on different sports-specific demands, such as aesthetics, optimal body types, speed, power, and endurance, nutrition can become a focal point for athletes, which poses risk for pathology. Estimates for prevalence of disordered eating and eating disorders meeting clinical criteria can range vastly among elite athletes (up to 19% of men and up to 45% of women) and may be three times as likely among some athletes than in general population [2, 16]. Co-occurring mental health disorders are common with eating disorders, with estimates of as high as 70% comorbidity [17]. Additionally, athletes may exhibit higher rates of post-traumatic stress disorder (PTSD) than the general population (13–25% in some subpopulations), and early identification of trauma symptoms may prevent escalation of symptoms to full-criteria PTSD [18].

Considered to be associated with a draw toward risk-taking and sensation-seeking, team sport athletes may be at higher risk for gambling disorders, associated problem gaming, and misuse of alcohol and other substances [19]. The substances most commonly used and misused by elite athletes across countries, sports, and genders are alcohol, caffeine, nicotine, cannabis/cannabinoids, stimulants, and anabolic androgenic steroids [20]. Athletes who are injured appear to be at greater risk of experiencing mental health disorders [10]. Attention to mental health of athletes appears to be gaining, but specific models of care have yet to be determined [10], and empirically grounded treatment and techniques, with a sound theoretical basis, are needed for optimizing the mental health treatment of elite athletes.

Mental Health Versus Mental Performance

Mental health treatment can be provided by a range of practitioners and can be conceptualized differently by the type of practitioner providing services [21]. Some practitioners are trained in both mental health and sport science while some are not. Areas of provider training and expertise, and specifics of the athlete presenting issues, should be given careful consideration by practitioners and by referrers or consumers.

Levels of treatment can range from more psychoeducational/counseling to general counseling to more intense clinical, longer-term work (Fig. 2.1). While distinctions may have pragmatic value with third-party reimbursement, practitioners are advised to consider these approaches more on a continuum, while also remembering to provide adequate informed consent and staying within areas of competence along the way [22]. Given that athletes may experience less stigma addressing performance than mental health, it may be common for athletes to initially seek mental performance services. However, as work evolves with the athlete, the focus may shift from sport to more clinical issues.

Mental Health Treatment Considerations: Concepts Across Theories

Several principles should be embedded into all forms of psychotherapy, even when they are often viewed as theories or techniques unto themselves. Active listening is a hallmark of most psychotherapeutic approaches. When done well, active listening can have athletes feeling like someone finally "gets them" so well, that as they hear themselves speak, they learn more about themselves in the process. "It sounds like you…" is a common way to begin an active listening reflective statement, and the power of it is embedded in the delivery. Without coming across as robotically reiterating what the client just said, the therapist might convey genuine warmth and compassion in saying something like, "It sounds like you didn't know how to respond to your coach, and that you felt both angry, and maybe powerless?"

Active listening incorporates the following counseling skills: encouraging gestures and words (such as head nodding), paraphrasing, summarizing, clarifying, and questioning [23]. Intentional use of verbal and nonverbal communication can help connection. Attending to the sport's subculture, systems of power/influence, and nuances in language can further help build a bridge [24].

Humanistic theories, such as person-centered psychotherapy, emphasize that the relationship is pivotal to enabling clients to change. As Ivey et al. [23] noted, clients do not want to tell a story to someone who is disinterested, cold, or unwelcoming. For change to occur, the practitioner must demonstrate (and the client must feel) empathy, genuineness, and unconditional positive regard [25, 26]. Williams [27] provides tips for clients seeking culturally competent therapists; these tips can also translate into best practices for therapists engaging in cross cultural work. In essence, she

Fig. 2.1 Continuum of care (reprinted with permission)

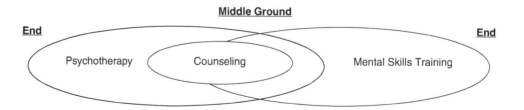

suggests: (1) don't shy away from topics such as oppression; (2) respond to these topics with appropriate concern; (3) demonstrate a working knowledge of identities that apply to your client (e.g., race, gender, sexual orientation, culture, and religion); and (4) express intention to learn more about any knowledge deficits. These tips may seem obvious; however, Terry [28] highlights how even well-intentioned therapists can easily get off track. Practitioner performance anxiety, given pressure to deliver quickly within an unfamiliar context, needs to be dealt with. Communication style should reflect what would be best received within another culture (e.g., Asians might experience Americans as being overly direct, whereas South Americans might experience Americans as being too reserved). Finally, a feminist perspective could be adopted, accepting that *values* are inherently a part of the psychotherapeutic process; practitioners can make a conscious choice to work in a manner that reduces shaming or conforming based on gender norms, and work to ensure that basic rights are applied to all, even if doing so can cause friction within a patriarchical culture [29].

Mental Health Treatment: Theories and Techniques

As stated in the International Olympic Committee consensus statement, "Psychotherapy is defined as the treatment of mental health symptoms or disorders or problems of living, and/or facilitation of personal growth, by psychological means; it is often based on therapeutic principles, structure and techniques" [2]. Research into the common factors of psychotherapy that facilitate change suggest that 30–70% of what contributes to change is the therapeutic alliance, whereas 15% of what facilitates change is the technique [30]. Utilizing psychotherapy theories and techniques in a manner that emphasizes the relationship and an appreciation of the person makes any approach more likely to be effective.

While not exhaustive, theories commonly used when working with athletes include: motivational interviewing (MI), cognitive behavioral therapy (CBT), third wave (mindfulness-based) cognitive behavioral therapies, and psychodynamic (attachment-oriented) psychotherapy. Many theories can shape practitioners' theoretical orientations, or lenses, through which they conceptualize and intervene with clients, and integrative or eclectic approaches are common [31]. While not discussed in detail within the current chapter, integrating elements of certain theories should be considered with athletes. Stillman et al. [7] suggest a systems-based approach incorporates an understanding of the individual athlete in the context of important others (e.g., family, coaches, teammates, National Governing Bodies, etc.). Solution-focused brief counseling (SFBC) is another per-

spective that intuitively seems a good fit for working with athletes, given athletic cultures that value expediency and concrete answers to concrete problems such as injury recovery [32]. With SFBC, there is a clear structure: (1) description of the problem, (2) development of well-formulated goals, (3) exploration for expectation, and (4) end-of-session feedback [33]. Elements of systems-based approaches and SFBC can mesh nicely with MI, CBT, third-wave CBTs, and psychodynamic approaches; these approaches can also be artfully integrated with each other.

Motivational Interviewing (MI) Theory

Motivational interviewing (MI) is commonly used to address substance misuse, and is applicable across a range of presenting problems and approaches. MI addresses ambivalence, acknowledging that one's potential to change depends largely on their stage of readiness [34]. The practitioner helps the client to acknowledge the part of oneself that wants to change a behavior and the part of oneself that does not. Rather than attempting to convince the client to change behavior, and likely eliciting resistance, the practitioner encourages verbalization of one's own inner conflict. In the process, the *client* thus takes greater ownership over decision-making, enhancing chances of long-term success. Athlete behavior change is elicited in a manner that taps into intrinsic motivation, and that fosters self-assurance, self-reliance, and self-efficacy as clients explore and resolve their own ambivalence [35, 36]. Understanding athletes' current stage of readiness can help inform a tailored use of motivational interviewing techniques, tapping into the client's priorities and their confidence that change is possible [37, 38]. Considerations of readiness are important for a wide variety of issues including, as just a few examples: deciding whether to adopt an ongoing breathing regimen to reduce performance anxiety; contemplating the reduction of drinking; and working to schedule activities that feel unappealing because of depression.

OARS Motivational Interviewing Techniques

"OARS" techniques exemplify MI. OARS is an acronym for: open-ended questions, affirmations, reflections, and summarizing [39, 40]. With *open-ended questions*, the athlete is encouraged to do most of the talking, as the practitioner learns what they care about, their values, and their goals. The therapist gives *affirmation* of their strengths and efforts, for instance, "You've really considered many approaches in tackling this problem." Every open-ended question is followed by approximately two to three *reflections*, whereby content and implicit meaning is rephrased to convey understanding. *Summarizing* is used along the way to ensure that the big picture is understood and that this understanding is mutual. The following example of summarizing can illustrate an OARS conversation:

> Okay, so if I'm hearing you right, you're saying that this injury is the hardest thing you've ever had to face (client nodding and continuing with affirming non-verbals and watery eyes). And, it sounds like you've wanted to escape this any way you can. Which makes sense, and at the same time...from what you're saying, it sounds like escaping hasn't really been working. And so it sounds like a part of you wants to keep hiding by drinking every night with your college friends, but it also sounds like an even bigger part of you wants to really engage your rehab, get your grades up, and think about long-term solutions?

Cognitive Behavioral Therapy (CBT) Theory

CBT emphasizes the link between cognitions, emotions, physiology, and behaviors, and has traditionally emphasized that if maladaptive thoughts can be controlled or suppressed, that one can ameliorate mental health symptoms. One assumption with cognitive-based theories and interventions is that lasting meaningful behavior changes are achieved by identifying problem situations, understanding how the situation is *interpreted* by the client, and modifying client responses [41]. CBT is commonly used with athletes because it is: (1) concrete in structure and application and thus, feels familiar to athletes with a dynamic that is akin to coaching; and (2) more easily researched than some theories. Thus, CBT is noted as an effective approach for common athlete concerns such as: substance use disorders, insomnia, anxiety, depression, anger/aggression, somatization, chronic pain, and general stress [7].

Cognitive Restructuring CBT Techniques

Different CBT theorists have created their own spin, and have used slightly different vocabulary, to describe their version of "cognitive restructuring" or "reframing" techniques (e.g., [42–45]). A common element between versions of the technique is to become more adept at recognizing the link between: (A) activating events (situations); (B) beliefs (automatic thoughts in the form of internally experienced words or pictures); and (C) consequences (mood and behavior). Traditional CBT approaches work to dismantle "maladaptive" [42] or "irrational" [44] beliefs by (D) disputing the belief (examining evidence and pros and cons of maintaining the belief). A newer twist on the technique, the mind–body ABCs, specifically addresses conducting this work with athletes [12]. The technique is applicable for addressing performance situations and/or mental health and places greater emphasis on recognizing cognition as influenceable (albeit not fully controllable), and it includes body sensations in the "Cs" (Consequences) and aims to bridge a divide between traditional CBT approaches and newer mindfulness-based approaches.

As an example, an athlete might experience depressive and anxiety symptoms associated with a thought such as, "My teammates hate me." Table 2.1 can serve as an example of using the mind–body ABCs approach. Note that the athlete may "try on" a few Bs before coming up with one that resonates, *feels* better, and leads to more adaptive behavior. In this example, "Maybe she is having a bad day? I can focus on me." leads to a more adaptive behavior. The drill aims at initially developing a new perspective retrospectively and developing a habit of thinking such that more adaptive appraisals can occur more seamlessly, in the moment, and with new situations.

Third Wave (Mindfulness-Based) Cognitive Behavioral Therapy (CBT) Theory

There has been a growing movement toward integrating mindfulness into psychology [46] and into the subdiscipline of sport psychology [47]. Contrary to traditional CBT, "third wave" CBTs emphasize that people do not have control over their thoughts, emotions, or physiology. Secularly pulling from Eastern traditions of mindfulness and acceptance, acceptance and commitment therapy (ACT) suggests that suffering stems from futile attempts at trying to control or avoid experiences that cannot be controlled. It suggests that problems arise out of experiential avoidance as one stays attached to thoughts such as, "I cannot handle this experience," and instead engages in behaviors such as disassociation, acting out, or substance misuse. ACT (and other third

Table 2.1 Mind–body ABCs approach to cognitive behavioral therapy with an athlete who believes her teammate hates her

Activating event	Belief (words and images)	Consequence (mood)	Consequence (body)	Consequence (behavior)
Teammate avoided eye contact in locker room	"My teammates hate me"	Sadness/anxiety	Low energy	Avoid making conversation. Withdraw from others
Teammate avoided eye contact in locker room	"What a jerk. They should treat me with more respect"	Anger	Heart racing, trap tension, fists clenched	Look for many ways in which I'm treated unjustly
Teammate avoided eye contact in locker room	"Maybe she is having a bad day? I can focus on me"	Empathy	Neutral. Long exhales	Ask teammate how she is if given opportunity. Engage others

wave CBTs such as dialectical behavior therapy) emphasizes engagement in valued behaviors while simultaneously fostering acceptance of experiences that are out of one's control. Another approach combining elements of mindfulness and cognitive therapy is mindfulness-based cognitive therapy (MBCT). There is growing interest in mindfulness and meditation as part of the techniques used with third wave theories and therapies [46, 47]. Traditional CBT exposure techniques address issues associated with avoidance; mindfulness-based techniques seek to build acceptance of internal experiences that one may attempt to avoid, and the problems that result from trying to avoid these experiences, such as substance misuse, interpersonal problems, anxiety, or depression.

ACT Cognitive Defusion Technique (Example: Silly Voices)

Whether experiencing performance anxiety or being absolutely consumed by depressive or anxious thoughts, one part of the problem can be that thoughts are experienced as defining reality rather than as passing experiences. ACT's cognitive defusion techniques can help athletes to consider thoughts as passing, that they come and go, without clinging to them, and without letting them dictate behaviors. To help illustrate this concept, a technique labeled "silly" voices might be used [48], whereby distressing thoughts may be imagined to have the voice and appearance of funny real or fictional characters, such as cartoon or television personas, e.g., an athlete's favorite cartoon character or favorite comedian. A practitioner can ask a client, "If 'Donald Duck' were to say, 'Nobody likes you,' would you take him seriously?" The answer often comes with a chuckle and a "no." By consistently practicing the technique on their own when distressing thoughts reappear, the client is empowered to more habitually defuse and cope with those thoughts more easily when situations arise.

Psychodynamic (Attachment-Oriented) Psychotherapy Theory

Originating from the work of Sigmund Freud, psychodynamic psychotherapies have become more palatable (e.g., less centered on unconscious sexual desires), and while theories are rich and often effective, their abstract structure make them more difficult to replicate and research than theories such as CBT. Nonetheless, these theories can be useful in conceptualizing interpersonal patterns and emphasize how faulty aspects of formative relationships (particularly with parents) dictate the manner in which one relates to others in the future, and whether one becomes stuck at certain stages of development (i.e., exhibiting pathology). Psychodynamic

psychotherapy aims to provide a corrective relationship, promoting healing from unconscious pain, reducing behavioral manifestations, and decreasing other symptoms in the process. In its traditional form, psychodynamic psychotherapy requires frequent meetings for long periods of time, and is perhaps less practical for work with athletes. Psychodynamic theory (and attachment theory in general) can be useful in conceptualizing athletes' relationships (e.g., is Coach regarded like Dad?), and adaptations (e.g., short-term psychodynamic psychotherapy) can be extremely useful in working with athletes and others who prioritize performance [2, 49, 50].

Psychodynamic Transference Interpretation Technique

According to psychodynamic theory, rational insight is not enough, and a corrective relationship is paramount for healing unconscious pain (Fairbairn, as cited in [51]). As Mitchell and Black [51] put it, "By encouraging the patient to report on all fleeting thoughts, the analyst hopes to get the patient to bypass the normal selection process that screens out the conflictual content" (p. 6). Often, that conflictual content can be aimed at the practitioner; this transference material can come in the form of expectations that develop within the relationship (e.g., the practitioner will be insensitive, judgmental, or disappointed; [51, 52]). Understanding the client interpersonally and helping them to relate to others better can come as practitioners interpret and respond effectively to transference. As transference is experienced, there may be some resistance to particular free associations (e.g., if the practitioner is the object of intense longing, love, or hate). Freud (as cited in [51]) indicated that these resistances were of the same kind of force that drove memories out of consciousness in the first place; thus, toward the aim of healing, it is important to analyze the client's transference. Interpreting resistance in the form of defense mechanisms such as suppression, repression, projection, sublimation, denial, displacement, and regression can unearth hidden feelings and memories. Conscious and unconscious defense mechanisms are exposed, identified, and dissolved. For example, the athlete may suppress the idea that the therapist would be insensitive to their needs. Dismantling this resistance could lead to more "real" discussion of mistrust toward Coach, and in other relationships. Denial of early impacts from relationships with one or both parents could be deconstructed, and emotions could be expressed, such that other relationships and sense of well-being improve, sometimes in an unconscious and seamless manner. According to Høglend and Gabbard [53], interpreting transference is less likely to work when the client suffers from a personality disorder. Practitioners should be advised, however, that over-pathologizing is ill-advised, and that impenetrable resistance could be partly cultural (e.g., a sport culture or culture of origin that over-emphasizes traditional masculinity) or stemming from a perception that anything done as part of sport psychology should always address sport performance in a linear, concrete, and face-valid manner. Embracing some of the considerations described early in the chapter (e.g., principles of person-centered therapy or motivational interviewing) may help enhance psychodynamic techniques, but practitioners may want to also consider utilizing other theories and techniques described in this chapter.

Conclusion

Elite athletes are, first and foremost, human and, like others, are at risk of experiencing mental health symptoms and disorders. Addressing sport performance first may help decrease stigma that can accompany mental health treatment. However, with more athletes being public about mental health, athletes may be becoming more direct about their needs. Good therapeutic work with athletes entails a clear understanding of why the athlete is seeking services. This knowledge assists the therapist with choosing a theoretical framework, and subsequent techniques, to best assist the athlete. Key considerations that cut across theories are establishing rapport, building a solid therapist–client relationship, deep and active listening, and multiculturalism. Commonly used theories when working with athletes for conceptualizing athletes and for interventions include, but are not limited to: motivational interviewing, cognitive behavioral therapy, third wave (mindfulness-based) therapies, and psychodynamic (attachment-oriented) psychotherapy. Other theoretical orientations that may have elements integrated into all approaches include person-centered, systems-based, solution-focused, multicultural, and feminist. At the heart of good work is the therapeutic alliance [26] and establishing rapport. Athletes want to be viewed as persons, not problems, receiving respect, genuine caring, and empathy from someone who is fully present.

References

1. Swann C, Moran A, Piggott D. Defining elite athletes: issues in the study of expert performance in sport psychology. Psychol Sport Exerc. 2015;16(1):3–14.
2. Reardon C, Hainline B, Aron C, Baron D, Baum A, Bindra A, Currie A. Mental health in elite athletes: International Olympic Committee consensus statement. Br J Sports Med. 2019;53(11):667–99.
3. Global Burden of Diseases, Injuries, and Risk Factors Study. Global, regional, and national incidence, prevalence, and years lived with disability for 354 diseases and injuries for 195 countries and territories, 1990–2017: a systematic analysis for the Global Burden of Disease Study 2017. Lancet. 2018;392(10159):1789–858.
4. ICD-11 for Mortality and Morbidity Statistics. 2021. https://icd.who.int/browse11/l-m/en#!/http%3A%2F%2Fid.who.int%2Ficd%2Fentity%2F334423054.
5. Glick ID, Horsfall JL. Psychiatric conditions in sports: diagnosis, treatment, and quality of life. Phys Sports Med. 2009;37(3):29–34. https://doi.org/10.3810/psm.2009.10.1726.
6. Wilson KG, Dufrene T. Mindfulness for two: an acceptance and commitment therapy approach to mindfulness in psychotherapy. Oakland: New Harbinger Publications; 2008.
7. Stillman MA, Glick ID, McDuff D, Reardon CL, Hitchcock ME, Fitch VM, Hainline BM. Psychotherapy for mental health symptoms and disorders in elite athletes: a narrative review. Br J Sports Med. 2019;53(12):767–71.
8. Rice SM, Gwyther K, Santesteban-Echarri O, Baron D, Gorczynski P, Gouttebarge V, Reardon CL, Hitchcock ME, Hainline B, Purcell R. Determinants of anxiety in elite athletes: a systematic review and meta-analysis. Br J Sports Med. 2019;53(11):722–30. https://doi.org/10.1136/bjsports-2019-100620.
9. World Health Organization. Depression: key facts. 2020. https://www.who.int/news-room/fact-sheets/detail/depression. Accessed September 30, 2021.
10. Rice SM, Purcell R, De Silva S, Mawren D, McGorry PD, Parker AG. The mental health of elite athletes: a narrative systematic review. Sports Med. 2016;46(9):1333–53. https://doi.org/10.1007/s40279-016-0492-2.
11. Belenky G, Wesensten NJ, Thorne DR, Thomas ML, Sing HC, Redmond DP, Balkin TJ. Patterns of performance degradation and restoration during sleep restriction and subsequent recovery: a sleep dose-response study. J Sleep Res. 2003;12(1):1–12.
12. Herzog T, Zavilla S, Dupee M, Stephenson M. Chapter 15: the psychophysiology of self-regulation. In: Cremades G, Mugford A, editors. Sport, exercise, and performance psychology: theories and applications. New York: Routledge; 2018.
13. Roberts SSH, Teo WP, Warmington SA. Effects of training and competition on the sleep of elite athletes: a systematic review and meta-analysis. Br J Sports Med. 2019;53(8):513–22.
14. Halson SL. Sleep monitoring in athletes: motivation, methods, miscalculations and why it matters. Sports Med. 2019;49(10):1487–97. https://doi.org/10.1007/s40279-019-01119-4.
15. Manber R, Edinger JD, Gress JL, San Pedro-Salcedo MG, Kuo TF, Kalista T. Cognitive behavioral therapy for insomnia enhances depression outcome in patients with comorbid major depressive disorder and insomnia. Sleep. 2008;31(4):489–95. https://doi.org/10.1093/sleep/31.4.489.
16. Sundgot-Borgen J, Torstveit M. Prevalence of eating disorders in elite athletes is higher than in the general population. Clin J Sport Med. 2004;14(1):25–32.
17. Hudson JI, Hiripi E, Pope HG Jr, Kessler RC. The prevalence and correlates of eating disorders in the National Comorbidity Survey Replication. Biol Psychiatry. 2007;61(3):348–58. https://doi.org/10.1016/j.biopsych.2006.03.040.
18. Aron CM, Harvey S, Hainline B, Hitchcock ME, Reardon CL. Post-traumatic stress disorder (PTSD) and other trauma-related mental disorders in elite athletes: a narrative review. Br J Sports Med. 2019;53(12):779–84.
19. Håkansson A, Kenttä G, Åkesdotter C. Problem gambling and gaming in elite athletes. Addict Behav Rep. 2018;8(2018):79–84.
20. McDuff D, Stull T, Castaldelli-Maia JM, et al. Recreational and ergogenic substance use and substance use disorders in elite athletes: a narrative review. Br J Sports Med. 2019;53:754–60.
21. Herzog T, Hays KF. Therapist or mental skills coach? How to decide. Sport Psychol. 2012;26(4):486–99.
22. Herzog T, Zito M. Chapter 7: ethics in sport and performance psychology: realities of practice in a multi-disciplinary field. In: Tod D, Krane V, Hodge K, editors. Routledge handbook of applied sport psychology. 2nd ed. New York: Routledge; in press.

23. Ivey AE, Ivey MB, Zalaquette CP. Intentional interviewing and counseling: facilitating client development in a multicultural society. 8th ed. Pacific Grove: Brooks/Cole; 2014.

24. Brown C. Contextual intelligence (CI): the key to successful consulting. Get your head in the game. 2012. https://headinthegame.net/resources/library/contextual-intelligence-ci-the-key-to-successful-consulting.

25. Rogers C. The necessary and sufficient conditions of therapeutic personality change. Psychotherapy. 2007;44:240–8. https://doi.org/10.1037/0033-3204.44.3.240.

26. Wampold BE. How important are the common factors in psychotherapy? An update. World Psychiatry. 2015;14(3):270–7. https://doi.org/10.1002/wps.20238.

27. Williams NE. How to find a culturally competent therapist who really makes you feel heard. SELF. 2021. https://www.self.com/story/find-culturally-competent-therapist. Accessed November 1 2021.

28. Terry PC. Chapter 7: strategies for reflective cultural sport psychology practice. In: Schinke RJ, Hanrahan SJ, editors. Cultural sport psychology. Champaign: Human Kinetics; 2009.

29. Kaschak E. What is feminist therapy? Why has it developed and continued? Psychology Today Blog. 2019. https://www.psychologytoday.com/us/blog/she-comes-long-way-baby/201905/what-is-feminist-therapy.

30. Imel ZE, Wampold BE. The importance of treatment and the science of common factors in psychotherapy. In: Brown SD, Lent RW, editors. Handbook of counseling psychology. 4th ed. Hoboken: Wiley; 2008. p. 249–62.

31. Norcross JC, Prochaska JO. A study of electric (and integrative) views revisited. Prof Psychol. 1988;19(2):170–4. https://doi.org/10.1037/0735-7028.19.2.170.

32. Gutkind SM. Using solution-focused brief counseling to provide injury support. Sport Psychol. 2004;18(1):75–88. https://doi.org/10.1123/tsp.18.1.75.

33. Høigaard R, Johansen BT. The Solution-focused approach in sport psychology. Sport Psychol. 2004;18(2):218–28. https://doi.org/10.1123/tsp.18.2.218.

34. Prochaska J, DiClemente C, Norcross J. In search of how people change: applications to addictive behaviors. Am Psychol. 1992;47:1102–14.

35. Outlaw KR, Toriello PJ. Off the court: helping African American athletes address behavioral health concerns while using motivational interviewing. J Hum Behav Soc Environ. 2014;24(5):557–64.

36. Sutcliffe JH, Greenberger PA. Identifying psychological difficulties in college athletes. J Allergy. 2020;8(7):2216–9. https://doi.org/10.1016/j.jaip.2020.03.006.

37. DiClemente C, Velasquez M. Motivational interviewing: preparing people for change. New York: Guildford Press; 2002.

38. Norcross JC, Krebs PM, Prochaska JO. Stages of change. J Clin Psychol. 2011;67(2):143–54. https://doi.org/10.1002/jclp.20758.

39. Hall K, Gibbie T, Lubman D. Motivational interviewing techniques: facilitating behaviour change in the general practice. Aust Fam Physician. 2012;41(9):660–7.

40. Miller WR, Rollnick S. Motivational interviewing: helping people change. 3rd ed. New York: Guilford Press; 2013.

41. Lenz AS, Hall J, Smith LB. Meta-analysis of group mindfulness-based cognitive therapy for decreasing symptoms of acute depression. J Special Group Work. 2015; https://doi.org/10.1080/01933922.2015.1111488.

42. Beck A. Cognitive therapy: basics and beyond. New York: Guilford; 1995.

43. Burns DD, Nolen-Hoeksema S. Coping styles, homework compliance, and the effectiveness of cognitive behavioral therapy. J Consult Clin Psychol. 1991;59(2):305–11. https://doi.org/10.1037/0022-006X.59.2.305.

44. Ellis A. Rational emotive behavior therapy and the mindfulness based stress reduction training of Jon Kabat-Zinn. J Ration Emot Cogn Behav Ther. 2006;24(1):63–78.

45. Meichenbaum D. Cognitive behaviour modification. Scand J Behav Ther. 1977;6(4):185–92. https://doi.org/10.1080/16506073.1977.9626708.

46. Goldberg SB, Tucker RP, Greene PA, Davidson RJ, Wampold BE, Kearney DJ, Simpson TL. Mindfulness for psychiatric disorders: a systematic review and meta-analysis. Clin Psychol Rev. 2018;29:52–60.

47. Zizzi S, Anderson M. Being mindful in sport and exercise psychology: pathways for practitioners and students. Morgantown: FIT; 2017.

48. Hayes S. n.d.. https://contextualscience.org/cognitive_defusion_deliteralization.

49. McCullough L. Desensitization of affect phobias in short-term dynamic psychotherapy. In: Solomon M, Neborsky R, McCullough L, Alpert M, Shapiro F, Malan D, editors. Short-term therapy for long-term change. New York: WW Norton & Co; 2001.

50. McCullough L, Osborn K. Short term dynamic psychotherapy goes to hollywood: the treatment of performance anxiety in cinema. J Clin Psychol. 2004;60(8):841–52.

51. Mitchell S, Black M. Freud and beyond. New York: Basic Books; 1995.

52. Anderson MB, Serra de Queiroz F. Chapter 17: psychodynamic models of therapy. In: Tod D, Krane V, Hodge K, editors. Routledge handbook of applied sport psychology. 2nd ed. New York: Routledge; in press.

53. Høglend P, Gabbard GO. When is transference work useful in psychodynamic psychotherapy? A review of empirical research. In: Levy RA, Ablon JS, Kächele H, editors. Psychodynamic psychotherapy research: evidence-based practice and practice-based evidence. New York: Springer; 2012. p. 449–67. https://doi.org/10.1007/978-1-60761-792-1_26.

General Approaches to Management of Mental Health in Elite Athletes: Pharmacological Treatment

Claudia L. Reardon

Introduction

Medications may be used to treat mental health symptoms and disorders in elite athletes, particularly when they are chronic in duration or moderate to severe in intensity [1]. Given how commonplace these symptoms and disorders are in athletes, as described in Chap. 1, all members of the athlete's health care team should have a working knowledge of the nuances of relevant pharmacological treatments.

While treatment of moderate to severe mental health symptoms and disorders with medications is an important option for elite athletes, there are numerous barriers that may impact an athlete's ability to get this type of treatment. Stigma, particularly prominent among athletes, is one such barrier [2]. Athletes reportedly are much more comfortable and willing to meet with a sports psychologist for the stated purpose of psychological performance enhancement than they are to seek treatment for mental health symptoms and disorders [3]. Additionally, elite athletes are often accustomed to having a team of providers to help with their medical conditions and treatments. Athletes may be less likely to attend psychiatry appointments, pick up psychiatric medication prescriptions, and take psychiatric medications regularly if they receive less support for this type of treatment compared to what they are used to with other physical ailments. Finally, other barriers for athletes when it comes to getting psychiatric treatment for mental health symptoms and disorders include lack of mental health literacy, negative past experiences with mental health help seeking, and busy athlete schedules [2, 4].

There are at least four important considerations when clinicians prescribe psychiatric medication to athletes: (1) potential negative impact on athletic performance; (2) potential therapeutic performance-enhancing effects (i.e., based on improvement in the condition the medication is designed to treat); (3) potential nontherapeutic performance-enhancing effects (i.e., ergogenic effects); and (4) potential safety risks [1]. Regarding the potential negative impact on performance, prescribers must keep in mind that even seemingly minor side effects can mean the difference between top achievement and lower levels of accomplishment. Side effects typically of greatest concern in this regard are sedation, weight gain, cardiac side effects (including changes in blood pressure or heart rate and abnormal heart rhythms), and tremor [5, 6]. Even an apparently minimal degree of sedation or undesired weight gain, for example, could slow down a runner's time by enough to meaningfully impact their performance. Other relevant side effects include impaired concentration, muscle rigidity, weight loss, blurred vision, anxiety or agitation, and insomnia [1, 5].

The distinction between therapeutic and ergogenic performance enhancement that may result from a psychiatric medication is important. For example, an athlete who is performing poorly because of anxiety may gain a *therapeutic* performance enhancement by taking a selective serotonin reuptake inhibitor (SSRI). However, there is no evidence that this class of medications provides ergogenic performance enhancement, and they are not prohibited substances at any level of sports competition [1, 7, 8]. With other medications, though, performance-enhancing effects are an important consideration. Many sports governing bodies, such as professional sports leagues, the U.S.'s National Collegiate Athletic Association (NCAA) [9], and the World Anti-Doping Agency (WADA) [8], prohibit medications that have been found to have nontherapeutic performance-enhancing effects. Stimulants are the main class of psychiatric drugs classified as prohibited substances by these organizations [8, 9]. Prescribers may be able to obtain a therapeutic use exception (TUE) from WADA or a professional sports league so as to be able to prescribe a prohibited medication such as a stimulant [10]. At the NCAA level, certain documentation may allow for use of stimulants [11]. However, some have argued that there are ethical issues to be considered in terms of if it is fair to prescribe such a medication, known to have

C. L. Reardon (✉)
Department of Psychiatry, University of Wisconsin School of Medicine and Public Health, Madison, WI, USA
e-mail: clreardon@wisc.edu

ergogenic effects, for an athlete, particularly those competing at the highest levels [12, 13].

Finally, safety risks that exist with certain psychiatric medications, when taken by athletes exercising at high intensity or with other unique physiological factors, are important. For example, some medications with blood levels that must be tightly regulated can be difficult to manage in athletes whose levels might be influenced by hydration status [1, 5, 6, 14]. Additionally, medications with any potential cardiac side effects may be of extra concern in heavily exercising athletes [7].

The degree of importance of the four considerations of prescribing medications to athletes varies by the particular sport and its demands, level of performance required, time frame within the athletic training/competition cycle, and anticipated duration of treatment [1, 5]. The end result is that clinicians prescribing psychiatric medication for athletes should tend toward relatively conservative prescribing practices. Thus, a psychiatric prescriber for athletes is well advised, if at all possible, not to simultaneously start multiple medications or escalate dosages quickly. Of course, there are always exceptions to these guidelines. In the case of severe mental health disorders, the athlete's health and well-being must be prioritized even if it means side effects emerge. There is a risk of undertreating mental health disorders in athletes, and care must be taken to avoid that circumstance as well, as ongoing, untreated mental health disorders are not conducive to high-level sports performance nor to life functioning.

Additionally, there are unique considerations within each category of psychiatric medications (e.g., antidepressants, antianxiety medications, etc.) when it comes to prescribing for athletes. Unfortunately, there is a paucity of research on the different classes of psychiatric medications that may be used in athletes. Studies that attempt to look at the impact of specific psychiatric medications on athletic performance tend to have several flaws, including small sample sizes, medications are not used in dosages or time frames that reflect their actual usage in the real world, populations studied are not high-level athletes, very few athletes who do not identify as male are studied, types of performance measures used (e.g., grip strength) in studies to determine if a medication has a negative impact on athletic performance may not be representative of real-world performance impact, and study subjects often do not have the mental health disorder that the medication is intended to treat [1, 12, 15]. With acknowledgment of the research limitations to date, the remainder of this chapter details what is known about medications prescribed for athletes within numerous major categories of mental health symptoms and disorders.

Pharmacological Treatments for Depression

Medications for depression in athletes have received some research attention. A small survey of sports psychiatrists noted that bupropion was a top choice of sports psychiatrists for depression, without comorbid anxiety, in athletes [6]. It can be speculated that the relatively energizing effect of this medication and lack of weight gain as a side effect may contribute to its top selection. However, this medication must not be prescribed in the presence of eating disorders that involve dietary restriction and/or purging because of an increased risk of seizures in such patients who take this medication [1]. Prescribers should be extra cautious about prescribing this medication, which generally may lower seizure threshold, in athletes with any potentially increased risk for seizures (e.g., because of significant alcohol use disorder) who are participating in sports where seizures could be especially dangerous (e.g., water sports).

It is important as well to note that bupropion is currently on WADA's *in-competition* monitored list, meaning that WADA is monitoring for patterns of misuse in sport [16]. Specifically, there is very preliminary evidence suggesting the possibility of performance enhancement for endurance athletes using bupropion as a single, high dose in warm climates [17]. Performance enhancement was not observed when the medication was dosed chronically [18], which is how it would be prescribed in actual clinical practice. A more recent study demonstrated performance enhancement with 300 mg dosing the night before and morning of a cycling time trial in warm climates, but no such enhancement was noted at doses less than 300 mg, and again, the medication was not studied when dosed chronically [19]. The sum of the research on bupropion preliminarily suggests that it may allow athletes to push themselves to higher core body temperatures and heart rates, thus allowing improved performance, especially when used at higher doses and in acute dosing time frames in warmer climates. However, such evidence is not to the level that WADA is prohibiting it at this point, and as such, it can be prescribed without restriction, the need for a TUE, or high degrees of concern about safety in most athletes, especially if athletes are taking it on a daily basis at dosages within approved ranges [1]. Given that it is among the most activating of antidepressants, though, it is often not a good choice for athletes with comorbid anxiety, as it may exacerbate the latter condition.

Fluoxetine is an SSRI antidepressant that has relatively more research in athletes than most other antidepressants, and specifically more research than any other SSRI to support that it does not have a negative impact on performance [20, 21]. In an earlier (2000) survey of sports psychiatrists, it had emerged as the top antidepressant choice for athletes [22]. Fluoxetine is also approved by the U.S.'s Food and

Drug Administration (FDA) for bulimia nervosa and thus may be a particularly reasonable choice for athletes with comorbid depression and bulimia nervosa or other binge/purge eating disorders. Regardless of the diagnosis for which it is used, fluoxetine has a significantly longer half-life than most other antidepressants [23], and thus can be a reasonable choice for athletes who may forget an occasional medication dosage in the context of busy and irregular travel schedules, as there will not be a sudden and precipitous drop in blood level of the medication—just what an athlete would not want during travel and competition—with an occasional forgotten dose. Sertraline and escitalopram are reasonable alternatives to fluoxetine if a different SSRI is desired [6]. Bleeding (e.g., gastrointestinal bleeding, excessive bruising, etc.) is an uncommon but well-described risk with most serotonergic antidepressants such as SSRIs [24]. While young and healthy populations are not generally at high risk for bleeding side effects, heavy use of nonsteroidal anti-inflammatory drugs (NSAIDs)—not an uncommon situation in athletes—synergistically increases the risk when these antidepressants are prescribed [24]; thus, athletes should be asked about NSAID use.

Serotonin norepinephrine reuptake inhibitors (SNRIs, e.g., venlafaxine, duloxetine, etc.), tricyclic antidepressants (e.g., nortriptyline, amitriptyline, etc.), mirtazapine, and other antidepressants have not been studied in athletes per se [1, 7]. SNRIs are sometimes regarded as relatively energizing and thus may make intuitive sense as a choice for athletes [7], but one small study suggested that a norepinephrine reuptake inhibitor (a class of related but different medications) may be performance limiting [25]. SNRIs may have potential pain-alleviating, including headache prophylactic, effects [26], such that they may have utility in the setting of sport-related postconcussion headaches comorbid with depression and/or anxiety, but they have received little study in this specific population.

Tricyclic antidepressants and mirtazapine may cause sedation and weight gain, which can be problematic for some athlete populations. That said, mirtazapine can have antinausea effects [27], which may create a niche for athletes who have significant gastrointestinal upset, with or without weight loss, in the context of depression with or without anxiety. Tricyclics, like SNRIs, are known to have pain-alleviating including headache prophylactic effects and have more of an established evidence base in this regard than do the SNRIs [28]. However, that evidence base must be weighed against the propensity to cause side effects [28] such as sedation and weight gain along with potential safety concerns in athletes pushing themselves to extremes. Specifically, supraventricular and ventricular arrhythmias have been described in young, healthy people taking tricyclics per very preliminary research [15]. Additionally, there is a theoretical risk that tricyclic blood levels could become toxic in athletes sweating heavily. One very small study demonstrated mild, temporary increases in tricyclic blood levels in exercising subjects. Though the authors concluded that the increases were unlikely to be dangerous, the subjects were not high-level athletes [14]. Finally, tricyclics are often regarded as contraindicated in the setting of eating disorders [29], which are disproportionately common in athletes [1].

Anxiety

There are important considerations when it comes to prescribing medications for anxiety in elite athletes as well. The medication that has emerged as sports psychiatrists' top choice for treatment of anxiety in athletes is the SSRI escitalopram [6]. That said, escitalopram has not been uniquely studied in athletes, and there is no research base to suggest that it is better tolerated in athletes relative to other SSRIs such as sertraline and fluoxetine, which also appear to be reasonable choices [6]. While FDA-approved for anxiety-related disorders, fluoxetine may initially be experienced as quite activating for athletes with anxious tendencies [23], and they should be warned of the potential for that often-temporary side effect.

Buspirone may be used as monotherapy or as an add-on to antidepressants (e.g., SSRIs or SNRIs) for anxiety. When added to SSRIs, it may also confer additional antidepressant effect [30]. One small study suggested performance impairment from buspirone, but only a single 45 mg dose of the medication was used [31], and that is a very large dose to be taken at any given time, nonreflective of real-world prescribing.

Medications are not indicated for anxiety that solely presents as sports performance anxiety and is thus not reflective of a broader anxiety disorder such as generalized anxiety disorder [1]. As-needed medications that would be used for situational anxiety such as performance anxiety could have detrimental effects on sports performance. For example, benzodiazepines have been shown to have a negative impact on performance [32, 33]. Such an impact is not surprising given this class's propensity to cause sedation, muscle relaxation, and slowed reaction time. Propranolol and other B-blockers should typically be avoided as well. As blood pressure medications, they may lower blood pressure and thus cause dizziness in athletes who already may have relatively low blood pressure. In endurance sports, they can problematically decrease cardiopulmonary capacity [34]. Moreover, they have been reported to improve fine motor control and are prohibited in certain sports, specifically rifle in the NCAA [9] and archery, automobile, billiards, darts, golf, shooting, some skiing/snowboarding, and some underwater sports at the WADA level [8]. The B-blocker prohibitions at the WADA level are *in-competition* only, except that in archery and shooting, they are also banned *out-of-competition* [8].

Insomnia

A major concern for athletes taking sleeping medications is potential sedation that carries over into the next morning, as this may have significant performance impact. Melatonin has emerged as a top choice of sports psychiatrists for insomnia [6], and it is the best-studied sleep medication in athletes [1, 7]. Melatonin, either in immediate release or extended release formulations, has not been shown to have a negative impact on performance [7, 33, 35]. A rare side effect of potential concern in athletes taking melatonin is a reduction in blood pressure [36].

Trazodone has been ranked as a second choice among sports psychiatrists for insomnia [6]. However, it is not FDA-approved for this purpose and has not been uniquely studied in athletes. Similarly, gabapentin and hydroxyzine are additional options for treating insomnia in athletes, though also not FDA-approved for sleep indications nor studied in this population [7]. Nonbenzodiazepine agonists, such as zolpidem and zopiclone, are additional options [7]. They have been shown to have less of a next-day sedation effect as compared to benzodiazepines (e.g., lorazepam, clonazepam) when performance effects have been studied [37–41]. Among the benzodiazepines, agents with longer half-lives have demonstrated a greater detrimental impact on next-day athletic performance compared with shorter-acting agents [32]. The latter finding must be considered alongside the fact that benzodiazepine with shorter half-lives (e.g., alprazolam) are more addictive [42].

Attention-Deficit/Hyperactivity Disorder

There are important considerations particular to athletes when prescribing medications for attention-deficit/hyperactivity disorder (ADHD) [43]. Stimulants have been shown to be performance-enhancing in sport via improved strength, acceleration, anaerobic capacity, time to exhaustion, and maximum heart rate [44]. Athletes taking stimulants may be able to exercise to higher core body temperatures without perceiving as much effort or thermal stress as they otherwise would [45]. This raises not only concerns about performance-enhancement, but also about safety, as athletes may be unaware of increasing heat stress [45]. Stimulants may be used for weight loss as a performance advantage in weight class sports (e.g., rowing, wrestling), those that may be aesthetic judged (e.g., gymnastics, artistic swimming), and

gravitational sports (e.g., distance running, cycling) and may be inappropriately used by athletes with an eating disorder to aid further weight loss [1]. These medications may also cause side effects, such as insomnia, anxiety, increased heart rate (athletes may perceive that they are starting workouts already closer to their maximum exertion, though there is not any evidence to support this as performance limiting), and an undesired decrease in appetite, all of which may interfere with performance [12, 46–49].

Higher levels of competition (e.g., collegiate, national that has the potential to ascend to international competition, international, elite, and professional) typically prohibit use of stimulants [43]. At the level of the NCAA, stimulants are only allowable for ADHD if institutions are able to submit the "NCAA Medical Exception Documentation Report to Support the Diagnosis of Attention Deficit Hyperactivity Disorder (ADHD) and Treatment with Banned Stimulant Medication" and supporting documentation to the NCAA in the event the athlete tests positive for stimulants [11]. This documentation must include: a summary of comprehensive clinical evaluation (referencing *Diagnostic and Statistical Manual* criteria and including family history, any indication of mood disorders, substance misuse, and previous history of ADHD treatment); blood pressure and pulse readings and comments; notation that alternative nonprohibited medications (e.g., atomoxetine) have been considered; diagnosis; medication(s) and dosage(s); and follow-up orders [11]. NCAA schools may differ in their internal requirements for validated ADHD psychological/neuropsychological testing and documentation. Of note, NCAA schools do not submit information to the NCAA until an athlete is actually tested and found to have evidence of a stimulant medication in their system.

At other higher levels of competition, stimulants typically are only allowable for ADHD with approved exemptions for therapeutic use [10]. TUE applications are available through professional sports leagues (e.g., the U.S.'s National Football League) or at the websites of individual countries' antidoping organizations (ADOs), e.g., the United States Anti-Doping Agency (USADA) [50]. Different entities have varying protocols for length of time for which TUEs are valid, and circumstances that would require resubmission of TUE application materials. In the case of ADOs, initial TUEs for stimulants are often granted for 12 months, while TUEs for a "well-documented, long standing" diagnosis of ADHD may be for up to 4 years [10]. Importantly, even if an athlete is granted a TUE for a particular stimulant, some countries may have prohibitions against travelers (athletes or otherwise) bringing certain medications such as particular stimulants within their borders.

Given these regulations, medication prescription for ADHD must be undertaken with great care. Behavioral interventions may be tried before prescriptions if symptoms are mild and/or if the athlete is not a student, in which case academic concerns would not be as paramount [12]. Nonstimulants should at least be considered, as articulated in the NCAA exceptions procedures, before stimulants in many cases [11]. Nonstimulant atomoxetine has emerged as a top medication choice for ADHD according to a small survey of sports psychiatrists, presumably owing to the drawbacks of stimulants [6]. Prescribers and athletes are advised to allow up to 2–3 months to see full benefit from atomoxetine [7], in contrast to the very rapid onset of effectiveness of stimulants. Nonstimulant bupropion has evidence as a treatment for ADHD [51], but has not received FDA approval for this purpose. As it is an antidepressant, it may be an especially reasonable choice if depression is comorbid with ADHD, the athlete does not have certain eating disorders and is otherwise not at increased risk for seizures, and stimulants are being avoided for any number of reasons.

If stimulants are used, many sports psychiatrists start with long-acting formulations, which are more convenient and less abusable. The top three stimulant choices of sports psychiatrists have been reported to be long-acting agents: lisdexamfetamine, long-acting methylphenidate, and long-acting mixed amphetamine salts [6]. However, another potentially reasonable stimulant prescribing strategy involves use of formulations and timing that allow for use during school, study, and work times only and not during practices and competition, thereby decreasing concerns about impact on performance and safety issues [12]. A final important consideration is that prescribers sometimes advise temporarily stopping the stimulant medication if the athlete is participating in endurance events in hot temperatures, given the described safety concerns [7].

Eating Disorders

Often even more so than with other mental health disorders, psychiatric medication prescribing for eating disorders in athletes should be undertaken only within the context of a multidisciplinary team [52]. Medical evaluation includes laboratory monitoring, physical examination, and consideration of electrocardiography and bone mineral density testing [52], all of which are typically ordered and/or conducted by the sports medicine or primary care physician or psychiatrist. Nutrition and psychotherapy are important aspects of treatment, in addition to any prescriptions for psychiatric medication. There are two medications FDA-approved for eating disorders in the United States [1, 52]. Fluoxetine is approved for bulimia nervosa, and by extension, all else being equal, tends to be a first-line medication used in the presence of any type of eating disorder if depression or anxiety are also present. That said, there is not a significant amount of research supporting its utility in anorexia nervosa alone, apart from any component of comorbid depression or anxiety [53].

Lisdexamfetamine is FDA-approved for binge eating disorder (BED), but this is a stimulant and thus is prohibited at higher levels of competition just as other stimulants are [8, 9]. As of the time of this publication, the NCAA and WADA do not have official, written policies specifically about the potential to apply for a TUE for use of this medication for a diagnosis of BED. While it is possible that an athlete might receive a TUE from USADA (or any other country's antidoping organization) for use of a stimulant to treat BED, they may not have it recognized by an International Federation or another country's ADO if it is not yet deemed an accepted practice world-wide. Thus, if an athlete plans to compete internationally, this could be a limiting factor.

Bipolar Disorder

Great care should be taken before making a diagnosis of bipolar disorder in anyone, and this assuredly includes athletes, as the indicated medications can cause significant side effects and safety concerns [54]. Medications are typically necessary to control this disorder, especially if it is the more severe form of the disorder (bipolar disorder type I). Lamotrigine and lithium are top choices of sports psychiatrists among mood stabilizing medications for athletes with bipolar spectrum disorders [6]. Lamotrigine is an unsurprising choice, given its favorable side effect profile. However, it is unreliable in preventing and treating mania and, rather, has more evidence for preventing and treating depression [6]. Thus, for athletes with full bipolar disorder type I, prescribers must use great caution and close monitoring if this is the sole mood stabilizing agent used. Lithium is a full-spectrum mood stabilizer, well established for management of both depression and mania. However, its blood levels can fluctuate with hydration status (e.g., due to athletes sweating heavily, dehydrating themselves for weigh-ins in certain sports, etc.). Thus, its use must occur only with close laboratory and clinical monitoring and insistence on adequate hydration [1, 7]. Many medications for bipolar disorder, apart from lamotrigine, can cause sedation, weight gain, and/or tremor. These include antipsychotic medications, valproic acid, and lithium [6]. Among the atypical antipsychotics, aripiprazole, lurasidone, and ziprasidone are relatively less likely to cause sedation and weight gain and thus might be preferable choices in athletes [6]. However, ziprasidone may cause a cardiac risk—QTc prolongation [55]—and thus may not be a first-line choice within this class for athletes, though it has not been studied in this population. Finally, it is worth noting that within the general population, antipsychotics such as quetiapine are sometimes used for sleep or anxiety (though not FDA-approved for these purposes), but for the athlete population in particular, in the absence of a bona fide bipolar or psychosis diagnosis, they should generally not be used for these purposes given the side effect burden that may be problematic in high-level sport [7].

Psychotic Disorders

It is important for members of athletes' health care teams to be aware of the signs and symptoms of psychotic disorders such as schizophrenia, as their peak age of onset coincides with typical peak ages of sport performance [54]. Early identification is important, as early treatment, including with medications, may favorably alter the course of these disorders. Presumably for the same reasons explained above, aripiprazole emerges as sports psychiatrists' top choice of medications for psychotic disorders in athletes [6]. So-called "typical" antipsychotics, e.g., haloperidol, appear to be infrequent choices for psychosis in athletes [6]. This latter class may cause significant sedation and movement side effects including, but not limited to, tremor, which can interfere with fine motor coordination [56]. Typical antipsychotics also appear more likely than most "atypical" antipsychotics (e.g., aripiprazole) to cause cardiac concerns [55].

Special Considerations: Supplements

Especially for athletes at higher levels of competition, care must be taken if any nonregulated/nonprescription supplements are taken to attempt to treat mental health symptoms or disorders. Athletes might be drawn to the idea of taking a "natural" product, especially given the stigma that exists regarding seeking of mental health treatment. However, supplements may be unknowingly tainted with prohibited substances [1]. Ignorance of ingredients or improper labeling is not typically regarded as a valid excuse for adverse analytical findings on drug tests [1]. If supplements are taken, they should be obtained from a reputable company [1]. Moreover, several supplements marketed for mental health symptoms and disorders may cause side effects such as sedation, insomnia, or gastrointestinal upset [57] that could be problematic for performing athletes. Cannabidiol (CBD) is one example of a supplement that has been widely marketed to athletes as helpful for anxiety, insomnia, pain, and postexercise recovery among other conditions, but it has not been the subject of rigorous study [58]. Additionally, athletes consuming it risk ingesting tetrahydrocannabinol, which may contaminate the product [58] and is prohibited at several levels of competition [8, 9].

Conclusion

Additional research on pharmacotherapy for mental health symptoms and disorders in athletes is severely needed. Studies with the following characteristics are particularly needed: large sample sizes across different sports and sexes; use of medications in dosing and duration representative of how they are used in the real world; studies of actual athletes competing at high levels of competition who have been diagnosed with the mental health disorder the medication is designed to treat; and study of the impact of medications on relevant performance metrics. New research of this type might allow more athletes with moderate to severe mental health disorders to be treated with needed medications in a manner that is safe, effective, and unlikely to negatively impact sport performance.

In conclusion, it is critical that prescribers of psychiatric medications for athletes be familiar with issues of relevance for this population, including safety risks, potential positive or negative impact on performance, and regulations surrounding use of certain medications. All treatment team members should be aware of and on the lookout for side effects that may limit performance. Importantly, though, it is a delicate balance between scrutinizing for side effects and not discouraging use of needed medication in mentally ill athletes. Additionally, all treatment team members should be aware of any medication prohibitions and documentation requirements within their athletes' leagues and levels of competition. Athletes should be reminded to always ask their prescribers if a given medication or substance is allowed in their sport, without extra documentation or preapproval needed, prior to ingesting it.

Athletes and their treatment teams do well to think of psychiatric medications as one potentially important part of a treatment plan, but rarely should they be the only part. An analogy to musculoskeletal injury is appropriate. With a musculoskeletal injury, athletes may need medication (e.g., to decrease pain or inflammation), but they also need to participate in rehabilitation exercises. Similarly, athletes with a mental health "injury" may need medication, but they also need to participate in rehabilitation exercises in the form of psychotherapy or other types of psychosocial support. It is critical that they have the support of all members of their health care team, just as they would for musculoskeletal injury, as they undertake any such treatment for mental health symptoms or disorders.

References

1. Reardon CL, Hainline B, Aron CM, Baron D, Baum AL, Bindra A, et al. Mental health in elite athletes: International Olympic Committee Consensus Statement. Br J Sports Med. 2019;53(11):667–99.

2. Castaldelli-Maia J, de Mello Gallinaro JG, Falcao RS, Gouttebarge V, Hitchcock ME, Hainline B, et al. Mental health symptoms and disorders in elite athletes: a systematic review on cultural influencers and barriers to athletes seeking treatment. Br J Sports Med. 2019;53(11):707–21.

3. Gabrilova Y. Concurrent mental health and sport performance enhancement in an athlete initiating behavioral intervention with no assessed pathology: a case examination supporting optimization. University of Nevada, Las Vegas Theses, Dissertations, Professionals Papers, and Capstones. 2016. Available from https://digitalscholarship.unlv.edu/cgi/viewcontent.cgi?article=3670&context=thesesdissertations. Accessed 9 May 2021.

4. Gorczynski P, Currie A, Gibson K, Gouttebarge V, Hainline B, Castaldelli-Maia JM, et al. Developing mental health literacy and cultural competence in elite sport. J Appl Sport Psychol. 2020. https://doi.org/10.1080/10413200.2020.1720045.

5. Johnston A, McAllister-Williams RH. Psychotropic drug prescribing. In: Currie A, Owen B, editors. Sports psychiatry. Oxford University Press: Oxford; 2016. p. 133–43.

6. Reardon CL, Creado S. Psychiatric medication preferences of sports psychiatrists. Phys Sports Med. 2016;44(4):397–402.

7. Reardon CL. The sports psychiatrist and psychiatric medications. Int Rev Psychiatry. 2016;28(6):606–13.

8. World Anti-Doping Agency. International standard prohibited list. 2021. Available from https://www.wada-ama.org/sites/default/files/resources/files/2021list_en.pdf. Accessed 10 May 2021.

9. NCAA Sport Science Institute. 2020-2021 NCAA banned substances. Available from https://www.ncaa.org/sport-science-institute/topics/2020-21-ncaa-banned-substances. Accessed 10 May 2021.

10. World Anti-Doping Agency. Therapeutic use exemptions. Available from https://www.wada-ama.org/en/what-we-do/science-medical/therapeutic-use-exemptions. Accessed 10 May 2021.

11. NCAA Sport Science Institute. Medical exceptions procedures. Available from: http://www.ncaa.org/sport-science-institute/medical-exceptions-procedures. Accessed 10 May 2021.

12. Reardon CL, Factor RM. Considerations in the use of stimulants in sport. Sports Med. 2016;46(5):611–7.

13. Garner AA, Hansen AA, Baxley C, Ross MJ. The use of stimulant medication to treat attention-deficit/hyperactivity disorder in elite athletes: a performance and health perspective. Sports Med. 2018;48(3):507–12.

14. de Zwaan M. Exercise and antidepressant serum levels. Biol Psychiatry. 1992;32:210–1.

15. Reardon CL, Factor RM. Sport psychiatry: a systematic review of diagnosis and medical treatment of mental illness in athletes. Sports Med. 2010;40(11):961–80.

16. World Anti-Doping Agency. Monitoring program. Available from https://www.wada-ama.org/en/resources/science-medicine/monitoring-program. Accessed 10 May 2021.

17. Watson P, Hasegawa H, Roelands B, Piacentini MF, Looverie R, Meeusen R. Acute dopamine/noradrenaline reuptake inhibition enhances human exercise performance in warm, but not temperate conditions. J Physiol. 2005;565(3):873–83.

18. Roelands B, Hasegawa H, Watson P, Piacentini MF, Buyse L, De Schutter G, et al. Performance and thermoregulatory effects of chronic bupropion administration in the heat. Eur J Appl Physiol. 2009;105(3):493–8.

19. Roelands B, Watson P, Cordery P, Decoster S, Debaste E, Maughan R, et al. A dopamine/noradrenaline reuptake inhibitor improves performance in the heat, but only at the maximum therapeutic dose. Scand J Med Sci Sports. 2012;22(5):93–8.

20. Meeusen R, Piacentini MF, van Den Eynde S, Magnus L, De Meirleir K. Exercise performance is not influenced by a 5-HT reuptake inhibitor. Int J Sports Med. 2001;22(5):329–36.

21. Parise G, Bosman MJ, Boeeker DR. Selective serotonin reuptake inhibitors: their effect on high-intensity exercise performance. Arch Phys Med Rehabil. 2001;82(7):867–71.

22. Baum AL. Psychopharmacology in athletes. In: Begel D, Burton RW, editors. Sport psychiatry. New York: W. W. Norton & Company; 2000. p. 249–59.

23. Marken PA, Munro JS. Selecting a selective serotonin reuptake inhibitor: clinically important distinguishing features. J Clin Psychiatry. 2000;2(6):205–10.

24. Bixby AL, VandenBerg A, Bostwick JR. Clinical management of bleeding risk with antidepressants. Ann Pharmacother. 2019;53(2):186–94.

25. Roelands B, Goekint M, Heyman E, Piacentini MF, Watson P, Hasegawa H, et al. Acute norepinephrine reuptake inhibition decreases performance in normal and high ambient temperature. J Appl Physiol. 2008;105:206–12.

26. Wang F, Wang J, Cao Y, Xu Z. Serotonin-norepinephrine reuptake inhibitors for the prevention of migraine and vestibular migraine: a systematic review and meta-analysis. Reg Anesth Pain Med. 2020;45(5):323–30.

27. Pae C. Low-dose mirtazapine may be successful treatment option for severe nausea and vomiting. Prog Neuro-Psychopharmacol Biol Psychiatry. 2006;30(6):1143–5.

28. Xu X, Liu Y, Dong M, Zou D, Wei Y. Tricyclic antidepressants for preventing migraine in adults. Medicine. 2017;96(22):e6989.

29. Marvanova M, Gramith K. Role of antidepressants in the treatment of adults with anorexia nervosa. Ment Health Clin. 2018;8(3):127–37.

30. Barowsky J, Schwartz TL. An evidence-based approach to augmentation and combination strategies for treatment-resistant depression. Psychiatry. 2006;3(7):42–61.

31. Marvin G, Sharma A, Aston W, Field C, Kendall MJ, Jones DA. The effects of buspirone on perceived exertion and time to fatigue in man. Exp Physiol. 1997;82(6):1057–60.

32. Charles RB, Kirkham AJ, Guyatt AR, Parker SP. Psychomotor, pulmonary, and exercise responses to sleep medication. Br J Clin Pharmacol. 1987;24(2):191–7.

33. Paul MA, Gray G, Kenny G, Pigeau RA. Impact of melatonin, zaleplon, zopiclone, and temazepam on psychomotor performance. Aviat Space Environ Med. 2003;74(12):1263–70.

34. Cowan DA. Drug abuse. In: Harries M, Williams C, Stanish WD, Micheli LJ, editors. Oxford textbook of sports medicine. Oxford: Oxford University Press; 1994. p. 314–29.

35. Atkinson G, Drust B, Reilly T, Waterhouse J. The relevance of melatonin to sports medicine and science. Sports Med. 2003;33(11):809–31.

36. Herman D, Macknight JM, Stromwall AE, Mistry DJ. The international athlete—advances in management of jet lag and anti-doping policy. Clin J Sport Med. 2011;30(3):641–59.

37. Grobler LA, Schwellnus MP, Trichard C, Calder S, Noakes TD, Derman WE. Comparative effects of zopiclone and loprazolam on psychomotor and physical performance in active individuals. Clin J Sport Med. 2000;10(2):123–8.

38. Holmberg G. The effects of anxiolytics on CFF. Pharmacopsychiatry. 1982;15(1):49–53.

39. Ito SU, Kanbayashi T, Takemura T, Kondo H, Inomata S, Szilagyi G, et al. Acute effects of zolpidem on daytime alertness, psychomotor and physical performance. Neurosci Res. 2007;59(3):309–13.

40. Tafti M, Besset A, Billiard M. Effects of zopiclone on subjective evaluation of sleep and daytime alertness and on psychomotor and physical performance tests in athletes. Neuropsychopharmacol Biol Psychiatry. 1992;16(1):55–63.

41. Maddock RJ, Casson EJ, Lott LA, Carter CS, Johnson CA. Benzodiazepine effects on flicker sensitivity: role of stimu-

lus frequency and size. Neuropsychopharmacol Biol Psychiatry. 1993;17(6):955–70.

42. Longo LP, Johnson B. Addiction: part I. Benzodiazepines – side effects, abuse risk, and alternatives. Am Fam Physician. 2000;61(7):2121–30.

43. Han DH, McDuff D, Thompson D, Hitchcock ME, Reardon CL, Hainline B. Attention-deficit/hyperactivity disorder in elite athletes: a narrative review. Br J Sports Med. 2019;53(12):741–5.

44. Chandler JV, Blair SN. The effect of amphetamines on selected physiological components related to athletic success. Med Sci Sports Exerc. 1980;12(1):65–9.

45. Roelands B, Hasegawa H, Watson P, Piacentini MF, Buyse L, De Schutter G, et al. The effects of acute dopamine reuptake inhibition on performance. Med Sci Sports Exerc. 2008;40(5):879–85.

46. Ciocca M, Stafford H, Laney R. The athlete's pharmacy. Clin J Sport Med. 2011;246(30):629–39.

47. Perrin AE, Jotwani VM. Addressing the unique issues of student athletes with ADHD. J Fam Pract. 2014;63:1–9.

48. Pujalte GGA, Maynard JR, Thurston MJ, Taylor WC III, Chauhan M. Considerations in the care of athletes with attention deficit hyperactivity disorder. Clin J Sport Med. 2019;29(3):245–56.

49. Putukian M, Kreher JB, Coppel DB, Glazer JL, McKeag DB, White RD. Attention deficit hyperactivity disorder and the athlete: an American Medical Society for Sports Medicine position statement. Clin J Sport Med. 2011;21(5):392–400.

50. U.S. Anti-Doping Agency. Apply for a therapeutic use exemption (TUE). Available from https://www.usada.org/substances/tue/apply/. Accessed 11 May 2021.

51. Verbeeck W, Bekkering GE, Van den Noortgate W, Kramers C. Bupropion for attention deficit hyperactivity disorder (ADHD) in adults. Cochrane Database Syst Rev. 2017;10:1–58.

52. Joy E, Kussman A, Nattiv A. 2016 update on eating disorders in athletes: a comprehensive narrative review with a focus on clinical assessment and management. Br J Sports Med. 2016;50(3):154–62.

53. American Psychiatric Association. Practice guideline for the treatment of patients with eating disorders, 3rd ed. American Psychiatric Association Publishing. Available from https://psychiatryonline.org/pb/assets/raw/sitewide/practice_guidelines/guidelines/eating-disorders.pdf. Accessed 11 May 2021.

54. Currie A, Gorczynski P, Rice S, Purcell R, McAllister-Williams RH, Hitchcock ME, et al. Bipolar and psychotic disorders in elite athletes: a narrative review. Br J Sports Med. 2019;53(12):746–53.

55. Beach SR, Celano CM, Noseworthy PA, Januzzi JL, Huffman JC. QTc prolongation, torsades de pointes, and psychotropic medications. Psychosomatics. 2013;54(1):1–13.

56. Macleod AD. Sport psychiatry. Aust N Z J Psychiatry. 1998;32(6):860–6.

57. Ravindran AV, Balneaves LG, Faulkner G. Canadian network for mood and anxiety treatments (CANMAT) 2016 clinical guidelines for the management of adults with major depressive disorder: section 5. Complementary and alternative medicine treatments. Focus. 2018;16(1):85–94.

58. Lachenmeier DW, Diel P. A warning against the negligent use of cannabidiol in professional and amateur athletes. Sports. 2019;7(12):251.

Creating an Environment That Supports Mental Well-Being and Resilience

Emily Kroshus

Introduction

Sports organizations are increasingly articulating a commitment to athlete mental health [1–4]. However, there is wide variability in how such organizational commitments are put into action. The differences include how mental health is operationalized, whether strategies adopted are evidence-informed, and the extent to which equity is prioritized. Ultimately, such choices determine the impact of organizational mental health initiatives, and this includes not just the extent of their impact, but also who benefits. Guided by a quality improvement (QI) perspective, the overarching goal of this chapter is to provide a framework for how sports organizations can work toward improving mental health. QI efforts tend to broadly follow iterative cycles of "Plan, Do, Study, Act" [5]. Reflecting on your organizational values as they pertain to equity and antiracism at the outset of this process can guide decision-making at key nodes. This will help guide your decision-making about who is involved in the planning process, whose needs are being prioritized, and who defines success.

Plan

Planning should be a reflexive process that engages a range of stakeholders in clarifying setting-specific needs and selecting interventions or strategies for improvement that address those needs. Oftentimes, this process is short-changed due to external pressures, such as compliance with an administrative mandate (e.g., from a sport governing body), or because decisions are made reactively or under time constraints. For example, after a high-profile crisis event, there may be a desire to quickly "do something." A low resource and high visibility approach might be an "awareness campaign." Such efforts often presume that increasing issue visibility will reduce stigma related to mental health symptoms and disorders, and thus encourage care seeking. This may in fact be a useful and setting-relevant strategy. However, it should be arrived at strategically rather than reactively or performatively. This means being clear about the needs of athletes and others in your organization, identifying the outcome you are trying to change, articulating the mechanisms or processes that contribute to that outcome, and identifying approaches to intervention that have the best chance of working. Below, questions are posed for reflection and to help guide a strategic planning process.

What Problem Are You Trying to Address? Knowing about the current needs of athletes served by your organization—problems, preferences, and priorities—is a necessary first step in the planning process. Before thinking about *how* to assess needs, it is critical that you reflect on *what* you are trying to answer through this process. This will determine the types of questions that you are asking, and from whom, which will determine the potential scope of what you might learn.

How Are You Defining Mental Health, and What Aspects of Mental Health Are You Prioritizing? What may first come to mind is the absence of symptomatology of mental health disorders. However, mental health is increasingly being conceptualized as occurring on dual continuums, including both the presence or absence of symptoms of mental health disorders, and the presence or absence of positive psychological functioning [6–9]; these are not mutually exclusive or opposite ends of the same continuum. A dual continuum approach to mental health sends important messages about what mental health means and for whom. Namely, it suggests that everyone can be taking steps to increase their subjective well-being, and that mental health is not a construct limited only to individuals struggling with

E. Kroshus (✉)
Seattle Children's Research Institute, Center for Child Health, Behavior and Development, Seattle, WA, USA

Department of Pediatrics, University of Washington, Seattle, WA, USA
e-mail: ekroshus@uw.edu

diagnosable mental health disorders. However, even if an organization's focus is on limiting pathology, reflection is needed on "which" disorders. The Diagnostic and Statistical Manual of Mental Disorders lists nearly 300 mental health disorders. "Internalizing" disorders (e.g., anxiety, depression) are among the most common mental disorders experienced by adolescents and young adults [10, 11]. However, also prevalent among adolescents and young adults in general, as well as among athletes, are "externalizing" disorders and eating disorders. Externalizing disorders may manifest as antisocial aggression or substance misuse. Successful transdiagnostic organizational initiatives are possible if they target common risk factors. Such initiatives might include improving access to licensed clinicians to help individuals with any mental health-related concern. However, the pathways through which specific disorders arise are not consistent across diagnoses, and sport setting messaging related to mental health may center some disorders to the exclusion of others. For example, messaging equating mental health with internalizing disorders may limit the willingness of individuals struggling with symptoms of externalizing disorders to engage with mental health supportive resources.

How Are You Defining Mental Health "Prevention" or "Promotion"? Concepts of primary, secondary, and tertiary prevention from the World Health Organization's prevention framework have been used as a broad framing for approaches to mental health intervention in the sport setting [12, 13]. Primary prevention refers to reducing new incidence of mental health disorders (primary prevention), secondary prevention to reducing harm through early detection and onset of treatment, and tertiary prevention to ensuring appropriate management across the duration of the disorder [14]. Asking questions specifically about each type of prevention during your needs assessment process can help determine which are the most appropriate opportunities for intervention. However, the decision to focus on one type of prevention over another may ultimately be a function of organizational values or priorities. Primary prevention is often a universal approach that shifts risk a small amount for a large number of people, whereas secondary and tertiary prevention tend to be indicated and targeted at individuals experiencing a specific event or need.

What Might Be Contributing to the Problem You Are Trying to Address? Interventions to improve mental health typically target factors upstream of health outcomes. Trying to identify these factors is a potentially overwhelming task. Below, theoretic perspectives that can help organize your thinking about what might be driving mental health differences for athletes in your setting are outlined. These frameworks can be used to help guide the questions you are asking

when conducting a needs assessment, and how you are organizing and interpreting the information you get back during this process.

Biology, Psychology, Context Biopsychosocial models broadly propose that mental health is a function of individual biology, psychological factors, and social/contextual factors [15]. Social and contextual factors can be understood as occurring at multiple levels, ranging from interpersonal interactions (e.g., with coaches, teammates, parents, health care providers), to the groups within which the athlete is embedded (e.g., team, family), to the broader administrative structures or organizations within which these groups are situated (e.g., athletic department, institution, community), all the way up to society broadly. Coaches, teammates, and organizations may influence mental health outcomes indirectly or directly. Teammates can potentially play an important role in limiting psychological distress if athletes are taking time aware from competition for illness, injury, or other reasons [16, 17]. Social support and social engagement are important determinants of subjective well-being, independent of their relationship with distress or mental health disorders [18]. The extent to which teammates feel empowered and encouraged to engage in such supportive practices is likely a function of how it is reinforced by their coach, and more broadly their organization. Coaches, for example, may make explicit negative comments about mental health disorders, or refer to people as being mentally weak; such communication may de-value care seeking and shape perceptions that it would be viewed negatively by the team's coach and potentially also team members [19–21]. On the other hand, explicit verbal messaging from coaches can help normalize and positively reinforce mental health care seeking [19], as well as ongoing treatment adherence [19, 22, 23]. Coaches may also directly modify stressors (e.g., scheduling practices at a time that allows for adequate sleep), and identify individuals who may require further evaluation and encourage or facilitate referral to a licensed mental health clinician. They can also help limit structural barriers to treatment adherence, for example, by making sure practice schedules or other sport responsibilities do not impede care seeking. Critically, coaches are part of broader sports organizations, and their actions—and the extent to which their actions lead to positive mental health outcomes—are constrained by organizational practices. For example, encouraging care seeking is only useful if athletes have access to licensed mental health care providers with appropriate competencies. Adopting a biopsychosocial perspective during the needs assessment process might lead you to ask questions specifically about barriers and facilitators to outcomes of interest in different interpersonal and organizational contexts.

Social Determinants of Health The World Health Organization Social Determinants of Health Framework [24] situates individual health outcomes, proximal biological, psychological, and material constraints, and access to health care, in social determinants of health (e.g., education, income), and then more broadly in structural determinants of health inequities (e.g., policies, racism). This is a more nuanced way of thinking about the contexts within which athletes are embedded and that shape their vulnerabilities and assets related to mental health. In the United States and many other countries, a key structural determinant of health inequities is ongoing systemic, institutional, interpersonal, and internalized racism; this contributes to inequitable risk of poor mental health among racial minority individuals [25], including athletes [26–30]. While different countries have different histories of racialization and racism, where such systemic factors exist, they are a critical—and often overlooked—influence on athlete mental health. Outside of sport there is a large body of evidence about how racial and ethnic minority populations often experience marginalization in health care settings, including not having their concerns taken seriously [31, 32]. Within the sport context, discussion about race, ethnicity, and mental health has tended to focus on differences in help seeking attitudes and behaviors. For example, the International Olympic Committee's consensus statement states, "Negative attitudes about mental health services are associated with several factors, including identification as male, younger age, and Black (versus Caucasian) race." [33] However, less often discussed is the systemic origin of differences in help seeking, such as lack of racial minority health care providers, and biases, and differences in communication and care in the sport and sports medicine setting. While sport-setting initiatives may have limited potential to change many structural determinants of health inequities, it is essential that this broad perspective be considered during the needs assessment process. It means considering how different athletes may enter the same sport setting with different vulnerabilities and assets that may impact the care that will meet their needs. It also means reflecting as an organization on whether organizational practices are exacerbating or maintaining inequities related to race or other structural or social determinants of health.

What Are Possible Approaches to Intervention? The right approaches to intervention will reflect setting-specific needs, priorities, and resource constraints. These will likely change over time. Broadly, the most impactful approaches to intervention tend to be changing organizational practices rather than intervening with individuals to change their behavior. Some potential organizational changes are discussed below.

Screening Implementing screening at an organizational level can help with secondary prevention: ensuring that individuals who may benefit from mental health care are identified. Screening could potentially be implemented during preparticipation physical examinations or clearance processes [34, 35], if those exist in a given sport setting. However, there may also be benefits to screening during the competitive season, given changes in sport-related stressors [36]. An important consideration with screening is ensuring there is a plan in place for what happens next. The United States Preventive Service Task Force specifies that organizations should only engage in screening if systems are in place for appropriate follow-up evaluation and care [37]. It is essential that the tools being used to screen are reliable and valid; partnering with a licensed mental health care provider can help with selecting appropriate measures and establishing a clinically relevant protocol for acting based on responses. Few questionnaire-based screening tools have been developed for athletes [34], meaning they may not adequately account for athlete-specific confounding symptomatology such as overtraining syndrome [38, 39]. Recently, a working group of the International Olympic Committee published a brief screening tool for athlete mental health problems: the Sport Mental Health Assessment Tool-1 (SMHAT-1) [40]. While validation work is ongoing, initial evidence suggests it is sensitive to problems that require further evaluation. It also contains guidance for clinicians on interpretation and disorder-specific screeners, making it relatively feasible to adopt and implement.

Mental Health Protocols Establishing a setting-specific protocol for what to do in routine and emergency mental health situations can help standardize responses [34]. Different stakeholders have different potential roles and responsibilities in terms of referral and management. Prior research finds that coaches are more confident in how to respond if an athlete is struggling with a mental health symptom or disorder if they are aware of their organization's mental health protocol [41].

Requirements Related to Clinician Licensure The National Collegiate Athletic Association's (NCAA's) Mental Health Best Practices outline the importance of individuals providing mental health care having relevant professional licensure [1]. This can include a potentially broad range of practitioners. Sometimes individuals with training in athletic performance enhancement, or sport psychology, are valued members of an athlete's or team's entourage but not licensed to provide mental health care. Organizations should review the NCAA's guidance and consider adopting it or something similar in their setting—reviewing who is currently supporting athletes with mental health concerns and establishing licensure criteria.

Staffing and Access to Licensed Clinicians Resource-related constraints and organizational structure will mean that different sport organizations will have different capacity to engage directly with mental health professionals. Some sports organizations will have the resources to employ mental health practitioners, while others will have relationships with community health care resources. Where resources allow, organizations should be mindful of the importance of adequate staffing to meet athlete needs and be open to creative solutions for staffing, including supervised clinical students. Where not possible to have dedicated staffing due to financial considerations or local availability, organizations can work to establish partnerships with community health providers (or in the case of universities, on campus providers) and/or explore telehealth. When hiring or identifying potential clinicians to whom athletes can be referred, organizations should consider prioritizing racial and ethnic diversity [42].

Clinician Competencies Organizations should also consider whether clinicians providing mental health care to athletes have received training related to trauma-informed and culturally competent care. In the United States, more than 40% of children experience at least one adverse childhood event [43]; experiencing such events is associated with worse mental health [44]. Rates are heightened among Black individuals, in part due to experiences of racism and racial trauma [45, 46]. Trauma-sensitive clinical care will not address the underlying systemic and structural causes of racism and other forms of trauma, but it can help ensure that clinical care is provided that best meets current mental health needs. Key practices include prioritizing safety, transparency, and empowerment, and limiting potential for re-traumatization [47]. Training in cultural competence, including understanding concepts of power and structural determinants of health inequities, are also important and can help ensure care is being provided that meets the needs of all athletes across diverse lived experiences and identities [47]. Organizations can consider encouraging or incentivizing continuing education trainings in trauma-informed care and cultural competence and prioritizing these competencies in the hiring process.

Stakeholder Education A dominant paradigm for education related to mental health is mental health first aid. Such approaches emphasize mental health literacy [48, 49], focusing on recognition of mental health symptoms and referral to appropriate sources of support, including evidence-based interventions [19, 48]. This can have an important place in organizational mental health initiatives, as prior research finds that many coaches are not sure what to do when it comes to supporting athletes with mental health symptoms [50] and are worried they will cause harm by doing the wrong thing [51].

Education has also been proposed as a strategy for addressing biases among sport-setting stakeholders, with the goal of reducing racism and other forms of discrimination [52]. There are many different approaches to bias-related education [53], with variable quality and limited evidence of effects persisting beyond a few hours or days [54]. One of the most promising interventions is the prejudice habit-breaking intervention [55], which has evidence of sustained impact on implicit bias [56]. Trainings that address the structural origins of biases [57] and that aim to support organizational change related to those structures tend to be the most impactful [58].

What is critical to emphasize is that such educational interventions—whether related to mental health broadly or bias specifically—must do more than just raise awareness [59]. They must provide concrete behavior change strategies and support oriented at those behaviors [60]. Considerations when deciding on educational approaches include the evidence base (is there a published evaluation about its effectiveness?) and delivery mechanism. Even the best-designed approaches to education will often be forgotten, so it is worth thinking about education as an ongoing process and determining when and how content will be refreshed and how it will be reinforced. How information is shared can impact the incidental information received by learners. For example, is the education being delivered via individual online learning? If so, individuals will not have the opportunity to observe peers endorsing these behaviors. On the other hand, when interventions are delivered in group settings, group processes may serve to undermine the messaging, for example via devaluing a given behavior or even just failing to support it explicitly [61, 62]. Organizations can help shape positive norms that reinforce educational messaging by attending explicitly to how education is delivered and whether there is a plan for supporting positive within-group dialogue.

What Data Are Being Used and Whose Voices Are Being Heard? Population-level data can provide a good start in identifying the types of mental health issues that are likely to be problematic in most sport settings and the types of mechanisms or factors that are related to those issues. For example, around one quarter of young adults will experience symptoms of depression and anxiety [11], with little differences between athletes and nonathletes at a population level [63]. Thus, it is likely that a nontrivial fraction of athletes in most elite sport settings will have needs related to symptoms of these and related internalizing disorders. Some sports organizations are collecting mental health surveillance data to inform organizational decision-making.

However, even accurate setting-specific prevalence estimates do not convey the extent to which these are the most pressing problems from the perspectives of athletes or the licensed mental health providers caring for athletes, or the setting-specific factors that are considered problematic. Stakeholder feedback can provide critical setting-specific information on problems. Information about needs can be elicited in a variety of ways, including interviews, surveys, or focus groups. Getting data from multiple sources and perspectives can help ensure that the conclusions being drawn reflect true needs in a given setting. However, it is important to think carefully about those from whom input is solicited, whether important voices are systematically being missed, and whether those present feel comfortable sharing their experiences and needs. For example, is feedback sought from individuals from historically under-represented and oppressed racial and ethnic groups in sufficient number? Is their feedback being sought in such a way that they feel comfortable sharing experiences and perspectives without fear of negative interpersonal interactions or recrimination? Options to consider include eliciting anonymous survey feedback, or convening one-on-one or small group listening sessions with homogeneous identities. Consider also that individuals sharing needs and experiences may benefit from support related to their disclosures. Organizations should partner with licensed mental health care providers throughout the needs assessment process.

What Are Your Organizational Values? A needs-assessment process will likely reveal many areas for potential change and many different perspectives on what is most important. With unlimited resources and time, all should be addressed. However, in practice, it is likely that hard decisions will have to be made about what to prioritize.

Clarifying organizational values can help guide this decision-making process.

Do

After deciding what steps to take, it is important to also think critically about how these steps will be put into action. This means identifying things that could get in the way of the plan happening the way that it needs to or having the desired impact. Below are some potential considerations to think through while making a plan to put a change strategy into action.

Clarify Roles and Responsibilities When implementing a new intervention or organizational change, it is important that everyone involved is clear on their roles, including what is required of them and their duration of responsibility. Continuing to engage a multidisciplinary group of stakeholders can help provide guidance on the type of messaging and support that is needed across roles.

Rehearse and Remind Some changes may require individuals to engage in specific behaviors in emergency situations, such as responding to a mental health emergency by following an established protocol. Practice can help make these behaviors automatic and accessible in situations of physiologic arousal. Information should also be repeated (e.g., across the sports season, rather than only addressing it once prior to the start of the season) so that it is more easily recalled.

Get Opinion Leaders on Board Opinion leaders can reinforce or undermine intervention approaches. In the case of educational programming for athletes, coach engagement is critical. Coaches do not have to be the ones leading educational sessions—and they do not have to be experts on mental health. Rather, they need to make explicit to athletes that they support the education being delivered. Coaches should also be encouraged to reflect on how they may be inadvertently undermining educational messaging. Getting coaches on board with this kind of self-reflection and engagement likely requires adopting a formal approach to coach education. Expecting all coaches to be ready and able to champion mental health initiatives is not realistic [13]. Thus, thinking about what support they are receiving, and what organizational incentives they are subject to, can help create a context for coaches to become champions for mental health initiatives.

Think About Incentives Organizational leaders should reflect on whether there are implied organizational values that may be undermining mental health initiatives. For example, an awareness campaign about mental health may be undermined if there is inadequate staffing; lack of staffing may send a message to athletes and coaches that the organization is not willing to invest necessary resources in mental health. Similarly, if coaches who win but are abusive or dismissive of mental health concerns are lauded and rewarded, athletes and other coaches may discount organizational messaging about mental health and well-being. Getting feedback from a diverse group of stakeholders and using a medium where they feel comfortable sharing their honest thoughts may help identify organizational blind spots or incongruence between stated and implied values.

Study

Often, health promotion efforts in sport settings are focused on compliance with sport governing body directives, or minimizing liability. While these are real and important imperatives, they do not guarantee that the approach being used is optimizing athlete health outcomes. Getting feedback on how things are going, and being willing to rapidly adjust, can help optimize mental health-related efforts. Below are some things to think through when deciding how you will study the impact of your program.

What Questions Are You Trying to Answer? What you study is directly linked to the questions you outlined during the planning process: what are you ultimately trying to impact, and what are you trying to change directly through your intervention? Your questions should be specific and measurable [64]. Do you anticipate changing mental health outcomes broadly, or are you focused on symptomatology of specific mental health symptoms or disorders? Are you measuring whether athletes have clinically relevant symptoms or a clinically diagnosed disorder [38]? Are you focusing on all athletes, or specific subgroups (e.g., sport, gender, race, or other identity or group factors)? Ultimately, athlete mental health outcomes will be difficult to shift on aggregate because they are influenced by a range of factors, only some of which are modifiable within a relatively short period of time and within the sport setting. Thus, to get information about the utility of the change you implemented, it is also useful to measure impact on *processes* or *behaviors* that are closely connected to the change you are implementing. For example, if you implemented a mental health protocol, you could measure process outcomes (did key stakeholder groups review the protocol, rehearse it, and remember what to do?) and behavioral outcomes (did they follow it if an emergency situation arose?).

Where Are You Getting Data? Where possible, using existing data sources will allow you to understand impact while limiting resource demands. In some settings, this might be data from electronic health records (attending to regulations and permissions related to confidentiality). The type of data needed will depend on the nature of the questions you are trying to answer (and the questions that you can answer depend on the data that you are able to access). If you are interested in changes in specific subgroups of athletes— or reducing differences between subgroups—then you need to make sure your data allow for subgroup analyses, both in terms of the information recorded and the number of people in each subgroup. As with the planning phase, be aware of those from whom you are seeking feedback, and who is involved in interpreting it, as this may reveal gaps in what you are learning based on the experiences and identities of individuals involved in the process.

What Is Your Timeframe? Quality improvement methods often use short cycles of intervention and study, making changes iteratively in response learnings [5, 65]. Rather than rolling out a comprehensive intervention and studying it over the course of a year, getting feedback shortly after any change has been implemented can help your organization course correct or optimize efforts to better meet athlete needs.

Act

Acting on what you find is a critical element of quality improvement processes. What you find might not necessarily provide a definitive answer about "effectiveness." You might learn that you need to ask questions a bit differently or address different barriers to implementation. Even if you find the changes you implemented were effective, needs will change over time, whether due to external or internal events or the composition of individuals in your setting. Taking a quality improvement perspective to organizational mental health-related efforts means assuming that there is always something to learn, and some way in which improvement or modification may be needed to meet the needs of stakeholders in your setting.

Conclusions

Creating an environment that supports mental health— whether minimizing symptoms of mental health disorders or optimizing subjective well-being—is an ongoing and evolving process for sports organizations. Taking a quality improvement approach to meeting organizational needs related to mental health promotion means being reflexive, intentional, and strategic in planning, implementing, and studying changes, and acting (e.g., course correcting) based on what you find. This process is, in large part, subjective. Organizations should clarify their values, and use these values to guide their quality improvement decision-making. To the extent these values include a commitment to equity, each stage of the quality improvement process should include reflection on whose voices are being heard, whose perspectives and preferences are being centered, and who is deciding what constitutes "success."

References

1. Mental Health Best Practices. 2016. https://www.ncaa.org/sites/default/files/HS_Mental-Health-Best-Practices_20160317.pdf.
2. Australia's winning edge 2012-2022. Australian Sport Commission. 2012. Accessed July 30, 2018. https://www.ausport.gov.au/__data/assets/pdf_file/0011/509852/Australias_Winning_Edge.pdf.

3. Leading the way on athlete mental health - Athlete365. Accessed January 24, 2022. https://olympics.com/athlete365/well-being/leading-the-way-on-athlete-mental-health/.

4. Liddle SK, Deane FP, Vella SA. Addressing mental health through sport: a review of sporting organizations' websites: addressing mental health through sport. Early Interv Psychiatry. 2017;11(2):93–103. https://doi.org/10.1111/eip.12337.

5. Harrison LM, Shook ED, Harris G, Lea CS, Cornett A, Randolph GD. Applying the model for improvement in a local health department: quality improvement as an effective approach in navigating the changing landscape of public health practice in Buncombe County, North Carolina. J Public Health Manag Pract. 2012;18(1):19–26. https://doi.org/10.1097/PHH.0b013e31822de37c.

6. Peter T, Roberts LW, Dengate J. Flourishing in life: an empirical test of the dual continua model of mental health and mental illness among Canadian university students. Int J Ment Health Promot. 2011;13(1):13–22. https://doi.org/10.1080/14623730.2011.9715646.

7. Franken K, Lamers SMA, Ten Klooster PM, Bohlmeijer ET, Westerhof GJ. Validation of the mental health continuum-short form and the dual continua model of well-being and psychopathology in an adult mental health setting: Franken et al. J Clin Psychol. 2018;74(12):2187–202. https://doi.org/10.1002/jclp.22659.

8. Eklund K, Dowdy E, Jones C, Furlong M. Applicability of the dual-factor model of mental health for college students. J Coll Stud Psychother. 2010;25(1):79–92. https://doi.org/10.1080/87568225.2011.532677.

9. Suldo SM, Shaffer EJ. Looking beyond psychopathology: the dual-factor model of mental health in youth. Sch Psychol Rev. 2008;37(1):52–68. https://doi.org/10.1080/02796015.2008.12087908.

10. Ghandour RM, Sherman LJ, Vladutiu CJ, et al. Prevalence and treatment of depression, anxiety, and conduct problems in US children. J Pediatr. 2019;206:256–67. https://doi.org/10.1016/j.jpeds.2018.09.021.

11. de Jonge P, Wardenaar KJ, Lim CCW, et al. The cross-national structure of mental disorders: results from the World Mental Health Surveys. Psychol Med. 2018;48(12):2073–84. https://doi.org/10.1017/S0033291717003610.

12. Kroshus E, Hainline B. Administering mental health: societal, coaching, and legislative approaches to mental health. In: Hong E, Rao AL, editors. Mental health in the athlete. New York: Springer; 2020. p. 245–59. https://doi.org/10.1007/978-3-030-44754-0_20.

13. Bissett JE, Kroshus E, Hebard S. Determining the role of sport coaches in promoting athlete mental health: a narrative review and Delphi approach. BMJ Open Sport Exerc Med. 2020;6(1):e000676. https://doi.org/10.1136/bmjsem-2019-000676.

14. Caplan G, Grunebaum H. Perspectives on primary prevention: a review. Arch Gen Psychiatry. 1967;17(3):331–46. https://doi.org/10.1001/archpsyc.1967.01730270075012.

15. Álvarez AS, Pagani M, Meucci P. The clinical application of the biopsychosocial model in mental health: a research critique. Am J Phys Med Rehabil. 2012;91(13):173–80. https://doi.org/10.1097/PHM.0b013e31823d54be.

16. Cassilo D, Sanderson J. From social isolation to becoming an advocate: exploring athletes' grief discourse about lived concussion experiences in online forums. Commun Sport. 2019;7(5):678–96. https://doi.org/10.1177/2167479518790039.

17. Putukian M. The psychological response to injury in student athletes: a narrative review with a focus on mental health. Br J Sports Med. 2016;50(3):145–8. https://doi.org/10.1136/bjsports-2015-095586.

18. Rice SM, Purcell R, De Silva S, Mawren D, McGorry PD, Parker AG. The mental health of elite athletes: a narrative systematic review. Sports Med Auckl N Z. 2016;46(9):1333–53. https://doi.org/10.1007/s40279-016-0492-2.

19. Gulliver A, Griffiths KM, Christensen H. Barriers and facilitators to mental health help-seeking for young elite athletes: a qualitative study. BMC Psychiatry. 2012;12(1):157. https://doi.org/10.1186/1471-244X-12-157.

20. Bauman NJ. The stigma of mental health in athletes: are mental toughness and mental health seen as contradictory in elite sport? Br J Sports Med. 2016;50(3):135–6. https://doi.org/10.1136/bjsports-2015-095570.

21. Breslin G, Shannon S, Haughey T, Donnelly P, Leavey G. A systematic review of interventions to increase awareness of mental health and well-being in athletes, coaches and officials. Syst Rev. 2017;6(1):177. https://doi.org/10.1186/s13643-017-0568-6.

22. López RL, Levy JJ. Student athletes' perceived barriers to and preferences for seeking counseling. J Coll Couns. 2013;16(1):19–31. https://doi.org/10.1002/j.2161-1882.2013.00024.x.

23. Watson JC. Student-athletes and counseling: factors influencing the decision to seek counseling services. Coll Stud J. 2006;40(1):35–42.

24. World Health Organization. Social determinants of health. Accessed August 30, 2021. https://www.who.int/westernpacific/health-topics/social-determinants-of-health.

25. Lipson SK, Kern A, Eisenberg D, Breland-Noble AM. Mental health disparities among college students of color. J Adolesc Health. 2018;63(3):348–56. https://doi.org/10.1016/j.jadohealth.2018.04.014.

26. Kroshus E, Davoren AK. Mental health and substance use of sexual minority college athletes. J Am Coll Heal. 2016;64(5):371–9. https://doi.org/10.1080/07448481.2016.1158179.

27. Ballesteros J, Tran AG. Under the face mask: racial-ethnic minority student-athletes and mental health use. J Am Coll Heal. 2020;68(2):169–75. https://doi.org/10.1080/07448481.2018.1536663.

28. Tran AG. Looking forward to student-athlete mental health: racial/ethnic trends from 2010 to 2015. J Am Coll Heal. 2020;2020:1–9. https://doi.org/10.1080/07448481.2020.1725018.

29. Rao AL, Asif IM, Drezner JA, Toresdahl BG, Harmon KG. Suicide in National Collegiate Athletic Association (NCAA) athletes: a 9-year analysis of the NCAA resolutions database. Sports Health Multidiscip Approach. 2015;7(5):452–7. https://doi.org/10.1177/1941738115587675.

30. Li H, Moreland JJ, Peek-Asa C, Yang J. Preseason anxiety and depressive symptoms and prospective injury risk in collegiate athletes. Am J Sports Med. 2017;45(9):2148–55. https://doi.org/10.1177/0363546517702847.

31. McGuire TG, Miranda J. New evidence regarding racial and ethnic disparities in mental health: policy implications. Health Aff. 2008;27(2):393–403. https://doi.org/10.1377/hlthaff.27.2.393.

32. Betancourt JR, Green AR, Carrillo JE, Ananeh-Firempong O. Defining cultural competence: a practical framework for addressing racial/ethnic disparities in health and health care. Public Health Rep. 2003;118(4):293–302. https://doi.org/10.1093/phr/118.4.293.

33. Reardon CL, Hainline B, Aron CM, et al. Mental health in elite athletes: International Olympic Committee consensus statement. Br J Sports Med. 2019;53(11):667–99. https://doi.org/10.1136/bjsports-2019-100715.

34. Rao AL, Hong ES. Understanding depression and suicide in college athletes: emerging concepts and future directions. Br J Sports Med. 2016;50(3):136–7. https://doi.org/10.1136/bjsports-2015-095658.

35. Trojian T. Depression is under-recognised in the sport setting: time for primary care sports medicine to be proactive and screen widely for depression symptoms. Br J Sports Med. 2016;50(3):137–9. https://doi.org/10.1136/bjsports-2015-095582.

36. McGuire LC, Ingram YM, Sachs ML, Tierney RT. Temporal changes in depression symptoms in male and female collegiate student-athletes. J Clin Sport Psychol. 2017;11(4):337–51. https://doi.org/10.1123/JCSP.2016-0035.

37. U.S. Preventive Services Task Force. Screening for depression in adults: U.S. Preventive Services Task Force recommendation statement. Ann Intern Med. 2009;151(11):784. https://doi.org/10.7326/0003-4819-151-11-200912010-00006.

38. Schuch FB. Depression in athletes or increased depressive symptoms in athletes? Curr Sports Med Rep. 2015;14(3):244. https://doi.org/10.1249/JSR.0000000000000151.

39. Bär KJ, Markser VZ. Sport specificity of mental disorders: the issue of sport psychiatry. Eur Arch Psychiatry Clin Neurosci. 2013;263(2):205–10. https://doi.org/10.1007/s00406-013-0458-4.

40. Gouttebarge V, Bindra A, Blauwet C, et al. International Olympic Committee (IOC) Sport Mental Health Assessment Tool 1 (SMHAT-1) and Sport Mental Health Recognition Tool 1 (SMHRT-1): towards better support of athletes' mental health. Br J Sports Med. 2021;55(1):30–7. https://doi.org/10.1136/bjsports-2020-102411.

41. Kroshus E, Coppel D, Chrisman SPD, Herring S. Coach support of high school student-athletes struggling with anxiety or depression. J Clin Sport Psychol. 2018;13:390–404.

42. Naoi A, Watson J, Deaner H, Sato M. Multicultural issues in sport psychology and consultation. Int J Sport Exerc Psychol. 2011;9(2):110–25. https://doi.org/10.1080/1612197X.2011.567101.

43. Adverse childhood experiences: national and state-level prevalence. Child Trends. https://www.childtrends.org/publications/adverse-childhood-experiences-national-and-state-level-prevalence. Accessed November 16, 2020.

44. Hughes K, Bellis MA, Hardcastle KA, et al. The effect of multiple adverse childhood experiences on health: a systematic review and meta-analysis. Lancet Public Health. 2017;2(8):356–66. https://doi.org/10.1016/S2468-2667(17)30118-4.

45. Liu JJ, Bao Y, Huang X, Shi J, Lu L. Mental health considerations for children quarantined because of COVID-19. Lancet Child Adolesc Health. 2020;4(5):347–9. https://doi.org/10.1016/S2352-4642(20)30096-1.

46. Heard-Garris NJ, Cale M, Camaj L, Hamati MC, Dominguez TP. Transmitting trauma: a systematic review of vicarious racism and child health. Soc Sci Med. 2018;199:230–40. https://doi.org/10.1016/j.socscimed.2017.04.018.

47. Racial trauma: theory, research, and healing: introduction to the special issue. Accessed August 12, 2021. https://psycnet.apa.org/fulltext/2019-01033-001.html.

48. Schinke RJ, Stambulova NB, Si G, Moore Z. International society of sport psychology position stand: athletes' mental health, performance, and development. Int J Sport Exerc Psychol. 2018;16(6):622–39. https://doi.org/10.1080/1612197X.2017.1295557.

49. Henriksen K, Schinke R, Moesch K, et al. Consensus statement on improving the mental health of high performance athletes. Int J Sport Exerc Psychol. 2019;1:1–8. https://doi.org/10.1080/1612197X.2019.1570473.

50. Kroshus E, Chrisman S, Coppel D, Herring S. Coach support of high school student-athletes struggling with anxiety or depression.

51. Mazzer KR, Rickwood DJ. Mental health in sport: coaches' views of their role and efficacy in supporting young people's mental health. Int J Health Promot Educ. 2015;53(2):102–14. https://doi.org/10.1080/14635240.2014.965841.

52. Marino KR, Vishnubala D, Ahmed OH, et al. Embrace your discomfort: leadership and unconscious bias in sport and exercise medicine. Br J Sports Med. 2021;55(6):303–4. https://doi.org/10.1136/bjsports-2020-103061.

53. Reducing implicit racial preferences: I. A comparative investigation of 17 interventions. PsycNET. https://psycnet.apa.org/doiLanding?doi=10.1037%2Fa0036260. Accessed May 18, 2021.

54. Lai CK, Skinner AL, Cooley E, et al. Reducing implicit racial preferences: II. Intervention effectiveness across time. J Exp Psychol Gen. 2016;145(8):1001–16. https://doi.org/10.1037/xge0000179.

55. Devine PG, Forscher PS, Austin AJ, Cox WTL. Long-term reduction in implicit race bias: a prejudice habit-breaking intervention. J Exp Soc Psychol. 2012;48(6):1267–78. https://doi.org/10.1016/j.jesp.2012.06.003.

56. Forscher PS, Mitamura C, Dix E, Cox W, Devine P. Breaking the prejudice habit: Mechanisms, time course, and longevity. J Exp Soc Psychol. 2017;72:133.

57. Cooley E, Lei RF, Ellerkamp T. The mixed outcomes of taking ownership for implicit racial biases. Personal Soc Psychol Bull. 2018;44(10):1424–34. https://doi.org/10.1177/0146167218769646.

58. Onyeador IN, Hudson S, Kiera TJ, Lewis NA. Moving beyond implicit bias training: policy insights for increasing organizational diversity. Policy Insights Behav Brain Sci. 2021;8(1):19–26. https://doi.org/10.1177/2372732220983840.

59. Kim J, Roberson L. I'm biased and so are you. What should organizations do? A content analysis of organizational Implicit Bias Training Programs. 2020.

60. Carter ER, Onyeador IN, Lewis NA. Developing & delivering effective anti-bias training: challenges & recommendations. Behav Sci Policy. 2020;6(1):57–70. https://doi.org/10.1353/bsp.2020.0005.

61. Kroshus E, Baugh CM, Hawrilenko M, Daneshvar DH. Pilot randomized evaluation of publically available concussion education materials: evidence of a possible negative effect. Health Educ Behav. 2015;42(2):153–62. https://doi.org/10.1177/1090198114543011.

62. Noelle-Neumann E. The spiral of silence a theory of public opinion. J Commun. 1974;24(2):43–51. https://doi.org/10.1111/j.1460-2466.1974.tb00367.x.

63. Gorczynski PF, Coyle M, Gibson K. Depressive symptoms in high-performance athletes and non-athletes: a comparative meta-analysis. Br J Sports Med. 2017;51(18):1348–54. https://doi.org/10.1136/bjsports-2016-096455.

64. Ogbeiwi O. Why written objectives need to be really SMART. Br J Healthc Manag. 2017;23(7):324–36. https://doi.org/10.12968/bjhc.2017.23.7.324.

65. Mascarenhas M, Beattie M, Roxburgh M, MacKintosh J, Clarke N, Srivastava D. Using the model for improvement to implement the critical-care pain observation tool in an adult intensive care unit. BMJ Open Qual. 2018;7(4):e000304. https://doi.org/10.1136/bmjoq-2017-000304.

Sleep Disorders and Sleep Concerns

Michael A. Grandner

Introduction

Sleep can be defined as "a naturally recurring, reversible state of perceptual disengagement, reduced consciousness, and relative immobility, the propensity of which is patterned by homeostatic and circadian factors [1]." It is a biological requirement for human life, alongside food, air, and water, one of the foundational elements of human biology. Yet, modern society often devalues sleep, leading to pressures toward worse sleep health [2]. For elite athletes, this can manifest as decreased time available for sleep due to other demands, sport-related activities impinging on sleep opportunity (such as early morning training or evening competitions), travel across multiple time zones, and frequent schedule disruptions [3]. In addition, athletes may suffer from any of a wide range of sleep disorders and disturbances that may require treatment [4].

Prevalence of Sleep Concerns in Elite Athletes

Sleep problems among elite athletes are relatively common. In a report by the PAC-12 athletics conference of the National Collegiate Athletic Association (NCAA), 66% of students indicated that lack of flexible time is the hardest thing about being an athlete—harder than the academic work [5]. This report also noted that sleep is the activity that students reported that their athletic time commitments most prevented them from doing. Other findings from this report support the discrepancy between perceived sleep needs among students and their opportunity for sleep. Among respondents, 77% reported that they perceive that they get less sleep than non-athletes at their institutions, and over 50% reported that if they had an extra hour of the day that it would be used for

sleep. Some athletes reported waking up at 5:00 AM or earlier to report to practice or training activities, which is inconsistent with developmental circadian rhythms [6]. Also noted in this report, when asked, many students reported that they needed a break of approximately 2–3 weeks just to catch up on sleep and relieve stress. Finally, this report noted that students requested that nonpractice hours be extended in order to make more time for sleep and studying [5].

Further data from the NCAA indicate that only about one in five student athletes achieve the recommended sleep duration of at least 8 h [7]. In addition, this same report found that approximately half of student athletes report 6 or fewer hours of sleep on a typical night, which is associated with a wide range of health and functional deficits [8]. This prevalence of insufficient sleep is greater than that seen in the general population, where approximately one-third of young adults age 18–30 report 6 or fewer hours [9].

A recent survey of collegiate varsity student athletes reported that 33% had received information about sleep difficulties from their college or university, but 52% wish that their institution provided more information. In this same study, 20% reported that sleep difficulties have been "traumatic or very difficult to handle" in the past 12 months, 28% reported extreme difficulty falling asleep or early morning awakenings at least 3 times per week, 61% reported excessive tiredness at least 3 days per week, and 33% reported going to bed because they could not maintain wakefulness at least 3 times per week [10, 11]. These data are supported by a meta-analysis across elite athlete populations reporting a prevalence of approximately 26% of sleep disturbances [12].

Regarding sleep disorders, prevalence estimates are not widely available. Insomnia disorder is present in about 10% of the general population [13], and indications are that this is comparable to rates seen in athletes. Sleep apnea is another common sleep disorder in the population [14], but since common risk factors include obesity, high blood pressure, and older age [15], rates are likely lower among athletes. Still, sleep apnea can occur in those with otherwise few risk factors. Some athlete populations, partially due to body size

M. A. Grandner (✉)
Department of Psychiatry, University of Arizona College of Medicine, Tucson, AZ, USA

and/or neck circumference, may present with high risk for sleep apnea. For example, 73% of professional (American) football players screened as high risk for sleep apnea, with over half of those later testing positive for the disorder [16, 17]. Other sleep disorders may be present in athletes as well, though it is not clear that rates are any different from those seen in the general population.

Overview of Basic Sleep–Wake Physiology

Basic Sleep Neurophysiology

Sleep is, physiologically, conceptualized in several different ways. One way to conceptualize sleep is through the neurophysiologic mechanisms that drive the three systems that interface with each other: the sleep system, the wake system, and the circadian system. The sleep system consists of structures primarily in the brainstem, the ventrolateral preoptic nucleus and other parts of the hypothalamus, the basal forebrain, and the subthalamus [18]. These populations of cells largely function by secreting gamma aminobutyric acid (GABA), which is an inhibitory neurotransmitter directed toward arousal centers, suppressing wake activity. The wake system involves a wider range of brain regions, including structures that are related to the reticular activating system— including the dorsal raphe (serotonergic cells), ventral tegmental area (dopaminergic cells), locus coeruleus (noradrenergic cells), laterodorsal tegmental nucleus (cholinergic cells), and pedunculopontine nucleus (cholinergic cells). These cells project to the cortex through a dorsal pathway that modulates thalamocortical pathways and a ventral pathway that goes through the lateral hypothalamus and tuberomammillary nucleus to the basal forebrain and frontal cortex. Stabilizing wakefulness and facilitating smooth and organized switching between sleep–wake states is accomplished through cells in the lateral hypothalamus that secrete orexin [18].

In parallel to this sleep–wake system is the circadian system. When light hits the retina of the eye, it activates several different sensors, including rods and cones, which contribute to vision. In addition to these cells, light—especially in the short wavelength range of approximately 440–540 nm (blue to green)—activates melanopsin-producing ganglion cells. These cells transmit signals in response to light exposure along the retinal-hypothalamic tract to the suprachiasmatic nucleus of the hypothalamus, located (as the name implies) directly behind the optic chiasm, where the optic nerves cross. These cells maintain an independent, endogenous rhythm of approximately 24 h. Light signals impact function of these cells, providing information about where in the 24-h day the external environment is suggesting the person is.

These cells then adapt to that information, shifting the internal clock earlier (if signals suggest that the time is earlier than presumed) or later (if signals suggest that the time is later). In this way, light, along with other environmental cues, can influence the endogenous central clock [19, 20]. This nucleus then projects to the paraventricular nucleus and then, through a route that goes through the spinal cord to the superior cervical ganglion, terminates at the pineal gland, which secretes melatonin [21, 22]. The pineal gland secretes melatonin as a signal of the biological night, in a regular 24-h rhythm dictated by the suprachiasmatic nucleus. This signal travels throughout the body, signaling to the rest of the body that it is nighttime. Although melatonin follows a 24-h rhythm that can be shifted with environmental light, acute light exposure during the night can acutely suppress melatonin secretion, which will recover to normal levels following removal of the light source. This central 24-h clock system is accompanied by a wide range of peripheral clocks in various tissues and cell types [23, 24]. These peripheral clocks exist in concert with the central 24-h clock and exist in nearly all tissues, including heart, lung, liver, muscle, adipose tissue, and other parts of the body.

These systems work in relation to each other. The circadian system informs a wide range of cellular and physiologic functions, including metabolic, immune, and neurologic functions and energy level, fatigue, and propensity for sleep or alertness. This system is rhythm-based, reflecting regular patterns within 24-h cycles. In parallel, the sleep–wake system operates according to homeostatic principles; upon the initiation of the wake phase, the sleep system is suppressed and wake is maintained. As wakefulness progresses, the pressure (i.e., "hunger") for sleep increases until the wake system can no longer remain stabilized, at which time sleep takes over. In the first hours of sleep, pressure for sleep remains high; this pressure discharges over the sleep period until it can no longer suppress the wake drive and the process begins again. This conceptualization—that a rhythmic circadian process operates in parallel with a homeostatic sleep–wake process—was originally conceptualized as the "two-process model of sleep–wake regulation."

Two-Process Model of Sleep–Wake Regulation

The two-process model, consisting of a circadian and a sleep–wake component, was first articulated by Borbely in 1982 [25]. Since that time, the two-process model has proven to be an immensely useful way to conceptualize the degree to which an individual is likely to be awake or asleep across 24 h. Under normal conditions, upon awakening, the sleep drive is at its lowest. It then proceeds to build throughout the day, such that levels needed to achieve sleep often occur approximately 16 h after awakening. Then, the individual falls asleep and the sleep drive dissipates until it is again depleted and the individual awakens. In parallel, the circadian drive toward alertness is still low upon awakening, though rising. It reaches a peak during the day and begins to diminish in the evening. At the point where a critical point is reached—the "sleep gate"—the sleep drive is high and the circadian wake signal is low. Then, the individual can fall asleep. The circadian wake signal remains low through the night and begins to rise again before awakening.

This model explains many aspects of sleep–wake behavior and function. It explains why a person may wake up despite still feeling tired (a wake signal overpowering a depleted sleep drive). It explains why activity peaks at certain times of the day (where the wake signals are strongest). It explains why awakenings in the second half of the night are more likely to become problematic or prolonged (due to depleted sleep drive). It also explains why napping too long or too late can make sleep onset more difficult, since these naps would serve to reduce sleep drive without enough time for it to sufficiently accumulate prior to the intended sleep period.

Sleep Stages and Sleep Cycles

One way to conceptualize sleep is through sleep stages and cycles. Sleep stages were originally characterized over 70 years ago, to describe the patterns of brain wave activity observed while individuals were asleep and connected to an electroencephalogram (EEG). The EEG device measures electrical activity at the scalp using electrodes placed in various parts of the head, in order to infer electrical activity occurring in the outer layers of the cortex around those electrodes. By sampling that electrical activity many times per second, tracings can be displayed that show the fluctuations in electrical activity over time. The EEG signal was eventually combined with an electromyography (EMG) signal to capture muscle activity, an electrooculography (EOG) signal to capture eye movements, an electrocardiography (ECG) signal to capture heart activity, and sensors to measure breathing rate and airflow, resulting in an assessment called polysomnography (PSG), comprising these and sometimes other signals to physiologically describe sleep. Sleep stages are captured using PSG, primarily based on EEG signals but with input from other signals as well.

The PSG signal during sleep can be split into two different states—Rapid Eye Movement (REM) sleep and non-REM sleep. Non-REM sleep can be further divided into three stages, N1, N2, and N3 [26]. N1 is generally considered light sleep. The EEG signal is characterized by low amplitude, fast frequency waveforms, similar to waking patterns, though these are slower than waking signals. N1 sleep only comprises a small percentage of the night in healthy sleepers and is generally seen at state transitions. It is very light sleep, and is where hypnic jerks occur (sudden jerking awake at the start of the sleep period, often with a falling sensation). Many people awakened from stage N1 deny that they were actually asleep. Stage N2 sleep is also characterized as light sleep but typically comprises about half of the night or more. It is not as light as N1 and much of the physiologic work of sleep can occur during N2. Stage N3 is often called "deep sleep" because it is associated with much lower muscle tone and individuals are much more difficult to awaken from this sleep stage. Stage N3 is also called "slow wave sleep" because the EEG signal shows much slower, large-amplitude waves suggesting an extremely high rate of cortical synchrony. Stage N3 is characterized by increased cellular and muscular recovery processes and, when individuals are deprived of N3 selectively, they will rebound when able. Stage N3 is also reflective of sleep pressure in general, as it mostly aggregates in the first few hours of the night, when sleep pressure is highest. REM sleep is quite different from the other sleep stages. Like stage N1, EEG activity is characterized by fast frequency, low amplitude signals, more similar to awake signals than those seen in deeper stages of sleep. However, muscle tone is even more reduced than stage N3; in fact, muscles are actively paralyzed, especially skeletal muscles. The EMG signal is weakest during REM sleep. Also during REM sleep, the eyes engage in rapid, seemingly coordinated movements (hence the name of the sleep stage), which are not seen in any other sleep stages. REM sleep seems especially important for memory and emotion function and is the primary sleep stage of dreams and nightmares. It tends to aggregate more toward the end of the night, with longer REM episodes (and more complex dreams) later in the night.

Sleep stages do not occur randomly across the night. When an individual falls asleep, they often quickly progress through stages N1 and N2 into N3, where they stay for a period of time. Then, they emerge back into N2, then to N1 and REM. Following a brief REM episode, they descend again through the sleep stages back to N3, where they remain for (typically) less time than before. They then progress back up from N2 to N1 to REM, where they remain for slightly longer than before. These cycles—progressing between deeper and lighter sleep—tend to last about 90 min each and persist across the night. As the cycles progress, deeper stages of sleep dissipate and REM episodes become longer. After the third or fourth cycle, it is not unusual for cycles to only consist of switching between stage N2 and REM. Thus, approximately 90-min cycles change across the night, transitioning from more deep to more REM sleep.

Sleep Continuity and Sleep Architecture

The structure of sleep stages as they cycle through the night is referred to as "sleep architecture." An alternative way to describe sleep is "sleep continuity." Sleep continuity refers to the pattern of sleep and wake across the night, regardless of PSG-derived sleep stage. Although sleep stages may provide information about physiologic processes taking place that change cortical signals, sleep continuity represents an individual's experience of sleep. As such, it is much more useful for assessing insomnia, sleep sufficiency, sleep timing, etc.

Sleep continuity represents the timeline of the night and is described using a set of metrics. The time that an individual gets into bed is usually referred to as time to bed (TTB), and the time they get out of bed at the end of the sleep period is often assessed as time out of bed (TOB). By subtracting TOB–TTB, the total amount of time of sleep opportunity is expressed as time in bed (TIB). Of note, some people get out of bed for periods of time during the night, but this metric is still often reported as "TIB" even if it includes some time not actually spent in bed. Once an individual is in bed, the amount of time it takes to fall asleep is usually quantified as Sleep Latency (SL). The number of awakenings that the person recalls during the night is often quantified as NWAK. The total amount of time spent awake during those awakenings is often quantified as wake after sleep onset (WASO). After an individual awakens for the last time, they may spend some time in bed, which is often quantified as early morning awakening (EMA) time. When expressed in minutes, an individual's total sleep time (TST) is computed based on their total sleep opportunity, minus the time spent awake: $TST = TIB - SL - WASO - EMA$. Another important metric obtained is sleep efficiency (SE%), characterized as $(TST/TIB) \times 100$. Thus, using sleep continuity metrics, one can ascertain the timing of sleep (TTB and TOB), the total sleep opportunity (TIB), the number of awakenings recalled (NWAK), the time spent awake during that period (SL at the start of the sleep period, WASO during the sleep period, and EMA at the end), the total amount of sleep obtained (TST), and the proportion of the sleep opportunity actually spent asleep (SE%). As a general rule of thumb, sleep efficiency values over 90% are considered high, and values <85% are typically considered low. Additionally, values for SL, WASO, or EMA over 30 min are generally considered high. Taken together, these metrics represent a way to quantify and characterize a single night or set of nights that reflect several aspects of sleep health.

Multidimensional Sleep Health

Sleep is not a unitary construct. Rather, sleep health represents a combination of features that may be assessed separately and may separately influence health and functioning.

Buysse [27] summarized these dimensions in the RU-SATED model that characterized sleep health along several components: regularity, satisfaction, alertness, timing, efficiency, and duration.

Regularity Sleep regularity refers to the predictability of the timing of the sleep period. For example, many athletes have irregular sleep periods due to scheduling demands. Early mornings and/or late nights on some nights but not others contribute to variability in sleep patterns. Studies have shown that irregularity of sleep itself may contribute to adverse health and performance outcomes [28, 29].

Satisfaction Some aspects of sleep cannot (yet) be assessed objectively. An individual's general sense of satisfaction with their sleep quality is still a reliable metric for predicting a wide range of mental health and other outcomes [30–33]. Many athletes report poor sleep quality, irrespective of other dimensions of sleep, and general sleep quality in athletes is associated with poor mental health [34].

Alertness As a counterpoint to the effects of sleep during the night, the degree to which a person is able to maintain alertness is often an indicator of sleep health. Problematic sleep can lead to increased sleep pressure during the day and decreased alertness, as well as an inability to stay awake. Of note, daytime symptoms are common in athletes and are associated with mental health and other outcomes [10, 34, 35].

Timing Sleep is most effective when it occurs during the biological night. Shift workers who sleep at times inconsistent with circadian physiology experience a wide range of functional and health problems [36, 37]. Many athletes are forced to sleep at times inconsistent with their natural sleep, whether it is due to activities scheduled into the night or beginning early in the morning, or due to sleeping while traveling, or napping due to insufficient sleep at night.

Efficiency In this model, efficiency refers to the collection of metrics described above as sleep continuity, especially sleep efficiency. Even if sleep is regular and at the right time, prolonged wakefulness during the night (leading to reduced sleep efficiency) is associated with a wide range of outcomes among athletes, including insomnia, poor mental health, and other outcomes.

Duration Sleep duration—which can be self-reported, computed as part of sleep continuity, or assessed objectively—refers to the total amount of sleep. It is recommended that young adults (the demographic most common among elite athletes) achieve 7–9 h of sleep [38, 39], with the possibility that they may require more [40]. Of note, this recommendation is meant to reflect retrospective self-report, which is often greater than computed values or objectively measured sleep duration. Therefore, if sleep as assessed with wearables is less than this amount, it may or may not be insufficient relative to the recommendations [41]. Insufficient sleep is a common and important concern for athletes, however, and is associated with more stress, worse mental health, and other adverse outcomes [34, 35, 42–44].

Sleep Health in Context

Sleep is not just a set of physiologic processes that exist out of context. In real-world situations, many factors influence sleep health. To conceptualize the role of sleep at the interface of downstream health factors and upstream social, behavioral, and environmental determinants, the Social-Ecological Model of Sleep Health was proposed [45] and later refined [1, 8]. This model depicts sleep health at the center with downstream influences on health domains including central factors (cognitive health, mental health, behavioral health) and peripheral factors (cardiovascular health, metabolic health, immune health). Upstream of sleep, the model depicts a set of embedded factors. Closest to sleep are the Individual-Level factors, including a person's own thoughts, feelings, behaviors, demographics, and genetics. These are the factors within the individual that influence sleep. These Individual-Level factors are embedded within a social level. Social-Level factors, which exist outside the individual but include the individual, include work, home, family, social networks, neighborhood, and religion/culture. These Social-Level factors are themselves embedded within Societal-Level factors such as globalization, 24/7 society, racism and discrimination, technology, policy, climate change, and the environment. Thus, the determinants of an individual's sleep represent the end result of a complex set of factors within and outside the individual.

For example, an individual athlete may be struggling with electronic media use at night. But that media use exists in the context of their sport and engagement with their fanbase/followers, which influences their success. Further, the only reason that this social network exists is because of societal-level changes in how we use technology and connect with each other. Thus, understanding the context of sleep health can lead to more nuanced insights about the underlying factors driving sleep health.

Assessment of Sleep Health

Polysomnography

As described above, PSG includes a range of sensors to capture physiologic changes that occur during sleep. It should be noted that PSG does not directly measure sleep, as that would require directly measuring activity in the brainstem and midbrain. Rather, PSG measures changes to other physiologic systems (e.g., cortex, muscles, heart, eyes) that occur during sleep in order to characterize sleep architecture. Although PSG is typically performed in a laboratory, there are ways to capture many of these signals outside of the laboratory using portable PSG equipment or newer headband devices that capture several (but not all) PSG signals [46, 47]. PSG is most useful for diagnosing sleep disorders (except for insomnia) and characterizing sleep stages. It should be noted that PSG sleep may or may not correlate with sleep continuity or subjective reports [48]. This is not necessarily a failure of subjective reports, which may capture elements of sleep not assessed by PSG.

Actigraphy and Wearables

Actigraphy refers to the use of movement sensing to characterize sleep and wake patterns. Wrist-based movement sensors have been used to estimate when an individual is awake or asleep since the 1970s [49–51], and the technology has progressed much since that time [52]. Currently, devices designed for scientific use have been used in many research studies in order to characterize sleep continuity in free-living conditions [53, 54]. Benefits include decreased burden and the ability to record for 24 h/day, across several days, weeks, or even months. Newer devices have incorporated other sensors in addition to movement (such as heart rate), and this may have improved sleep–wake detection. Many devices have been previously examined, though not all devices on the market have demonstrated accuracy in recording sleep [55]. Further, although devices have typically been evaluated regarding ability to discern sleep versus wake, not only are those performance evaluations often limited to otherwise good sleepers (so they may be less accurate for individuals with atypical or disordered sleep), but they typically do not include other metrics that devices nevertheless report (such as recovery metrics or sleep stages). Therefore, even if a device has demonstrated good performance at discerning sleep versus wake, other metrics obtained by the device may not be as reliable or accurate.

Sleep Diaries

Sleep diaries are the gold standard strategy for assessing sleep continuity, prospectively [56]. This is especially the case for insomnia and related complaints, which are often not well detected using objective methods. Sleep diaries are typically completed in the morning by the individual upon awakening, recording sleep continuity metrics such as TTB, SL, NWAK, WASO, EMA, and TOB. Typically, these values are used to compute TIB, TST, and SE%. Sleep diaries may also collect daily ratings of sleep satisfaction, naps, caffeine and alcohol use, or other daily metrics that may influence sleep.

Retrospective Questionnaires

There are many validated retrospective questionnaires frequently used for assessing sleep. Although these tend to lack temporal precision, they can be useful as screening tools to detect problems or quantify constructs related to sleep. The Athlete Sleep Screening Questionnaire (ASSQ [57]) was specifically developed to determine whether athletes are at high, moderate, or low risk for a possible sleep disorder. Those identified as high risk by this questionnaire are recommended to follow up with a qualified clinician for evaluation. Those at moderate risk should be examined further or be provided education or other support to improve sleep, and those at low risk likely sleep well and may be able to further optimize their sleep.

Other questionnaires have not yet been validated specifically in athletes but may prove useful. General sleep disorders screening questionnaires include the sleep disorders symptom check list (SDSCL [58]), the general sleep assessment questionnaire (GSAQ [59]), and the SLEEP-50 Questionnaire [60]. The structured clinical interview for sleep disorders (SCISD [61]) also can be administered by clinicians to identify sleep disorders. Insomnia is often measured with the insomnia severity index (ISI [62]), though other insomnia questionnaires exist [63]. Sleep apnea risk can be evaluated with the Berlin Questionnaire (BQ [64]) or STOP-BANG questionnaire [15], though these include items like high blood pressure that are less relevant for athletes. Other sleep disorders can be assessed using questionnaires such as the Swiss Narcolepsy Scale (SNS [65]) or the international restless legs syndrome scale (IRLS [66]).

The Epworth Sleepiness Scale (ESS [67]) is a standard assessment of inability to stay awake, whereas the fatigue severity scale (FSS [68]) is a measure of general fatigue. The functional outcomes of sleep questionnaire (FOSQ [69]) assesses the impact of sleep on daytime functioning, and the PROMIS scales for sleep disturbance and daytime dysfunction [70] are useful outcome measures. The Sleep Timing Questionnaire (STQ [71]) and Self-Assessment of Sleep Scale (SASS [72]) can capture typical sleep timing and continuity from a retrospective lens.

To assess circadian rhythms, it may be useful to employ the Munich Chronotype Questionnaire [73, 74] (CITE) or the Morningness-Eveningness Questionnaire (MEQ [75]), though the Circadian Energy Scale (CIRENS [76]) is a brief scale that can be used with athletes.

Other scales that may be useful to assess aspects of sleep health might include the Dysfunctional Beliefs and Attitudes about Sleep (DBAS [77]) scale to determine whether people have unrealistic or unhealthy attitudes about sleep. The sleep beliefs scale (SBS [78]) also assesses unhelpful beliefs. The brief index of sleep control (BRISC [79]) assesses the degree to which an individual perceives control over their ability to sleep. The assessment of sleep environment (ASE [80]) can identify which elements of the sleep environment are adversely impacting sleep. The Sleep Practices and Attitudes Questionnaire (SPAQ [81]) can assess a wide range of sleep-related factors, including sleep beliefs, ways of coping with poor sleep, knowledge about sleep, perceptions of sleep, and impacts on sleep.

Sleep Disorders and Problems in Elite Athletes

Athletes may present with a wide range of sleep-related problems. Some of these may fall under the broad category of "sleep disorders" and some may represent subclinical—but still relevant—disturbances. Sleep disorders are primarily defined by the International Classification of Sleep Disorders (ICSD [82]), which is published by the American Academy of Sleep Medicine. These disorders are very consistent with other classification systems including the American Psychiatric Association Diagnostic and Statistical Manual (DSM [83]) and the International Classification of Disease (ICD), though there are some mostly minor differences. For the purposes of consistency, the ICSD definitions of sleep disorders are used in this chapter. Sleep disorders are typically categorized into several groups: (1) Insomnia Disorder and related conditions, (2) Circadian Rhythm Sleep–Wake Disorders, (3) Sleep-Disordered Breathing, (4) Hypersomnia Disorders, (5) Sleep-Related Movement Disorders, and (6) Parasomnias. Other sleep problems relevant to athletes that are not disorders include insufficient sleep and sleep deprivation, poor sleep quality, daytime sleepiness, and circadian rhythm problems.

Insomnia Disorder

The most common sleep disorder is Insomnia Disorder. This condition is diagnosed when patients present with persistent difficulty falling asleep or staying asleep, or awakening and being unable to resume sleep, for at least three nights per week, lasting at least 3 months. In addition, this needs to exist in the context of adequate opportunity to sleep and must cause some sort of daytime disturbance. Typically, those who take at least 30 min to fall asleep or are awake for at least 30 min during the night or early morning unable to fall asleep would be considered to experience clinically significant insomnia symptoms. Insomnia can arise from many sources, including stress, discomfort, life events, or even mis-timed sleep opportunity. However, once an individual meets criteria for an Insomnia Disorder, this is considered an independent diagnosis, not secondary to the original cause.

This is because chronic insomnia typically reflects a conditioned arousal to the bed, bedroom, and/or falling asleep. This conditioned arousal is brought about because, over time, sleep becomes predictably difficult to initiate or maintain. The stress associated with not being able to sleep becomes conditioned to the act of trying to fall asleep; thus, simply trying to fall asleep (or resume sleep) becomes stressful, resulting in the very activation that itself precludes sleep. The predominant model used to conceptualize insomnia pathogenesis is the Spielman 3-P model [84]. In this model, individuals have a relatively stable set of predisposing factors, including genetics and other factors that bestow an individual with an amount of risk for insomnia. Some individuals are more susceptible to insomnia, and these traits tend not to change over time. The second element in the model is the precipitating factors that cause the acute insomnia. Whatever those precipitants are, they lead an individual to become unable to sleep. Over time, those factors wane in importance as the individual habituates to them or they resolve. When insomnia becomes chronic, the precipitating factors are typically no longer the primary drivers of the insomnia symptoms. At this stage, it is the perpetuating factors that maintain the conditioned arousal, precluding healthy sleep. Typically, these perpetuating factors are comprised of maladaptive coping strategies that sustain the conditioned arousal, leading to chronic sleep problems. For this reason, most treatments for insomnia tend to target these perpetuating factors in order to effectively resolve chronic insomnia [85].

The recommended first-line treatment for insomnia is Cognitive Behavioral Therapy for Insomnia (CBTI). CBTI is a multicomponent treatment that includes a core set of techniques, as well as several other tools and approaches for improving sleep [86, 87]. The way CBTI works is to increase natural homeostatic drive for sleep, regulate circadian sleep opportunity, de-condition arousal associated with sleep, create a positive sleep association with the bed, promote relaxation, and optimize the individual's natural ability to sleep. This approach has proven effective in meta-analyses [88, 89], including in patients with comorbid conditions such as pain and depression [90, 91], and has proven to be as effective or more effective than pharmacotherapy in comparative meta-analysis [92]. CBTI differs from sleep hygiene, which consists of behavioral instructions for removing obvious barriers to sleep [93–95]. Sleep hygiene is often incorporated into CBTI, but it often is insufficient to ameliorate insomnia symptoms. For these reasons, CBTI is recognized as first-line treatment of adult insomnia [86, 96]. Of note, CBTI tends to avoid the performance-impairing side effects commonly seen with sedative medications.

When CBTI is infeasible, pharmacotherapy for insomnia is sometimes warranted. Melatonin—a hormone that can be taken as a supplement—is typically secreted by the pineal gland to signal nighttime to the body. When taken as a supplement, melatonin can improve sleep health [97, 98] and may be effective for athletes [99–101]. This is especially the case because melatonin does not impair performance. Still, it is frequently insufficient for resolving insomnia [102]. Other medications include sedative hypnotics, which can improve insomnia symptoms but typically come at a cost to daytime performance [102]. This is especially relevant to athletes because these medications are associated with significant injury risks [103–105].

Circadian Rhythm Sleep–Wake Disorders

Circadian Rhythm Sleep–Wake Disorders (CRSWDs) represent a group of conditions wherein an individual experiences "a chronic or recurrent pattern of sleep-wake rhythm disruption primarily due to alteration of the endogenous circadian timing system or misalignment between the endogenous circadian rhythm and the sleep-wake schedule desired or required by an individual's physical environment or social/work schedules [82]." These conditions can lead to excessive sleeplessness, sleepiness, or both, and cause significant distress or impairment in social, physical, or other important areas of functioning. Thus, these conditions arise when a person's circadian rhythms are out of alignment with their schedules.

Most common among young adults, including athletes, is a delayed circadian rhythm [106]. In this case, the individual's "biological night" (the portion of the 24-h day where that individual's endogenous rhythm is predisposed to sleep) starts and ends later than is needed. These individuals may be "night owls" that have rhythms that predispose them to staying up late and waking late. This can be problematic when individuals need to get to sleep early or wake up early (which is common among athletes). Naturally delayed rhythms are most common among adolescents and young adults [107], and these individuals experience difficulties when they try to go to sleep earlier than that to which their physiology is predisposed, and their physical and mental performance is significantly impaired if they need to wake up much earlier than that to which their physiology is predisposed. Endogenous rhythms can often be adjusted with specific doses and timing of bright light and/or melatonin [108], and these approaches can be used to treat this condition effectively.

Less common among young adults is advanced circadian rhythm. In contrast to delayed circadian rhythm, this is where individuals' physiology is predisposed to going to sleep early and waking early. Among athletes, this can help facilitate early morning training activities but may interfere with performance during evening competitions. Treatment approaches are similar (light and melatonin) but reversed in terms of timing. Rather than attempting to shift rhythms earlier, the approach is to shift rhythms later [109].

Other CRSWDs may also present in athletes. Irregular sleep–wake rhythm occurs when there is no discernable day-night pattern. Non-24-Hour Sleep–Wake Rhythm is a condition where the individual's circadian rhythm is unable to be reset by light to the circadian system and is running at >24 h. If an individual is living in a non-24-h day, their rhythm will shift slightly later each day. This can often be treated with melatonin or medication. Shift Work Disorder is a CRSWD that is typically seen in occupational settings; it consists of insomnia and/or excessive sleepiness, accompanied by reduced sleep duration, leading to significant daytime impairments, where the disruption is due to the individual needing to be awake during hours when their physiology is predisposed to be asleep. It is possible that athletes who need to train and/or compete at hours incompatible with natural circadian rhythms may develop a form of shift work disorder. Finally, Jet Lag Disorder is also a CRSWD that can be seen in athletes. This condition is represented by a complaint of insomnia and/or excessive sleepiness, accompanied by reduced sleep duration, associated with travel across multiple time zones. This condition often is associated with daytime impairments, as well as general malaise or somatic symptoms within one to two days after travel. It can be treated using light and melatonin, as well as strategies for shifting rhythms faster and promoting healthy sleep. To reduce the burden of jet lag, strategies for optimizing travel might include beginning to shift schedules before departure, timed light exposure to stimulate a day signal and avoidance of light to stimulate a night signal, melatonin, and morning physical activity [110].

Sleep-Disordered Breathing

There are several sleep disorders that fall under the category of sleep-disordered breathing [82]. The most common of these are obstructive and central sleep apnea. Sleep apnea often presents as any combination of fatigue, depression, lethargy, complaints of restless sleep or sudden awakenings, loud snoring, early morning awakenings, and occasionally witnessed or experienced breathing pauses during sleep. Typical risk factors include factors often uncommon in elite athletes, such as obesity, hypertension, large neck circumference, and advanced age. However, many cases of sleep apnea occur even in normal weight and otherwise healthy individuals [14]. The diagnosis of sleep apnea is made using an objective recording that includes sensors to measure respiratory flow, respiratory effort, and blood oxygen saturation, though these recordings typically also assess sleep architec-

ture, movement, and other parameters. These recordings can determine if an individual experiences a respiratory event due to an airway obstruction (obstructive event), a respiratory event reflected by decreased effort in the absence of an obstruction (central event), or a mixed event. Respiratory events are categorized as apneas (respiratory signal drop of at least 90%, for at least 10 s, resulting in a reduction in blood oxygen) or a hypopnea (respiratory signal drops by at least 30%, also lasting at least 10 s and resulting in a concomitant drop in blood oxygen) [82]. The number of apneas and/or hypopneas per hour of recording is quantified as the Apnea–Hypopnea Index (AHI), and sleep apnea conditions are classified as mild (AHI 5 to <15), moderate (AHI 15 to <30), or severe (AHI 30 or greater). If the primary type of event is obstructive, the condition is diagnosed as Obstructive Sleep Apnea (OSA), and if the type of event is predominantly central, they are diagnosed as Central Sleep Apnea (CSA).

Sleep apnea is a serious condition that can result in significant cognitive, mental health, and general medical (especially cardiometabolic) risks [8, 111–120]. Untreated sleep apnea is a major health concern and can lead to premature death [121–124], including in elite athletes [125]. Some sports, such as American Football, are especially predisposed to sleep apnea due to body type [114]. Of note, sleeping at altitude (where many athletes train) can cause central respiratory events or CSA in otherwise healthy people [126, 127]. Therefore, it may be inadvisable to have athletes sleep at high altitudes, as the benefits of training at altitude may be undone by the disturbed sleep.

The primary treatment for sleep apnea is positive airway pressure (PAP) therapy, most commonly Continuous Positive Airway Pressure (CPAP) [128]. PAP therapies work by having patients wear a mask, which is attached to a machine that blows a cushion of air into the airway, during sleep in order to prevent collapse. PAP therapies are extremely effective and improve daytime functioning when used, but adherence can be problematic [128]. Other therapies exist, especially for milder cases, which are more common in athletes. These include dental devices [129], positional therapies [130], surgeries [131, 132], and other approaches [133].

Hypersomnia Disorders

Rather than experiencing insomnia, some patients experience Hypersomnia Disorders. Patients with these conditions present with periods of an unavoidable need to sleep, or daytime lapses into sleep, for at least 3 months [82]. These individuals often have extreme daytime sleepiness not caused by another condition. They may need to take multiple naps during the day or they may experience "sleep attacks" that consist of a sudden urge/need to lay down to sleep. There are several conditions that fall under the category of Hypersomnia Disorders.

Narcolepsy is the main Hypersomnia Disorder. Like others, it presents with extreme difficulty making it through the day without multiple sleep periods, either planned naps or "sleep attacks." Narcolepsy is an autoimmune condition, where orexin-producing cells in the hypothalamus are no longer functional. It tends to arise in adolescence or young adulthood. Because of the loss of this neurotransmitter function, these individuals have difficulty staying awake during the day and difficulty staying asleep at night. The boundaries between sleep and wake can become blurred. Further, the boundaries among sleep, non-REM, and REM can also become blurred. These patients may also frequently experience sleep paralysis (where the muscle atonia of REM sleep persists into awakening, sometimes associated with disturbing dream-like sensations), and/or hypnogogic hallucinations (auditory or visual hallucinations around sleep onset)or hypnopompic hallucinations (auditory or visual hallucinations after awakening). These patients may also experience cataplexy, which is a sudden loss of muscle tone in response to a strong emotional stimulus. This can be experienced as a localized loss of muscle tone (e.g., dropping things or knees buckling) up to a complete, full-body loss of muscle tone, where the individual appears to be asleep. It should be noted that cataplexy is often portrayed in the media as unpredictable and sudden initiation of otherwise normal sleep; rather it is brought on by specific extreme emotional reactions leading to atonia and a REM-like state but the individual often remains conscious.

Narcolepsy is typically diagnosed with a Multiple Sleep Latency Test (MSLT), which begins with a PSG in a lab, followed by four to five nap opportunities spaced 2 h apart, across the day [134]. As soon as the patient falls asleep during these nap opportunities, they are awakened by staff. The outcome of the MSLT is the mean sleep latency across all naps, as well as whether any of the naps included REM sleep in the first few minutes (since REM sleep should not initiate until about 90 min of sleep). If the mean sleep latency is short (eight or fewer minutes) and the patient experienced REM episodes around sleep onset, they could receive a diagnosis of narcolepsy, either type-1 (with cataplexy) or type-2 (without cataplexy). Narcolepsy is a chronic condition that is managed medically, using medications that consolidate sleep at night and/or consolidate wakefulness during the day [135, 136]. Of note, many of these medications may be prohibited substances and/or performance-enhancing for athletes.

Idiopathic Hypersomnia can be diagnosed when an individual experiences narcolepsy-like symptoms and demonstrates a short MSLT sleep latency but does not demonstrate REM episodes around sleep onset [82]. These patients also may be less likely to experience other REM-related symptoms such as sleep paralysis and/or sleep-related hallucinations. In the absence of a short mean MSLT sleep latency of eight or fewer minutes, the diagnosis can be made if documented sleep in these individuals takes at least 11 of 24 h. There are medical treatments for Idiopathic Hypersomnia, but similar to those for narcolepsy, they may be performance-enhancing for athletes, since they improve ability to stay awake during the day.

Sleep-Related Movement Disorders

Restless Legs Syndrome (RLS) is a sleep-related movement disorder characterized by frequent periods of uncomfortable or unpleasant, nonpainful sensations in limbs (usually legs), which typically occurs at night or when laying down, accompanied by a strong urge to move those limbs to alleviate that sensation [82]. In addition, in RLS, this movement alleviates the uncomfortable sensation. It occurs during wakefulness but can interfere with sleep. This condition typically represents a neuromuscular issue that is treated medically [137] but can also be treated nonpharmacologically [138]. Pharmacologic treatments include anticonvulsant and dopamine agonist medications. Of note, RLS can also be caused by iron deficiency, and blood tests showing ferritin levels below 75 ng/ml may warrant iron supplementation [139].

A common movement disorder that occurs during sleep is Periodic Limb Movement Disorder (PLMD). This is within the larger family of sleep-related myoclonus conditions, where, during sleep, involuntary muscle twitches occur [82]. These can sometimes disturb sleep, even if the individual does not know that they are occurring. They are frequently seen in untreated sleep apnea, but they can occur on their own as well. These can also be treated medically. Of note, the medical treatments may include benzodiazepines, which can impair performance.

Other common sleep-related movement disorders include nocturnal leg cramps and sleep-related bruxism. Nocturnal leg cramps are painful muscle contractions that can occur around sleep onset or during sleep. Frequency tends to increase with age, and frequent leg cramps are associated with other dimensions of poor sleep, as well as impaired daytime function [140]. Bruxism (teeth-grinding) during sleep is also common and can be exacerbated by stress [141, 142]. It can lead to wearing of the teeth, as well as jaw/facial pain. Dental devices are often successfully used to treat bruxism, but sometimes medications such as muscle relaxants, which may interfere with athletic performance, are used.

Parasomnias

There are two types of parasomnias—those that predominantly occur in non-REM sleep and those that predominantly occur in REM sleep. Non-REM parasomnias are represented by recurrent episodes of "incomplete awakening from sleep." This refers to the patient engaging in wake-like behavior but being neurophysiologically asleep [82]. The prototypical non-REM parasomnia is sleepwalking, but there are other variations. In all cases, these episodes are typically accompanied by the patient being unresponsive or minimally responsive to others trying to intervene or redirect them during the event, limited or absent cognition or dream imagery during the event, and partial or complete lack of memory for the episode. In addition to sleepwalking (engaging in ambulation or other complex behaviors), some patients experience sleep-talking (often comprehensible but relatively nonsensical speech), sleep-eating (sometimes leading to unsafe behaviors such as turning on a stove or consuming nonfood items), or sleep-sex (engaging in any of a wide range of sexual activities while asleep). Sleep terrors, which are often confused with nightmares, are actually a non-REM parasomnia such that it occurs during sleep, not during a dream, and the individual has no memory of the event. Unlike a typical sleep-walking episode, a sleep terror can include screaming, flailing, or other extreme behaviors, even though the individual is asleep. These episodes tend to be very distressing for anyone sleeping in the same place, but the individual does not have any memory, even if their eyes were open and they interacted with another individual.

Non-REM parasomnias are relatively common in children but typically abate prior to adolescence. However, some individuals continue to experience these into adulthood, especially later adolescence and young adulthood (the age of many elite athletes). In particular, stress, sleep disruption, sleeping in an unfamiliar place, substance use, and/or schedule disruptions can trigger these episodes, especially in young adults who experienced non-REM parasomnias as children. Treatment usually involves helping to keep the individual safe and redirecting them gently to bed. Sometimes, these can be treated medically, though this can include sedatives, which impact athletic performance.

The most common REM parasomnias are nightmare disorder and REM sleep behavior disorder. Nightmare disorder can be diagnosed when the patient presents with recurrent nightmares that cause often extreme distress and impairment in mood, sleep, cognitive, physical, or other domains [143]. Treatments for nightmares, including medications [144] and nonpharmacologic therapies, exist [145, 146]. REM sleep behavior disorder occurs when the muscle atonia of REM sleep fails and the individual begins to act out their dreams [82]. This often results in relatively violent behaviors during the night and can cause injuries to the patient and/or the bedpartner. REM sleep behavior disorder is common in older adults (especially men) and is rare in younger adults. It often reflects a neurodegenerative condition that typically results in eventual Parkinsonism or other neurodegenerative conditions [147–149]. Symptoms can often be treated with medications, including benzodiazepines, but no cure yet exists. Of note, not all occurrences of individuals acting out dreams are REM behavior disorder, and evaluation with PSG may be warranted.

Sleep Problems and Disturbances

In addition to sleep disorders, many athletes experience subclinical sleep disturbances. Of note, although sleep disorders are relatively well-characterized in terms of available treatments, subclinical sleep problems have received less attention. Still, recommendations can be made.

Sleep Deprivation and Insufficient Sleep Sleep deprivation refers to the acute experience of loss of sleep, resulting in impairments in daytime functioning. Insufficient sleep, on the other hand, refers to the chronic experience of accumulated sleep loss, resulting in more chronic impairments across multiple domains. According to recommendations [38, 39], adults should get about 7–8 h of sleep per night in order to perform optimally. Adolescents and younger adults may need more than 8 h for optimal functioning [38, 150], as may elite athletes. Still, there are individual differences in sleep needs, and it is possible that some individuals do not experience decrements in performance with less sleep [151]. On average, though, insufficient sleep of 6 or fewer hours is associated in general adult samples with weight gain and obesity, metabolic disorders like diabetes, cardiovascular disease, hypertension, immune system dysfunction, substance use problems, mental health symptoms and disorders, performance deficits, and shorter lifespan [8, 117, 118, 152–156]. Signs of insufficient sleep include daytime sleepiness and/or fatigue, cognitive problems, and decreased energy. Among athletes, insufficient sleep can be caused by increased time demands, travel, timing of practices/competitions in a way that interferes with sleep opportunity, social pressures, and other factors.

Daytime Sleepiness and Fatigue Daytime sleepiness refers to the inability to maintain wakefulness during the day. People with excessive daytime sleepiness often fall asleep at inappropriate times or places, especially if they stop moving. This is in contrast to fatigue, which is a psychophysiologic state of feeling that there are insufficient resources to meet demands. Many people with fatigue have no difficulty maintaining wakefulness, and many people who experience daytime sleepiness do not realize how impaired they are and do not feel very fatigued [157]. However, these symptoms, though different, often co-occur. Common causes of excessive sleepiness in athletes includes insufficient sleep at night, untreated sleep disorder, pain or other physical discomfort during the night, medication/substance side effects, and environmental disturbances.

Poor Sleep Quality Sleep quality is typically a subjective appraisal of the degree to which sleep was refreshing and/or restorative, whether sleep was sufficient to perform its functions, and the degree to which sleep was, overall, "good" or "bad." Sleep quality is a somewhat general, subjective term that, nevertheless, remains a valuable metric [4, 158, 159]. "Good" sleep quality is typically reflected in sleep being restful, restorative, regenerative, and recuperative, that it was easy enough to obtain and keep during the night, that it was not excessively interrupted or obstructed, that it allowed for sufficient daytime functioning, that it was satisfying and not worrisome, and that it was a generally pleasant experience. Despite these nonspecific definitions, general sleep quality seems to represent an aspect of sleep health that is not captured by other metrics, yet is related to outcomes as diverse as mental health [32, 160], cardiometabolic health [30, 161], and immune function [162]. Athletes may experience poor sleep quality when their sleep is disturbed by factors that lead to insomnia symptoms or when medical or environmental conditions keep sleep shallow and nonrestorative. Athletes may not know why their sleep does not feel refreshing, just that it is not refreshing. This is especially common during recovery after injury, when pain can disrupt sleep quality, sleeping immediately before or after a competition, or sleeping in an unfamiliar environment.

Addressing Sleep Problems Although there is less scientific evidence for strategies targeted at nonclinical sleep disturbances, sleep hygiene recommendations may be especially useful in these cases. By removing barriers to sleep, it is possible to allow athletes to obtain their best sleep possible and perhaps reduce the burden of insufficient sleep, daytime sleepiness/fatigue, and/or poor sleep quality. Several key sleep hygiene recommendations include:

- *Keep a regular schedule*: By keeping as regular a schedule as possible, time can become an element that helps promote healthy sleep. For example, by going to bed at the same time each night, this can help the body anticipate the time for sleep. In addition, a regular wake time may help the body anticipate not only when to have energy during the day, but also it may help predict the onset of sleep approximately 16 h later. The more regular a person's sleep schedule, the more sleep can become predictable and entrained. This is often a problem for athletes who have irregular schedules or may travel across time zones. To accommodate this, athletes should still try to make their schedule as predictable as possible. In addition, a regular bedtime routine may help build portable regularity and predictability even during periods of travel.
- *Obtain enough bright light during the day and avoid bright light at night*: Bright light at night, especially in the blue-green spectrum, sends a daytime signal to the supra-

chiasmatic nucleus in the hypothalamus, which may alter the circadian clock and delay bedtime. Conversely, light in the daytime, especially the morning, can have an alerting effect and promote increased energy during the day, as well as increased mood. Further, bright light exposure during the day may reduce the adverse impact of light at night. For athletes, this may be possible via morning outdoor activities, as well as use of blue-blocking glasses at night.
- *Keep the sleeping environment cool, quiet, and comfortable*: The sleeping environment may be an overlooked opportunity for optimizing sleep quality. People tend to sleep better in cooler environments, so climate control during the night may improve sleep. In addition, as mentioned above, light at night may impede sleep. For this reason, bedrooms should be sufficiently dark to promote sleep, though some individuals find that a sleeping environment that is too dark may disrupt sleep, perhaps due to anxiety. Although there is surprisingly little research on sleeping surfaces, consideration should be given regarding the mattress, in terms of softness/firmness, as well as bedcoverings and pillows.
- *Avoid excessive liquids at night*: Consuming excessive liquids at night can increase the frequency of nocturia and associated awakenings. Although hydration is important for athletes, perhaps sufficient hydration should be a focus earlier in the day.
- *Refrain from consuming too much food close to sleep*: Excessive food intake close to sleep may be more likely to be unnecessary metabolically and, worse, may lead to unwanted weight gain and metabolic dysregulation. Further, eating heavy or spicy meals may contribute to nocturnal reflux symptoms that can interfere with sleep.
- *Put down screens before getting ready for bed*: Electronic media use can interfere with sleep quality, timing, and duration in a number of ways [163]. First, the light from devices may lead to circadian dysregulation and delaying of bedtime. Second, the mental activation from electronic media use can have strong, independent effects on sleep quality. Third, electronic media use can be very distracting, leading to excessive time displacement—where individuals lose sense of the passage of time and become very distracted. Evening electronic media use may therefore delay onset of sleep and lead to more shallow sleep. Studies show that athletes using electronic media during the sleep period may experience next-day performance decrements, especially if they do not typically use media at night [164].
- *Avoid caffeine within 10 h of sleep*: Caffeine is an important substance for athletes—it is perhaps the most potent performance enhancer that is not prohibited across most sports. Caffeine can interfere with sleep even after several hours following ingestion [165].

- *Avoid alcohol prior to sleeping*: Alcohol, a sedative, may cause an individual to fall asleep faster and may even contribute to deeper sleep in the early part of the night. However, as the alcohol is metabolized, it becomes an alerting substance that can make sleep more shallow and cause awakenings. For this reason, alcohol is more likely to impair sleep quality than improve it [166].
- *Do not go to bed angry, worried, or upset*: Frequently, people take their concerns to bed with them. The problem with this is that the bed becomes associated with these thoughts and worries. This can lead to a conditioned arousal to the bed. To counteract this, the bed should be primarily used for sleeping, and if an individual is in bed engaged in an activity that is not compatible with sleep (e.g., thinking and worrying), that activity should be taken out of bed. Removing nonsleep activities from bed is a key aspect of stimulus control therapy, a core component of CBTI [167]. For athletes who have limited options in terms of where to go when out of bed (e.g., sleeping in a dormitory, hotel room, or vehicle), the individual can at least take a position that is incompatible with sleep. For example, sitting up in bed, especially in a part of the bed not used for sleeping, such as the foot of the bed, can accomplish this goal as well.
- *Pay less attention to the clock*: Most people check the clock when they awaken during the night. Sometimes, this can lead to distress and worry about not having slept long enough or not being able to resume sleep quickly enough. For these individuals, it is recommended to turn the clock around or make it somewhat inaccessible so that it can be viewed in emergencies but not with a simple glance. This may reduce the impact of the clock on increased arousal during awakenings, thereby facilitating return to sleep.
- *Do not nap too long or too late*: Naps can be helpful for increasing physical and mental performance, as well as cognitive function [158, 168]. Naps can also be used—especially in adolescents and younger adults—to counteract adverse effects of sleep deprivation. Athletes can use naps to improve performance [158]. However, naps that are too long or too late in the day can interfere with sleep homeostasis and lead to worse sleep and worse performance. For that reason, naps should be kept relatively brief and relatively early in the day, under most circumstances.

Although it is unlikely that these will completely ameliorate all subclinical sleep problems, they represent a starting point for sleep health education programs and recommendations. In addition, many of these recommendations may be difficult in the context of athlete schedules and time demands.

Importance of Sleep Health in Elite Athletes

This chapter is focused on introducing basic concepts of sleep science, clinical sleep concerns, and applications to athletes. A complete overview of all of the ways that sleep is important for health and performance in athletes is beyond the scope of this chapter. Several recent reviews have explored these issues in detail [3, 4, 7, 44, 158].

Many previous studies have documented adverse effects of poor sleep on physical performance. Sleep restriction, in particular, has been associated with both cardiorespiratory and neurobehavioral effects both in the short term and over periods of days to weeks [3]. Mechanisms of this relationship are still being explored. For example, physical performance following sleep restriction may require greater physiologic output, leading to more rapid exhaustion [169]. This is supported by work showing that maximal power output is reduced following sleep restriction [170, 171]. Other studies have shown that sleep restriction impairs tennis serving accuracy [172, 173], treadmill running distance [174], sprint speed [175], isometric force [176], and testosterone levels [177, 178]. Sleep restriction impairs muscle glycogen recovery [179] and contributes to overtraining.

Poor sleep is also a risk factor for injury among athletes. Elite athletes screened for subclinical sleep concerns were followed for 1 year. Those that reported daytime sleepiness or insomnia symptoms at baseline were more likely to experience a concussion in the subsequent year, and these predictors outperformed more standard concussion risk factors including gender, sport played, and prior concussion history [180, 181]. This work is consistent with other research showing that athletes who reported shorter sleep were more likely to experience an injury [182].

Insomnia is a reliable predictor of depression and other mental health symptoms and disorders [160, 183]. In particular, poor sleep is associated with a tripling of suicide risk [184]. This is especially alarming because suicide is among the leading causes of death among young adults, including athletes. In particular, being awake during the night, when the brain is predisposed to sleep, may lead to a neurophysiologic cascade that leads to unhealthy decision making, including suicide [185, 186]. Among collegiate student athletes, shorter sleep duration was associated with greater perceived stress and higher depression scores [34]. In this sample, worse overall sleep quality was also associated with more stress, depression, and anxiety, as were insomnia symptoms and fatigue. In addition, decreased social support was experienced by athletes who slept less and experienced worse sleep quality. Decreased social support was also reported by student athletes who reported a delayed sleep–wake phase, and this decreased social support partially explained relationships to depression [187]. Among a national sample of collegiate student athletes, sleep-related distress and insufficient sleep were associated with a greater likelihood of suicide ideation [35].

Elements of a Sleep Program in Athletics

The Sleep and Wellness task force of the NCAA recommended that athletics programs should incorporate five key elements: (1) an annual time demands survey, (2) sleep screening to be included in preparticipation exams, (3) education programs for athletes, (4) education programs for coaches/staff, and (5) efforts to ensure that any wearables and sleep tracking technology adhere to appropriate privacy standards (7). The International Olympic Committee (IOC) consensus statement on mental health in elite athletes suggests that athletics programs should include screening for primary sleep disorders and provision of sleep improvement programs for those that present with sleep problems [188]. The international consensus recommendations for athlete sleep programs [158] advise that athletics programs engage in four types of activities to promote sleep health: (1) sleep education for athletes, (2) regular, systematic screening for sleep problems and sleep concerns, (3) encouragement of naps—especially brief naps in the middle of the day—to improve performance, and (4) banking sleep, defined as accumulating periods of optimal sleep to buffer against planned periods of poor sleep (e.g., before competition). Taken together, these different sets of recommendations consist of multiple common themes.

Screening and Assessment

Screening and assessment of sleep is a key concern for athletics programs, for several reasons. First, untreated sleep disorders need to be identified so that they can be appropriately treated. As mentioned above, sleep disorders can have profound impacts on athlete performance and well-being, though they frequently remain underdiagnosed. In addition to the identification of sleep disorders, screening tools can identify problem areas, subclinical sleep problems, and barriers to healthy sleep experienced by athletes. A typical approach is a triaging strategy where athletes are screened into categories of high risk (referred for further diagnosis and treatment), medium risk (provided education and troubleshooting of sleep problems), and low risk (provided education towards optimization and performance improvement). Earlier in this chapter, a wide range of screening instruments was described.

One aspect of sleep assessment that is highly relevant to sport is the use of wearable and other sleep tracking technologies. Wearable movement-based sleep tracking technol-

ogies have been in use for research since the 1970s [189]. Since that time, the technology has been more fully developed and expanded such that movement-based estimations of sleep–wake patterns have come to make use of complex, multiaxial accelerometry [54]. These devices are frequently used in research and typically demonstrate approximately 85% accuracy relative to PSG in determinations of sleep versus wake. More recently, optical photoplethysmography signals have been added to these wearables in order to incorporate heart-rate signals into sleep–wake detection [190]. Recent evidence suggests that this may significantly improve the performance of wearables in detecting sleep versus wake, increasing accuracy to over 90% for many devices [54]. Additional devices have been dubbed "nearables" because they are not worn but sense movement and other signals at the bedside, above or under the mattress, or even embedded within the mattress. These devices tend to demonstrate sleep–wake detection similar to wearables [54]. EEG-based wearables that are incorporated into headbands have also begun to permeate the market and demonstrate relatively good accuracy relative to PSG in determining sleep versus wake [46]. Detecting if an individual is asleep or awake seems to be the greatest strength of sleep wearables (and nearables). Other metrics, though, are less well studied. Devices that obtain heart rate data can estimate PSG sleep stages using the combination of movement, heart rate, and other signals. Accuracy of these sleep stage estimates is moderate but not high [54, 55]. This is significant for athletes who may wish to optimize sleep states that promote recovery. These devices cannot yet determine sleep stages accurately enough. Other metrics obtained by these devices (e.g., recovery metrics, sleep need) are even less well studied and may not be reliable or valid. Caution should be exercised when interpreting these results.

Referral and Treatment

When athletes are identified as being high risk for sleep disorders, athletics programs should refer to a qualified sleep specialist in order to diagnose and treat those conditions. There are multiple types of sleep specialists that may be helpful, based on the presenting problem.

Sleep Physicians These are medical doctors who have special training and certification in the field of sleep medicine. They are qualified to diagnose and treat nearly all sleep disorders, though these specialists typically primarily work with sleep apnea patients. Of note, they are also an important resource for medical treatment of sleep disorders. Although some physicians may claim to be sleep specialists, those who are board-certified in sleep medicine are the most qualified.

Behavioral Sleep Medicine Specialists These are typically clinical psychologists but can represent other specialties such as nursing or social work. Clinicians who specialize in behavioral sleep medicine should become board-certified in behavioral sleep medicine by taking the examination offered by the Board of Behavioral Sleep Medicine. The field of Behavioral Sleep Medicine includes licensed clinicians who can diagnose and treat most sleep disorders. One key difference with this group is that they typically do not prescribe medications or medical devices and use nonmedication strategies to treat sleep disorders. These specialists may have experience with a wide range of sleep disorders but tend to be especially well-qualified for working with insomnia. As mentioned above, the recommended first-line therapy for insomnia is a nonpharmacologic approach (CBTI). These specialists may also be uniquely qualified to assess mental health impacts on sleep and impacts of sleep on performance.

Education and Culture

In addition to screening and assessment, athletics programs should provide education to athletes, coaches, and other staff who may benefit from this information. The NCAA recommendations suggest that education programs should contain information on best sleep practices, information about the role of sleep in athlete physical and mental performance, and strategies for addressing barriers to sleep. Through education and support from coaches and other staff, the athletics program should promote a culture that values sleep health. Practices that support the ability of athletes to get the best sleep possible should be encouraged. Viewing sleep as part of athletic training and recovery should similarly be encouraged, and individuals who promote attitudes and beliefs about sleep that devalue it should be corrected. Athletes should feel that they have permission to leverage sleep health as part of their athletics performance optimization strategy.

Sleep Optimization Programs

In addition to identifying and ameliorating problems and providing education, athletics programs can provide useful supports for optimizing sleep health among athletes to improve performance. Although there is still relatively little data on specific programs and how they may be applied, several recommendations can be made. For example, these programs may include the use of wearables to track sleep, identify emerging problems, and use sleep metrics to predict how an athlete will perform. Sleep skills trainings can help athletes improve their ability to be in control of their sleep when they want, where they want, and for as long as they want. Stimulus control can be an important element of these programs. Athletics programs can also carefully consider scheduling of trainings, practices, travel, and pre- and postcompetition activities in order to optimize performance. Providing support for individuals with sleep struggles (and sleep disorders) may ameliorate problems as they arise. Providing incentives for achieving good quality sleep may counterbalance the incentives for staying awake later and getting less sleep. Although few comprehensive programs have been evaluated, preliminary results from a multicomponent program that included education, tracking, support, and incentives are promising, including positive impacts on sleep health, mental well-being, and perceived mental, general physical, social, and athletic performance [191, 192].

Conclusions and Recommendations

Sleep health is important for athletes. Sleep is fundamental to many physiologic processes, and healthy sleep in athletes can promote well-being, better cardiometabolic and immune health, improved cognition, reduced injury risk, faster and more efficient recovery, and improved mental health. Yet, sleep disorders and sleep concerns are highly prevalent in athletics populations. This may be due to risk factors associated with sport and being an athlete, and these may also be due to social and environmental constraints. For these reasons, sleep concerns should be prioritized by athletics programs. Promoting sleep health in athletes includes four components: (1) screening and assessment in order to identify and triage problems, (2) referral and treatment to address sleep disorders, (3) education and culture change in order to empower athletes to strategically prioritize sleep, and (4) sleep training programs that can optimize sleep among athletes. To assist with these efforts, it is recommended that athletics programs refer to published statements and guidelines [7, 158, 188, 193] to develop programs, reviews (3, 4) to conceptualize the role of sleep in athletics, and qualified sleep specialists to assist in addressing sleep concerns.

References

1. Grandner MA, Fernandez FX. The translational neuroscience of sleep: a contextual framework. Science. 2021;374(6567):568–73.
2. Henry D, McClellen D, Rosenthal L, Dedrick D, Gosdin M. Is sleep really for sissies? Understanding the role of work in insomnia in the US. Soc Sci Med. 2008;66(3):715–26.
3. Charest J, Grandner MA. Sleep and athletic performance: impacts on physical performance, mental performance, injury risk and recovery, and mental health. Sleep Med Clin. 2020;15(1):41–57.
4. Brauer AA, Athey AB, Ross MJ, Grandner MA. Sleep and health among collegiate student athletes. Chest. 2019;156(6):1234–45.

5. Penn Schoen Berland Student-athlete time demands. Penn Schoen Berland; 2015.

6. Carskadon MA. Sleep in adolescents: the perfect storm. Pediatr Clin N Am. 2011;58(3):637–47.

7. Kroshus E, Wagner J, Wyrick D, Athey A, Bell L, Benjamin HJ, et al. Wake up call for collegiate athlete sleep: narrative review and consensus recommendations from the NCAA Interassociation Task Force on Sleep and Wellness. Br J Sports Med. 2019;53(12):731–6.

8. Grandner MA. Sleep, health, and society. Sleep Med Clin. 2020;15(2):319–40.

9. Grandner MA, Schopfer EA, Sands-Lincoln M, Jackson N, Malhotra A. Relationship between sleep duration and body mass index depends on age. Obesity. 2015;23(12):2491–8.

10. Turner RW, Vissa K, Hall C, Poling K, Athey A, Alfonso-Miller P, et al. Sleep problems are associated with academic performance in a national sample of collegiate athletes. J Am Coll Heal. 2019;2019:1–8.

11. Athey A, Grandner MA. Student athletes' access to healthy sleep information on campus: how does it relate to other types of health information and sleep difficulties? Sleep. 2017;40:451.

12. Gouttebarge V, Castaldelli-Maia JM, Gorczynski P, Hainline B, Hitchcock ME, Kerkhoffs GM, et al. Occurrence of mental health symptoms and disorders in current and former elite athletes: a systematic review and meta-analysis. Br J Sports Med. 2019;53(11):700–6.

13. Ohayon MM. Epidemiology of insomnia: what we know and what we still need to learn. Sleep Med Rev. 2002;6(2):97–111.

14. Peppard PE, Young T, Barnet JH, Palta M, Hagen EW, Hla KM. Increased prevalence of sleep-disordered breathing in adults. Am J Epidemiol. 2013;177:1006–14.

15. Chung F, Subramanyam R, Liao P, Sasaki E, Shapiro C, Sun Y. High STOP-Bang score indicates a high probability of obstructive sleep apnoea. Br J Anaesth. 2012;108(5):768–75.

16. George CF, Kab V, Kab P, Villa JJ, Levy AM. Sleep and breathing in professional football players. Sleep Med. 2003;4(4):317–25.

17. George CF, Kab V, Levy AM. Increased prevalence of sleep-disordered breathing among professional football players. N Engl J Med. 2003;348(4):367–8.

18. Joiner WJ. The neurobiological basis of sleep and sleep disorders. Physiology. 2018;33(5):317–27.

19. Allada R, Bass J. Circadian mechanisms in medicine. N Engl J Med. 2021;384(6):550–61.

20. Tahkamo L, Partonen T, Pesonen AK. Systematic review of light exposure impact on human circadian rhythm. Chronobiol Int. 2019;36(2):151–70.

21. Reiter RJ, Tan DX, Fuentes-Broto L. Melatonin: a multitasking molecule. Prog Brain Res. 2010;181:127–51.

22. Cermakian N, Boivin DB. The regulation of central and peripheral circadian clocks in humans. Obes Rev. 2009;10(2):25–36.

23. Ruben MD, Wu G, Smith DF, Schmidt RE, Francey LJ, Lee YY, et al. A database of tissue-specific rhythmically expressed human genes has potential applications in circadian medicine. Sci Transl Med. 2018;10:458.

24. Anafi RC, Francey LJ, Hogenesch JB, Kim J. CYCLOPS reveals human transcriptional rhythms in health and disease. Proc Natl Acad Sci U S A. 2017;114(20):5312–7.

25. Borbely AA. A two process model of sleep regulation. Hum Neurobiol. 1982;1(3):195–204.

26. American Academy of Sleep Medicine. The AASM manual for the scoring of sleep and associated events. 6th ed. Darien: AASM; 2020.

27. Buysse DJ. Sleep health: can we define it? Does it matter? Sleep. 2014;37(1):9–17.

28. Phillips AJK, Clerx WM, O'Brien CS, Sano A, Barger LK, Picard RW, et al. Irregular sleep/wake patterns are associated with poorer academic performance and delayed circadian and sleep/wake timing. Sci Rep. 2017;7(1):3216.

29. Nakanishi-Minami T, Kishida K, Funahashi T, Shimomura I. Sleep-wake cycle irregularities in type 2 diabetics. Diabetol Metab Syndr. 2012;4(1):18.

30. St-Onge MP, Grandner MA, Brown D, Conroy MB, Jean-Louis G, Coons M, et al. Sleep duration and quality: impact on lifestyle behaviors and cardiometabolic health: a scientific statement from the American Heart Association. Circulation. 2016;134(18):367–86.

31. Grandner MA, Jackson NJ, Pak VM, Gehrman PR. Sleep disturbance is associated with cardiovascular and metabolic disorders. J Sleep Res. 2012;21(4):427–33.

32. Hertenstein E, Feige B, Gmeiner T, Kienzler C, Spiegelhalder K, Johann A, et al. Insomnia as a predictor of mental disorders: a systematic review and meta-analysis. Sleep Med Rev. 2019;43:96–105.

33. Baglioni C, Battagliese G, Feige B, Spiegelhalder K, Nissen C, Voderholzer U, et al. Insomnia as a predictor of depression: a meta-analytic evaluation of longitudinal epidemiological studies. J Affect Disord. 2011;135(1-3):10–9.

34. Grandner MA, Hall C, Jaszewski A, Alfonso-Miller P, Gehrels J, Killgore WDS, et al. Mental health in student athletes: associations with sleep duration, sleep quality, insomnia, fatigue, and sleep apnea symptoms. Athl Train Sports Health Care. 2021;13:4.

35. Khader WS, Tubbs AS, Haghighi A, Athey AB, Killgore WDS, Hale L, et al. Onset insomnia and insufficient sleep duration are associated with suicide ideation in university students and athletes. J Affect Disord. 2020;274:1161–4.

36. Mendlewicz J. Disruption of the circadian timing systems: molecular mechanisms in mood disorders. CNS Drugs. 2009;23:15–26.

37. Barnard AR, Nolan PM. When clocks go bad: neurobehavioural consequences of disrupted circadian timing. PLoS Genet. 2008;4(5):1000040.

38. Hirshkowitz M, Whiton K, Alpert SM, Alessi C, Bruni O, DonCarlos L, et al. National Sleep Foundation's updated sleep duration recommendations: final report. Sleep Health. 2015;1:233–43.

39. Watson NF, Badr MS, Belenky G, Bliwise DL, Buxton OM, Buysse D, et al. Recommended amount of sleep for a healthy adult: a joint consensus statement of the American Academy of Sleep Medicine and Sleep Research Society. Sleep. 2015;38(6):843–4.

40. Watson NF, Badr MS, Belenky G, Bliwise DL, Buxton OM, Buysse D, et al. Joint Consensus Statement of the American Academy of Sleep Medicine and Sleep Research Society on the recommended amount of sleep for a healthy adult: methodology and discussion. J Clin Sleep Med. 2015;11(8):931–52.

41. Kurina LM, McClintock MK, Chen JH, Waite LJ, Thisted RA, Lauderdale DS. Sleep duration and all-cause mortality: a critical review of measurement and associations. Ann Epidemiol. 2013;23(6):361–70.

42. Ramsey T, Athey A, Ellis J, Tubbs AS, Turner R, Killgore WDS, et al. Dose-response relationship between insufficient sleep and mental health symptoms in collegiate student athletes and non-athletes. Sleep. 2019;42:362.

43. Biggins M, Cahalan R, Comyns T, Purtill H, O'Sullivan K. Poor sleep is related to lower general health, increased stress and increased confusion in elite Gaelic athletes. Phys Sports Med. 2018;46(1):14–20.

44. Simpson NS, Gibbs EL, Matheson GO. Optimizing sleep to maximize performance: implications and recommendations for elite athletes. Scand J Med Sci Sports. 2017;27(3):266–74.

45. Grandner MA, Patel NP, Hale L, Moore M. Mortality associated with sleep duration: the evidence, the possible mechanisms, and the future. Sleep Med Rev. 2010;14:191–203.

46. Arnal PJ, Thorey V, Debellemaniere E, Ballard ME, Bou Hernandez A, Guillot A, et al. The Dreem headband compared to polysomnography for electroencephalographic signal acquisition and sleep staging. Sleep. 2020;43(11):97.

47. Chambon S, Thorey V, Arnal PJ, Mignot E, Gramfort A. DOSED: a deep learning approach to detect multiple sleep micro-events in EEG signal. J Neurosci Methods. 2019;321:64–78.

48. Grandner MA, Perlis ML. Pharmacotherapy for insomnia disorder in older adults. JAMA Netw Open. 2019;2(12):1918214.

49. Kupfer DJ, Detre TP, Foster G, Tucker GJ, Delgado J. The application of Delgado's telemetric mobility recorder for human studies. Behav Biol. 1972;7(4):585–90.

50. Foster FG, Kupfer D, Weiss G, Lipponen V, McPartland RJ, Delgado J. Mobility recording and cycle research in neuropsychiatry. J Interdisc Cycle Res. 1972;3(1):61–72.

51. Kripke DF, Mullaney DJ, Messin S, Wyborney VG. Wrist actigraphic measures of sleep and rhythms. Electroencephalogr Clin Neurophysiol. 1978;44(5):674–6.

52. Ancoli-Israel S, Martin JL, Blackwell T, Buenaver L, Liu L, Meltzer LJ, et al. The SBSM guide to actigraphy monitoring: clinical and research applications. Behav Sleep Med. 2015;13:4–38.

53. Grandner MA, Lujan MR, Ghani SB. Sleep-tracking technology in scientific research: looking to the future. Sleep. 2021;44:5.

54. Lujan MR, Perez-Pozuelo I, Grandner MA. Past, present, and future of multisensory wearable technology to monitor sleep and circadian rhythms. Front Digit Health. 2021;3:721919.

55. Chinoy ED, Cuellar JA, Huwa KE, Jameson JT, Watson CH, Bessman SC, et al. Performance of seven consumer sleep-tracking devices compared with polysomnography. Sleep. 2021;44(5):291.

56. Carney CE, Buysse DJ, Ancoli-Israel S, Edinger JD, Krystal AD, Lichstein KL, et al. The consensus sleep diary: standardizing prospective sleep self-monitoring. Sleep. 2012;35(2):287–302.

57. Bender AM, Lawson D, Werthner P, Samuels CH. The clinical validation of the athlete sleep screening questionnaire: an instrument to identify athletes that need further sleep assessment. Sports Med Open. 2018;4(1):23.

58. Klingman KJ, Jungquist CR, Perlis ML. Introducing the sleep disorders symptom checklist-25: a primary care friendly and comprehensive screener for sleep disorders. Sleep Med Res. 2017;8(1):17–25.

59. Roth T, Zammit G, Kushida C, Doghramji K, Mathias SD, Wong JM, et al. A new questionnaire to detect sleep disorders. Sleep Med. 2002;3(2):99–108.

60. Spoormaker VI, Verbeek I, van den Bout J, Klip EC. Initial validation of the SLEEP-50 questionnaire. Behav Sleep Med. 2005;3(4):227–46.

61. Taylor DJ, Wilkerson AK, Pruiksma KE, Williams JM, Ruggero CJ, Hale W, et al. Reliability of the structured clinical interview for DSM-5 sleep disorders module. J Clin Sleep Med. 2018;14(3):459–64.

62. Bastien CH, Vallieres A, Morin CM. Validation of the insomnia severity index as an outcome measure for insomnia research. Sleep Med. 2001;2(4):297–307.

63. Schutte-Rodin S, Broch L, Buysse D, Dorsey C, Sateia M. Clinical guideline for the evaluation and management of chronic insomnia in adults. J Clin Sleep Med. 2008;4(5):487–504.

64. Netzer NC, Stoohs RA, Netzer CM, Clark K, Strohl KP. Using the Berlin questionnaire to identify patients at risk for the sleep apnea syndrome. Ann Intern Med. 1999;131(7):485–91.

65. Bargiotas P, Dietmann A, Haynes AG, Kallweit U, Calle MG, Schmidt M, et al. The Swiss narcolepsy scale (SNS) and its short form (sSNS) for the discrimination of narcolepsy in patients with hypersomnolence: a cohort study based on the bern sleep-wake Database. J Neurol. 2019;266(9):2137–43.

66. Walters AS, LeBrocq C, Dhar A, Hening W, Rosen R, Allen RP, et al. Validation of the International Restless Legs Syndrome Study Group rating scale for restless legs syndrome. Sleep Med. 2003;4(2):121–32.

67. Johns MW. A new method for measuring daytime sleepiness: the Epworth sleepiness scale. Sleep. 1991;14(6):540–5.

68. Krupp LB, LaRocca NG, Muir-Nash J, Steinberg AD. The fatigue severity scale. Application to patients with multiple sclerosis and systemic lupus erythematosus. Arch Neurol. 1989;46(10):1121–3.

69. Chasens ER, Ratcliffe SJ, Weaver TE. Development of the FOSQ-10: a short version of the functional outcomes of sleep questionnaire. Sleep. 2009;32(7):915–9.

70. Buysse DJ, Yu L, Moul DE, Germain A, Stover A, Dodds NE, et al. Development and validation of patient-reported outcome measures for sleep disturbance and sleep-related impairments. Sleep. 2010;33(6):781–92.

71. Monk TH, Buysse DJ, Kennedy KS, Pods JM, DeGrazia JM, Miewald JM. Measuring sleep habits without using a diary: the sleep timing questionnaire. Sleep. 2003;26(2):208–12.

72. Dietch JR, Sethi K, Slavish DC, Taylor DJ. Validity of two retrospective questionnaire versions of the consensus sleep diary: the whole week and split week self-assessment of sleep surveys. Sleep Med. 2019;63:127–36.

73. Ghotbi N, Pilz LK, Winnebeck EC, Vetter C, Zerbini G, Lenssen D, et al. The microMCTQ: an ultra-short version of the Munich ChronoType questionnaire. J Biol Rhythm. 2020;35(1):98–110.

74. Roenneberg T, Wirz-Justice A, Merrow M. Life between clocks: daily temporal patterns of human chronotypes. J Biol Rhythm. 2003;18(1):80–90.

75. Horne JA, Ostberg O. A self-assessment questionnaire to determine morningness-eveningness in human circadian rhythms. Int J Chronobiol. 1976;4(2):97–110.

76. Ottoni GL, Antoniolli E, Lara DR. The Circadian Energy Scale (CIRENS): two simple questions for a reliable chronotype measurement based on energy. Chronobiol Int. 2011;28(3):229–37.

77. Morin CM, Vallieres A, Ivers H. Dysfunctional beliefs and attitudes about sleep (DBAS): validation of a brief version (DBAS-16). Sleep. 2007;30(11):1547–54.

78. Adan A, Fabbri M, Natale V, Prat G. Sleep beliefs scale (SBS) and circadian typology. J Sleep Res. 2006;15(2):125–32.

79. Grandner MA, Olivier K, Gallagher R, Hale L, Barrett M, Branas C, et al. Quantifying impact of real-world barriers to sleep: the brief index of sleep control (BRISC). Sleep Health. 2020;6(5):587–93.

80. Olivier K, Gallagher RA, Killgore WDS, Carrazco N, Alfonso-Miller P, Gehrels J, et al. Development and initial validation of the assessment of sleep environment: a novel inventory for describing and quantifying the impact of environmental factors on sleep. Sleep. 2016;39:367.

81. Patel NP, Jackson NJ, Grandner MA. Development and initial validation of a questionnaire to assess sleep-related practices, attitudes, and beliefs. Sleep. 2012;35:425–6.

82. American Academy of Sleep Medicine. International classification of sleep disorders. 3rd ed. Darien: American Academy of Sleep Medicine; 2014.

83. American Psychiatric Association. Diagnostic and statistical manual of mental disorders: DSM-5-TR. 5th ed. Washington: American Psychiatric Association Publishing; 2022.

84. Perlis ML, Shaw P, Cano G, Espie C. Models of insomnia. In: Kryger M, Roth T, Dement WC, editors. Principles and practice of sleep medicine. 5th ed. Philadelphia: Elsevier; 2010. p. 850–65.

85. Ebben MR, Narizhnaya M. Cognitive and behavioral treatment options for insomnia. Mt Sinai J Med. 2012;79(4):512–23.

86. Edinger JD, Arndt JT, Bertisch SM, Carney CE, Harrington JJ, Lichstein KL, et al. Behavioral and psychological treatments for chronic insomnia disorder in adults: an American Academy

of Sleep Medicine clinical practice guideline. J Clin Sleep Med. 2021;17(2):255–62.

87. Edinger JD, Arnedt JT, Bertisch SM, Carney CE, Harrington JJ, Lichstein KL, et al. Behavioral and psychological treatments for chronic insomnia disorder in adults: an American Academy of Sleep Medicine systematic review, meta-analysis, and GRADE assessment. J Clin Sleep Med. 2021;17(2):263–98.

88. Okajima I, Komada Y, Inoue D. A meta-analysis on the treatment effectiveness of cognitive behavioral therapy for primary insomnia. Sleep Biol Rhythms. 2011;9(1):24–34.

89. Morin CM, Culbert JP, Schwartz SM. Nonpharmacological interventions for insomnia: a meta-analysis of treatment efficacy. Am J Psychiatry. 1994;151(8):1172–80.

90. Gebara MA, Siripong N, DiNapoli EA, Maree RD, Germain A, Reynolds CF, et al. Effect of insomnia treatments on depression: a systematic review and meta-analysis. Depress Anxiety. 2018;35(8):717–31.

91. Wu JQ, Appleman ER, Salazar RD, Ong JC. Cognitive behavioral therapy for insomnia comorbid with psychiatric and medical conditions: a meta-analysis. JAMA Intern Med. 2015;175(9):1461–72.

92. Smith MT, Perlis ML, Park A, Smith MS, Pennington J, Giles DE, et al. Comparative meta-analysis of pharmacotherapy and behavior therapy for persistent insomnia. Am J Psychiatry. 2002;159(1):5–11.

93. Moorcroft WH. Sleep hygiene. In: Butkov N, Lee-Chiong T, editors. Fundamentals of sleep technology. New York: Lippincott Williams and Wilkins; 2007.

94. Attarian HP. Sleep hygiene. In: Attarian HP, editor. Clinical handbook of insomnia. Current clinical neurology. Totowa: Humana; 2004. p. 99–106.

95. Riedel BW. Sleep hygiene. In: Lichstein KL, Morin CM, editors. Treatment of late-life insomnia. Thousand Oaks: Sage; 2000. p. 125–46.

96. Qaseem A, Kansagara D, Forciea MA, Cooke M, Denberg TD. Clinical guidelines committee of the American College of P. Management of Chronic Insomnia Disorder in adults: a clinical practice guideline from the American College of Physicians. Ann Intern Med. 2016;165(2):125–33.

97. Fatemeh G, Sajjad M, Niloufar R, Neda S, Leila S, Khadijeh M. Effect of melatonin supplementation on sleep quality: a systematic review and meta-analysis of randomized controlled trials. J Neurol. 2022;269(1):205–16.

98. Low TL, Choo FN, Tan SM. The efficacy of melatonin and melatonin agonists in insomnia - An umbrella review. J Psychiatr Res. 2020;121:10–23.

99. Halson SL. Sleep in elite athletes and nutritional interventions to enhance sleep. Sports Med. 2014;44:13–23.

100. Reardon CL, Creado S. Psychiatric medication preferences of sports psychiatrists. Phys Sportsmed. 2016;44(4):397–402.

101. Creado S, Reardon C. The sports psychiatrist and performance-enhancing drugs. Int Rev Psychiatry. 2016;28(6):564–71.

102. Sateia MJ, Buysse DJ, Krystal AD, Neubauer DN, Heald JL. Clinical practice guideline for the pharmacologic treatment of chronic insomnia in adults: an American Academy of Sleep Medicine clinical practice guideline. J Clin Sleep Med. 2017;13(2):307–49.

103. Garbarino S, Lanteri P, Bragazzi NL, Gualerzi G, Ricco M. Occupational injuries and use of benzodiazepines: a systematic review and metanalysis. Front Hum Neurosci. 2021;15:629719.

104. Tom SE, Wickwire EM, Park Y, Albrecht JS. Nonbenzodiazepine sedative hypnotics and risk of fall-related injury. Sleep. 2016;39(5):1009–14.

105. Treves N, Perlman A, Kolenberg Geron L, Asaly A, Matok I. Z-drugs and risk for falls and fractures in older adults-a systematic review and meta-analysis. Age Ageing. 2018;47(2):201–8.

106. Roenneberg T, Kuehnle T, Pramstaller PP, Ricken J, Havel M, Guth A, et al. A marker for the end of adolescence. Curr Biol. 2004;14(24):1038–9.

107. Roenneberg T, Kuehnle T, Juda M, Kantermann T, Allebrandt K, Gordijn M, et al. Epidemiology of the human circadian clock. Sleep Med Rev. 2007;11(6):429–38.

108. Morgenthaler TI, Lee-Chiong T, Alessi C, Friedman L, Aurora RN, Boehlecke B, et al. Practice parameters for the clinical evaluation and treatment of circadian rhythm sleep disorders. An American Academy of Sleep Medicine report. Sleep. 2007;30(11):1445–59.

109. Sack RL. Clinical practice. Jet lag. N Engl J Med. 2010;362(5):440–7.

110. Bin YS, Postnova S, Cistulli PA. What works for jetlag? A systematic review of non-pharmacological interventions. Sleep Med Rev. 2019;43:47–59.

111. Chasens ER, Imes CC, Kariuki JK, Luyster FS, Morris JL, DiNardo MM, et al. Sleep and metabolic syndrome. Nurs Clin North Am. 2021;56(2):203–17.

112. Wickwire EM. Value-based sleep and breathing: health economic aspects of obstructive sleep apnea. Fac Rev. 2021;10:40.

113. Tubbs AS, Khader W, Fernandez F, Grandner MA. The common denominators of sleep, obesity, and psychopathology. Curr Opin Psychol. 2020;34:84–8.

114. Rogers AJ, Xia K, Soe K, Sexias A, Sogade F, Hutchinson B, et al. Obstructive sleep apnea among players in the National Football league: a scoping review. J Sleep Disord Ther. 2017;6(5):278.

115. King S, Cuellar N. Obstructive sleep apnea as an independent stroke risk factor: a review of the evidence, stroke prevention guidelines, and implications for neuroscience nursing practice. J Neurosci Nurs. 2016;48(3):133–42.

116. Baltzis D, Bakker JP, Patel SR, Veves A. Obstructive sleep apnea and vascular diseases. Compr Physiol. 2016;6(3):1519–28.

117. Grandner MA, Alfonso-Miller P, Fernandez-Mendoza J, Shetty S, Shenoy S, Combs D. Sleep: important considerations for the prevention of cardiovascular disease. Curr Opin Cardiol. 2016;31(5):551–65.

118. Grandner MA, Seixas A, Shetty S, Shenoy S. Sleep duration and diabetes risk: population trends and potential mechanisms. Curr Diab Rep. 2016;16(11):106.

119. Gupta MA, Simpson FC. Obstructive sleep apnea and psychiatric disorders: a systematic review. J Clin Sleep Med. 2015;11(2):165–75.

120. Franklin KA, Lindberg E. Obstructive sleep apnea is a common disorder in the population-a review on the epidemiology of sleep apnea. J Thorac Dis. 2015;7(8):1311–22.

121. Lee YC, Chang KY, Mador MJ. Racial disparity in sleep apnea-related mortality in the United States. Sleep Med. 2022;90:204–13.

122. Pepin JL, Bailly S, Rinder P, Adler D, Benjafield AV, Lavergne F, et al. Relationship between CPAP termination and all-cause mortality: a French nationwide database analysis. Chest. 2022;2:13.

123. Lechat B, Appleton S, Melaku YA, Hansen K, McEvoy RD, Adams R, et al. Co-morbid insomnia and obstructive sleep apnoea is associated with all-cause mortality. Eur Respir J. 2021;2:2101958.

124. Bae E, Kwak N, Choi SM, Lee J, Park YS, Lee CH, et al. Mortality prediction in chronic obstructive pulmonary disease and obstructive sleep apnea. Sleep Med. 2021;87:143–50.

125. Iso Y, Kitai H, Kyuno E, Tsunoda F, Nishinaka N, Funato M, et al. Prevalence and significance of sleep disordered breathing in adolescent athletes. ERJ Open Res. 2019;5(1):29.

126. Sargent C, Schmidt WF, Aughey RJ, Bourdon PC, Soria R, Claros JC, et al. The impact of altitude on the sleep of young elite soccer players (ISA3600). Br J Sports Med. 2013;47:86–92.

127. Chatila W, Krachman S. Sleep at high altitudes. In: Lee-Chiong TL, editor. Sleep: a comprehensive handbook. Hoboken: Wiley; 2006. p. 933–7.

128. Patil SP, Ayappa IA, Caples SM, Kimoff RJ, Patel SR, Harrod CG. Treatment of adult obstructive sleep apnea with positive airway pressure: an American Academy of Sleep Medicine clinical practice guideline. J Clin Sleep Med. 2019;15(2):335–43.

129. Ramar K, Dort LC, Katz SG, Lettieri CJ, Harrod CG, Thomas SM, et al. Clinical practice guideline for the treatment of obstructive sleep apnea and snoring with oral appliance therapy: an update for 2015. J Clin Sleep Med. 2015;11(7):773–827.

130. de Vries N, Ravesloot M, van Maanen JP. Positional therapy in obstructive sleep apnea. Cham: Springer; 2015.

131. Kent D, Stanley J, Aurora RN, Levine CG, Gottlieb DJ, Spann MD, et al. Referral of adults with obstructive sleep apnea for surgical consultation: an American Academy of Sleep Medicine systematic review, meta-analysis, and GRADE assessment. J Clin Sleep Med. 2021;17(12):2507–31.

132. Kent D, Stanley J, Aurora RN, Levine C, Gottlieb DJ, Spann MD, et al. Referral of adults with obstructive sleep apnea for surgical consultation: an American Academy of Sleep Medicine clinical practice guideline. J Clin Sleep Med. 2021;17(12):2499–505.

133. Morgenthaler TI, Kapen S, Lee-Chiong T, Alessi C, Boehlecke B, Brown T, et al. Practice parameters for the medical therapy of obstructive sleep apnea. Sleep. 2006;29(8):1031–5.

134. Kirsch D, Adusumilli J. Multiple sleep latency test and maintenance of wakefulness test. Sleep Med Clin. 2009;4:385–92.

135. Maski K, Trotti LM, Kotagal S, Robert Auger R, Swick TJ, Rowley JA, et al. Treatment of central disorders of hypersomnolence: an American Academy of Sleep Medicine systematic review, meta-analysis, and GRADE assessment. J Clin Sleep Med. 2021;17(9):1895–945.

136. Maski K, Trotti LM, Kotagal S, Robert Auger R, Rowley JA, Hashmi SD, et al. Treatment of central disorders of hypersomnolence: an American Academy of Sleep Medicine clinical practice guideline. J Clin Sleep Med. 2021;17(9):1881–93.

137. Aurora RN, Kristo DA, Bista SR, Rowley JA, Zak RS, Casey KR, et al. Update to the AASM clinical practice guideline: "The treatment of restless legs syndrome and periodic limb movement disorder in adults-an update for 2012: practice parameters with an evidence-based systematic review and meta-analyses". Sleep. 2012;35(8):1037.

138. Yeh P, Walters AS, Tsuang JW. Restless legs syndrome: a comprehensive overview on its epidemiology, risk factors, and treatment. Sleep Breath. 2012;16(4):987–1007.

139. Gossard TR, Trotti LM, Videnovic A, St Louis EK. Restless legs syndrome: contemporary diagnosis and treatment. Neurotherapeutics. 2021;18(1):140–55.

140. Grandner MA, Winkelman JW. Nocturnal leg cramps: prevalence and associations with demographics, sleep disturbance symptoms, medical conditions, and cardiometabolic risk factors. PLoS One. 2017;12(6):e0178465.

141. Huynh NT, Emami E, Helman JI, Chervin RD. Interactions between sleep disorders and oral diseases. Oral Dis. 2014;20(3):236–45.

142. Huynh N, Lavigne GJ, Okura K, Yao D, Adachi K. Sleep bruxism. In: Montagna P, Chokroverty S, editors. Sleep disorders. Handbook of clinical neurology. Edinburgh: Elsevier; 2011. p. 901–11.

143. Spoormaker VI, Schredl M, van den Bout J. Nightmares: from anxiety symptom to sleep disorder. Sleep Med Rev. 2006;10(1):19–31.

144. Kung S, Espinel Z, Lapid MI. Treatment of nightmares with prazosin: a systematic review. Mayo Clin Proc. 2012;87(9):890–900.

145. Casement MD, Swanson LM. A meta-analysis of imagery rehearsal for post-trauma nightmares: effects on nightmare frequency, sleep quality, and posttraumatic stress. Clin Psychol Rev. 2012;32(6):566–74.

146. Perlis ML, Aloia M, Kuhn BR. Behavioral treatments for sleep disorders: a comprehensive primer of behavioral sleep medicine interventions. Boston: Academic; 2011. p. 389.

147. Korotun M, Quintero L, Hahn SS. Rapid eye movement behavior disorder and other parasomnias. Clin Geriatr Med. 2021;37(3):483–90.

148. Chokroverty S, Billiard M. Sleep medicine: a comprehensive guide to its development, clinical milestones, and advances in treatment. New York: Springer; 2015.

149. Mahowald MW, Schenck CH. REM sleep behaviour disorder: a marker of synucleinopathy. Lancet Neurol. 2013;12(5):417–9.

150. Paruthi S, Brooks LJ, D'Ambrosio C, Hall WA, Kotagal S, Lloyd RM, et al. Pediatric sleep duration consensus statement: a step forward. J Clin Sleep Med. 2016;12(12):1705–6.

151. Lundholm KR, Honn KA, Skeiky L, Muck RA, Van Dongen HPA. Trait interindividual differences in the magnitude of subjective sleepiness from sleep inertia. Clocks Sleep. 2021;3(2):298–311.

152. Ben Simon E, Vallat R, Barnes CM, Walker MP. Sleep loss and the socio-emotional brain. Trends Cogn Sci. 2020;24(6):435–50.

153. Koren D, Taveras EM. Association of sleep disturbances with obesity, insulin resistance and the metabolic syndrome. Metabolism. 2018;84:67–75.

154. Grandner MA. Sleep and obesity risk in adults: possible mechanisms; contextual factors; and implications for research, intervention, and policy. Sleep Health. 2017;3(5):393–400.

155. Liu TZ, Xu C, Rota M, Cai H, Zhang C, Shi MJ, et al. Sleep duration and risk of all-cause mortality: a flexible, non-linear, meta-regression of 40 prospective cohort studies. Sleep Med Rev. 2017;32:28–36.

156. Palmer CA, Alfano CA. Sleep and emotion regulation: an organizing, integrative review. Sleep Med Rev. 2017;31:6–16.

157. Van Dongen HP, Baynard MD, Maislin G, Dinges DF. Systematic interindividual differences in neurobehavioral impairment from sleep loss: evidence of trait-like differential vulnerability. Sleep. 2004;27(3):423–33.

158. Walsh NP, Halson SL, Sargent C, Roach GD, Nedelec M, Gupta L, et al. Sleep and the athlete: narrative review and 2021 expert consensus recommendations. Br J Sports Med. 2020;55(7):356–68.

159. Ohayon M, Wickwire EM, Hirshkowitz M, Albert SM, Avidan A, Daly FJ, et al. National Sleep Foundation's sleep quality recommendations: first report. Sleep Health. 2017;3(1):6–19.

160. Spiegelhalder K, Regen W, Nanovska S, Baglioni C, Riemann D. Comorbid sleep disorders in neuropsychiatric disorders across the life cycle. Curr Psychiatry Rep. 2013;15(6):364.

161. Grandner MA. Addressing sleep disturbances: an opportunity to prevent cardiometabolic disease? Int Rev Psychiatry. 2014;26(2):155–76.

162. Irwin MR, Olmstead R, Carroll JE. Sleep disturbance, sleep duration, and inflammation: a systematic review and meta-analysis of cohort studies and experimental sleep deprivation. Biol Psychiatry. 2016;80(1):40–52.

163. Snyder CK, Chang A. Mobile technology, sleep, and circadian disruption. In: Grandner MA, editor. Sleep and health. London: Academic; 2019. p. 159–70.

164. Jones JJ, Kirschen GW, Kancharla S, Hale L. Association between late-night tweeting and next-day game performance among professional basketball players. Sleep Health. 2019;5(1):68–71.

165. Roehrs T, Roth T. Caffeine: sleep and daytime sleepiness. Sleep Med Rev. 2008;12(2):153–62.

166. Ebrahim IO, Shapiro CM, Williams AJ, Fenwick PB. Alcohol and sleep I: effects on normal sleep. Alcohol Clin Exp Res. 2013;37(4):539–49.

167. Perlis ML, Junquist C, Smith MT, Posner D. Cognitive behavioral treatment of insomnia: a session-by-session guide. New York: Springer; 2005.

168. Ficca G, Axelsson J, Mollicone DJ, Muto V, Vitiello MV. Naps, cognition and performance. Sleep Med Rev. 2010;14(4):249–58.

169. Mougin F, Davenne D, Simon-Rigaud ML, Renaud A, Garnier A, Magnin P. Disturbance of sports performance after partial sleep deprivation. C R Seances Soc Biol Fil. 1989;183(5):461–6.

170. Mougin F, Simon-Rigaud ML, Davenne D, Renaud A, Garnier A, Kantelip JP, et al. Effects of sleep disturbances on subsequent physical performance. Eur J Appl Physiol Occup Physiol. 1991;63(2):77–82.

171. Mougin F, Bourdin H, Simon-Rigaud ML, Didier JM, Toubin G, Kantelip JP. Effects of a selective sleep deprivation on subsequent anaerobic performance. Int J Sports Med. 1996;17(2):115–9.

172. Schwartz J, Simon RD Jr. Sleep extension improves serving accuracy: a study with college varsity tennis players. Physiol Behav. 2015;151:541–4.

173. Reyner LA, Horne JA. Sleep restriction and serving accuracy in performance tennis players, and effects of caffeine. Physiol Behav. 2013;120:93–6.

174. Oliver SJ, Costa RJ, Laing SJ, Bilzon JL, Walsh NP. One night of sleep deprivation decreases treadmill endurance performance. Eur J Appl Physiol. 2009;107(2):155–61.

175. Skein M, Duffield R, Edge J, Short MJ, Mundel T. Intermittent-sprint performance and muscle glycogen after 30 h of sleep deprivation. Med Sci Sports Exerc. 2011;43(7):1301–11.

176. Ben Cheikh R, Latiri I, Dogui M, Ben SH. Effects of one-night sleep deprivation on selective attention and isometric force in adolescent karate athletes. J Sports Med Phys Fitness. 2017;57(6):752–9.

177. Cote KA, McCormick CM, Geniole SN, Renn RP, MacAulay SD. Sleep deprivation lowers reactive aggression and testosterone in men. Biol Psychol. 2013;92(2):249–56.

178. Leproult R, Van Cauter E. Effect of 1 week of sleep restriction on testosterone levels in young healthy men. JAMA. 2011;305(21):2173–4.

179. Costill DL, Flynn MG, Kirwan JP, Houmard JA, Mitchell JB, Thomas R, et al. Effects of repeated days of intensified training on muscle glycogen and swimming performance. Med Sci Sports Exerc. 1988;20(3):249–54.

180. Raikes AC, Athey A, Alfonso-Miller P, Killgore WDS, Grandner MA. Author response: concussion assessment tools - a possible measure of sleepiness? Sleep Med. 2020;66:260–1.

181. Raikes AC, Athey A, Alfonso-Miller P, Killgore WDS, Grandner MA. Insomnia and daytime sleepiness: risk factors for sports-related concussion. Sleep Med. 2019;58:66–74.

182. Milewski MD, Skaggs DL, Bishop GA, Pace JL, Ibrahim DA, Wren TA, et al. Chronic lack of sleep is associated with increased sports injuries in adolescent athletes. J Pediatr Orthop. 2014;34(2):129–33.

183. Gupta R, Lahan V. Insomnia associated with depressive disorder: primary, secondary, or mixed? Indian J Psychol Med. 2011;33(2):123–8.

184. Pigeon WR, Pinquart M, Conner K. Meta-analysis of sleep disturbance and suicidal thoughts and behaviors. J Clin Psychiatry. 2012;73(9):e1160–7.

185. Perlis ML, Grandner MA, Brown GK, Basner M, Chakravorty S, Morales KH, et al. Nocturnal wakefulness as a previously unrecognized risk factor for suicide. J Clin Psychiatry. 2016;77(6):726–33.

186. Perlis ML, Grandner MA, Basner M, Chakravorty S, Brown GK, Morales KH, et al. When accounting for wakefulness, completed suicides exhibit an increased likelihood during circadian night. Sleep. 2014;37:268–9.

187. Wills C, Ghani S, Tubbs A, Fernandez FX, Athey A, Turner R, et al. Chronotype and social support among student athletes: impact on depressive symptoms. Chronobiol Int. 2021;2021:1–11.

188. Reardon CL, Hainline B, Aron CM, Baron D, Baum AL, Bindra A, et al. Mental health in elite athletes: International Olympic Committee consensus statement (2019). Br J Sports Med. 2019;53(11):667–99.

189. Sadeh A, Hauri PJ, Kripke DF, Lavie P. The role of actigraphy in the evaluation of sleep disorders. Sleep. 1995;18(4):288–302.

190. Depner CM, Cheng PC, Devine JK, Khosla S, de Zambotti M, Robillard R, et al. Wearable technologies for developing sleep and circadian biomarkers: a summary of workshop discussions. Sleep. 2020;43:2.

191. Athey A, Alfonso-Miller P, Killgore WD, Grandner MA. Preliminary results of a sleep health intervention in student athletes: perceived changes to sleep, performance, and mental and physical well-being. Sleep. 2017;40:450.

192. Alfonso-Miller P, Athey A, Grandner MA. Evaluation of a sleep health intervention in student athletes: Insights for intervention development. Sleep. 2017;40:450.

193. Reardon CL, Hainline B, Aron CM, Baron D, Baum AL, Bindra A, et al. Infographic: mental health in elite athletes. An IOC consensus statement. Br J Sports Med. 2020;54(1):49–50.

Major Depressive Disorder and Depressive Symptoms

Paul Gorczynski

Introduction

In professional sport, the mental health of elite athletes is a major concern [1]. The term *elite athlete* has variably been used to refer to athletes on a continuum of competition, ranging from semi-elite (e.g. highly competitive youth programs, collegiate sport, professional top-level leagues) to world-class elite (e.g. Olympics, world championships, international-level competition) [2]. In recent years, several narrative and systematic reviews and meta-analyses have demonstrated the high rate of prevalence and severity of various mental health symptoms and disorders amongst elite athletes [3–8]. Such epidemiological evidence has also demonstrated the different consequences that mental health symptoms and disorders may have on athletes and sporting organizations [1, 9]. For athletes, consequences can be experienced physically (e.g. decreased performance, increased risk of injury), cognitively (e.g. loss of interest or pleasure), behaviourally (e.g. increased risk of exit from sport, increased risk taking), relationally (e.g. fragmented team dynamics and coaching relationships, tensions with family and friends), and financially (e.g. loss of sponsorship, inability to earn an income) and include a worsened state of mental health (e.g. other mental health symptoms may be exacerbated). For sporting organizations, the unmanaged mental health needs of athletes can result in reputational damage and financial losses with potential legal ramifications where duty of care was neglected. Also in recent years, several position statements on the topic of mental health in elite sport have confirmed the need to address the growing concerns with mental health symptoms and disorders amongst athletes (for a review, see: [10]). Researchers recommended providing assistance with raising awareness about mental health symptoms and disorders; providing on-going and culturally appropriate mental health literacy training; providing and using comprehensive, valid, and reliable strategies to identify and diagnose mental health symptoms and disorders; and creating and using clear care pathways to support athletes so that they may be able to receive treatment in a timely manner. Ultimately, provisions need to be established to help athletes begin a process of recovery. Such provisions are not only needed for current athletes, but also those who have retired or otherwise exited from professional sport [6].

Given its high prevalence and the potential for multifaceted and severe consequences, major depressive disorder is one of the greatest concerns with respect to the mental health of elite athletes. The purpose of this chapter is to provide a review of major depressive disorder and depressive symptoms within the elite sport research literature. Along with information on the epidemiology of depressive symptoms, risk and protective factors will also be examined. Strategies to enhance diagnosis, treatment, management, and recovery, including culturally situated mental health literacy, will also be discussed. The chapter will conclude with suggestions for future research and clinical and organizational intervention.

Major depressive disorder is typically characterized by low or depressed mood, along with a loss of interest or pleasure in most activities and accompanying physical, psychological, and cognitive symptoms over a continuous period of at least 2 weeks [11]. Most symptoms must be present most of the day and on a daily basis for this period of time. Although a diagnosis of major depressive disorder requires the individual to experience at least five symptoms over a 2-week period, of which at least one symptom must be a depressed mood or a loss of interest or pleasure in most activities, individuals may experience depressive symptoms without a major depressive disorder diagnosis. For a diagnosis of major depressive disorder, symptoms must have clearly worsened when compared to the individual's pre-episode condition, and symptoms must have caused significant distress or impairment in social, educational, occupational, or (as extrapolated to elite

P. Gorczynski (✉)
School of Human Sciences, University of Greenwich, London, UK
e-mail: Paul.Gorczynski@greenwich.ac.uk

Table 6.1 Diagnostic criteria for major depressive disorder episode

Diagnostic criteria for major depressive disorder episode [11]
- Five or more of the following symptoms must be present, including at least a low or depressed mood or a loss of interest or pleasure in most activities
- Depressed mood (in children and adolescents, this may be present as an irritable mood)
- Loss of interest or pleasure in most activities
- Significant unintentional weight changes (+/− weight change of >5% per month) or increased or decreased appetite
- Disturbance in sleep (insomnia or hypersomnia)
- Severe psychomotor changes (agitation or retardation)
- Fatigue or loss of energy
- Feelings of worthlessness or excessive or inappropriate guilt
- Difficulties with thinking, concentrating, or making decisions
- Recurring thoughts of death or suicide, or suicide attempts
- Symptoms have caused significant distress or impairment in social, educational, occupational, or sport areas of functioning
- Symptoms have not been related to the physiological effects of a substance or another medical condition
- Manic or hypomanic episodes have never occurred
- Symptoms may not be better described by schizophrenia spectrum or other psychotic disorders

athletes) sport areas of functioning. Additionally, it must be shown that symptoms are not related to the physiological effects of a substance or another medical condition, and are not better described by schizophrenia spectrum or other psychotic disorders. Lastly, manic or hypomanic episodes must have never occurred. Full details of diagnostic criteria for major depressive disorder are listed in Table 6.1.

Epidemiology of Depressive Symptoms

Epidemiological evidence suggests the prevalence of depressive symptoms amongst elite athletes ranges from 4% [12] to 68% [13]. Prevalence ratings of depressive symptoms consistently have been reported to be higher for athletes who identify as female, and ratings are similar to non-athletes in the general population [4, 5]. Comparisons between active and retired athletes have shown that those who have retired have lower rates of prevalence of depressive symptoms [6]. Given most epidemiological studies that examined depressive symptoms within elite sport generally lacked clinical diagnosis and oversight and used a variety of methods to assess depressive symptoms, including different questionnaires with different cut-off values for severity, as well as varying sample sizes of different athletic levels and sports, caution must be taken with any epidemiological results, especially when any direct comparisons between populations are made [4, 5]. Most literature within sport has focused on athletes who have self-reported depressive symptoms, rather than athletes living with diagnoses of major depressive disorder.

Risk Factors for Depressive Symptoms

There are many risk factors that may cause or exacerbate depressive symptoms in elite athletes (for a review, see [14]). Risk factors for depressive symptoms can be mapped along an ecological framework, spanning intrapersonal, interpersonal, and environmental levels [15–21]. The ecological model also allows for a broader understanding of risk factors, including how factors may interconnect, and at times, collectively exacerbate depressive symptom severity. Furthermore, the ecological model also serves as a reminder to explore mental health from a holistic lifespan perspective [22, 23], where an athlete is understood to be multidimensional with both athletic and non-athletic lived experiences.

Intrapersonal-level risk factors include the physical and psychological characteristics of an individual. For example, this would include female sex [13], injury [24], surgery [25], concussion [26], adverse/critical life events [25], greater demonstrated need for psychotherapy [27], osteoarthritis [28], pain [29], age younger than 25 years [30], chronic stress [31], burnout [31], perfectionism [32], competitive anxiety [32], poor sleep [33], negative attribution after failure [34], negative coping strategies [35], negative stress-recovery strategies [35], career dissatisfaction [36], contemplating retirement [30], competitive failure [37], and athletic identity [38]. Some athletes will have a family history or a genetic predisposition to experiencing major depressive disorder or depressive symptoms [1, 39, 40].

Interpersonal-level risk factors include interactions with other individuals, either in sport or outside of sport. This may include family, friends, teammates, coaches, referees/officials, athletic directors, organizational personnel, healthcare professionals, and fans. Evidence of poor, strained, or unsupportive interpersonal relationships has implications for athletes experiencing depressive symptoms. For example, this would include low social support from teammates [41], coach conflict [42], and relationship difficulties within families, such as separation or divorce [42]. Some athletes have also demonstrated that social phobias may increase the risk of depressive symptoms [32].

Environmental-level risk factors are broadly defined and incorporate various aspects of a sporting institution or organization. This would include the physical environments where sport is practiced and played, the sport's cultural practices and norms, and regulatory policies at local, national, and international levels. For example, this would include participating in individual (versus team) sports [30], aesthetic or fine motor sport [12], less match experience [27], position (e.g. forwards, goalies) [42], level of play [42], forced/involuntary retirement [43], and experiencing non-accidental violence [44].

The majority of research in sport concerning risk factors pertaining to depressive symptoms amongst athletes has focused on the individual, specifically situated within the intrapersonal level. To a degree, parts of this body of literature have constructed a form of *life-style theory of disease* narrative within sport [16, 45], where depressive symptoms may be the result of some form of personal occurrence or personal failure. Considerably less research has investigated risk factors at the interpersonal or environmental levels. This lack of research at these two levels means we do not understand well the interaction of multiple risk factors that may cause depressive symptoms. Ultimately, this lack of research limits the types of interventions that may be designed to prevent or eliminate multiple risk factors associated with depressive symptoms. Unfortunately, the *life-style theory of disease* narrative often contributes to perceptions that depressive symptoms may only be addressed by the athlete, rather than by interpersonal or environmental means. This can partially be addressed through exploration of protective factors associated with depressive symptoms.

Protective Factors Against Depressive Symptoms

Protective factors, like risk factors, can be mapped along an ecological framework. Intrapersonal-level protective factors include male sex [13], older age [30], and career satisfaction [36]. Interpersonal-level protective factors have included having social support from significant others and teammates [41], having support from coaches [42], and having supportive family [42]. The establishment of positive therapeutic relationships with mental health practitioners may be associated with fewer depressive symptoms, but further research is needed [46]. Environmental-level protective factors have included participating in team sports [30], employment status [47], and ending one's career on one's own terms [43].

Non-functional Overreaching and Overtraining and Depressive Symptoms

Effective and optimal performance is enhanced through careful training and planned rest or recovery, and this requires attention paid to training load in terms of frequency, intensity, time, and type [48, 49]. An increased training load with insufficient rest or recovery may result in physiological and psychological symptoms that may decrease short- or long-term performance or result in a form of injury [1, 50, 51]. Non-functional overreaching is defined as a short-term decrease in performance and results from an accumulation of increased training load, insufficient rest or recovery, and non-training stressors [51]. Non-training stressors may include environmental factors (e.g. adjustment difficulties to heat, cold, humidity, or altitude), occupational or sport related challenges, poor nutrition, sleep disturbances, general poor health, and interpersonal challenges [51]. Decreased performance may last from several days to several weeks. Overtraining is considered a more severe form of non-functional overreaching, where decreased performance may last longer, spanning from several weeks to several months [51, 52]. Overtraining is also associated with more severe physiological and psychological symptoms than non-functional overreaching. Both non-functional overreaching and overtraining are associated with depressive symptoms, including low or depressed mood, loss of pleasure, loss of motivation, irritability, fatigue, poor concentration, sleep disturbances, changes in weight, and changes in appetite [48, 51–55]. Definitions or diagnostic criteria of non-functional overreaching and overtraining are not standardized, and recommendations for recovery remain limited [51]. Athletes should rest to address non-functional overreaching and overtraining. In certain cases, a reduced training load may be sufficient to alleviate depressive symptoms.

Suicide

Suicide is defined as a death that was caused by an injury to oneself where the intention was to die [56]. In sport, suicide has far reaching consequences and is a tragedy that affects families, friends, teams, sporting organizations, and fans [57]. A better understanding of and treatment options for mental health symptoms and disorders, especially depressive symptoms, is key to preventing suicide. Recurring thoughts of death or suicide, or suicide attempts, are symptoms of major depressive disorder, and research has shown that individuals with major depressive disorder are at a higher risk of suicide ideation, suicide planning, and suicide attempts than those without a diagnosis of major depressive disorder [58].

When compared to non-athletes, athletes are at a lower risk of suicide. For instance, an analysis of suicides amongst National Collegiate Athletic Association (NCAA) collegiate athletes found a rate of suicide of 0.93/100,000 per year [59]. In comparison, in 2019, females aged 15–24 years in the United States had a suicide rate of 5.5/100,000 per year, while males aged 15–24 years had a suicide rate of 22.0/100,000 [60]. Within the sporting environment, there are a number of risk factors for suicide. These factors include: male sex; middle and older age; white race; risk taking behaviours; bullying and hazing; experiencing sexual assault; financial difficulties; injury; concussion; taking performance enhancement drugs; and retirement from sport [57].

With respect to suicide prevention, several steps can help athletes. For instance, strategies can help identify and manage stress, distress, and other mental health symptoms and disorders, like major depressive disorder [61, 62]. Mental health literacy strategies can help raise awareness of risk factors associated with suicide amongst athletes, coaches, support staff who work with athletes, and parents. Social support structures should be built within the lives of athletes and should include support from family and friends, teammates, other athletes, coaches, and other staff [63–65]. Understanding environmental stressors is also key, including setting and establishing expectations within sport, addressing financial concerns, and providing assistance with transition to retirement [57].

Diagnosis and Management

A recent scoping review of depressive symptom assessment tools in sport research revealed that 28 different tools have been used with athletes [66]. Some of the most frequently used tools have included the Beck Depression Inventory (BDI) (all versions, including BDI—Fast Screen, BDI—II, BDI-Short Form) (n = 46 studies) [67], the Center for Epidemiologic Studies Depression Scale (CES-D) (all versions, including CES-D-10 (short version), CES-DC (for children), CESD-R (revised)) (n = 37 studies) [68], and the Patient Health Questionnaire (PHQ) (all versions, PHQ-2 and PHQ-9) (n = 19) [69]. Although each of these tools has been validated, researchers have argued that depressive symptom questionnaires should be validated specifically for athletes. Both the Baron Depression Screener for Athletes [70, 71] and the Stress Response Scale for Athletes - depression scale [72] have been designed specifically for athletes. Currently, the PHQ-9, found within the IOC Sport Mental Health Assessment Tool 1 (SMHAT-1), [73] a standardized assessment tool developed to help identity elite athletes 16 years or older at risk of or already experiencing distress and various mental health symptoms and disorders, has been adapted for use with athletes. The PHQ-9 was chosen for the SMHAT-1 given it is a commonly used depressive symptom questionnaire that has been used in research with elite athletes and has been found to be valid across multiple languages.

Treatment

Psychotherapy

The treatment of major depressive disorder consists of psychotherapy and often includes psychiatric medication [1]. Psychotherapy involves the use of psychological methods, with each method rooted in various therapeutic principles, structures, and techniques, in order to help an individual experience personal growth through the exploration of their own behaviours, needs, beliefs, thoughts, and emotions [1, 74, 75]. Psychotherapy can be essential in helping athletes manage both subclinical and clinical mental health symptoms. Individuals who are qualified to deliver psychotherapy can include psychiatrists, clinical psychologists, social workers, and licenced mental health counsellors [76]. Following evaluation and diagnosis, the athlete and the mental health professional must establish treatment goals [77]. Treatment goals help establish a therapeutic alliance—a collaborative relationship between the athlete and mental health professional—where an agreement on outcomes for treatment is established, a course of action is refined, and commitment to treatment is discussed [77, 78]. Research has suggested that the therapeutic alliance between clients and mental health professionals acts as an important mediator associated with helping reduce symptoms [78].

There are different types of psychotherapy, including individual psychotherapy, couple/family psychotherapy, and group psychotherapy [74, 75]. Individual psychotherapy is delivered in a one-on-one setting between the athlete and mental health professional. Psychotherapy can also be delivered virtually, through Zoom, Skype or other communications software [79]. Cognitive behaviour therapy, delivered in an individual setting, may be appropriate for athletes who are experiencing depressive symptoms. The structure of cognitive behaviour therapy, one rooted in self-directed practice, is similar to athletic training and exercise [80]. Cognitive behaviour therapy explores connections between thoughts, emotions, and behaviours, and is designed to help individuals identify and change their thoughts, beliefs, attitudes, and behaviours in order to improve emotional regulation [81].

Couple/family psychotherapy involves the inclusion of partners, significant others, and family members of athletes in the psychotherapeutic process [74, 75, 82]. Couple/family psychotherapy helps athletes and their significant others better understand how their relationship may be affecting their own and collective mental health. Group psychotherapy for major depressive disorder has been assessed in the general population and shown to be efficacious when compared to untreated controls [83]. Further research is needed in better understanding this modality of treatment for major depressive disorder in athletes.

Psychiatric Medication

With respect to psychiatric medication prescription to athletes, clinicians must consider the side effects of the medication and any physical performance impairments it may cause, any safety concerns (given athletes will train and perform at high intensities of exercise), and any potential performance enhancement properties and whether the medication is on the Prohibited List of the World Anti-Doping Agency (WADA) or other governing body for a particular sport [1, 84–86]. For major depressive disorder, without anxiety or bipolar disorder, sport psychiatrists generally prefer bupropion [85]. Bupropion is a norepinephrine-dopamine-reuptake inhibitor (NDRI) and is commonly used to treat major depressive disorder [87]. Bupropion is considered an energizing medication that is not associated with weight gain and does not impair performance [1, 85, 86]. Bupropion is included in the WADA 2021 Monitoring Program and is not considered a prohibited substance. Currently, further evidence is being collected on its performance enhancement properties [84]. Bupropion should not be prescribed for athletes with eating disorders that involve restricting and/or purging as it may increase the risk of seizures [1, 86, 88]. Other preferred psychiatric medications prescribed for major depressive disorder in athletes include selective serotonin reuptake inhibitors (SSRIs) (e.g. escitalopram, fluoxetine, sertraline) and serotonin-norepinephrine reuptake inhibitors (SNRIs) (e.g. venlafaxine) [1, 85, 86].

Mental Health Literacy

Mental health literacy is a key strategy to better understanding, recognizing, preventing, treating, and managing mental health symptoms and disorders in athletes [89, 90]. Mental health literacy focuses on knowledge, beliefs, and attitudes of mental health and mental health symptoms and disorders that ultimately facilitate symptom recognition, address public- and self-mental health stigma, and help individuals set intentions to seek and maintain support [91]. Mental health literacy incorporates several cognitive and social skills that are used to not only help individuals seek out the support they need, but also help organizations establish key policies that will help prevent and manage mental health symptoms and disorders [90, 92, 93]. Ultimately, mental health literacy can be seen as a form of individual and collective empowerment, whereby individuals advocate for their own mental health and collectively for the mental health of others [94]. Research in mental health literacy in sport has shown that interventions were associated with improved knowledge of mental health symptoms and disorders, increased professional knowledge, reduced stigma, improved referral confidence, and improved intentions to seek support [95–98].

Within elite sport, progressive mental health literacy strategies need to be further established, to raise awareness of mental health symptoms and disorders amongst athletes, help battle stigma, create clear pathways to support, and establish policies to address interpersonal and environmental risk factors of mental health symptoms and disorders. Given the prevalence and consequences of depressive symptoms amongst athletes, mental health literacy strategies need to be focused in this particular area. This requires collective action and coordination amongst various mental health professionals, educators, families, and sport staff; early and on-going pedagogically sound training about mental health, including depressive symptoms; mental health literacy interventions that are culturally and contextually appropriate to the sport; and designing interventions that reduce public and self-mental health stigma [89, 90, 99].

Discussion and Summary

There are several areas that require further research to help mental health researchers and practitioners better understand, prevent, and treat major depressive disorder and depressive symptoms in athletes. This will require focused and rigorous research in the areas of descriptive and analytical epidemiology, diagnosis, treatment and management, and mental health literacy. Strategies should aim to prevent major depressive disorder and find ways to better facilitate recovery and return to play.

Epidemiology is concerned with the study of the distribution, patterns, and determinants of health and illness within clearly defined populations [100]. The key goals of epidemiology are not only to identity the causes of illness but also to prevent and/or treat them in the most effective ways. Epidemiological research must evolve from descriptive epidemiological studies (i.e. understanding the prevalence and incidence of illness) to analytical epidemiology (i.e. understanding the risk factors of illness) [101, 102]. To date, most research that has explored depressive symptoms in athletes has been cross-sectional, based on self-report questionnaires, and heavily reliant on student or collegiate populations [66]. Further research needs to be conducted longitudinally, involve both self-report questionnaires as well as confirmed diagnoses of major depressive disorder, and examine elite athletes from various sports, levels of play, times of season, transitions, ages, and cultures. Further research should also investigate major depressive disorder and depressive symptoms amongst individuals with various definitions of gender, sexualities, socioeconomic classes, races, ethnicities, (dis) abilities, and geographic locations (e.g. low- and middle-income countries) [90, 103]. Furthermore, consistent use of self-report or clinician-administered questionnaires, with expanded and detailed demographic collection forms, is essential to allow comparisons across sports and populations and better understand not only sport-related factors but also broader cultural factors associated with major depressive disorder and depressive symptoms. The creation of the SMHAT-1 will hopefully help facilitate this type of data collection and analysis across cultures [73]. Clear guidelines on improvements to methods of recording and reporting epidemiological data on injury and illness in sport have recently been established by a consensus group organized by the International Olympic Committee (for a review, see: [104]).

With respect to treatment and management of major depressive disorder and depressive symptoms, continued research into both psychotherapy and psychiatric medication is essential. This will involve formulating research programs that rely on confirmed diagnoses of major depressive disorder amongst athletes, as well as examinations of different modalities of treatment with carefully constructed therapeutic alliances against appropriate controls. Additionally, designing and evaluating mental health literacy strategies, which focus on athletes and organizations, will require appropriate design considerations of unique cultural factors, adequate sample sizes, valid and reliable questionnaires, and rigorous evaluations [90]. Strategies will need to be developed to help athletes feel knowledgeable, confident, and comfortable in seeking support [105]. Rigorous randomized controlled studies are needed to facilitate treatment, management, and prevention of mental health symptoms and disorders amongst athletes [106]. Collective action amongst mental health researchers and practitioners, as well as athletes, coaches, staff, and their families, can help drive continual improvements in the prevention and treatment of major depressive disorders and depressive symptoms.

References

1. Reardon CL, Hainline B, Miller Aron C, Baron D, Baum AL, Bindra A, et al. Mental health in elite athletes: International Olympic Committee consensus statement. Br J Sports Med. 2019;53(11):667–99. https://doi.org/10.1136/bjsports-2019-100715.

2. Swann C, Moran A, Piggott D. Defining elite Athletes: issues in the study of expert performance in sport psychology. Psychol Sport Exerc. 2015;16(1):3–14. https://doi.org/10.1016/j.psychsport.2014.07.004.

3. Currie A, Gorczynski P, Rice SM, Purcell R, McAllister-Williams RH, Hitchcock ME, et al. Bipolar and psychotic disorders in elite athletes: a narrative review. Br J Sports Med. 2019;53(12):746–53. https://doi.org/10.1136/bjsports-2019-100685.

4. Golding L, Gillingham RG, Perera NKP. The prevalence of depressive symptoms in high-performance athletes: a systematic review. Phys Sports Med. 2020;48(3):247–58. https://doi.org/10.1080/00913847.2020.1713708.

5. Gorczynski PF, Coyle M, Gibson K. Depressive symptoms in high-performance athletes and non-athletes: a comparative meta-analysis. Br J Sports Med. 2017;51(18):1348–54. https://doi.org/10.1136/bjsports-2016-096455.

6. Gouttebarge V, Castaldelli-Maia JM, Gorczynski P, Hainline B, Hitchcock M, Kerkhoffs GM, et al. Occurrence of mental health symptoms and disorders in current and former elite athletes: a systematic review and meta-analysis. Br J Sports Med. 2019;53(11):700–6. https://doi.org/10.1136/bjsports-2019-100671.

7. Rice SM, Gwyther K, Santesteban-Echarri O, Baron D, Gorczynski P, Gouttebarge V, et al. Determinants of anxiety in elite athletes: a systematic review and meta-analysis. Br J Sports Med. 2019;53(11):722–30. https://doi.org/10.1136/bjsports-2019-100620.

8. Rice SM, Purcell R, De Silva S, Mawren D, McGorry PD, Parker AG. The mental health of elite Athletes: a narrative systematic review. Sports Med. 2016;46(9):1333–53. https://doi.org/10.1007/s40279-016-0492-2.

9. Mountjoy M, Brackenridge C, Arrington M, Blauwet C, Carska-Sheppard A, Fasting K, et al. International Olympic Committee consensus statement: harassment and abuse (non-accidental violence) in sport. Br J Sports Med. 2016;50(17):1019–29. https://doi.org/10.1136/bjsports-2016-096121.

10. Vella S, Sutcliffe J, Swann C, Schweickle M. A systematic review and meta-synthesis of mental health position statements in sport: scope, quality and future directions. Psychol Sport Exerc. 2021;55(4):101946. https://doi.org/10.1016/j.psychsport.2021.101946.

11. American Psychiatric Association. Diagnostic and statistical manual of mental disorders (DSM-5). Washington, DC: American Psychiatric Publishing; 2013.

12. Schaal K, Tafflet M, Nassif H, Thibault V, Pichard C, Alcotte M, et al. Psychological balance in high level athletes: gender-based differences and sport-specific patterns. PLoS One. 2011;6(5):e19007. https://doi.org/10.1371/journal.pone.0019007.

13. Hammond T, Gialloreto C, Kubas H, Hap Davis H. The prevalence of failure-based depression among elite athletes. Clin J Sport Med. 2013;23(4):273–2777. https://doi.org/10.1097/JSM.0b013e318287b870.

14. Kuettel A, Larsen CH. Risk and protective factors for mental health in elite athletes: a scoping review. Int Rev Sport Exerc Psychol. 2020;13(1):231–65. https://doi.org/10.1080/1750984X.2019.1689574.

15. Bronfenbrenner U. Toward an experimental ecology of human development. Am Psychol. 1977;32(7):513–31. https://doi.org/10.1037/0003-066X.32.7.513.

16. McLeroy KR, Bibeau D, Steckler A, Glanz K. An ecological perspective on health promotion programs. Health Educ Q. 1988;15(4):351–77. https://doi.org/10.1177/109019818801500401.

17. McLaren L, Hawe P. Ecological perspectives in health research. J Epidemiol Community Health. 2005;59(1):6–14. https://doi.org/10.1136/jech.2003.018044.

18. Reupert A. A socio-ecological framework for mental health and well-being. Adv Ment Health. 2017;15(2):105–7. https://doi.org/10.1080/18387357.2017.1342902.

19. Schinke RJ, Stambulova NB, Si G, Moore Z. International society of sport psychology position stand: Athletes' mental health, performance, and development. Int J Sport Exerc Psychol. 2018;16(6):622–39. https://doi.org/10.1080/1612197X.2017.1295557.

20. Scarneo-Miller S, Kerr Z, Kroshus E, Register-Mihalik J, Hosokawa Y, Stearns R, et al. The Socioecological framework: a multifaceted approach to preventing sport-related deaths in high school sports. J Athl Train. 2019;54(4):256–360. https://doi.org/10.4085/1062-6050-173-18.

21. Purcell R, Gwyther K, Rice SM. Mental health in elite athletes: increased awareness requires an early intervention framework to respond to athlete needs. Sports Med Open. 2019;5:46. https://doi.org/10.1186/s40798-019-0220-1.

22. Stambulova N, Wylleman P. Athletes' career development and transitions. In: Papaioannou AG, Hackfort D, editors. Routledge companion to sport and exercise psychology: Global perspectives and fundamental concepts. New York: Routledge; 2014. p. 605–20.

23. Wylleman P, Reints A, De Knop P. A developmental and holistic perspective on athletic career development. In: Sotiaradou P,

Bosscher VD, editors. Managing high performance sport (foundations of sport management). New York: Routledge; 2013. p. 159–82.

24. Appaneal RN, Levine BR, Perna FM, Roh JL. Measuring postinjury depression among male and female competitive athletes. J Sport Exerc Psychol. 2009;31(1):60–76. https://doi.org/10.1123/jsep.31.1.60.

25. Schuring N, Kerkhoffs G, Gray J, Gouttebarge V. The mental wellbeing of current and retired professional cricketers: an observational prospective cohort study. Phys Sports Med. 2017;45(4):463–9. https://doi.org/10.1080/00913847.2017.1386069.

26. Du Preez EJ, Graham KS, Gan TY, Moses B, Ball C, Kuah DE. Depression, anxiety, and alcohol use in elite rugby league players over a competitive season. Clin J Sport Med. 2017;27(6):530–5. https://doi.org/10.1097/JSM.0000000000000411.

27. Junge A, Prinz B. Depression and anxiety symptoms in 17 teams of female football players including 10 German first league teams. Brit J Sport Med. 2019;53(8):471–7. https://doi.org/10.1136/bjsports-2017-098033.

28. Schuring N, Aoki H, Gray J, Kerkhoffs GMMJ, Lambert M, Gouttebarge V. Osteoarthritis is associated with symptoms of common mental disorders among former elite athletes. Knee Surg Sports Traumatol Arthrosc. 2017;25(10):3179–85. https://doi.org/10.1007/s00167-016-4255-2.

29. Yang J, Peek-Asa C, Corlette JD, Cheng G, Foster DT, Albright J. Prevalence of and risk factors associated with symptoms of depression in competitive collegiate student athletes. Clin J Sport Med. 2007;17(6):481–7. https://doi.org/10.1097/JSM.0b013e31815aed6b.

30. Beable S, Fulcher M, Lee AC, Hamilton B. SHARPSports mental health awareness research project: prevalence and risk factors of depressive symptoms and life stress in elite athletes. Aust J Sci Med Sport. 2017;20(12):1047–52. https://doi.org/10.1016/j.jsams.2017.04.018.

31. Frank R, Nixdorf I, Beckmann J. Analyzing the relationship between burnout and depression in junior elite athletes. J Clin Sport Psychol. 2017;11(4):287–303. https://doi.org/10.1123/JCSP.2017-0008.

32. Jensen SN, Ivarsson A, Fallby J, Dankers S, Elbe AM. Depression in Danish and Swedish elite football players and its relation to perfectionism and anxiety. Psychol Sport Exerc. 2018;36:147–55. https://doi.org/10.1016/j.psychsport.2018.02.008.

33. Gerber M, Holsboer-Trachsler E, Pühse U, Brand S. Elite sport is not an additional source of distress for adolescents with high stress levels. Percept Mot Skills. 2011;112(2):581–99. https://doi.org/10.2466/02.05.10.PMS.112.2.581-599.

34. Nixdorf I, Frank R, Beckmann J. Comparison of athletes' proneness to depressive symptoms in individual and team sports: research on psychological mediators in junior elite athletes. Front Psychol. 2016;7:893. https://doi.org/10.3389/fpsyg.2016.00893.

35. Nixdorf I, Frank R, Hautzinger M, Beckmann J. Prevalence of depressive symptoms and correlating variables among German elite athletes. J Clin Psychol. 2013;7(4):313–26. https://doi.org/10.1123/jcsp.7.4.313.

36. Foskett RL, Longstaff F. The mental health of elite athletes in the United Kingdom. J Sci Med Sport. 2018;21(8):765–70. https://doi.org/10.1016/j.jsams.2017.11.016.

37. Reardon CL. Psychiatric comorbidities in sports. Neurol Clin. 2017;35(3):537–46. https://doi.org/10.1016/j.ncl.2017.03.007.

38. Sanders G, Stevinson C. Associations between retirement reasons, chronic pain, athletic identity, and depressive symptoms among former professional footballers. Eur J Sport Sci. 2017;17(10):1311–8. https://doi.org/10.1080/17461391.2017.1371795.

39. Sullivan PF, Neale MC, Kendler KS. Genetic epidemiology of major depression: review and meta-analysis. Am J Psychiatr. 2000;157(1):1552–62. https://doi.org/10.1176/appi.ajp.157.10.1552.

40. Bigdeli T, Ripke S, Peterson R, Trzaskowski M, Bacanu S-A, Abdellaoui A, et al. Genetic effects influencing risk for major depressive disorder in China and Europe. Transl Psychiatry. 2017;7:e1074. https://doi.org/10.1038/tp.2016.292.

41. Gouttebarge V, Frings-Dresen MH, Sluiter JK. Mental and psychosocial health among current and former professional footballers. Occup Med. 2015;65(3):190–6. https://doi.org/10.1093/occmed/kqu202.

42. Prinz B, Dvořák J, Junge A. Symptoms and risk factors of depression during and after the football career of elite female players. BMJ Open Sport Exerc Med. 2016;2:e000124. https://doi.org/10.1136/bmjsem-2016-000124.

43. Wippert PM, Wippert J. The effects of involuntary athletic career termination on psychological distress. J Clin Sport Psychol. 2010;4(2):133–49. https://doi.org/10.1123/jcsp.4.2.133.

44. Mountjoy M, Brackenridge C, Arrington M, et al. International Olympic Committee consensus statement: harassment and abuse (non-accidental violence) in sport. Br J Sports Med. 2016;50:1019–29. https://doi.org/10.1136/bjsports-2016-09612.

45. Tesh S. Disease causality and politics. J Health Polit Policy Law. 1981;6(3):369–90. https://doi.org/10.1215/03616878-6-3-369.

46. Doherty S, Hannigan B, Campbell MJ. The experience of depression during the careers of elite male athletes. Front Psychol. 2016;7:1069. https://doi.org/10.3389/fpsyg.2016.01069.

47. Gouttebarge V, Aoki H, Verhagen E, Kerkhoffs G. Are level of education and employment related to symptoms of common mental disorders in current and retired professional footballers? Asian J Sports Med. 2016;7(2):e28447. https://doi.org/10.5812/asjsm.28447.

48. Birrer D. Rowing over the edge: Nonfunctional overreaching and overtraining syndrome as maladjustment-diagnosis and treatment from a psychological perspective. Case Stud Sport Exercise Psychol. 2019;3(1):50–60. https://doi.org/10.1123/cssep.2019-0006.

49. Gabbett TJ. The training-injury prevention paradox: should athletes be training smarter and harder? Br J Sports Med. 2016;50(5):273–80. https://doi.org/10.1136/bjsports-2015-095788.

50. Halson SL, Jeukendrup AE. Does overtraining exist? An analysis of overreaching and overtraining research. Sports Med. 2004;34(14):967–81. https://doi.org/10.2165/00007256-200434140-00003.

51. Meeusen R, Duclos M, Foster C, Fry A, Gleeson M, Nieman D, et al. Prevention, diagnosis, and treatment of the overtraining syndrome: joint consensus statement of the European College of Sport Science and the American College of Sports Medicine. Med Sci Sports Exerc. 2013;45(1):186–205. https://doi.org/10.1249/MSS.0b013e318279a10a.

52. Roy B. Overreaching/overtraining. ACSMs Health Fitness J. 2015;19(2):4–5. https://doi.org/10.1249/FIT.0000000000000100.

53. Armstrong LE, Van Heest JL. The unknown mechanism of the overtraining syndrome—clues from depression and psychoneuroimmunology. Sports Med. 2002;32(3):185–209. https://doi.org/10.2165/00007256-200232030-00003.

54. Kreher JB. Diagnosis and prevention of overtraining syndrome: an opinion on education strategies. J Sports Med. 2016;7:115–22. https://doi.org/10.2147/OAJSM.S91657.

55. Richardson SO, Andersen M, Morris T. Overtraining athletes: personal journeys in sport. Champaign: Human Kinetics; 2008.

56. Centers for Disease Control and Prevention, National Center for Injury Prevention and Control. Facts about suicide. https://www.cdc.gov/suicide/facts/index.html. Accessed November 26, 2021.

57. Rao AL. Athletic suicide. In: Hong E, Rao AL, editors. Mental health in the athlete. London: Springer Nature; 2020. p. 39–56.

58. Cai H, Xie X-M, Zhang Q, Cui X, Lin J-X, Sim K, et al. Prevalence of suicidality in major depressive disorder: a systematic review and meta-analysis of comparative studies. Front Psych. 2021;12:690130. https://doi.org/10.3389/fpsyt.2021.690130.

59. Rao AL, Asif IM, Drezner JA, Toresdahl BG, Harmon KG. Suicide in National Collegiate Athletic Association (NCAA) athletes: a 9-year analysis of the NCAA resolutions database. Sports Health. 2015;7(5):452–7. https://doi.org/10.1177/1941738115587675.

60. National Institute of Mental Health. Suicide. Available from https://www.nimh.nih.gov/health/statistics/suicide#part_2557. Accessed November 26, 2021.

61. Mann JJ, Apter A, Bertolote J, Beautrais A, Currier D, Haas A, et al. Suicide prevention strategies: a systematic review. JAMA. 2005;294(16):2064–74. https://doi.org/10.1001/jama.294.16.2064.

62. Patel V. Talking sensibly about depression. PLoS Med. 2017;14:e1002257. https://doi.org/10.1371/journal.pmed.1002257.

63. Hirsch JK, Barton AL. Positive social support, negative social exchanges, and suicidal behavior in college students. J Am Coll Heal. 2011;59(5):393–8. https://doi.org/10.1080/07448481.2010.515635.

64. Schroeder PJ. Changing team culture: the perspectives of ten successful head coaches. J Sport Behav. 2010;33(1):63–88.

65. Macalli M, Tournier M, Galéra C, Montagni I, Soumare A, Côté SM, et al. Perceived parental support in childhood and adolescence and suicidal ideation in young adults: a cross-sectional analysis of the i-Share study. BMC Psychiatry. 2018;18(1):373. https://doi.org/10.1186/s12888-018-1957-7.

66. Tahtinen RE, Shelley J, Morris R. Gaining perspectives: a scoping review of research assessing depressive symptoms in athletes. Psychol Sport Exerc. 2021;54:101905. https://doi.org/10.1016/j.psychsport.2021.101905.

67. Beck AT, Ward CH, Mendelson M, Mock J, Erbaugh J. An inventory for measuring depression. Arch Gen Psychiatry. 1961;4(6):561–71. https://doi.org/10.1001/archpsyc.1961.01710120031004.

68. Radloff LS. The CES-D scale: a self-report depression scale for research in the general population. Appl Psychol Meas. 1977;1(3):385–401. https://doi.org/10.1177/014662167700100306.

69. Kroenke K, Spitzer RL. The PHQ-9: a new depression diagnostic and severity measure. Psychiatr Ann. 2002;32(9):509–15. https://doi.org/10.3928/0048-5713-20020901-06.

70. Baron DA, Baron SH, Tompkins J, Polat A. Assessing and treating depression in athletes. In: Baron DA, Reardon C, Baron SH, editors. Clinical sports psychiatry: an international perspective. Chichester: Wiley; 2013. p. 65–78.

71. Polat A, Cakir U, Karabulut U, Tural U, Baron D. Reliability and validity of Turkish form of baron depression screener for athletes. Bull Clin Psychopharmacol. 2015;25(1):134.

72. Hagiwara G, Iwatsuki T, Isogai H, Van Raalte JL, Brewer BW. Relationships among sports helplessness, depression, and social support in American College student-athletes. J Phys Educ Sport. 2017;17(2):753–7. https://doi.org/10.7752/jpes.2017.02114.

73. Gouttebarge V, Bindra A, Blauwet C, Campriani N, Currie A, Engebretsen L, et al. International Olympic Committee (IOC) Sport Mental Health Assessment Tool 1 (SMHAT-1) and Sport Mental Health Recognition Tool 1 (SMHRT-1): towards better support of athletes' mental health. Br J Sports Med. 2021;55(1):30–7. https://doi.org/10.1136/bjsports-2020-102411.

74. Stillman MA, Glick ID, McDuff D, Reardon CL, Hitchcock ME, Fitch VM, et al. Psychotherapy for mental health symptoms and disorders in elite athletes: a narrative review. Br J Sports Med. 2019;53(12):767–71. https://doi.org/10.1136/bjsports-2019-100654.

75. Stillman MA, Farmer H. Psychotherapeutic approaches to addressing mental health problems among elite athletes. In: Taiar R, editor. Contemporary advances in sports science. London: IntechOpen Limited; 2021. https://doi.org/10.5772/intechopen.96978.

76. Glick ID, Kamis D, Stull T. The ISSP manual of sports psychiatry. New York: Routledge; 2018.

77. McDuff DR, Garvin M. Working with sports organizations and teams. Int Rev Psychiatry. 2016;28(6):595–605. https://doi.org/10.1080/09540261.2016.1212820.

78. Baier AL, Kline AC, Feeny NC. Therapeutic alliance as a mediator of change: a systematic review and evaluation of research. Clin Psychol Rev. 2020;82:101921. https://doi.org/10.1016/j.cpr.2020.101921.

79. Humer E, Stippl P, Pieh C, Schimböck W, Probst T. Psychotherapy via the internet: what programs do psychotherapists use, how well-informed do they feel, and what are their wishes for continuous education? Int J Environ Res Public Health. 2020;17(21):8182. https://doi.org/10.3390/ijerph17218182.

80. Hays KF. Working it out: using exercise in psychotherapy. Washington: American Psychological Association; 2009.

81. Fenn K, Byrne M. The key principles of cognitive behavioural therapy. InnovAiT. 2013;6(9):579–85. https://doi.org/10.1177/1755738012471029.

82. Stillman MA, Brown T, Ritvo EC, Glick I. Sport psychiatry and psychotherapeutic intervention, circa 2016. Int Rev Psychiatry. 2016;28(6):614–22. https://doi.org/10.1080/09540261.2016.1202812.

83. McDermut W, Miller IW, Brown RA. The efficacy of group psychotherapy for depression: A meta-analysis and review of the empirical research. Clin Psychol. 2006;8(1):98–116. https://doi.org/10.1093/clipsy.8.1.98.

84. World Anti-Doping Agency. List of prohibited substances and methods. 2021. Available from https://www.wada-ama.org/sites/default/files/resources/files/2021list_en.pdf. Accessed November 27, 2021.

85. Reardon CL, Creado S. Psychiatric medication preferences of sports psychiatrists. Phys Sports Med. 2016;44(4):397–402. https://doi.org/10.1080/00913847.2016.1216719.

86. Reardon CL. Managing psychiatric disorders in athletes. In: Hong E, Rao AL, editors. Mental health in the athlete. London: Springer; 2020. p. 57–67.

87. Patel K, Allen S, Haque MN, Angelescu I, Baumeister D, Tracy DK. Bupropion: a systematic review and meta-analysis of effectiveness as an antidepressant. Therap Adv Psychopharm. 2016;6(2):99–144. https://doi.org/10.1177/2045125316629071.

88. Davidson J. Seizures and bupropion: a review. J Clin Psychiatry. 1989;50(7):256–61.

89. Gorczynski P, Gibson K, Thelwell R, Harwood C, Papathomas A, Kinnafick F. The BASES expert statement on mental health literacy in elite sport. Sport Exerc Sci. 2019;59:6–7.

90. Gorczynski P, Currie A, Gibson K, Gouttebarge V, Hainline B, Castaldelli-Maia JM, Mountjoy M, Purcell R, Reardon CL, Rice S, Swartz L. Developing mental health literacy and cultural competence in elite sport. J Appl Sport Psychol. 2021;33(4):387–401. https://doi.org/10.1080/10413200.2020.1720045.

91. Jorm AF, Korten AE, Jacomb PA, Christensen H, Rodgers B, Pollitt P. "Mental health literacy": a survey of the public's ability to recognise mental disorders and their beliefs about the effectiveness of treatment. Med J Aust. 1997;166(4):182–6. https://doi.org/10.5694/j.1326-5377.1997.tb140071.x.

92. Canadian Alliance on Mental Illness and Mental Health (CAMIMH). Mental health literacy in Canada: phase one report mental health literacy project. Ottawa: CAMIMH; 2007.

93. Kutcher S, Wei Y, Coniglio C. Mental health literacy: past, present, and future. Can J Psychiatr. 2016;61(3):154–8. https://doi.org/10.1177/0706743715616609.

94. Jorm AF. Mental health literacy: empowering the community to take action for better mental health. Am Psychol. 2012;67(3):231–43. https://doi.org/10.1037/a0025957.

95. Breslin G, Shannon S, Haughey T, Leavey G. A systematic review of interventions to increase awareness of mental health and well-being in athletes, coaches and officials. Syst Rev. 2017;6:177. https://doi.org/10.1186/s13643-017-0568-6.

96. Chow GM, Bird MD, Gabana NT, Cooper BT, Swanbrow Becker MA. A program to reduce stigma toward mental illness and promote mental health literacy and help-seeking in National Collegiate Athletic Association Division I student-athletes. J Clin Sport Psychol. 2021;15:21.

97. Bu D, Chung PK, Zhang CQ, Liu J, Wang X. Mental health literacy intervention on help-seeking in athletes: a systematic review. Int J Environ Res Public Health. 2020;17(19):7263. https://doi.org/10.3390/ijerph17197263.

98. Oftadeh Moghadam S, Gorczynski P. Mental health literacy, help-seeking, and mental health outcomes in women rugby players. Women Sport Phys Act J. 2021. https://doi.org/10.1123/wspaj.2020-0066

99. McCabe T, Peirce N, Gorczynski P, Heron N. Narrative review of mental illness in cricket with recommendations for mental health support. BMJ Open Sport Exerc Med. 2021;7:e000910. https://doi.org/10.1136/bmjsem-2020-000910.

100. Porta M. A dictionary of epidemiology. 6th ed. New York: Oxford University Press; 2014.

101. Merikangas KR, Nakamura EF, Kessler RC. Epidemiology of mental disorders in children and adolescents. Dialogues Clin Neurosci. 2009;11(1):7–20. https://doi.org/10.31887/DCNS.2009.11.1/krmerikangas.

102. Gorczynski P, Webb T. Developing a mental health research agenda for football refees. Soccer Soc. 2021;22(6):655–62. https://doi.org/10.1080/14660970.2021.1952695.

103. Gorczynski P, Fasoli F. LGBTQ+ focused mental health research strategy in response to COVID19. Lancet Psychiatry. 2020;7(8):E56. https://doi.org/10.1016/S2215-0366(20)30300-X.

104. Bahr R, Clarsen B, Derman W, Dvorak J, Emery CA, Finch CF, et al. International Olympic Committee consensus statement: methods for recording and reporting of epidemiological data on injury and illness in sport 2020 (including STROBE Extension for Sport Injury and Illness Surveillance (STROBE-SIIS)). Br J Sports Med. 2020;54(7):372–89. https://doi.org/10.1136/bjsports-2019-101969.

105. Coyle M, Gorczynski P, Gibson K. "You have to be mental to jump off a board any way": elite divers' conceptualizations and perceptions of mental health. Psychol Sport Exerc. 2017;29:10–8. https://doi.org/10.1016/j.psychsport.2016.11.005.

106. Chang C, Putukian M, Aerni G, Diamond A, Hong G, Ingram Y, et al. Mental health issues and psychological factors in athletes: detection, management, effect on performance and prevention: American Medical Society for Sports Medicine Position Statement-Executive Summary. Br J Sports Med. 2020;54(4):216–20. https://doi.org/10.1136/bjsports-2019-101583.

Anxiety and Related Disorders

7

Rosemary Purcell, Courtney C. Walton,
Claudia L. Reardon, and Simon M. Rice

Introduction

It is common, if not ubiquitous, for elite athletes to experience some degree of anxiety during their competitive careers. Understanding and managing the performative anxiety experienced by athletes has been a focus of sport psychology for decades, but only more recently has enquiry turned to the more *clinical* forms of anxiety, viewed from a mental health perspective. Anxiety disorders are characterized by intense and excessive fear, worry or apprehension, and/or avoidance of real or perceived threats, to an extent that is persistent and debilitating. They are the most commonly reported mental health disorders in the community [1, 2] with an estimated 12-month prevalence ranging between 2.4% and 29.8%, depending on the type of anxiety disorder [3]. Research shows that they are also among the most studied and reported mental health symptoms and disorders in elite athletes [4–7]. This chapter examines the anxiety disorders commonly encountered in elite sport, namely generalized anxiety disorder (GAD), panic disorder and social anxiety disorder, as well as the related conditions of obsessive-compulsive disorder (OCD) and performance anxiety. The risk factors for these symptoms or disorders in elite athletes are examined, along with literature regarding diagnosis and clinical management of these conditions within the context of high-performance sport.

R. Purcell (✉) · C. C. Walton · S. M. Rice
Elite Sport and Mental Health, Orygen, Melbourne, VIC, Australia

Centre for Youth Mental Health, The University of Melbourne, Melbourne, VIC, Australia
e-mail: rosie.purcell@orygen.org.au;
courtney.walton@orygen.org.au; simon.rice@orygen.org.au

C. L. Reardon
Department of Psychiatry, University of Wisconsin School of Medicine and Public Health, Madison, WI, USA
e-mail: clreardon@wisc.edu

Epidemiology of Anxiety Disorders

Anxiety disorders have a significantly earlier age of onset than other high-prevalence mental disorders, with an estimated median onset of 6 years, compared to 13 years for mood/affective disorders and 15 years for substance use disorders [8]. This is important to consider in relation to the duration and persistence of anxiety symptoms that athletes may experience. Within the anxiety disorders, specific phobias and social anxiety tend to emerge earlier than panic disorder and GAD, with the onset of the latter disorders more likely in early to mid-adulthood [9]. Anxiety disorders are differentiated by the types of objects or situations that induce fear or anxiety, along with associated cognitive (e.g., rumination), behavioral (e.g., avoidance), or physiological (e.g., hyperventilation, nausea, fainting) consequences. Anxiety disorders commonly co-occur with other mental health disorders, particularly depression and somatic conditions [10], and sex is a significant risk factor, with females approximately twice as likely to be diagnosed with an anxiety disorder compared to males [3, 11]. The etiology of anxiety disorders is complex, inclusive of a range of biopsychosocial factors such as genetic predisposition, temperament, learning and psychological patterns, personality (such as high neuroticism traits), as well as neurobiological and neuropsychological vulnerabilities [12].

Anxiety Disorders in Elite Athletes

While an appropriate degree of anxiety can facilitate performance by increasing athletes' cognitive and physiological preparedness for action and response [13], anxiety symptoms and disorders have also been shown to have a detrimental impact on sport performance. Anxiety is known to affect various domains pertinent to elite competition, including attention, executive function, muscle tension and information selection, processing, and appraisal [4]. The association between anxiety and *injury* in sport is one of the most established correlates of this form of mental ill-health [14].

The prevalence of anxiety symptoms and disorders in elite athletes, like the general population, varies considerably. In one of the most rigorous and comprehensive studies to date, Schaal and colleagues [15] examined the 12-month and lifetime prevalence of anxiety disorders (via clinical review of psychological consultations) in a large sample of young French elite athletes (mean age = 18.5 years; SD = 4.9 years). The 12-month prevalence of any anxiety disorder was 9%, which is largely consistent with the rates observed in the general population (11–12%; [16], while the lifetime prevalence was 12.1%. Rice and colleagues' [17] subsequent meta-analysis suggested that, broadly defined, anxiety *symptoms* in elite athletes do not differ significantly in terms of their nature and severity from that of the general population (although it should be noted that the comparative prevalence of anxiety *disorders* in elite athletic populations is generally lacking). Consistent with the general population, anxiety symptoms and disorders in athletes commonly co-occur with other forms of mental health symptoms and disorders, particularly depression and eating disorders [18–21], with the latter form of psychopathology disproportionately prevalent among elite athletes [19, 20].

Rice et al.'s systematic review and meta-analysis of determinants of anxiety in elite athletes [17] indicated that female sex, younger age, and the reporting of adverse life events were significantly associated with higher reporting of anxiety symptoms (usually based on self-report measures of generalized anxiety symptoms, including scales assessing mixed depression/anxiety). Sports injury is a specific risk factor for anxiety among athletes, including in the context of fear of re-injury, and isolation and alienation from others (e.g., teammates, coaches) [22]. Evidence regarding the association between *type* of sport and anxiety is inconsistent, including whether individual sports confer a higher risk than team sports [17], which is hypothesized on the basis of individual sport athletes being more likely to internalize failure after loss, set intense personal goals and have less access to social support, among other risk factors [23]. There is some evidence that among specific sports, those which are subjectively judged (including a number of "aesthetic" sports, such as gymnastics or figure skating) correlate with the highest rates of anxiety. It is thought that this may reflect athletes' perceptions of being under pressure to differentiate themselves from the competition in order to excel and win judges' approval [13].

The general and sport-specific risk factors associated with an increased likelihood of reporting anxiety symptoms or disorders should be considered in the context of the complex interplay between the individual athlete and their wider environment. This warrants careful and comprehensive assessment by sports mental health practitioners to determine the optimal management strategies within the high-performance context (see the following section). This includes not only focusing on interventions at the individual-athlete level, but also taking into account the wider "ecology" of sport [24] that may be contributing or perpetuating factors (e.g., team-building exercises that promote "mental toughness" via exposure to risk-taking behaviors, or coaching styles that humiliate or mock). The tendency to "pathologise" the individual athlete, when wider environmental factors may contribute to anxiety symptomatology, is an important pitfall to avoid.

The following sections explore the literature regarding specific anxiety disorders in elite athletes.

Generalized Anxiety Disorder (GAD)

GAD is characterized by excessive anxiety and worry about a range of events or activities, which may be both related and unrelated to sport, that is out of proportion to the actual likelihood or impact of the occurrence. Within elite sport, GAD is the most extensively researched of the anxiety disorders.

The prevalence of GAD among athletes appears to be largely consistent with the general population, ranging from 6.0% based on clinical review/diagnostic criteria [15] to 14.6% using self-report [25]. It should be noted that there is considerable variation in *self-reported* prevalence among athletes, with 1% of Swiss first league players scoring above the threshold for GAD [26] compared to 22% of elite Chinese collegiate athletes [27]. These differences likely reflect measurement issues (e.g., timing of assessments) as well as cohort differences. The key risk factors for all forms of anxiety that are observed in elite athletes are mirrored in relation to GAD, with female sex [38–44], younger age [28], injury [29], and aesthetic sport participation conferring the highest risks [15]. Non-sport-related stressors are also associated with increased GAD symptomatology, including unstable housing, relationship stressors, interpersonal loss, humiliation, and role change/disruption [30].

Social Anxiety Disorder

Social anxiety disorder refers to fear, anxiety, or avoidance of social interactions or situations that involve the perceived possibility of being scrutinized, negatively evaluated, embarrassed, humiliated, or rejected. The lifetime prevalence of social anxiety in young athletes based on clinical review and diagnostic criteria in Schaal et al.'s study [15] was 1.3% (similar across sex), with 0.8% reporting current distress. These rates are lower than studies utilizing self-report thresholds to determine "caseness" (clinically significant symptoms), where 14.7% of participants, irrespective of sex, met criteria [29], which is more consistent with rates in the general population [31].

When considering social anxiety in elite athletes, it is important to assess whether patterns of negative appraisal or fear of social evaluation occur outside of performance contexts, since some degree of fear of negative appraisal or scrutiny by others *within* sport is relatively normative, and more likely to reflect competitive or performative anxiety. Athletes who experience social anxiety disorder may feel heightened anxiety in, and therefore seek to avoid—or tolerate under subjective duress—noncompetitive contexts such as team meetings or group sessions or services (the latter including interactions such as sharing meals, team networking functions, or group rehabilitation). Social anxiety, and its accompanying cognitive distortions that focus on the self, has been shown to negatively impact competitive performance [32].

Panic Disorder

Panic disorder is characterized by panic attacks, which are abrupt, unexpected surges of intense fear or discomfort that are accompanied by physical and/or cognitive symptoms that may or may not occur in relation to specific triggers. Recurrent panic attacks give rise to maladaptive changes in behavior or avoidance due to the fear of further attacks ("anticipatory anxiety"). The lifetime prevalence for panic disorder in elite athletes is estimated at 2.8% (females: 4.4%, males: 1.9%), while the current prevalence ranges from 1.2% [15] to 4.5% [29], the latter based on self-report and largely consistent with the rates in the general population [31]. These two studies constitute the only research on panic disorder in elite sport to date. Like social anxiety, panic disorder should be differentiated from competition/performance anxiety on the basis of the context in which the panic occurs (with elite athletes in some sports describing competition as "controlled panic attacks"). Given an association between vigorous exercise and panic attacks in general (nonsport) clinical samples [33], which likely reflects the physical sensations of tachycardia and breathlessness mimicking panic symptoms, this warrants consideration and clinical enquiry as to whether an athlete's experience of panic is exacerbated during exercise and training.

Obsessive-Compulsive Disorder (OCD)

OCD is characterized by repetitive, intrusive and unwanted thoughts, urges, or images (obsessions) and/or repetitive behaviors or mental acts that the individual feels driven to perform in response to an obsession or according to rules that must be applied rigidly (compulsions). Diagnosis of OCD requires that the obsessions and/or compulsions are time consuming (typically at least 1 h/day) and cause significant distress or impairment in daily functioning [34]. While OCD is now classified by the American Psychiatric Association under Obsessive-Compulsive and Related Disorders, it is included here given the anxiety phenomenology. Only one study to date has examined the rates of OCD in elite collegiate athletes, where 5.2% of the sample met the diagnostic criteria on the basis of self-reported symptoms, but over a third (35%) reported experiencing OCD *symptoms* [35].

It is critical to differentiate OCD from the far more common superstitious rituals or performance routines that athletes often engage in before, during, or after competition [36–38]. Such behaviors (e.g., putting clothing on in a particular order, or entering the field of competition in a specific sequence) are common in sport and do not warrant a diagnosis of OCD in the absence of significant distress and/or functional impairment. However, clinicians should consider the possibility of OCD if rituals and routines are time consuming, or cause the athlete distress if they cannot be performed (e.g., due to time or other constraints) or extend outside of sport [20]. OCD can negatively impact upon sport performance if intrusive thoughts interfere with attention or reaction, or if the athlete is unable to inhibit their symptoms to perform [32].

Competitive Performance Anxiety

Performance anxiety refers to fear than an athlete experiences in the context of their sport participation, especially competition, that they will not be able to perform as hoped or planned or that the situation/competition will be too challenging or even dangerous. Such anxiety is accompanied by cognitive distortions (e.g., "I *can't* deal with this"), behavioral responses, and/or physiological arousal. Key risk factors include female sex, younger age, athlete perceptions of coaching as being controlling (as opposed to autonomy-supporting [39]), and engagement with social media preceding or even during competition [40].

Distinguishing between normal hyperarousal associated with competition, clinical anxiety disorders (e.g., panic disorder) and competitive performance anxiety can be challenging for sports mental health practitioners. Reardon and colleagues [6] described various symptom characteristics—such as onset, duration, and severity—that can be used to differentiate these three possibilities (Table 7.1). Given that performance anxiety can overlap with specific anxiety disorders (such as GAD or panic disorder), a comprehensive evaluation is required to determine the appropriate diagnosis and corresponding clinical management.

Table 7.1 Distinguishing normal competition-induced hyperarousal, competitive performance anxiety, and specific anxiety disorders

	Normal competition-induced hyperarousal	Competitive performance anxiety	Anxiety disorder (e.g., GAD)
Pattern of symptom onset	Mild hyperarousal symptoms (e.g., feeling mildly nervous) typically starting during the day before/of or during sport performance	Hyperarousal symptoms starting any time before or during sport performance	Anxiety symptoms present most days irrespective of performance times (though symptoms might become even worse before/during performance). In GAD, symptoms have been present at least 6 months
Source of worry	Performance in sport	Performance in sport	Worries that are often multiple (in the case of GAD) and that are not solely sport-related
Duration	Typically, <24 h	Variable; can be up to a week or more before performances	Ongoing
Severity	No negative impact on functioning or significant distress, and arousal to a certain degree may optimize performance according to the "inverted-U" hypothesis	Detrimental impact on sport performance and/or significant distress	Detrimental impact on life functioning outside of (and sometimes within) sport and/or significant distress

This modified table is reproduced with permission from Reardon et al. [6]

The experience of competitive performance anxiety can cause significant distress and functional impairment for athletes and should not be regarded as a "common feature" of elite sport. It can lead to acute or prolonged performance difficulties that may be accompanied by significant (and harmful) public scrutiny or self-criticism, which themselves could give rise to impaired mental well-being.

Assessment of Anxiety Symptoms and Disorders in Elite Athletes

Ideally, sports mental health practitioners that work with elite athletes will operate within comprehensive mental health frameworks or systems that both *promote* athlete mental health and well-being and emphasize *early intervention* for athletes who are at risk of developing, or already experiencing mental health symptoms or disorders [24]. Early detection of mental health symptoms is critical, but to date,

there are no validated athlete-specific anxiety screening tools to aid in this regard. The International Olympic Committee's Sports Mental Health Assessment Tool 1 (SMHAT-1; 41) includes a range of screening tools to assess psychopathology, including the GAD-7 [42] for general anxiety symptoms. Other measures such as the Beck Anxiety Inventory [43] are suitable for screening for panic symptoms, or the Yale-Brown Obsessive Compulsive Scale [44] for symptoms of OCD. The Sport Anxiety Scale-2 has been developed specifically to screen for competitive performance anxiety [45]. For a more structured clinical (as opposed to self-report) assessment of anxiety disorders, the Anxiety and Related Disorders Interview Schedule for DSM-5 (ADIS-5; Adult Version; [46]) is a comprehensive tool that can guide assessment, including comorbidities and the impacts of anxiety on functional impairment. Finally, in any comprehensive assessment of anxiety in elite athletes, sports mental health practitioners should consider potential medical conditions that may contribute to or mimic the physiological symptoms of anxiety, such as asthma (breathlessness), thyroid dysfunction (fatigue, palpitations), or excessive caffeine intake (tachycardia) among others [6].

Clinical Management of Anxiety in Elite Athletes

When considering the most appropriate treatments or interventions for anxiety disorders in elite athletes, sport-specific contextual factors must be taken into account. For example, medications and their side effects may impair performance or athlete safety [47] making it prudent to consider other treatments such as psychotherapies as first-line treatments where clinically indicated. Mental health professionals working in elite sport also have a role to play in advocating for preventative or "environmental" interventions that may contribute to the risk of anxiety, such as efficient and effective processes to manage harassment or abuse of athletes [48].

Psychotherapy is recommended as the first-line treatment for mild to moderate anxiety symptoms and disorders both in the general population and in athletes [7, 49]. The efficacy of various cognitive behavioral therapy (CBT) techniques for anxiety disorders—such as cognitive restructuring for GAD, guided exposure for panic disorder, and response prevention for OCD—are well established in the general population, and such evidence-based approaches should be utilized with athletes, despite a lack of controlled trials in this population. There is emerging evidence of the effectiveness of CBT for general mental health symptoms (e.g., depression and anxiety) in elite athletic cohorts [50], and CBT may be more acceptable to elite athletes than the general population, given athletes' familiarity with self-monitoring (e.g., biofeedback) and "homework" (e.g., memorizing strategies or plays). "Third wave" CBT approaches such as mindfulness-based therapies also show promise in elite athletes [51], particularly in relation to stress management and other anxiety-related symptoms, as does acceptance and commitment therapy (ACT) [52]. Compassion-focused interventions are also gaining attention in high-performance contexts such as elite sport [53, 54], given the emphasis with this approach of addressing high levels of self-attacking cognitions or shame, which can often accompany loss, rejection, or unfulfilled expectations.

Beyond specific therapies or interventions, psychological factors that can aid both high-performance and anxiety symptom management can also be a focus of treatment, such as emotion regulation, adaptive coping strategies (including overcoming phobic avoidance behavior), and relaxation techniques (such as breathing retraining) [6].

Pharmacotherapies, either as stand-alone treatment or adjunctive to CBT approaches, should be considered for athletes with moderate to severe anxiety disorders (and/or those for whom cognitive approaches are not suitable or have not been effective). Antidepressant medications, specifically the selective serotonin reuptake inhibitors fluoxetine, escitalopram, and sertraline, are preferred for this cohort [47] given their efficacy and side effect profiles (although only fluoxetine has been studied in elite athletic samples). While tricyclic antidepressants are sometimes used for anxiety disorders (such as OCD) in the general population, there is little literature on their use in athletes, and their side effects make this class of antidepressant likely to be unsuitable for many athletes, and one to be considered with caution [6]. Benzodiazepines are associated with significant side effects that may impair athletic performance [55] and come with the risk of dependence.

Medications are not indicated for managing competitive performance anxiety [7], and agents such as the beta-blocker propranolol are prohibited by the World Anti-Doping Agency for athletes in specific sports (both in and out of competition depending on the sport [6]). CBT and related therapies are recommended for equipping athletes with the self-management skills to effectively cope with competition anxiety. The use of nonregulated "supplements" to manage anxiety (and/or aid performance) in elite athletes is an area of significant concern, and mental health professionals should assist athletes (and high-performance support staff/teams) to understand the risks that such substances may pose to their health, as well as their careers. Supplements may contain prohibited substances [6] and/or substances with unknown long-term side effects.

Finally, a key ingredient in the management of anxiety symptoms and disorders in elite athletes is the treating clinician's skills and experience. Elite athletes typically engage best with clinicians who have an understanding of the culture and demands of elite sport, and who can connect with the athletes' needs to manage their anxiety in the context of their sporting career. This includes being mindful of the non-sport-related factors that may be precipitating or sustaining anxiety symptoms or disorders. Developing a shared understanding of the athlete's anxiety (including the role of potential "ecological" or environmental factors) as well as shared treatment goals that can be measured, monitored, and revised are critical factors for the therapeutic alliance with the elite athlete, as the general client.

Conclusion

Elite athletes may experience a range of anxiety symptoms and disorders that, left untreated, could impact their mental well-being, psychosocial functioning, and sporting performance. Anxiety disorders often have an early age of onset and chronic course of illness, making them among the more intractable forms of mental illness. While anxiety is ubiquitous in elite sport, it should not be regarded as "part of" high-performance sport to be tolerated or endured. Instead, anxiety symptoms should be identified and managed as early as possible to enable the provision of evidence-based treatment to alleviate athletes of this form of distress.

References

1. Slade T, Johnston A, Oakley Browne MA, Andrews G, Whiteford H. 2007 national survey of mental health and wellbeing: methods and key findings. Aust N Z J Psychiatry. 2009;43(7):594–605.
2. Kessler RC, Chiu WT, Demler O, Walters EE. Prevalence, severity, and comorbidity of 12-month DSM-IV disorders in the National Comorbidity Survey Replication. Arch Gen Psychiatry. 2005;62(6):617–27.
3. Baxter AJ, Scott KM, Vos T, Whiteford HA. Global prevalence of anxiety disorders: a systematic review and meta-regression. Psychol Med. 2013;43(5):897.
4. Rice SM, Gwyther K, Santesteban-Echarri O, et al. Determinants of anxiety in elite athletes: a systematic review and meta-analysis. Br J Sports Med. 2019;53(11):722–30.
5. Rice SM, Purcell R, De Silva S, et al. The mental health of elite athletes: a narrative systematic review. Sports Med. 2016;46(9):1333–53.
6. Reardon CL, Gorczynski P, Hainline B, et al. Anxiety disorders in athletes: a clinical review. Adv Psychiatry Behav Health. 2021;1:149–60.
7. Reardon CL, Hainline B, Aron CM, et al. Mental health in elite athletes: International Olympic Committee consensus statement. Br J Sports Med. 2019;53(11):667–99. https://doi.org/10.1136/bjsports-2019-100715.
8. Merikangas KR, He J, Burstein M, et al. Lifetime prevalence of mental disorders in US adolescents: results from the National Comorbidity Study-Adolescent Supplement (NCS-A). J Am Acad Child Adolesc Psychiatry. 2010;49(10):980–9.
9. Lijster JM, Dierckx B, Utens EM, et al. The age of onset of anxiety disorders. Can J Psychiatr. 2017;62(4):237–46.

10. Penninx BW, Pine DS, Holmes EA, Reif A. Anxiety disorders. Lancet. 2021;397:914–27.

11. Remes O, Brayne C, Van Der Linde R, Lafortune L. A systematic review of reviews on the prevalence of anxiety disorders in adult populations. Brain Behav. 2016;6(7):e00497.

12. Craske MG, Stein MB, Eley TC, et al. Anxiety disorders. Nat Rev Dis Primers. 2017;4(3):17024.

13. Mellalieu SD, Hanton S, Fletcher D. A competitive anxiety review: recent directions in sport psychology research. Lit Rev Sport Psychol. 2006;2006:1–45.

14. Ford JL, Ildefonso K, Jones ML, Arvinen-Barrow M. Sport-related anxiety: current insights. Open Access J Sports Med. 2017;8:205–12.

15. Schaal K, Tafflet M, Nassif H, et al. Psychological balance in high level athletes: gender-based differences and sport-specific patterns. PLoS One. 2011;6:e19007.

16. Somers JM, Goldner EM, Waraich P, et al. Prevalence and incidence studies of anxiety disorders: a systematic review of the literature. Can J Psychiatr. 2006;51:100–13.

17. Rice SM, Gwyther K, Santestebanecha O, et al. Determinants of anxiety in elite athletes: a systematic review and meta-analysis. Br J Sports Med. 2019;53:722–30.

18. Gouttebarge V, Aoki H, Verhagen EA, et al. A 12-month prospective cohort study of symptoms of common mental disorders among European professional footballers. Clin J Sport Med. 2017;27:487–92.

19. Hulley AJ, Hill AJ. Eating disorders and health in elite women distance runners. Int J Eat Disord. 2001;30:312–7.

20. Reardon CL. Psychiatric comorbidities in sports. Neurol Clin. 2017;35:537–46.

21. Junge A, Prinz B. Depression and anxiety symptoms in 17 teams of female football players including 10 German first league teams. Br J Sports Med. 2019;53:471–7.

22. Forsdyke D, Smith A, Jones M, Gledhill A. Psychosocial factors associated with outcomes of sports injury rehabilitation in competitive athletes: a mixed studies systematic review. Br J Sports Med. 2016;50(9):537. https://doi.org/10.1136/bjsports-2015-094850.

23. Nixdorf I, Frank R, Beckmann J. Comparison of athletes' proneness to depressive symptoms in individual and team sports: research on psychological mediators in junior elite athletes. Front Psychol. 2016;7:893.

24. Purcell R, Gwyther K, Rice SR. Mental health in elite athletes: Increased awareness requires an early intervention framework to respond to athlete needs. Sports Med Open. 2019;5(1):46–54.

25. Du Preez EJ, Graham KS, Gan TY, Moses B, Ball C, Kuah DE. Depression, anxiety, and alcohol use in elite rugby league players over a competitive season. Clin J Sport Med. 2017;27(6):530.

26. Junge A, Feddermann-Demont N. Prevalence of depression and anxiety in top-level male and female football players. BMJ Open Sport Exerc Med. 2016;19:e000087.

27. Li C, Fan R, Sun J, Li G. Risk and protective factors of generalized anxiety disorder of elite collegiate athletes: a cross-sectional study. Front Public Health. 2021;9:607800.

28. Akesdotter C, Kentta G, Eloranta S, Franck J. The prevalence of mental health problems in elite athletes. Aust J Sci Med Sport. 2020;23(4):329–35.

29. Gulliver A, Griffiths KM, Mackinnon A, Batterham PJ, Stanimirovic R. The mental health of Australian elite athletes. Aust J Sci Med Sport. 2015;18(3):255–61.

30. McLoughlin E, Fletcher D, Slavich GM, Arnold R, Moore LJ. Cumulative lifetime stress exposure, depression, anxiety, and well-being in elite athletes: a mixed-method study. Psychol Sport Exerc. 2020;52:101823.

31. Bandelow B, Michaelis S. Epidemiology of anxiety disorders in the 21st century. Dialogues Clin Neurosci. 2015;17:327–35.

32. Chang CJ, Putukian M, Aerni G, et al. Mental health issues and psychological factors in athletes: detection, management, effect on performance, and prevention: American Medical Society for Sports Medicine Position Statement. Clin J Sport Med. 2020;30(2):e61–87.

33. Cameron OG, Hudson CJ. Influence of exercise on anxiety level in patients with anxiety disorders. Psychosomatics. 1986;27:720–3.

34. American Psychiatric Association. Diagnostic and statistical manual of mental disorders. 5th ed. Arlington: APA; 2013.

35. Cromer L, Kaier E, Davis J, Stunk K, Stewart SE. OCD in college athletes. Am J Psychiatr. 2017;174(6):595–7.

36. Bleak JL, Frederick CM. Superstitious behavior in sport: levels of effectiveness and determinants of use in three collegiate sports. J Sport Behav. 1998;21:1–15.

37. Dömötör Z, Ruíz-Barquín R, Szabo A. Superstitious behavior in sport: a literature review. Scand J Psychol. 2016;57:368–82.

38. Rupprecht AG, Tran US, Gröpel P. The effectiveness of pre-performance routines in sports: a meta-analysis. Int Rev Sport Exerc Psychol. 2021;2021:1–26.

39. Cho S, Choi H, Youngsook K. The relationship between perceived coaching behaviors, competitive trait anxiety, and athlete burnout: a cross-sectional study. Int J Environ Res Public Health. 2019;16(8):1424.

40. Encel K, Mesagno C, Brown H. Facebook use and its relationship with sport anxiety. J Sports Sci. 2017;35(8):756–61.

41. Gouttebarge V, Bindra A, Blauwet C, et al. International Olympic Committee (IOC) sport mental health assessment tool 1 (SMHAT-1) and sport mental health recognition tool 1 (SMHRT-1): towards better support of athletes' mental health. Br J Sports Med. 2020;55:30–7.

42. Spitzer RL, Kroenke K, Williams JBW, et al. A brief measure for assessing generalized anxiety disorder: The GAD-7. Arch Intern Med. 2006;166:1092–7.

43. Beck AT, Steer RA. Beck anxiety inventory manual. San Antonio: Psychological Corporation; 1993.

44. Goodman WK, Price LH, Rasmussen SA, et al. The yale-brown obsessive compulsive scale: I. Development, use, and reliability. Arch Gen Psychiatry. 1989;46(11):1006–11.

45. Smith RE, Smoll FL, Cumming SP, et al. Measurement of multidimensional sport performance anxiety in children and adults: the sport anxiety scale-2. J Sport Exerc Psychol. 2006;28(4):479–501.

46. Brown TA, Barlow DH. Anxiety and related disorders interview schedule for DSM-5 (ADIS-5). Oxford: Oxford University Press; 2014.

47. Reardon CL, Factor RM. Sport psychiatry: a systematic review of diagnosis and medical treatment of mental illness in athletes. Sports Med. 2010;40:961–80.

48. Mountjoy M, Brackenridge C, Arrington M, et al. International Olympic Committee consensus statement: harassment and abuse (non-accidental violence) in sport. Br J Sports Med. 2016;50(17):1019.

49. Stillman MA, Glick ID, McDuff D, et al. Psychotherapy for mental health symptoms and disorders in elite athletes: a narrative review. Br J Sports Med. 2019;53(12):767–71.

50. Purcell R, Chevroulet C, Pilkington V, Rice S. What works for mental health in sporting teams? An evidence guide for best practice in mental health promotion and early intervention. Melbourne: Orygen; 2020.

51. Moreton A, Wahesh E, Schmidt CD. Indirect effect of mindfulness on psychological distress via sleep hygiene in division I college student athletes. J Am Coll Heal. 2020;2020:1–5.

52. Henriksen K, Hansen J, Larsen CH. Mindfulness and acceptance in sport: How to help athletes perform and thrive under pressure. London: Routledge; 2019.

53. Mosewich AD, Ferguson LJ, McHugh T-LF, Kowalski KC. Enhancing capacity: integrating self-compassion in sport. J Sport Psychol Action. 2019;10(4):235–43.

54. Walton CC, Baranoff J, Gilbert P, Kirby J. Self-compassion, social rank, and psychological distress in athletes of varying competitive levels. Psychol Sport Exerc. 2020;50:101733.

55. Johnston A, McAllister-Williams RH. Psychotropic drug prescribing. In: Currie A, Owen B, editors. Sports psychiatry. Oxford: Oxford University Press; 2016. p. 133–43.

Post-traumatic Stress Disorder and Other Trauma-Related Disorders

Cindy Miller Aron and Sydney Marie LeFay

Introduction

Given particular risk factors, elite athletes may experience trauma-related disorders at a higher rate than the typical population. A distinguishing risk factor from the general population is the likelihood of orthopedic injury and concussion. Institutional abuses and lifetime traumas (childhood trauma, sexual assault, and other all-cause trauma) add to the likelihood of the development of trauma-related disorders in athletes [1]. Trauma-related disorders may manifest differently or appear "masked" for the sport population compared to the general population by virtue of adaptive coping strategies and physiologic adaptations endemic to sport [1]. Underappreciation of trauma-related disorders in athletes may lead to significant impairment in social, occupational, and sport function, as well as long-term mental health consequences of chronic disorders including post-traumatic stress disorder (PTSD) [2–4]. The extent of trauma-related disorders in athletes is still a growing field of research, with efforts being made to develop athlete-specific screening tools and algorithms for intervention on both individual and institutional levels [1, 5, 6]. This chapter seeks to expand on the neurobiological underpinnings of trauma and its relationship with the psychological and physiological adaptations of athletes, describe coping schemes that may "mask" trauma-related symptoms, and explore methods to identify and intervene for the benefit of athletes who may be suffering from trauma-related disorders.

Understanding Trauma

Athletes can experience trauma in a variety of ways. It may occur prior to sport participation, as a result of sport, and outside of sport during their sport careers [1]. There is speculation that transition from sport for some can be experienced traumatically. Trauma can occur for a multiplicity of reasons: a catastrophic event such as injury, persistent verbal, physical, and/or sexual abuse within or outside of sport, cultural marginalization, racialized trauma, transgenerational trauma, and many others.

To better make sense of trauma-related presentations, whether somatic, performance breakdowns, inconsistent play, behavior problems, and/or mood dysregulation, it is useful to understand the neurobiological underpinnings.

Trauma and the Brain

Trauma is not well understood. It has a jolting impact on the brain, activating our brain stem into survival mode. This transpires within a split second; stress hormones are secreted to defend against the threat. Bessel Van der Kolk [7] describes this process as the primary job of the brain: ensuring survival, everything else being secondary. The nature of traumatic memory is that it is "fixed and static," unlike other memories, which are "mutable and dynamically changing over time" [8]. Unmanaged trauma can lead individuals to easily become overwhelmed when triggered.

Bruce Perry's "Tree of Regulation [9]" outlines what happens when sensory information "triggers" the athlete. In order for that sensory information to reach the rational part of our brain (cortex), it must travel through the diencephalon, which filters the sensory information, sending it on to other parts of the brain. The limbic system, which is responsible for the behavioral and emotional responses, includes the amygdala, which attaches emotions to memories. This process determines how robustly these memories are stored. Fearful memories tend to "stick" and can be formed after

C. M. Aron
Clinical Services, Ascend, Consultation in Health Care, LLC, Chicago, IL, USA

S. M. LeFay (✉)
Department of Psychiatry, Samaritan Health Services, Corvallis, OR, USA

only a small number of repetitions. Our bodies are designed to remember danger. By the time the sensory information that was first processed by the brain stem reaches the rational part of our brain, our system is already put into action, as if there is an "enemy to fight." In individuals exposed to extreme or prolonged distress (e.g., physical, emotional, sexual abuse) or unpredictable and uncontrollable stress (e.g., poverty, environmental trauma, racialized trauma, transgenerational trauma), the response systems can become "sensitized," meaning the individuals' baseline state is overactive, which sets the stage for an overly anxious (and/or inappropriate) reaction to a simple request or task. Additionally, with less "cortex" available, the athlete's ability to learn can be diminished [9].

The athlete keeps trying to manage these unbearable sensations, perpetuating the body's natural responses. Stress hormones are secreted to protect the individual from the imagined "enemy." The athlete is often confused by the performance, somatic, and/or behavioral issues that transpire, as a result of being controlled by this, essentially, unconscious biological process.

It is advantageous for sports medicine team members to look at an athlete's presentation through a trauma-informed lens. Once trauma is properly diagnosed, treatment needs to maximize the power of neurobiological healing. A variety of therapeutic approaches can increase the athlete's "window of tolerance" [10] for the discomfort they are experiencing. This process develops tools for managing arousal when it transpires, as well as positions the brain to develop new neural pathways. Relationships are placed at the center of understanding trauma.

Polyvagal Theory helps practitioners appreciate the centrality of relationships, especially when a traumatic event has occurred. Polyvagal Theory helps us value the biology of safety and danger [11, 12]. A soothing voice from an important person can have a dramatic effect upon the traumatized individual, interrupting their sense of aloneness [12]. The co-regulation that can transpire, creating a "felt sense" of safety in the present moment, is foundation to the curative process. Being dismissed, ignored, or having an experience trivialized has the potential to incite rage and/or emotional collapse. Polyvagal Theory supports the notion of relationships being front and center to healing [13].

Humans are highly attuned to subtle facial and/or body movements and tone of voice, all in the service of environmental assurance or threat [13]. A traumatized individual will scan the environment for safety with a rigor that a non-traumatized person will not automatically use. The more actively the athletic team or department or sports medicine team works to create a relationship-driven culture, the more the stage is set to mitigate traumatic experiences, whether past, present, or in the future. Supportive social systems are protective, as well as necessary for recovery. This is consis-tent with the encouragement within the International Olympic Committee (IOC) Consensus Statement on Mental Health in Elite Athletes for the creation of environments that support athlete resilience and well-being, with particular emphasis on the coaches who are often central interpersonal figures in an athlete's life [14].

Diagnosis

Trauma references can be found descriptively for thousands of years, yet trauma only became the core component of a recognized psychiatric diagnosis in 1980. At that time, it was categorized under anxiety disorders. In 2013, trauma was given its own Diagnostic and Statistical Manual of Mental Disorders 5th edition (DSM-5) [15] category, "Trauma- and Stressor-Related Disorders." Understanding the diagnosis of PTSD requires the conceptual differentiation between exposure to trauma and the psychological response to it [16]. Athletes may not meet full criteria for a diagnosis of PTSD but may struggle with many of the affective and regulatory symptoms.

The diagnosis of PTSD and other trauma-related disorders in athletes can be distinctly complicated compared to other populations. It is key to look at acute and persistent symptoms, both mental and other physical symptoms, through the PTSD frame of reference that includes individual developmental factors, family systems factors, and a diagnosis based upon the DSM-5 [1]. Investigating presenting symptoms through a "developmentally informed/trauma lens" [17] can increase the potential for diagnostic accuracy, which then can inform treatment approaches.

The DSM-5 requires assessment of several categories of trauma-related symptoms for establishment of a trauma-related disorder diagnosis: intrusion, negative mood/cognitions, dissociative symptoms, alterations in arousal/reactivity, and avoidance [15]. A diagnosis of PTSD requires the presence of a traumatic stressor, at least one intrusion symptom, at least one avoidance symptom, two or more negative alterations in cognition or mood, and alteration in arousal and reactivity, with functionally impairing symptoms present for more than 1 month [15]. Acute stress disorder may be diagnosed if symptoms are present less than 1 month and may or may not progress to a diagnosis of PTSD [5].

Athletes may come to the attention of teams or medical professionals with behaviors resulting from trauma, which may not be immediately obvious as a mental health disorder; some concerns may include increased and unusual somatic complaints, persistent physical complaints beyond the expected recovery for an injury, avoidance of sport or events reminding the athlete of past trauma, increased interpersonal conflict, or sudden diminished/inconsistent performance [11, 18].

Athletes whose trauma-related disorders go unrecognized may suffer negative outcomes specific to sport. Trauma-related disorders resulting from injury may result in decreased participation in physical rehabilitation, avoidance of training with full intensity, and physiologically reduced immune function and healing [19, 20]. Athletes who are suffering from trauma-related symptoms may struggle with affective regulation, concentration/focus, and reactivity, negatively affecting their participation on the team [1]. Athletes suffering from these symptoms may be interpreted by teams and coaches as apathetic, "lazy," irritable, or unreliable. Additionally, studies have shown that people in racial minority groups are less likely to be identified with trauma-related symptoms for a variety of reasons [11]. For example PTSD appears to be more common in the African American population in the United States, yet this group is less likely to be diagnosed with the disorder [11, 21]. Cross-cultural assessments bear strong consideration, paying particular attention to the "idioms of distress" (culturally influenced methods of coping, describing, and displaying distress), which may differ from the culture of the clinician doing the assessment [11]. Early diagnosis of trauma-related disorders opens the opportunity for interventions that may mitigate morbidity, including the progression from acute stress disorder to more chronic trauma-related disorders [1]. Institutional interventions, including trauma-informed debriefing, clear pathways to access mental health support, and a nonjudgmental environment can improve treatment outcomes; conversely, institutional cultures that are passive or dismissive of trauma, blaming of those experiencing symptoms, or that actively attempt to cover up trauma, may worsen treatment outcomes [2–4].

Several screening tools have been developed to more easily identify patients with a likely diagnosis of PTSD, including the Primary Care PTSD Screen for DSM-5 (PC-PTSD-5), Trauma Screening Questionnaire (TSQ), Startle, Physically upset by reminders, Anger, and Numbness (SPAN), and the Short Post-Traumatic Stress Disorder Rating Interview (SPRINT) [11]. These screening tools were developed for general use and are often utilized in primary care clinics. Work has been done to create sport-specific screening tools due to the unique complicating factors of identifying mental health disorders in athletes.

The IOC Mental Health in Elite Athletes Toolkit is a document that provides a framework for addressing the overall mental health of athletes, including exploring the appropriate roles for members of the athlete's health care team, and highlighting common mental health symptoms and disorders that may indicate a need for further intervention [6]. This toolkit is meant to create a jumping off point for individuals supporting athletes and their institutions to create environments that holistically support the health of athletes. Athlete-specific screening tools for mental health disorders have also been developed through the International Olympic Committee [6]. The Sport Mental Health Assessment Tool 1 (SMHAT-1) and the Sport Mental Health Recognition Tool 1 (SMHRT-1) create a framework to assist in the early identification of mental health disorders in elite athletes [5]. The SMHAT-1 is intended for use by licensed health professionals [5]. It includes broad screening for mental health conditions with athlete-specific questions, screening tools specific for major mental health disorders (generalized anxiety disorder, major depressive disorder, alcohol use disorder, sleep disorders, and eating disorders), and a structured clinical assessment format. This assessment is best carried out in the pre-competition period and followed up during the mid- and end-season periods; it can also be repeated following a significant illness, injury, change in performance, or other events of concern that may affect the athlete's mental health. Individuals who are not licensed health professionals (including friends, family, coaches, etc.) can use the SMHRT-1 as a tool to help identify athletes who may be suffering from mental health symptoms or disorders, and if positive, should be followed up with a formal evaluation by a licensed health professional [5].

It should be noted that screening for trauma-related disorders may be necessary for those who have witnessed trauma or experienced "vicarious trauma." Studies of vicarious trauma within sport teams have shown that witnessed trauma may lead to experiences of fear, horror, helplessness, re-experiencing, numbing, and impaired function, as well as the potential for "injury contagion" wherein the injury of one teammate leads to additional injuries in other teammates beyond expected levels [3, 22]. Team-based interventions including skilled debriefings may be an important intervention to address this aspect of trauma-informed care [11].

Clinical Practice Considerations

Establishing timely, standardized interventions may prevent progression of acute symptoms into chronic trauma-related disorders, though evidence-based algorithms specific to the athlete population have yet to be firmly established [11]. Athletes' high tolerance for discomfort can contribute to mental health symptoms being masked by perfectionism, compartmentalization, and dissociation [1].

Perfectionism

Perfectionism can be adaptive as well as nonadaptive in sport, manifesting in psychological, emotional, and behavioral tendencies. Adaptive perfectionism is expressed by the athlete who is deriving satisfaction from sport and their intensive training combined with the ability to tolerate their own imperfections without excessive self-criticism [1]. Perfectionism can become maladaptive when the athlete establishes unrealistic personal standards. There is evidence that perfectionism can be a powerful driver and motivator for achievement, though is not necessarily a positive experience for the athlete. Though there is a paucity of research, one study on perfectionism and PTSD in the general population found that there is a significant correlation. It found that rumination was a significant mediator of the relationship between "concern over mistakes" and PTSD [23]. Additionally, perfectionism, particularly over-concern about mistakes, could be a manifestation of obsessive-compulsive disorder, which can be comorbid with trauma-related disorders. Without proper management, the long-term impact for athletes with perfectionism could be overt mental health symptoms or disorders [1]. Finally, athletes with "lost movement syndrome" ("yips") involving a loss of sport-related fine and/or gross motor skills often report a history of significant life events, such as traumatic loss of a loved one or traumatic injury [24]. Individuals with high levels of perfectionism can be more susceptible to the negative consequences of traumatic life events. Unhealthy perfectionism combined with a high perceived stress response puts an athlete at greater risk for experiencing performance breakdown (e.g., lost movement syndrome) as a traumatic event in itself [1].

Compartmentalization

Compartmentalization can be a psychological defense or a conscious (intentional) strategy. A psychological defense operates on an unconscious level, allowing individuals to live with irreconcilable conflicts, which in turn help the person avoid cognitive dissonance. Compartmentalization is used as a mental strategy to maintain, for example, a separation of the athlete's sporting life from their personal life [11, 25]. It is a mental skill that can help increase focus during competition. When used as a conscious defense strategy, athletes can modify painful memories by compartmentalizing thoughts regarding the event. This could mask underlying trauma, essentially protecting the athlete from the reality of the problem. An athlete can then be stuck in a stage of avoidance or intrusion, which can interfere with adaptive processing of traumatic events during the acute phase, setting the stage for a pathological response to the inciting event [1]. It is likely that high-performing athletes may compartmentalize in order to manage their emotions, which in turn can conceal mental health symptoms [1, 26]. A subjective sense of compartmentalization regarding the traumatic event can develop and lead to a fragmentation or emotional detachment from the event [1, 26]. This over-regulation of affect could allow the athlete to continue to practice and compete. However, this is potentially at the cost of a prolonged recovery [1].

Olympic swimmers in a 2015 study [27] reported using the pool and their training as a way to cope with and avoid adverse experiences. Being immersed in the water, a world unto itself, was experienced as a refuge and a comfort. Over time, these efforts were no longer adaptive. They began to experience more intrusive thoughts and emotional suffering. Through the process of recognizing the need to confront the traumatic experiences and receive support, personal growth followed. This was expressed by superior performances, enhanced relationships, and prosocial behavior [11].

Case: Unmasking Symptoms in a Semi-Professional Cyclist

Hine (not her real name) is a 28-year-old Māori/New Zealand European woman with a history of major depressive episodes in her early 20s who presented to an inpatient psychiatric facility with increased intensity of suicidal ideation and self-injurious (cutting) behaviors.

Hine had been seen by the mental health community team for approximately 2 months prior to her presentation. Hine reported symptoms of depression, anxiety, nightmares, re-experiencing phenomena, and dissociative symptoms beginning approximately 9 months prior to presentation. She admitted to using cutting to cope with unwanted emotions when she was a teenager, but prior to this episode had not cut in over 10 years. Hine struggled to describe any triggers for her decompensation, citing that she had recently obtained a new job she liked in education and was caring for her two children, who appeared to be protective. Two years prior she had broken up with a partner who had been physically assaultive, resulting in legal action. She did not connect this event to her current mental state, indicating that she felt this was "old news" and that she had "dealt with" the fallout from that relationship already. Community mental health intervened with cognitive behavioral therapy (CBT) and medication adjustments for depression. Nonetheless, Hine's symptoms worsened, resulting in time off from work and her aunt moving into her apartment to care for her children. Diagnostic considerations by outpatient providers included bipolar disorder and borderline personality disorder. Precise diagnosis was unclear at the time of her admission to inpatient psychiatry.

On admission, Hine was withdrawn and minimally able to participate in the diagnostic interview. She had difficulty naming her emotions or connecting her thoughts, feelings, and behaviors. She admitted to significant "numbing" of her emotions, which made it difficult for her to express herself or understand her own emotional state; this was cited as a primary reason for her cutting behaviors. She responded well to cultural support and began to open up with the assistance of the ward kaumautua (Māori elder). Hine's Māori heritage was an aspect of herself that was newly important; her mother, who was Māori, died when she was 3 years old, and she had only recently been in touch with some of her Māori whānau (family). Hine had been raised by her father and stepmother of New Zealand-European descent, who were unsure how to support Hine on her cultural journey. Hine had reached out to her local marae (communal sacred space) in the past year, but hesitated to become involved with that community due to her lack of experience.

In the course of exploring her cultural background, Hine admitted that she had experienced trauma throughout her lifetime, including her mother leaving when she was young, sexual assault as a teenager, and intimate partner violence as an adult. She mentioned that one of the "saving graces" of her life had been her semi-professional career in cycling, something she had not discussed with her community treatment team as it "didn't seem relevant."

On further exploration, Hine explained that she took up cycling in her late teens and had competed in races throughout New Zealand. She had never qualified for the Olympics, but had been moving her cycling career in that direction during her early 20s, ultimately limited by her finances and family responsibilities. Hine continued to take her training very seriously, spending most of her free time training for races. Hine suffered an ACL tear while weight training approximately 1 year prior to her psychiatric decompensation, and had not been back on her bike since. She initially was highly engaged in treatment for her ACL tear, including via physical therapy, but her engagement waned in the weeks following her injury; she reported feeling fatigued, apathetic, and unable to fully participate in caring for her injury. As her depressive and trauma-related symptoms emerged, she disengaged from her sport and focused solely on her work as an educator and a mother. At the time of inpatient admission, she reported that she had "given up" on cycling, that she was getting "too old anyway," and had not made any plans to resume sport involvement. Her cycling teammates and coach had not been in touch with her for months.

Hine's narrative around her cultural background and involvement in sport assisted the inpatient psychiatric team in reframing Hine's clinical presentation. By history, Hine did not appear to have the enduring traits of a person with borderline personality disorder. Hine had long-standing relationships with coaches, friends, and at work prior to her decompensation, and was able to function well in those systems. Her difficulty accessing her emotions and "numbing" appeared less like the dissociative features of a personality disorder, and more consistent with unmasking of chronically untreated trauma-related symptoms, which were less apparent when she was engaged in her sport. Hine relied on coping strategies including compartmentalization and perfectionism, and used cycling as an outlet for these coping strategies. Despite Hine's history of multiple traumatic experiences in her lifetime, including distance from her cultural background and supports, she had never been diagnosed with PTSD. Nightmares, other re-experiencing phenomenon, and dissociative symptoms were not clinically apparent while Hine was actively engaged with cycling, and she had not sought mental health contact since her teen years.

In Hine's case, there may have been opportunities to intervene earlier in her care. Hine showed evidence of declining engagement in physical therapy during recovery from her injury, and dropped out of her cycling team altogether in the weeks following her ACL tear. These behaviors in a previously highly active member of a team can be an indication of underlying psychiatric distress. Hine had difficulty identifying this for herself until symptoms worsened to the point of suicidal ideation. In this case, Hine's tendency to distance herself from her emotions made it more difficult for her to self-recognize symptoms. Once engaged in community mental health services, Hine still found it difficult to connect events and behaviors with her emotional state, and ultimately benefited from culturally sensitive support in forming a narrative of events leading up to her psychiatric decompensation. Cultural support allowed her to talk more openly about her history with sport and her connection to her Māori heritage. These findings assisted the inpatient team in developing a whole-person approach to care, which included ward cultural support in connecting with her local marae, development of a plan to re-engage with physical therapy, ultimately re-introduction of exercise as a component of her recovery, and trauma-related therapeutic interventions to support her wellness. Hine found the framing of her narrative useful, eagerly engaged in these interventions by the time of her discharge from inpatient psychiatry, and carried the treatment plan forward into the community.

Dissociation

Dissociation is another psychological defense commonly associated with trauma. The traumatic memory is 'set apart' from consciousness by this process. Dissociation can be an adaptive, active mental skill that athletes use to enhance performance. This psychological strategy helps the athlete focus their attention externally in order to distract from internal feelings of pain or fatigue [1, 28]. Endurance athletes in particular utilize dissociative skills. Partial dissociative states are often described as "flow" or "in the zone." These can be described as "normative" or "creative" dissociation versus maladaptive dissociation [29].

Compartmentalization can be a feature of dissociation, though dissociation involves an altered state and detachment from the environment [11, 30]. It is essentially an observational position that separates the athlete from their internal discomfort. This disruption in consciousness can also become a disruption in the conscious ability to observe oneself, which can be nonadaptive when stress demands are low

[11, 24]. Although this can be potentially helpful with performance, it is not to be ignored, as it could be masking a serious mental health disorder [1]. If the feeling of being disconnected from one's body is perceived by the athlete as "normal," it could be minimized or dismissed when the athlete is asked about symptoms in a mental health screening or evaluation [11, 31]. Shuer and Dietrich's [32] research showed that chronically injured athletes develop posttraumatic symptoms and coping strategies similar to people traumatized by natural disasters. They found this to be the case in intrusive thoughts and avoidance subscales. Their avoidance subscales included dissociation as an active defense mechanism. Active use of dissociation could minimize the extent and nature of injuries. The dissociative experience of detachment, operating at times adaptively, unfortunately can also numb the athlete from positive feelings of joy and pleasure. Inappropriate numbing to dangerous future circumstances can also be an outcome of this inability to "feel." It is believed that acute dissociative responses predict chronic PTSD [11].

Secondary Trauma

Secondary trauma—the witnessing of a traumatic event or of disturbing descriptions of traumatic events by a survivor—can transpire within sport teams. This can include witnessing physical injury or death or witnessing abusive dynamics including sexual and other forms of abuse within teams [1]. Secondary trauma can affect teammates, coaches, and athletic trainers in a silent, less-than-conscious manner, which left unaddressed can develop into mental health symptoms for individuals as well as the team as a whole, similar to those in PTSD. Having trauma-informed personnel working with athletes promotes a culture of safety, healing, and empowerment for the affected individuals.

Case: The Unwanted Legacy of Nonaccidental Violence

A 17-year-old elite male athlete, Lyle, presents for outpatient treatment as a result of unresolved somatic issues inhibiting play and performance. He had been a participant in an Olympic Development Program (ODP) in his sport for 5 years. During the course of these years, Lyle was relentlessly bullied, emotionally and physically, by teammates, as well as targeted and routinely humiliated by coaches. His determination to be "the best" in the sport compelled him to continue, in spite of feeling miserable, sad, and alone. His parents encouraged him to speak up to the coaches, which he did, but to no avail. His parents repeatedly asked if he would like to stop participating in the ODP. Lyle said "no," that his sport was his entire life. Lyle developed a remarkable ability to compartmentalize his experience, as well as dissociate, describing himself as an "observer of my own experiences."

He reported "watching" the bullying, rather than experiencing it directly. Over time, he began to experience somatic symptoms in addition to the typical sport-related injuries. The somatic complaints could not find medical explanations, yet had significant impact on his ability to "feel" the lower half of his body, as he often described himself as "numb" from the waist down.

Lyle presented for treatment 2 years after his experience with OPD ended. He continued to play on his high school and club teams. He was a top player, though often unavailable to play because of "injury." In addition to his anxiety presentation, he continued to describe an inability to feel his lower body, and when he could experience sensation, it was a "heaviness." His physical therapist reported that his "glute muscles were not working at all." These somatic compromises became the primary obstacle to successfully competing. This was adaptive in the sense that it "protected" him from being on the field, potentially subject to more humiliation and performance breakdowns. Simultaneously, the somatic issues were maladaptive, as they prevented any possibility of reparative experiences on the field as a player and with teammates or coaches, which could have included ending his relationship with them.

Lyles' treatment involved intensive psychotherapy, a combination of CBT to manage obsessive thinking, psychoeducation about trauma and the brain, and psychodynamic approaches that addressed the different levels of consciousness to be managed. Lyle was psychologically minded, highly motivated, and intrigued by the intellectual puzzle of treatment. He expressed relief at having the opportunity to be understood around this most devastating and destructive part of his life. It was recommended that he have a sports psychiatric medication consultation to help with his anxiety and obsessive thinking. A selective serotonin reuptake inhibitor (SSRI) was prescribed, which provided symptom relief. The medication and psychotherapy, combined with the work of a skilled athletic acupuncturist and physical therapist, restored feeling and function to his lower body. During the spring of his senior year in high school, he competed successfully on his club and high school teams but began experiencing performance breakdowns as a result of emotional triggering of the trauma. When triggered by a "look" or "comment," Lyle would find himself in a "black hole" of mental abuse. At times he would develop somatic symptoms, and when addressed in therapy, they would quickly resolve. Lyle ambivalently accepted a college scholarship in his sport. He looked forward to this opportunity, but was "scared that the history would repeat itself."

Once college began, the hope of an interpersonally reparative experience was high. The first week was successful. During the second week, at an informal practice, Lyle was picked last to be on a team. This incited emotional triggers that resulted in punitive intrusive/obsessive thoughts that he could not quiet. At times he was briefly able to manage these thoughts, only to be retriggered by seemingly small exchanges or events. His overall experience on the team and at college was clouded by his developing depression and a profound sense of inadequacy. He became increasingly socially isolated, and his motivation and performance dropped athletically. As the season progressed, he could identify that his internal experience did not "match" his positive value on the team, which was expressed by his coach as well as teammates. His inability to experience joy or positive feedback, in spite of intensive efforts therapeutically, positioned him to consider a medical retirement from sport as a result of trauma history in sport. This is not the outcome that was hoped for, but he ultimately decided to medically retire from sport. He is working to decide how to transition from active sport and what his relationship to the sport that has defined his life will be.

Management

Once an athlete is identified as suffering from trauma-related symptoms, evidence-based management should include a multipronged treatment approach tailored to the needs of the client. Research has primarily focused on PTSD and consistently supports psychotherapeutic and psychoeducational interventions that may be used alongside pharmacologic treatment where necessary [33, 34]. The nature of the interventions used should be guided by the athlete's severity of symptoms and impairment as well as personal treatment engagement/preferences. There are efforts to create athlete-specific interventions; however, an algorithmic guideline has not yet been established. Most interventions stem from research in the general population; we will highlight some athlete-specific interventions later in this section.

There is strong support for the use of psychotherapy in trauma-related disorders, including a wide variety of modalities. Robust evidence has been demonstrated for prolonged exposure therapy (PE), cognitive processing therapy (CPT), and trauma-focused cognitive behavioral therapy (TF-CBT). These interventions are structured and time-limited (typically 16 sessions or less) and may be used for athletes whose symptoms range from mild-moderate to severe [33–35]. There is growing evidence to support the use of eye movement desensitization and reprocessing therapy (EMDR), though the evidence is not quite as abundant or robust as the evidence for CPT, PE, or TF-CBT [35]. These therapies can all be practiced on an individual basis; there are protocols to utilize CBT and EMDR in group settings [35].

Additional psychotherapeutic modalities have been utilized in the treatment of PTSD; the Agency for Healthcare Research and Quality reviewed protocols for Seeking Safety, Trauma Affect Regulation, Brief Eclectic Psychotherapy, and Image Rehearsal Therapy, finding that these interventions may be helpful but have a lower strength of evidence than CBT [34]. Other interventions, including mindfulness/meditation, somatic therapies, and supportive interventions such as case management, may also provide some treatment benefit to engaged and interested patients [7, 33, 36].

While some psychotherapeutic interventions have lower strength of evidence than others when analyzing large swaths of data, weight should be given to therapeutic "fit" and patient preference in regard to selecting the appropriate intervention. A systematic review published by the *Journal of the American Medical Association* examined the effects of patient preference for psychological interventions, finding that patients whose preferences were met had lower dropout rates and higher therapeutic alliance scores, both key factors in successful treatment [37]. Therapeutic alliance has a strong effect on reducing dropout rates, increasing treatment adherence, and likely improving outcomes, and should be taken into account when a client is seeking treatment [38–40]. Therapeutic alliance with the treating provider may also impact effective prescribing [40]. This is supported in the treatment of trauma-related disorders by neurobiological research on the importance of relationships in healing from trauma [9, 13].

In cases where an athlete is suffering significant functional impairment, severe symptoms, and/or symptoms that present a barrier to psychological interventions, medications may be a necessary component of holistic treatment. Combination treatment with psychotherapy and medications is common and shows positive treatment outcomes [33–35]. Medications may be initiated by a primary care provider or sports medicine provider in most cases; in cases with complicating factors such as general medical comorbidity (including traumatic brain injury), psychiatric comorbidity, treatment-resistant symptoms, or diagnostic uncertainty, consultation with a specialist should be considered. Patients with a history of or positive screening for bipolar disorder should be carefully managed, as antidepressants may increase the risk of mania [41]. First-line medications for athletes with trauma-related disorders are similar to those for nonathletes, with some additional considerations due to the physiologic demands of sport. First-line treatment for PTSD is well documented and includes SSRIs or serotonin and norepinephrine reuptake inhibitors (SNRIs) [34]. Sertraline and paroxetine are U.S. Food and Drug Administration-approved for the treatment of PTSD, though all SSRI and SNRI medications may be considered for the treatment of PTSD. Systematic reviews of medications for PTSD have shown some support for the use of venlafaxine, paroxetine, or fluoxetine over other SSRIs and SNRIs [34, 42]. Factors impacting the selection of the pharmacologic agent should include past responses to medications, side effect profile, and sport-specific research in the area. Sertraline, fluoxetine, and escitalopram have been studied and/or recommended for use in the athlete population and may be reasonable options in the absence of other factors [43]. Paroxetine may present challenges in the athlete population due to side effects that include significant fatigue, weight gain, and other anticholinergic-related side effects.

Pharmacologic treatment of hyperarousal symptoms, nightmares, and re-experiencing phenomena in PTSD has been explored at some length. Alpha-blocking agents including prazosin, clonidine, doxazosin, and others have historically been used, particularly for nightmares, which often cause patients significant distress. Evidence supporting the use of alpha-blockers has been called into question as efficacy may not be as substantial as once believed [33, 34, 44], though they are still fairly commonly used. Reviews including those by the Agency for Healthcare Research and Quality have found this evidence to be weak or "low." These agents are often tried in severe cases, as there may be a subset of patients who experience benefit from their use. Athletes' physiologic adaptations to sport often include lower baseline blood pressure and heart rate; thus, practitioners considering the use of these alpha-blockers should carefully monitor vital signs to detect any problematic decrease in heart rate and blood pressure.

Further pharmacologic interventions have included antipsychotics such as quetiapine, risperidone, or olanzapine, as well as anticonvulsants such as lamotrigine. These interventions have a low strength of evidence; however, there may be additional factors that lead to the use of these agents, including comorbid bipolar disorder, psychotic symptoms, or severe affective instability [34, 42]. Antipsychotic agents carry side effects including extrapyramidal symptoms, metabolic syndrome (including weight gain), and sedation; the risks and benefits of these agents should be collaboratively discussed with the athlete in the context of their symptoms.

Institutional, team-based approaches to the care of athletes directly or indirectly affected by trauma may provide further effective interventions for the athlete population. The IOC Mental Health in Elite Athletes Toolkit provides detailed information on a broad range of mental health conditions affecting athletes, along with a framework for holistic support of athletes through institutions and individuals on an athlete's team, such as their coaches, clubs, and entourage [6]. A sports psychologist or integrated sports psychotherapist may be positioned to provide skilled debriefing of traumatic events to teams, reducing the stigma of seeking help and addressing the phenomenon of vicarious trauma [3, 24]. The creation of a trauma-informed, nonjudgmental, destigmatizing culture within institutions may be instrumental in mitigating the broader complications of shared traumatic events and increase an athlete's likelihood of receiving early interventions [2, 24]. Institutions should be encouraged to create clear and supportive pathways to access support, ide-

ally incorporating known sports and mental health practitioners who have training and experience with the nuances of the athlete population and trauma-informed care. Institutions promoting early interventions and trauma-informed cultures may aid in reducing the morbidity of traumatic experiences affecting athletes, including reducing the likelihood of progression of acute stress disorder to PTSD [45]. Systems-level interventions have the potential to create environments that not only reduce suffering, but also promote post-traumatic growth [1, 46].

Promoting Post-Traumatic Growth/Wisdom

Post-traumatic growth and ultimately wisdom is central to successful outcomes for trauma-affected athletes. Post-traumatic growth refers to the manner in which a traumatic event can be an impetus for change. Given the exposure to biopsychosocial trauma an athlete can face, there is a need for understanding how these lived experiences not only resonate with PTSD but also post-traumatic growth. Research demonstrates athletes can grow from trauma if proper support is provided [47].

As interventional practitioners, there is opportunity to respond in ways that promote post-traumatic growth, including by being open to and aware of the how the inciting event can be a profound experience of helplessness, uncontrollability, and life threat. Trauma can be a life-changing circumstance in which the athletes' assumptive world is challenged [46]. This can bring core beliefs into question. The younger the athlete is when the trauma occurs, the greater the risk there is for acute responses that can become chronic. The assumptions of safety and comfort are gone. It is common for feelings of shame to accompany trauma. Athletes can find themselves struggling with existential concerns and a loss of illusions, which can be more traumatic for the athlete, particularly if it involves interpersonal and/or institutional betrayals [11]. These losses need to be mourned.

Working with trauma is not for the "faint of heart." It challenges the practitioner to be able to "stay present," while managing their own activation, fears of being consumed by the trauma, tendency to dissociate for fear of experiencing vicarious trauma, and worry about re-traumatizing the athlete. It is important to be a compassionate witness, to help the athlete "experience" the sensations they feel in their bodies, and to not rush to "explain it."

Clinical efforts need to focus on psychosocial growth and development of resilience beyond the athlete's pre-traumatic state, resulting in a more integrated and functioning individual, as well as a superior performer [11]. Post-traumatic wisdom results from the athlete's ability to take what they have learned from their experience to view the world differently, and to not have their perspective decimated by the trauma.

With help, they are able to alchemize the unbearable suffering into power that propels them forward in their lives [8].

Summary

Trauma-related disorders appear to be more prevalent in the athlete population compared to the general population, with the potential for athletes to experience trauma before, during, and as a result of sport. Athletes may elude diagnosis in the absence of a trauma-informed approach due to coping and masking strategies borne out of their psychological and physiologic adaptations as a result of their sport participation.

Untreated trauma, as a result of missed diagnoses, can lead to a wide array of untoward outcomes for the athlete, including complications in recovery from injuries, inconsistencies in performance, interpersonal conflicts, and overall psychological morbidity. Early interventions may prevent complications arising from trauma-related symptoms and mitigate progression of acute symptoms to chronic trauma-related disorders. Available research suggests a multipronged approach, including creating a trauma-informed team culture, skilled team debriefings following traumatic incidents, validated screening of athletes who appear at risk of trauma-related disorders, and prompt, evidence-based treatment of athletes exhibiting mental health disorders, which may include psychotherapy, medications, or a combination thereof. Future research on systematic approaches to identifying at-risk athletes may help address the challenges in identifying athletes whose coping schemes increase their diagnostic complexity.

References

1. Aron CM, Harvey S, Hainline B, Hitchcock ME, Reardon CL. Post-Traumatic stress disorder (PTSD) and other trauma-related mental disorders in elite athletes: a narrative review. Br J Sports Med. 2019;53(12):779–84.
2. Wenzel T, Zhu L. Post traumatic stress in athletes. In: Baron D, Reardon C, Baron S, editors. Clinical sports psychiatry: an international perspective. 1st ed. New York, NY: Wiley; 2013. p. 102–14.
3. O'Neill D. Injury contagion in alpine ski racing: the effect of injury on teammates' performance. J Clin Sport Psychol. 2008;2(3):278–92.
4. Mountjoy M, Brackenridge C, Arrington M, Blauwet C, Carska-Sheppard A, Fasting K, Kirby S, Leahy T, Marks S, Martin K, Starr K, Tiivas A, Budgett R. International Olympic Committee consensus statement: harassment and abuse (non-accidental violence) in sport. Br J Sports Med. 2016;50(17):1019–29.
5. Gouttebarge V, Bindra A, Blauwet C, Campriani N, Currie A, Engebretsen L, Hainline B, Kroshus E, McDuff D, Mountjoy M, Purcell R, Putukian M, Reardon CL, Rice SM, Budgett R. International Olympic Committee (IOC) Sport Mental Health Assessment Tool 1 (SMHAT-1) and Sport Mental Health Recognition Tool 1 (SMHRT-1): towards better support of athletes' mental health. Br J Sports Med. 2021;55(1):30–7.
6. Burrows K, Cunningham L, Raukar-Herman C. IOC mental health in athletes toolkit. In: Athlete 365. Lausanne: International Olympic Committee; 2021.
7. Van der Kolk BAI, Stone L, West J, Rhodes A, Emerson D, Suvak M, Spinazzola J. Yoga as an adjunctive treatment for posttraumatic stress disorder: a randomized controlled trial. J Clin Psychiatry. 2014;75(6):559–65.
8. Levine PA. Trauma and memory: brain and body in a search for the living past: a practical guide for understanding and working with traumatic memory. Berkeley, CA: North Atlantic Books; 2015.
9. Perry BD, Jackson AL. Trauma-informed leadership. In: Leadership in child and family practice. London: Routledge; 2018. p. 125–41.
10. Siegel DJ. An interpersonal neurobiology approach to psychotherapy: awareness, mirror neurons, and neural plasticity in the development of well-being. Psychiatr Ann. 2006;36(4):248–56.
11. Miller Aron CM, Lefay SM. Best practices for diagnosis and management of trauma-related disorders in athletes. In: Marks DR, Wolanin AT, Shortway KM, editors. The Routledge handbook of clinical sport psychology. London: Routledge; 2021. p. 306–20.
12. Porges SW. Polyvagal theory: a primer. In: Porges SW, Dana D, editors. Clinical applications of the polyvagal theory: the emergence of polyvagal-informed therapies. New York, NY: WW Norton; 2018. Chapter 4.
13. Geller SM, Porges SW. Therapeutic presence: neurophysiological mechanisms mediating feeling safe in therapeutic relationships. J Psychother Integr. 2014;24(3):178.
14. Reardon CL, Hainline B, Aron CM, Baron D, Baum AL, Bindra A, Budgett R, Campriani N, Castaldelli-Maia JM, Currie A, Derevensky JL, Glick ID, Gorczynski P, Gouttebarge V, Grandner MA, Han DH, McDuff D, Mountjoy M, Polat A, Purcell R, Putukian M, Rice S, Sills A, Stull T, Swartz L, Zhu LJ, Engebretsen L. Mental health in elite athletes: International Olympic Committee consensus statement (2019). Br J Sports Med. 2019;53(11):667–99.
15. DSM: American Psychiatric Association. Diagnostic and statistical manual of mental disorders. 5th ed. Arlington, VA: American Psychiatric Publishing; 2013.
16. North CS, Surís AM, Smith RP, King RV. The evolution of PTSD criteria across editions of DSM. Ann Clin Psychiatry. 2016;28(3):197–208.
17. Winfrey O, Perry BD. What happened to you?: Conversations on trauma, resilience, and healing. New York, NY: Flatiron Books; 2021.
18. Thomson P, Jaque V. Visiting the muses: creativity, coping, and PTSD in talented dancers and athletes. Am J Play. 2016;8(3):363–78.
19. Putukian M, Echemendia RJ. Psychological aspects of serious head injury in the competitive athlete. Clin Sports Med. 2003;22(3):617–30.
20. Bateman A, Morgan K. The postinjury psychological sequelae of high-level Jamaican athletes: exploration of a posttraumatic stress disorder–self-efficacy conceptualization. J Sport Rehabil. 2017;28:144–52.
21. Roberts AL, Gilman SE, Breslau J, Breslau N, Koenen KC. Race/ethnic differences in exposure to traumatic events, development of post-traumatic stress disorder, and treatment-seeking for post-traumatic stress disorder in the United States. Psychol Med. 2011;41(1):71–83.
22. Day MC, Bond K, Smith B. Holding it together: coping with vicarious trauma in sport. Psychol Sport Exerc. 2013;14(1):1–11.
23. Egan SJ, Hattaway M, Kane RT. The relationship between perfectionism and rumination in post traumatic stress disorder. Behav Cogn Psychother. 2014;42(2):211–23.
24. Bennett J, Rotherham M, Hays K, et al. Yips and lost move syndrome: assessing impact and exploring levels of perfectionism, rumination, and reinvestment. Sport Exerc Psychol Rev. 2016;12:1.
25. Poucher ZA, Tamminen KA. Maintaining and managing athletic identity among elite athletes. Revista de psicología del deporte. 2017;26(4):63–7.

26. Lanius RA, Vermetten E, Loewenstein RJ, et al. Emotion modulation in PTSD: clinical and neurobiological evidence for a dissociative subtype. Am J Psychiatry. 2010;167:640–7.

27. Howells K, Fletcher D. Sink or swim: adversity-and growth-related experiences in Olympic swimming champions. Psychol Sport Exerc. 2015;16:37–48.

28. Silva JM, Appelbaum MI. Association-dissociation patterns of United States Olympic marathon trial contestants. Cogn Ther Res. 1989;13(2):185–92.

29. Warr M, Henriksen D, Mishra P. Creativity and expressive arts, performance, physicality and wellness: a conversation with Dr. Paula Thomson and Dr. Victoria Jaque. TechTrends. 2019;63(2):102–7.

30. Spitzer C, Barnow S, Freyberger HJ, et al. Recent developments in the theory of dissociation. World Psychiatry. 2006;5:82–6.

31. Leahy T, Pretty G, Tenenbaum G. A contextualized investigation of traumatic correlates of childhood sexual abuse in Australian athletes. Int J Sport Exerc Psychol. 2008;6:366–84.

32. Shuer ML, Dietrich MS. Psychological effects of chronic injury in elite athletes. West J Med. 1997;166:104–9.

33. American Psychiatric Association Guideline, Ursano RJ, Bell C, Eth S, Friedman M, Norwood A, Pfefferbaum B, Pynoos JD, Zatzick DF, Benedek DM, McIntyre JS, Charles SC, Altshuler K, Cook I, Cross CD, Mellman L, Moench LA, Norquist G, Twemlow SW, Woods S, Yager J, Work Group on ASD and PTSD; Steering Committee on Practice Guidelines. Practice guideline for the treatment of patients with acute stress disorder and posttraumatic stress disorder. Am J Psychiatry. 2004;161:3.

34. Hoffman V, Middleton JC, Feltner C, Gaynes BN, Weber RP, Bann C, Viswanathan M, Lohr KN, Baker C, Green J. Psychological and pharmacological treatments for adults with posttraumatic stress disorder: a systematic review update 2018 comparative effectiveness review no. 207. Am J Psychiatry. 2018;161(11 Suppl):3–31.

35. American Psychological Association Guideline: Guideline Development Panel for the Treatment of PTSD in Adults. Clinical practice guideline for the treatment of Posttraumatic Stress Disorder (PTSD) in adults (PDF). Washington, DC: American Psychological Association; 2017. p. ES–2.

36. Bremner JD, Mishra S, Campanella C, Shah M, Kasher N, Evans S, Fani N, Shah AJ, Reiff C, Davis LL, Vaccarino V, Carmody J. A pilot study of the effects of mindfulness-based stress reduction on post-traumatic stress disorder symptoms and brain response to traumatic reminders of combat in Operation Enduring Freedom/Operation Iraqi Freedom combat veterans with post-traumatic stress disorder. Fron Psychiatry. 2017;8:157.

37. Windle E, Tee H, Sabitova A, Jovanovic N, Priebe S, Carr C. Association of patient treatment preference with dropout and clinical outcomes in adult psychosocial mental health interventions: a systematic review and meta-analysis. JAMA Psychiatry. 2020;77(3):294–302.

38. Baier AL, Kline AC, Feeny NC. Therapeutic alliance as a mediator of change: a systematic review and evaluation of research. Clin Psychol Rev. 2020;82:101921.

39. Krupnick JL, Sotsky SM, Elkin I, Moyer J, Pilkonis PA. The role of the therapeutic alliance in psychotherapy and pharmacotherapy outcome: findings in the National Institute of Mental Health Treatment of Depression Collaborative Research Program. J Lifel Learn Psychiatry. 2006;IV(2):269–77.

40. Sijercic I, Liebman RE, Stirman SW, Monson CM. The effect of therapeutic alliance on dropout in cognitive processing therapy for posttraumatic stress disorder. J Trauma Stress. 2021;34(4):819–28.

41. Howland RH. Induction of mania with serotonin reuptake inhibitors. J Clin Psychopharmacol. 1996;16(6):425–7.

42. Management of Post-Traumatic Stress Working Group. VA/DoD clinical practice guideline for management of post-traumatic stress, version 3.0. Washington, DC: Department of Veterans Affairs and Department of Defense; 2017.

43. Reardon CL, Creado S. Psychiatric medication preferences of sports psychiatrists. Phys Sportsmed. 2016;44(4):397–402.

44. Raskind MA, Peskind ER, Chow B, Harris C, Davis-Karim A, Holmes HA, Hart KL, McFall M, Mellman TA, Reist C, Romesser J, Rosenheck R, Shih MC, Stein MB, Swift R, Gleason T, Lu Y, Huang GD. Trial of prazosin for post-traumatic stress disorder in military veterans. N Engl J Med. 2018;378(6):507–17.

45. Rothbaum B, et al. Early intervention may prevent the development of posttraumatic stress disorder: a randomized pilot civilian study with modified prolonged exposure. Biol Psychiatry. 2012;72(11):957–63.

46. Hammer C, Podlog L, Wadey R, Galli N, Forber-Pratt A, Newton M. From core belief challenge to posttraumatic growth in para sport athletes: moderated mediation by needs satisfaction and deliberate rumination. Disabil Rehabil. 2019;41:2403–11.

47. Vann SE, Moore DM, Freiburger K, Johnson H. The end is not the injury: posttraumatic growth after sport injuries. J Amateur Sport. 2019;4(2):87–102.

Eating Disorders

Elizabeth Joy

Introduction

Eating disorders are devastating diseases that are experienced by athletes and nonathletes, all genders, children, adolescents, and adults. Among athletes, eating disorders have long been recognized in females who seek to optimize their performance by manipulating their dietary intake and in turn body size, shape, and weight. Taken to the extreme, this can have negative impacts on health and performance [1]. Increasingly, we are observing eating disorders in athletes across genders, and similar to females, as an attempt to improve sport performance [2].

Eating disorders often result in a state of "low energy availability" (low EA, to be described later), which in turn causes disruption of reproductive physiology. In females, low EA manifests in oligo- or amenorrhea, hypoestrogenism, and low bone mineral density (BMD). Referred to as the Female Athlete Triad (Triad), this scenario increases the likelihood of sport-related bone stress injuries (BSIs) [3].

More recently, the Male Athlete Triad has been defined. Similar to what is observed in females who, through dietary restriction and/or excessive exercise, develop a state of low EA, males experience hypogonadotropic hypogonadism, resultant low bone mineral density, and an increase in the risk of sport-related BSIs [4].

While some may consider BSIs to be a minor inconvenience, they can be a season-ending, or worse yet, career-ending, life-altering injury. Imagine the scenario of the athlete with a tension side femoral neck stress fracture, who, despite pain, continues to train until she suffers a fatigue fracture resulting in the placement of a femoral rod or need for a hip replacement.

It is critically important that sports medicine providers (physicians, athletic trainers, physical therapists, sports dietitians) understand the athlete at risk for eating disorders, recognize behaviors, symptoms, and signs of an eating disorder, and within their scope of practice, intervene as early as possible to prevent adverse consequences to health and performance.

Epidemiology

Eating disorders are defined by the *Diagnostic and Statistical Manual of Mental Disorders 5th edition* (Table 9.1). While binge-eating disorder is most common in the general population (3.5% of women and 2.0% of men, or three times anorexia nervosa and bulimia nervosa combined) [6], the concern among athletes is typically for anorexia nervosa and bulimia nervosa. A study of US high school female athletes found that 41.5% reported disordered eating [7]. A survey of US college female athletes revealed that 25.5% reported subclinical eating disorder symptoms [8].

Females

It is estimated that nearly 1 in 20 females are affected by an eating disorder (anorexia nervosa, bulimia nervosa, binge-eating disorder) [9]. The proportion of female athletes affected varies by several factors including age, sport, and level of competition. While any athlete may develop an eating disorder, athletes participating in sports where leanness confers a competitive advantage, aesthetic sports, and weight category sports are often affected at higher rates [10].

Males

While females are more likely to be affected by eating disorders, increasingly, males are engaging in pathologic eating behaviors. In the United States, it is estimated that eating disorders (anorexia nervosa, bulimia nervosa, binge-eating disorder) affect 2.2% of males [9, 11]. The sports in which

E. Joy (✉)
Wellness & Nutrition, Intermountain Healthcare,
Salt Lake City, UT, USA
e-mail: Liz.joy@imail.org

Table 9.1 Eating disorders as defined in the *Diagnostic and Statistical Manual of Mental Disorders 5th edition (DSM-5)* [5]

Eating disorder	Diagnostic criteria	Types	Severity
Anorexia nervosa	• Restriction of dietary intake leading to low body weight for age, sex, growth, and health	• Restricting type—no binge eating; includes those who achieve weight loss through excessive exercise	Adults (for children and adolescents, corresponding BMI *percentiles* should be used):
	• Intense fear of weight gain or becoming fat, despite low body weight	• Binge-eating/purging type—includes those who engage in recurrent binge/ purge behaviors	• Mild: BMI $\geq$17 kg/m^2
	• Disturbance in how body size, shape, and weight is experienced, and persistent lack of recognition of how low body weight is impacting health		• Moderate: 16–16.99 kg/m^2
			• Severe: 15–15.99 kg/m^2
			• Extreme: <15 kg/m^2
Bulimia nervosa	• Recurrent binge eating, and a lack of control over eating		• Mild: 1–3 episodes of compensatory behaviors/ week
	• Regular use of compensatory behaviors such as self-induced vomiting, use of laxatives, diuretics, fasting, and/or excessive exercise		• Moderate: 4–7 episodes/ week
			• Severe: 8–13 episodes/ week
			• Extreme: 14 or more episodes/week
Binge-eating disorder	• Recurrent binge eating, and a lack of control over eating		• Mild: 1–3 binge eating episodes/week
	• Eating more rapidly than normal, until uncomfortably full, consuming large amounts of food, eating alone (due to embarrassment over eating), feeling disgusted and shame after bingeing		• Moderate: 4–7 episodes/ week
	• Binge eating occurs at least 1 time/week		• Severe: 8–13 episodes/ week
	• Not associated with compensatory behaviors		• Extreme: 14 or more episodes/week
Avoidant/restrictive food intake disorder	• More often observed in children		
	• Results in eating/feeding avoidance as a result of apparent lack of interest in eating, of concern about a negative experience associated with eating, e.g., dysphagia, nausea, abdominal pain, or of avoidance based on the sensory characteristics of food		
	• Results in a failure to meet nutrition and energy needs in support of growth, function, and health		
Unspecified or other specified feeding or eating disorder	• These terms largely replace the former "Eating Disorder Not Otherwise Specified—EDNOS"		
	• Used when an individual presents with behaviors that do not meet the full diagnostic criteria of other defined eating disorders (e.g., an athlete with "atypical anorexia nervosa" who technically has a normal BMI—perhaps because of high muscle mass—but otherwise meets criteria for anorexia nervosa)		

BMI body mass index

males are most likely to be affected by eating disorders are similar to those in which females are most likely to be affected.

Para Athletes, Racial and Ethnic Minorities, LGTBQ Athletes

Less is known about the risk and prevalence of eating disorders (and the Female and Male Athlete Triads) in diverse populations of athletes. A study of US elite male and female para athletes (*n* = 260) examined nutrition, menstrual function, bone health, and awareness of the Female Athlete Triad. Few respondents reported an eating disorder (3.1%), although 32.4% had elevated Eating Disorder Examination Questionnaire (EDE-Q) pathologic behavior subscale scores,

and a majority of respondents reported efforts to change their weight and body composition to improve performance. Over 9% reported BSIs, and 54% reported low BMD. Less than 10% were aware of the Triad [12].

While eating disorders have long been thought of as disorders affecting upper middle class white females, that is in fact far from the truth. Hispanic and Black teenagers are more likely to suffer from bulimia nervosa compared to white teens [13], and people of color with eating disorders are significantly less likely to receive help for their eating disorder [14]. There remains a significant gap in our understanding of eating disorders in racial and ethnic minority athletes.

Eating disorders are observed at higher rates among gay males [15, 16] and transgender college students [17]. Eating disorder rates among LGBTQ athletes are unknown.

Health and Sport Consequences of Eating Disorders: A Systems Approach

Eating disorders can affect many aspects of human physiology. Among athletes, this can demonstrably impact performance due to acute injury, nonhealing injury, or as a result of other altered physiologic functions.

Reproductive and Endocrine

Eating disorders result in hypogonadotropic hypogonadism in females and males. The relationship between low EA (from dietary restriction, excessive exercise, and/or other purging behaviors), menstrual dysfunction leading to hypoestrogenism, and low BMD is known as the Female Athlete Triad [3]. More recently, the relationship between low EA, hypogonadotropic hypogonadism, and low BMD in males has been referred to as the Male Athlete Triad [4].

In females, the Triad may result in reversible infertility. In males, the Triad may result in decreased libido and oligospermia. The degree of energy deficiency necessary to cause these reproductive/endocrine consequences appears to be greater among males compared to females.

Importantly, in the Female and Male Athlete Triads, low EA and its consequences may occur with or without an eating disorder. Although the exact prevalence of eating disorders as part of the Triads is unknown, clinical observation would suggest that it is a majority—meaning that low EA is a consequence of intentional dietary restriction, excessive exercise, purging behaviors, or some combination. EA is defined as the amount of energy (kilocalories) that remains after subtracting average daily exercise energy expenditure from average daily dietary energy intake, then normalizing (dividing) by the person's fat-free mass (FFM). The formula looks like this:

$$\text{Energy availability}(\text{kcal}) = \frac{\text{Avg Daily Energy Intake}(\text{kcal}) - \text{Avg Daily Exercise Energy Expenditure}(\text{kcal})}{\text{Fat Free Mass}(\text{kg})}$$

Components of the Female Athlete Triad vary depending on sport and competitive level. Rates of disordered eating are observed in as high as 70% of elite athletes. Likewise, the prevalence of menstrual dysfunction among athletes where leanness is emphasized can be as high as 69%. Finally, the prevalence of osteopenia among female athletes ranges between 22% and 50% [18]. An athlete with any one component of the Triad should be thoroughly evaluated for the other components.

Beyond abnormalities of reproductive physiology, a multitude of hormonal abnormalities result from eating disorders, especially anorexia nervosa [19]. In women with low weight from anorexia nervosa, total T3 tends to be low, and free T4 and TSH vary from normal to low normal. These changes are not reflective of thyroid disease but are an adaptive response to decreases in metabolic rate and energy expenditure. Cortisol levels are almost universally elevated in women with anorexia nervosa and can result in Cushing's-like symptoms (e.g., low bone mineral density, truncal fat accumulation with weight regain). Elevated antidiuretic hormone can result in hyponatremia. Interestingly, anorexia nervosa-related alterations in the levels of estrogen, androgens, and cortisol are associated with higher measures of anxiety and depression [19].

Musculoskeletal

The combination of low bone mineral density and weight bearing or sport-related bone stress can lead to BSI—stress reactions or stress fractures. The mechanism for low bone mineral density is an imbalance between osteoblasts and osteoclasts brought on by decreased lean mass and hormonal alterations [20, 21]. Low bone density may result from inadequate acquisition of bone mineral density during periods of growth, the loss of bone mineral density, or both. Resultant BSIs are most commonly observed in weight bearing athletes such as runners, dancers, and soldiers. In decreasing order of frequency, BSIs occur in the metatarsals, tibia, tarsals, femur, fibula, and pelvis [22]. Upper extremity focused sports may develop BSIs of the ribs or humerus.

Neuropsychiatric

A study of more than 2400 individuals hospitalized for an eating disorder found that 94% of the participants had a co-occurring mood disorder, with 92% of those in the sample struggling with a depressive disorder [23]. Also common are obsessive-compulsive disorder (OCD) [24] and post-traumatic stress disorder (PTSD) [25]. Anorexia nervosa has a mortality rate of 10%, and it is estimated that one in five deaths is by suicide [26]. According to the National Center on Addiction and Substance Abuse, up to 50% of individuals with eating disorders misused alcohol or illicit drugs, a rate five times higher than in the general population [27]. In a study of women with bulimia nervosa, 31% had a history of alcohol abuse and 13% had a history of alcohol dependence (using prior DSM terminology) [28]. Less is understood about the risk of substance use disorders in athletes with concurrent eating disorders.

Cardiopulmonary [29]

Cardiac consequences of anorexia nervosa and bulimia nervosa result from dietary restriction, fluid restriction, excessive exercise, weight loss, and electrolyte disturbances. Arrhythmias can include bradycardia and tachycardia. Electrocardiography abnormalities can include prolonged Q-T intervals and low voltage. Echocardiograms may show cardiac hypoplasia and mitral valve prolapse. Hemodynamic problems include hypotension, orthostasis, near syncope, and syncope.

Sports medicine physicians should consider a cardiology consultation for patients demonstrating resting heart rate <40 beats/min, prolongation of the Q-T interval, evidence of anatomical abnormalities (e.g., valvular heart disease, congestive heart failure), or syncope; during ongoing cardiology consultation, participation in training and competition should be prohibited.

Oropharyngeal

Oropharyngeal manifestations of eating disorders are typically observed in those who engage in self-induced vomiting (SIV). Specifically, these manifestations include dental enamel erosion and recurrent sore throats. Efforts to reduce dental erosion include rinsing the oral cavity with a solution of baking soda and water immediately after vomiting to neutralize hydrochloric acid. Individuals actively engaged in SIV should be cautioned to NOT brush their teeth immediately after purging as this can further expose the teeth and gums to gastric acid.

Other oropharyngeal consequences include mouth sores, perleche, cracked lips, parotid gland enlargement, dental decay and loss of teeth, and bleeding gums.

Gastrointestinal [30]

Gastrointestinal (GI) complications of eating disorder behaviors are quite common and can be very impactful. Constipation is the most frequent GI consequence among patients with either bulimia nervosa or anorexia nervosa. Recurrent SIV results in scarring and dysfunction of the gastroesophageal (GE) junction and subsequent GE reflux (GERD), regurgitation, and esophagitis. Forceful SIV can result in acute injury, tears, and bleeding at the GE junction, known as a Mallory–Weiss tear. Patients abusing laxatives will experience diarrhea and are at higher risk of hemorrhoids and rectal prolapse.

Chronic dietary restriction may result in paradoxical satiety as well as functional gastroparesis. Patients will complain of significant bloating, discomfort, and nausea with minimal oral intake, resulting in further dietary restriction. Significant weight loss resulting in decreased visceral fat can lead to superior mesenteric artery syndrome, and abdominal pain that worsens with eating.

Renal [31]

Renal abnormalities may occur as a result of restriction or purging. Chronic hypokalemia can lead to irreversible chronic kidney disease. Restriction of fluid intake increases the risk of nephrolithiasis.

Clinical Best Practice in Screening, Evaluation, Treatment, and Return to Sport

All members of the athlete care team have a role in the identification, care, and safe return to sport for athletes affected by eating disorders.

Screening

Although the US Preventive Services Task Force recently concluded that the current evidence is insufficient to assess the balance of benefits and harms of screening for eating disorders in adolescents and adults, providing an "I" statement, the task force did acknowledge the higher prevalence of eating disorders among athletes and other high-risk groups [32].

Recognizing the higher risk of eating disorders among athletes, screening for eating disorders in athletes has long been recommended and is often initiated during the sports preparticipation evaluation. The *Preparticipation Physical Evaluation* (PPE) Monograph, now in its 5th edition [33], developed by six medical professional organizations in the United States, includes questions to screen for eating disorders and related consequences:

- Do you worry about your weight?
- Are you trying to or has anyone recommended that you gain or lose weight?
- Are you on a special diet or do you avoid certain types of foods or food groups?
- Have you ever had an eating disorder?

And for females:

- Have you ever had a menstrual period?
- How old were you when you had your first menstrual period?
- When was your most recent menstrual period?
- How many periods have you had in the past 12 months?

The International Olympic Committee (IOC) Periodic Health Examination includes the following relevant questions [34]:

Nutrition questions:

- Do you worry about your weight or body composition?
- Are you satisfied with your eating pattern?
- Are you a vegetarian?
- Do you lose weight to meet weight requirements for your sport?
- Does your weight affect the way that you feel about yourself?
- Do you worry that you have lost control over how much you eat?
- Do you make yourself sick when you are uncomfortably full?
- Do you ever eat in secret?
- Do you currently suffer, or have you ever suffered in the past with an eating disorder?

And for females:

- Have you ever had a menstrual period?
- What was your age at your first menstrual period?
- Do you have regular menstrual cycles?
- How many menstrual cycles did you have in the last year?
- When was your most recent menstrual period?
- Have you had a stress fracture in the past?
- Have you ever been identified as having a problem with your bones such as low bone density (osteopenia or osteoporosis)?

- Are you presently taking any female hormones (estrogen, progesterone, birth control pills)?

Once completed, the sport preparticipation history form is reviewed by the sports medicine physician and oftentimes the athlete care team to determine if further evaluation and treatment is necessary.

Evaluation and Treatment

If an athlete is identified as at risk for an eating disorder, is demonstrating signs and symptoms of an eating disorder, or is active in their eating disorder, they should undergo evaluation and treatment by members of a multidisciplinary team. Athlete-centered care is the goal, leveraging both expertise and trusted relationships between the athlete and the care team. Figure 9.1 demonstrates the relationships between the athlete and their care team:

The bi-directional arrows in Fig. 9.1 represent the importance of information sharing between members of the multidisciplinary care team. This provides for comprehensive assessment and development of a collaborative, cohesive treatment plan.

Each member of the team has their domain of expertise, but there is cross-over between disciplines. For example, the *sports medicine physician* is not only managing health consequences of an eating disorder, but also assessing dietary intake and mental well-being. The *sports dietitian* is most effective as a "nutrition therapist," understanding the emotional connections between food, eating, and body image, and applying evidence-based behavior change. The role of the *mental health professional* is critical, and expertise in eating disorder care is essential. Suicide is the second lead-

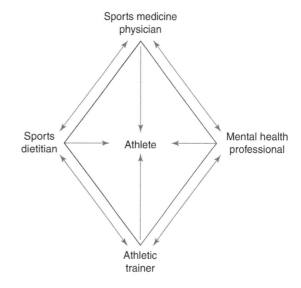

Fig. 9.1 Multidisciplinary care of athletes with eating disorders

Table 9.2 Roles and responsibilities of the multidisciplinary athlete care team

Role	Screening/identification	Evaluation	Treatment
Sports medicine physician	• During the preparticipation physical evaluation • Any time presenting with signs and symptoms • Referral from other members of athlete care team	• History and physical examination, including detailed mental health assessment • Laboratory testing • Other diagnostic testing as indicated (electrocardiogram, bone density testing)	• Refer to other members of multidisciplinary team • Prescribe pharmacotherapy when indicated • Treat associated conditions (e.g., mood and anxiety disorders) and injuries (e.g., bone stress injuries) • Responsible for clearance and return to play decision-making
Sports dietitian	• Same as sports medicine physician (in some settings, athletes routinely undergo screening with a registered dietitian as part of the preparticipation physical evaluation)	• Detailed dietary history, including pathologic eating and exercise behaviors	• Provide medical nutrition therapy
Mental health professional	• Same as sports medicine physician (In some settings athletes routinely undergo screening with a mental health professional as part of the preparticipation physical evaluation)	• Detailed psychological and behavioral history with a focus on body image, psychosomatic reactions, physiology, past and ongoing physical and psychological trauma, assessing the current situation, taking a psychological approach for the assessment of comorbid conditions (e.g., mood and anxiety disorders)	• Provide psychotherapy (most often cognitive behavioral therapy) • Prescribe and monitor pharmacotherapy when indicated (in the case of psychiatry)
Athletic trainer	• The "eyes and ears" of the athlete care team • Often are the first to identify the athlete who is struggling from the effects of an eating disorder • May observe pathologic eating and exercise behaviors	• Initial assessment of eating disorder-related conditions (e.g., bone stress injuries)	• Support the athlete in staying engaged in treatment • Perform physician directed biometric assessments (e.g., weight, heart rate, blood pressure) • Assist in the rehabilitation of associated injuries • Help to keep the athlete engaged with the team if participation is restricted • Work with coaching staff to reengage the athlete with training when cleared by sports medicine physician

ing cause of death for individuals with anorexia nervosa—a rate that is 18 times higher than age and gender matched comparison groups. Between a quarter and a third of those with anorexia nervosa or bulimia nervosa have considered suicide, and a quarter have attempted suicide [35]. Finally, the *athletic trainer* often is the "eyes and ears" of the athlete care team. They are the healthcare professionals who spend the most time with the athlete and are more likely to observe aberrant eating behaviors, excessive exercise, or hear from team members concerns about eating disorder behaviors at home and on the road.

The odds of developing an eating disorder after sexual violence are substantial; a history of rape increases the odds for lifetime incidence of eating disorder by nearly 22-fold. Similarly, among women with eating disorders, there is a much higher likelihood of experiencing sexual violence [36].

Given the relationship between sexual violence and eating disorders, it bears mention that sports medicine physicians and mental health professionals should ascertain whether an athlete with an eating disorder has experienced or is experiencing sexual violence.

Table 9.2 provides a summary of the roles and responsibilities of each member of the athlete care team when caring for an individual with an eating disorder.

Treatment of eating disorders exists on a continuum (outpatient to residential) based on severity of illness and involves each member of the multidisciplinary team. Ideally, patients/athletes are able to safely and adequately receive care in outpatient settings, where they are regularly seen by their physician, dietitian, and psychotherapist. The focus of treatment is psychotherapy and nutrition therapy. The goal of treatment is to address attitudes and beliefs about food, weight, eating, and body image, improve behaviors (i.e., involving eating, exercise, weighing), and normalize weight. Among athletes, sport is often a strong motivator to engage in treatment and recover. It is important that members of the treatment team understand the physical/psychological demands of an athlete's sport to inform treatment goals and safe return to sport.

Although the primary treatment for eating disorders is nutrition therapy and psychotherapy, patients/athletes may benefit from pharmacotherapy for their eating disorder and/or related co-morbidities. Only two medications in the United States have a Food and Drug Administration (FDA) indication for the treatment of eating disorders: fluoxetine for bulimia nervosa, and lisdexamfetamine for binge eating disorder [37]. Importantly, stimulants such as lisdexamfetamine are typically prohibited or tightly regulated in sport at the collegiate or higher levels and may require therapeutic use exemptions in order to be used. While other psychotropic medications are often prescribed, it is typically an off-label application, or alternatively to treat mental health co-morbidities and physical health consequences of an eating disorder. Table 9.3 is a non-exhaustive list of medications that may be used or should be avoided in the treatment of athletes affected by an eating disorder and related consequences.

Table 9.3 Pharmacotherapy of eating disorders and related symptoms or disorders

Condition/medication	Notes
Eating disorder	
Fluoxetine	Indicated for the treatment of bulimia nervosa.
Vyvanse	Indicated for the treatment of binge eating disorder.
Depression, anxiety, and insomnia	
Selective serotonin reuptake inhibitors (SSRIs)	Often a first choice in the treatment of depression and anxiety.
Mirtazapine	Indicated for the treatment of depression. Associated with weight gain (which may or may not be desirable). Sedating.
Bupropion	**Avoid** in patients with a history of seizures.
	Avoid in patients with an eating disorder involving restricting or purging. In combination with electrolyte disturbances, it is more likely to lower seizure threshold.
Benzodiazepines	**Use with caution**. Can cause tolerance and dependence. Sedating. Do not use in close relationship to training or competition.
Trazodone	Sedating. Can cause orthostatic hypotension.
	Avoid in athletes who participate in sports with significant postural changes (e.g., gymnastics, diving).
Thought disturbance	
Atypical antipsychotics	There is some evidence of positive effects on depression, anxiety, and core eating disordered psychopathology in patients with anorexia nervosa [38].
	Associated with weight gain (which may or may not be desirable).
	Use with caution in athletes where weight gain may adversely affect performance or safety (e.g., sports dependent on positive strength to weight ratios, sports where athletes must carry weight over distance, sports with weight class requirements).
Amenorrhea	
Estrogen patch + oral progesterone	**Preferred treatment** in athletes with low BMD, one or more low risk or one high risk stress fracture, and persistent amenorrhea despite 1 year of nonpharmacologic treatment [39].
Etonogestrel and ethinyl estradiol ring (NuvaRing)	Consider for hormone replacement therapy in athletes with a need for contraception [39].
Combined oral contraceptive pills	**Avoid** in athletes with hypothalamic hypogonadism, as first pass metabolism in the liver may adversely affect hormones in support of bone health [39].
Low bone mineral density	
Calcium	Ensure adequate dietary intake of calcium or supplement 1000–1300 mg daily.
Vitamin D	Supplement if indicated.
Bisphosphonates	Consider in athletes with nonhealing stress fracture.
Teriparatide	Consider in athletes with nonhealing stress fracture.
Gastrointestinal symptoms	
Proton pump inhibitors	Consider for athletes with symptoms of gastroesophageal reflux as a result of current or past self-induced vomiting.
H2 blockers	Consider for athletes with symptoms of gastroesophageal reflux as a result of current or past self-induced vomiting.
Erythromycin	Acts as a promotility agent. Consider in the athlete with constipation.
Metclopramide	Promotility agent. Consider in the athlete with symptoms of gastroparesis. Has significant drug interactions. May be sedating.
Miralax	Osmotic-type laxative. Consider in the athlete with constipation.

BMD bone mineral density

Recovery From Eating Disorders

A review of 119 studies, including nearly 6000 patients, found that approximately half of eating disorder survivors recovered, one-third improved, and 20% remained chronically ill. Predictors of recovery were younger age at onset and longer duration of follow-up [40]. A 22-year follow-up study of patients with anorexia nervosa or bulimia nervosa found that approximately two-thirds were recovered. Notably a third had persistent disease [41]. Few studies have examined eating disorder recovery in athletes. A 2014 study of 47 current and former US collegiate athletes who completed an online questionnaire examined factors associated with recovery. At the time of the study, 77% had fully recovered, and 33% had relapsed. A third of respondents indicated that their desire to recover was facilitated by a desire to regain their strength and ability to fully participate in their sport. Over a quarter of respondents reported that changing values and beliefs and support from others were key to their recovery [42].

Return to Sport

Decisions regarding return to sport ultimately lie with the team physician, but it is often the collective assessment of the multidisciplinary team that determines the athlete's readiness to return to training and competition. One of the first guides for return to sport came from the Female Athlete Triad Coalition in their publication, *2014 Female Athlete Triad Coalition Consensus Statement on Treatment and Return to Play of the Female Athlete Triad: 1st International Conference held in San Francisco, California, May 2012 and 2nd International Conference held in Indianapolis, Indiana, May 2013* [39]. This publication provides physicians with a Cumulative Risk Assessment tool for female athletes affected by the Triad, and Clearance and Return-to-Play (RTP) Guidelines based on their medical risk stratification. Notably, the guidelines state, "It is the recommendation of the Consensus Panel that athletes diagnosed with anorexia nervosa who have a body mass index (BMI) <16 kg/m^2 or with moderate-to-severe bulimia nervosa (purging >4 times/week) should be categorically restricted from training and competition. Future participation is dependent on treatment of their eating disorder, including ascertainment of BMI > 18.5 kg/m^2, cessation of bingeing and purging and close interval follow-up with the multidisciplinary team."

While developed for females, a 2019 study examined the predictability of the Cumulative Risk Assessment tool in 156 male collegiate distance runners. Using the risk assessment categories of low energy availability, low BMI, BMD, and prior BSI, investigators found that prior BSI was associated with a 57% higher risk of prospective BSI, and every one-point increase in the cumulative risk score was associated with a 37% increase in prospective BSI [43].

Athletes who are identified as being at moderate to high risk based on the Cumulative Risk Assessment tool should be provided with a written contract that clearly describes expectations of the treatment team, the responsibilities of the athlete in their recovery, and the criteria for safe return to training and competition.

Even upon return to sport, it is critical that the athlete have regular follow-up with members of the multidisciplinary team to ensure adherence to recommended guidelines for safe participation.

Some athletes will be unable to resolve their eating disorder sufficiently to safely return to sport, and some will require a higher level of care (e.g., intensive outpatient programs, partial hospitalization programs, hospitalization, or residential care) to recover. It is incumbent on the sports medicine physician to know when a higher level of care is necessary, and what resources for such care are available within the community to facilitate timely referrals to expert care. Beware of the athlete restricted from training and competition who isolates and restricts their dietary intake to such an extent that their life is at risk. Anorexia nervosa has the second highest mortality rate (opioid use disorder being first) of any mental health disorder [44]. Athletic trainers can play a key role in checking in with the restricted athlete and ensuring that they are actively participating in recommended treatment.

Prevention of Eating Disorders

Recognizing the risks of developing an eating disorder inherent in sport (some sports more than others), it behooves all members of the athlete care team and sports administrators to engage in efforts to prevent eating disorders. This includes education of athletes, parents, and coaches, as well as ensuring members of the athlete care team have the necessary expertise. A 1-year school-based intervention within Norwegian Elite High Schools that aimed to decrease eating disorders and disordered eating behaviors in elite adolescent female and male athletes was successful in the prevention of eating disorders and a reduction in disordered eating behaviors [45].

Educational resources have been developed by the US National Collegiate Athletic Association (https://www.ncaa.org/sports/2014/11/4/mind-body-and-sport-eating-disorders.aspx), by the International Olympic Committee (https://olympics.com/ioc/healthy-body-image), and by the Female and Male Athlete Triad Coalition (https://www.femaleandmaleathletetriad.org/). Sports medicine physicians, sports dietitians, and athletic trainers should all be trained to recognize the athlete who is either at risk for development of an eating disorder or is early in their disease, to prevent worsening health consequences. Early intervention is associated with better outcomes [46].

Summary

Athletes are at risk for the development of eating disorders due to pressures applied/perceived to optimize their body weight/composition to improve sport performance. Additionally, athletes face unique pressures due to sport, as a result of attempting to balance academic demands and sport, and like others, may experience traumatic events, all of which may trigger eating disordered behaviors. The consequences of eating disorders are extensive and affect nearly every system of the body. Resultant low energy availability adversely affects reproductive physiology across genders. In turn, hypogonadotropic hypogonadism may result in low bone mineral density, increasing the risk of BSI—a constellation of conditions referred to as either the Female Athlete Triad or Male Athlete Triad.

Each member of the athlete care team has a role in the prevention, screening, evaluation, and treatment of athletes affected by the Triad. The sports medicine physician is responsible for screening (during the preparticipation physical evaluation), evaluation, treatment, and return to sport decisions. Evidence-based guidance on clearance and return to play is available for female athletes and can inform decision-making for athletes across genders. The sports dietitian has a critical role in helping the athlete achieve adequate caloric and nutrient intake to restore normal physiology. Mental health professionals with experience in eating disorder care (and preferably athlete care) are essential in the treatment of an athlete with an eating disorder [47]. Finally, athletic trainers are often closest to the athlete and may observe concerning eating and exercise behaviors, overhear comments about body size, shape, or weight, and are often the first people to whom a concerned teammate or coach may reach out.

References

1. El Ghoch M, Soave F, Calugi S, Dalle GR. Eating disorders, physical fitness and sport performance: a systematic review. Nutrients. 2013;5(12):5140–60.
2. Glazer JL. Eating disorders among male athletes. Curr Sports Med Rep. 2008;7(6):332–7.
3. Nattiv A, Loucks AB, Manore MM, Sanborn CF, Sundgot-Borgen J, Warren MP, American College of Sports Medicine. American College of Sports Medicine position stand. The female athlete triad. Med Sci Sports Exerc. 2007;39(10):1867–82.
4. Nattiv A, De Souza MJ, Koltun KJ, Misra M, Kussman A, Williams NI, Barrack MT, Kraus E, Joy E, Fredericson M. The male athlete triad-a consensus statement from the female and male athlete triad coalition part 1: definition and scientific basis. Clin J Sport Med. 2021;31(4):335–48.
5. American Psychiatric Association. Desk reference to the diagnostic criteria from DSM-5 (R). Washington, DC: American Psychiatric Association Publishing; 2013.
6. Hudson JI, Hiripi E, Pope HG Jr, Kessler RC. The prevalence and correlates of eating disorders in the National Comorbidity Survey Replication. Biol Psychiatry. 2007;61(3):348–58.
7. Jankowski C. Associations between disordered eating, menstrual dysfunction, and musculoskeletal injury among high school athletes. Yearbook Sports Med. 2012:394–5.
8. Greenleaf C, Petrie TA, Carter J, Reel JJ. Female collegiate athletes: prevalence of eating disorders and disordered eating behaviors. J Am Coll Heal. 2009;57(5):489–96.
9. Duncan AE, Ziobrowski HN, Nicol G. The prevalence of past 12-month and lifetime DSM-IV eating disorders by BMI category in US men and women. Eur Eat Disord Rev. 2017;25(3):165–71.
10. Martinsen M, Sundgot-Borgen J. Higher prevalence of eating disorders among adolescent elite athletes than controls. Med Sci Sports Exerc. 2013;45(6):1188–97.
11. Tenforde AS, Barrack MT, Nattiv A, Fredericson M. Parallels with the Female Athlete Triad in Male Athletes. Sports Med. 2016;46(2):171–82.
12. Brook EM, Tenforde AS, Broad EM, et al. Low energy availability, menstrual dysfunction, and impaired bone health: a survey of elite para athletes. Scand J Med Sci Sports. 2019;29:678–85.
13. Swanson SA, Crow SJ, Le Grange D, Swendsen J, Merikangas KR. Prevalence and correlates of eating disorders in adolescents. Results from the national comorbidity survey replication adolescent supplement. Arch Gen Psychiatry. 2011;68(7):714–23.
14. Marques L, Alegria M, Becker AE, Chen C, Fang A, Chosak A, Diniz JB. Comparative prevalence, correlates of impairment, and service utilization for eating disorders across U.S. ethnic groups: implications for reducing ethnic disparities in health care access for eating disorders. Int J Eat Disord. 2011;44(5):412–20.
15. Strother E, Lemberg R, Stanford SC, Turberville D. Eating disorders in men: underdiagnosed, undertreated, and misunderstood. Eat Disord. 2012;20(5):346–55.
16. Feldman MB, Meyer IH. Eating disorders in diverse lesbian, gay, and bisexual populations. Int J Eat Disord. 2007;40:218–26.
17. Diemer EW, Grant JD, Munn-Chernoff MA, Patterson DA, Duncan AE. Gender identity, sexual orientation, and eating-related pathology in a national sample of college students. J Adolesc Health. 2015;57(2):144–9.
18. Nazem TG, Ackerman KE. The female athlete triad. Sports Health. 2012;4(4):302–11.
19. Schorr M, Miller KK. The endocrine manifestations of anorexia nervosa: mechanisms and management. Nat Rev Endocrinol. 2017;13(3):174–86.
20. Misra M, Klibanski A. Bone health in anorexia nervosa. Curr Opin Endocrinol Diab Obes. 2011;18(6):376–82.
21. Fazeli PK, Klibanski A. Effects of anorexia nervosa on bone metabolism. Endocr Rev. 2018;39(6):895–910.
22. May T, Marappa-Ganeshan R. Stress fractures. In: StatPearls. Treasure Island, FL: StatPearls Publishing; 2022. https://www.ncbi.nlm.nih.gov/books/NBK554538/. Accessed 27 Mar 2022.
23. Tagay S, Schlottbohm E, Reyes-Rodriguez ML, Repic N, Senf W. Eating disorders, trauma, PTSD, and psychosocial resources. Eat Disord. 2014;22(1):33–49.
24. Mandelli L, Draghetti S, Albert U, De Ronchi D, Atti AR. Rates of comorbid obsessive-compulsive disorder in eating disorders: a meta-analysis of the literature. J Affect Disord. 2020;277:927–39.
25. Rijkers C, Schoorl M, van Hoeken D, Hoek HW. Eating disorders and posttraumatic stress disorder. Curr Opin Psychiatry. 2019;32(6):510–7.

26. Arcelus J, Mitchell AJ, Wales J, Nielsen S. Mortality rates in patients with Anorexia Nervosa and other eating disorders. Arch Gen Psychiatry. 2011;68(7):724–31.

27. The National Center on Addiction and Substance Abuse (CASA) at Columbia University. Food for thought: substance abuse and eating disorders. New York, NY: The National Center on Addiction and Substance Abuse (CASA), Columbia University; 2003.

28. Gregorowski C, Seedat S, Jordaan GP. A clinical approach to the assessment and management of co-morbid eating disorders and substance use disorders. BMC Psychiatry. 2013;13(1):289.

29. Casiero D, Frishman WH. Cardiovascular complications of eating disorders. Cardiol Rev. 2006;14(5):227–31.

30. Santonicola A, Gagliardi M, Pier Luca Guarino M, Siniscalchi M, Ciacci C, Iovino P. Eating disorders and gastrointestinal diseases. Nutrients. 2019;11:3038.

31. Li Cavoli G, Mulè G, Rotolo U. Renal Involvement in psychological eating disorders. Nephron Clin Pract. 2011;119:c338–41.

32. Screening for Eating Disorders in Adolescents and Adults. US Preventive Services Task Force recommendation statement, US Preventive Services Task Force. JAMA. 2022;327(11):1061–7.

33. American Academy of Pediatrics, American Academy of Family Physicians, American College of Sports Medicine, American Medical Society for Sports Medicine, American Medical Society for Sports Medicine, American Orthopaedic Society for Sports Medicine, and American Osteopathic Academy of Sports Medicine. Preparticipation physical evaluation. 5th ed. Itasca, IL: American Academy of Pediatrics; 2019.

34. Ljungqvist A, Jenoure PJ, Engebretsen L, Alonso JM, Bahr R, Clough AF, de Bondt G, Dvorak J, Maloley R, Matheson G, Meeuwisse W, Meijboom EJ, Mountjoy M, Pelliccia A, Schwellnus M, Sprumont D, Schamasch P, Gauthier JB, Dubi C. The International Olympic Committee (IOC) consensus statement on periodic health evaluation of elite athletes. Clin J Sport Med. 2009;19(5):347–65.

35. Smith AR, Zuromski KL, Dodd DR. Eating disorders and suicidality: what we know and what we don't know, and suggestions for future research. Curr Opin Psychol. 2018;22:63–7.

36. Hailes HP, Yu R, Danese A, Fazel S. Long-term outcomes of childhood sexual abuse: an umbrella review. Lancet Psychiatry. 2019;6(10):830–9.

37. Bello NT, Yeomans BL. Safety of pharmacotherapy options for bulimia nervosa and binge eating disorder. Expert Opin Drug Saf. 2018;17(1):17–23.

38. McKnight RF, Park RJ. Atypical antipsychotics and anorexia nervosa: a review. Eur Eat Disord Rev. 2010;18(1):10–21.

39. De Souza MJ, Nattiv A, Joy E, et al. Female Athlete Triad Coalition Consensus Statement on Treatment and Return to Play of the Female Athlete Triad: 1st International Conference held in San Francisco, California, May 2012 and 2nd International Conference held in Indianapolis, Indiana, May 2013. Br J Sports Med. 2014;48:289.

40. Steinhausen HC. The outcome of anorexia nervosa in the 20th century. Am J Psychiatry. 2002;159(8):1284–93.

41. Eddy KT, Tabri N, Thomas JJ, et al. Recovery from anorexia nervosa and bulimia nervosa at 22-year follow-up. J Clin Psychiatry. 2017;78(2):184–9.

42. Arthur-Cameselle JN, Quatromoni PA. Eating disorders in collegiate female athletes: factors that assist recovery. Eat Disord. 2014;22(1):50–61.

43. Kraus E, Tenforde AS, Nattiv A, Sainani KL, Kussman A, Deakins-Roche M, Singh S, Kim BY, Barrack MT, Fredericson M. Bone stress injuries in male distance runners: higher modified Female Athlete Triad Cumulative Risk Assessment scores predict increased rates of injury. Br J Sports Med. 2019;53(4):237–42.

44. Chesney E, Goodwin GM, Fazel S. Risks of all-cause and suicide mortality in mental disorders: a meta-review. World Psychiatry. 2014;13(2):153–60.

45. Martinsen M, Bahr R, Børresen R, Holme I, Pensgaard AM, Sundgot-Borgen J. Preventing eating disorders among young elite athletes: a randomized controlled trial. Med Sci Sports Exerc. 2014;46(3):435–47.

46. Austin A, Flynn M, Shearer J, et al. The first episode rapid early intervention for eating disorders - upscaled study: clinical outcomes. Early Interv Psychiatry. 2022;16:97–105.

47. Rice SM, Purcell R, De Silva S, Mawren D, McGorry PD, Parker AG. The mental health of elite athletes: a narrative systematic review. Sports Med. 2016;46(9):1333–53.

Attention-Deficit/Hyperactivity Disorder

Doug Hyun Han

Attention-Deficit/Hyperactivity Disorder in Sports

Most athletes require a heightened level of attention while competing. However, several factors including physical fatigue, general life stress, the pressure of competition, and environmental factors prohibit sportspeople—even elite athletes—from focusing on performance. Elite athletes are defined as those competing at the professional, Olympic, Paralympic, or collegiate/university levels. These prohibitive factors notwithstanding, some elite athletes with attention-deficit/hyperactivity disorder (ADHD) become disappointed with their performance, which may be affected by frequent errors and impulsive behavior even when they have trained intensively. In cases in which disenchanted athletes stop exercising because of such experiences, a diagnosis of ADHD should be considered.

ADHD is a common developmental disorder of the brain with the essential features of a persistent pattern of age-inappropriate inattention and/or hyperactivity–impulsivity. These characteristics cause dysfunction before the age of 12 years in multiple settings, including in academic, work, and sporting life, and in interpersonal relationships [1].

ADHD symptoms occur across a person's life span, but unique symptoms are observed during developmental stages. Among preschool- and school-aged children, individuals with ADHD show behavioral disturbances, poor social interactions, academic difficulty, and poor peer acceptance. Adolescents with ADHD display low self-esteem, poor social interaction, impulsivity, academic difficulty, and substance misuse, while adults with ADHD exhibit low self-esteem, frequent errors in everyday life, unemployment or under-employment, mood instability, and driving issues [2].

D. H. Han (✉)
Department of Psychiatry, Chung Ang University Hospital, Seoul, South Korea

Diagnosis of ADHD in Elite Athletes

A formal diagnosis of ADHD made in the general population draws on clinical symptoms and history, and is based on the criteria in the *Diagnostic and Statistical Manual of Mental Disorders 5th edition (DSM-5)* [3]. Individuals with ADHD present a persistent pattern of inattention and/or hyperactivity–impulsivity that is associated with functioning or development. At least six symptoms from the "inattention" or "hyperactivity and impulsivity" domains must persist for at least 6 months to establish the diagnosis [3].

The nine symptoms of inattention are that the individual often: (1) fails to pay close attention to details or makes careless mistakes, (2) has difficulty sustaining attention in tasks or play, (3) does not listen when spoken to directly, (4) cannot follow through on instruction and fails to finish schoolwork, chores, or workplace duties, (5) has difficulty organizing tasks and activities, (6) has difficulty engaging in tasks that require sustained mental effort, (7) loses things, (8) is easily distracted by extraneous stimuli (or by unrelated thoughts in older adolescents and adults), and (9) is forgetful in daily activities. The symptoms of hyperactivity and impulsivity include that the individual often: (1) fidgets or taps hands or feet, or squirms in seat, (2) leaves seat in situations when remaining seated is expected, (3) runs about or climbs in inappropriate circumstances, (4) is unable to play or engage quietly in leisure activities, (5) is "on the go," acting as if "driven by a motor," (6) talks excessively, (7) blurts out an answer before a question has been completed, (8) has difficulty waiting their turn, and (9) interrupts or intrudes upon others.

Additional laboratory or neurocognitive tests can support a diagnosis of ADHD, rule out other conditions, or both. Testing of executive function including planning, spatial and verbal working memory, response inhibition, and vigilance is recommended as a common neurocognitive function test for ADHD [4]. Laboratory testing is not routinely employed for the diagnosis of ADHD. However, laboratory tests are useful to differentiate substance misuse from ADHD as some symptoms of substance misuse mimic those in individuals with ADHD [5].

Neuroimaging as a diagnostic tool for ADHD is not routinely recommended because of inconclusive evidence. Reduced brain volume within the basal ganglia, cerebellum, and frontal lobe is observed in ADHD in brain volumetric measurements [6–8]. In resting-state functional magnetic resonance imaging, the functional activity of the default mode and cognitive control networks are less anticorrelated (inversely correlated) compared to normally developed individuals, indicating that the function of the cognitive control network is disrupted in individuals with ADHD [9, 10]. Delayed thinning of cortical thickness indicates individuals with ADHD may experience a delay in brain maturation [11].

In sum, the diagnostic process in ADHD among elite athletes is similar to that in the general population. The clinical symptoms of daily life and athletic competition provide primary evidence for the diagnosis of ADHD. Several neurocognitive function tests support this diagnostic process. Neuroimaging findings may be considered as an experimental approach. However, the fame and advanced athletic skills of elite athletes can influence the diagnostic decision of clinicians, who must remain cautious and objective when assessing the clinical symptoms of elite athletes.

Prevalence of ADHD in Elite Athletes

The prevalence of ADHD is 5.0–7.1% in children and 2.5–5.0% in adults in the general population [1, 12]. ADHD has been historically perceived as a childhood-onset neurodevelopmental disorder [13]. However, the concept of adult ADHD as a continuum of childhood ADHD is controversial [14]. Approximately 65% of children with ADHD were reported to experience continuation of functional impairment from ADHD symptoms into adulthood [15]. A considerable proportion of adult patients with ADHD had no history of diagnosed childhood ADHD [16].

Few studies have examined the prevalence of ADHD in elite athletes. The powerful stigma of psychiatric assessment may prohibit the estimation of the true prevalence of ADHD in elite athletes [1]. For this reason, the prevalence of ADHD in elite athletes is extrapolated from data in the general population and from the limited amount of information specific to athletes.

In a systematic review of ADHD studies, the prevalence of ADHD in young athletes ranged from 4.2% to 14.1% [17]. In a report published annually by Major League Baseball in the United States, the annual number of players who received a Therapeutic Use Exemption (TUE) for ADHD ranged from 91 to 119 athletes from 2008 to 2019 (105–119 per year in 2008–2016, 103 in 2017, 101 in 2018, and 91 in 2019) [18,

19]. In a report by the National Football League, 8.1% of former players were described as suffering symptoms of ADHD [20].

Preliminarily, then, the prevalence of ADHD in the athlete population (4.2–14.1%) is higher than that observed in the general population (2.5–7.1%). While definite reasons for the high prevalence of ADHD among athletes have not been identified, some scholars believe that the positive reinforcing effect of physical activity that makes exercise rewarding in the ADHD population is a key factor [21].

Differential Diagnosis and Comorbidity of ADHD in Elite Athlete

In the general population, differential diagnosis and assessment of comorbidities in those with apparent ADHD are critical to diagnosis and treatment. Common comorbid conditions or those that mimic ADHD include major depressive disorder (MDD), bipolar disorders, anxiety and related disorders, intellectual and learning disorders, oppositional defiant disorder, autism spectrum disorder (ASD), substance use disorders, and concussion.

Individuals with ADHD and those with MDD are unable to concentrate. Differentiation of conditions is difficult when individuals with MDD display mild depressive symptoms and irritable behavior. However, individuals with MDD exhibit inattention only during depressive episodes, while individuals with ADHD are continuously inattentive.

Many clinicians have difficulty differentiating ADHD and bipolar disorder when assessing pediatric patients [22]. Features common to ADHD and bipolar disorder are irritability, hyperactivity, accelerated speech, increased activity, impulsivity, and distractibility [23]. However, individuals with bipolar disorder exhibit elevated mood and grandiosity in episodes that last a minimum of several days, while individuals with ADHD who display considerable mood changes—from elation to depression—do so within the same day.

Several genetic and neuropsychological studies suggest that ADHD and ASD are pathogenetically related. Individuals with ADHD and those with high functional ASD in particular share remarkably similar symptoms including inattention, social dysfunction, and behavioral outbursts. Individuals with ASD display behavioral outbursts and social dysfunction due to an inability to tolerate changes from their expected course of events, while individuals with ADHD reveal these symptoms as a result of impulsivity or poor self-control.

Concussions are frequently reported in athletes with ADHD. Individuals with a history of frequent concussion showed symptoms of poor concentration, possible memory deficit, regular fatigue, mood fluctuation, and anxiety [24–26]. McCrory et al. [27] reported that athletes with ADHD had a greater history of concussions than those without ADHD [27]. Moreover, ADHD may be associated with recovery delay following sport-related concussions in athletes [28]. Given the common and normative sport-related hyperactivity in athletes, clinicians should be cautious distinguishing ADHD from concussion [29].

The Effects of ADHD Symptoms on Sports Performance in Elite Athletes

Neurocognitive deficits and labile mood may be associated with a lack of focus and concentration, oppositional behavior, argumentative attitude, frustration, and lowered self-esteem. These symptoms negatively correlate with athletic performance [30]. Thus, poor focus, low tolerance of frustration in response to failure, low self-esteem, and frequent argumentativeness prohibit the effective performance of elite athletes. In addition to exercise performance, neurocognitive deficits including poor concentration and memory deficits influence the academic proficiency of student athletes with ADHD [30].

During complex sports play, athletes require implicit memory, distributive attention, and working memory. Implicit memory in adults with ADHD is relatively unaffected while explicit memory is impaired [31]. However, Pedersen and Ohmann [32] reported that adults with ADHD showed reduced efficiency in the inhibition of incorrect responses in implicit sequence learning. Implicit memory is related to the procedure of exercise.

Elite athletes require excellent distributive attention and working memory—features essential for effective performance during a game. Han, et al. [33] studied Korean professional baseball rookies over three seasons from 2009 to 2011. Elite players with a high draft ranking showed better working memory and distributive attention compared to players ranked in the lowest 30% of drafted players. Moreover, these players had increased activation in the frontal cortex in response to the working memory task.

Other comorbid conditions such as mood disorders, anxiety, and substance use disorders in ADHD may negatively affect sports performance [30]. Along with dysfunction in neurocognition and social relationships, patients with ADHD may display anxiety and unstable mood (which may or may not be part of a comorbid depressive disorder or bipolar disorder) [34, 35]. Regnart, et al. [36] observed that mood and substance use disorders or the co-occurrence of these disorders are commonly reported in adult athletes with ADHD [36]. Overlapping symptoms of these disorders create barriers to the accurate diagnosis and effective treatment of ADHD [37]. Emotional fluctuation or dysregulation are distinctive features in adults with ADHD, which can be misdiagnosed as a bipolar disorder or personality problems [37]. A meta-analysis of 71 studies in 18 countries suggested that

7.95% of adults with ADHD were also diagnosed with bipolar disorder, while 17.11% of adults with bipolar disorder were also diagnosed with ADHD [38].

In addition, medical doctors are not as familiar with ADHD in adults as they are with conditions such as mood and anxiety disorders. This lack of familiarity may lead to misdiagnosis, under-diagnosis, and under-treatment of ADHD in adult populations [38–40]. Conversely, clinicians should verify whether apparent bipolarity, emotional dysregulation, and anxiety in elite athletes result from undiagnosed and untreated ADHD [41].

ADHD symptoms affect the safety of individuals with the condition. High impulsivity and recklessness increase the risk of substance misuse and the incidence of traffic citations and vehicular accidents [14, 42]. Aggressive behavior in elite athletes with ADHD is occasionally misunderstood as a manifestation of substance use [41]. Serious ADHD symptoms and poor performance in attention tasks are associated with traffic violations, and ADHD symptoms are associated with traffic accidents [43]. In addition, adults with ADHD visit the emergency room and are hospitalized more frequently than healthy adults [44]. Thus, clinicians should consider the significant risks of ADHD to the overall health and safety of athletes.

The Reciprocal Effects of ADHD Characteristics and Sports

Several aspects of ADHD may be advantageous to athletic performance. The quick movements and reactive decision-making due to the inherent impulsivity characteristic of ADHD can positively impact performance in baseball and basketball [45].

Hyperfocus can occur in situations in which the athlete is goal-oriented, receives immediate feedback in response to activity stimulation, and performs without distraction from immaterial information [46, 47]. Individuals with ADHD "hyperfocus" on activities in which they are interested [48]. The hyperfocus trait allows elite athletes with ADHD to disregard irrelevant distractions during practice and competition. According to Hartmann's hunter theory of ADHD [49], the ADHD traits of hunter-gatherers—constant monitoring of the environment, flexibility, immediate responsiveness—are easily transferrable to sports, translating into elevated energy, effective monitoring of plays, and immediate reaction to stimuli [46].

Cognitive characteristics of ADHD may play an important role in deciding on a sports career during early development. Implicit procedure memory appears unaffected, while deficits in explicit memory are found in adults with ADHD [31, 50]. In the theory of the mind, explicit memory is associated with academic abilities [51]. Therefore, children with

ADHD seeking vocational fields in which they may be successful may consider sports because athletics require implicit procedure memory, while academic performance in school mainly requires explicit memory.

In personality studies, high novelty-seeking (NS) traits in individuals with ADHD are associated with superior performance in elite athletes [52]. In a cohort study of Korean professional baseball players including rookies to star players, elite players showed higher NS traits and reward dependence scores than general players [53]. Individuals with high temperamental traits of NS frequently show high impulsivity and hyperactivity, and display exhilaration and excitement in response to cues for potential rewards [54].

Several studies suggest that physical activity and sports improve ADHD symptoms including inattention, depressive mood, anxiety, and impaired cognition. Physical activity improves overall attitude and academic performance in adolescents [55]. Active participation in sports by children with ADHD can reduce anxiety and depressive symptoms [56], and control emotion and stress [57].

Brain imaging studies support the influence of sports on symptom improvement via changes in brain activity. Choi, et al. [58] observed that improved clinical symptoms of ADHD in response to routine exercises are associated with increased brain activity within the prefrontal cortex. In the clinical setting, the combination treatment of 6 weeks of exercise and medication treatment significantly increased brain activity within the prefrontal cortex in adolescents with ADHD [58]. In addition, equine-assisted physical training improved ADHD symptoms of inattention, unbalanced gait, and connectivity between the frontal lobe and the cerebellum in children with ADHD [45].

ADHD Treatment in Elite Athletes

The treatment of ADHD is generally divided into two domains: psychosocial interventions and medication. Stimulant medication with or without psychosocial intervention is commonly the first-line treatment for ADHD. However, sports clinicians and other healthcare providers insist that psychosocial intervention should be the foundation of medical management, if necessary [21, 59]. Psychosocial intervention has similar effects to medications for athletes with mild functional impairment [60]. Some clinicians recommend psychosocial interventions as an alternative to medication for athletes with ADHD [61–63].

The age and educational level of athletes with ADHD should be considered when applying psychosocial intervention. Types of psychosocial interventions include behavioral therapy, cognitive behavioral therapy, and psychoeducation [64]. Cognitive behavioral therapies include brief group therapy, metacognitive therapy, and group rehabilitation [65–67].

Dialectical behavioral group therapy is a form of cognitive behavioral therapy that consists of modules covering interpersonal skills, tolerance of discomfort, regulation of emotions, and mindfulness [68]. Psychosocial intervention is important because individuals with ADHD face challenges and dysfunction in daily life, including in academic performance and behavior at school, and in relationships with peers and family members.

Preliminary studies suggest that neurofeedback or biofeedback using an electroencephalogram is an alternative in the management of ADHD symptoms in those experiencing adverse effects from medications. However, the biological mechanism of neurofeedback is not fully understood, and this modality is not supported by evidence in athletes [69].

Pharmacological management for ADHD consists of stimulants and nonstimulants. Stimulants are the primary pharmacological treatment for ADHD in the general population and in elite athletes [21, 62]. Stimulants work via the activation of dopamine and noradrenergic systems, which are responsible for improving attention and concentration [70]. Most stimulants have a rapid 1-h onset, while duration of action varies depending on formulation. Stimulants can cause side effects that interfere with athletic performance and produce symptoms—such as increased heart rate and blood pressure, abdominal pain, headache, anorexia, weight loss, nervousness, and constipation—that can threaten the athlete's safety [70, 71]. Occasionally, sudden death from cardiac arrest due to a lowered threshold for cardiac arrhythmias has been described in elite athletes taking stimulants [72]. Clinicians should be careful to verify personal and family history of cardiac symptoms, and should monitor blood pressure and heart rate before starting stimulant medications while also ensuring a sufficient follow-up period with repeat measurements of blood pressure and heart rate. Additionally, athletes prescribed stimulants must be vigilant when participating in endurance events in hot temperatures due to the increased risk of heat illness [73]. Stimulants interfere with thermoregulation, with a higher core temperature increasing the risk of sudden death [74].

Athletes with ADHD taking stimulants experience side effects comparable to those observed in the general ADHD population. Side effects beyond those potentially impacting safety as described above, and which may further impact sports performance, include: lack of creativity, lack of spontaneity, palpitations, sweating, and irritability [75]. Stimulants frequently cause sleep disturbance [76], which leads to several negative effects on sports performance including skill execution, submaximal strength, muscular and anaerobic power weakness, easy fatigue, and delayed decision-making [77].

Stimulants are occasionally used off-label by athletes for nonmedical reasons such as performance enhancement and weight loss [78, 79]. Similar to other ergogenic aids, stimulants mask the symptoms of fatigue [80]. Some athletes competing in sports that require leanness or include weight classes abuse stimulants to lose weight or to secure a performance advantage [29, 75]. A recent study reported a stimulant misuse rate of 17% among college students [81]. The misuse of stimulants can increase the risk of psychosis, seizure, and cardiovascular crisis [82].

To ensure safety and prevent misuse, a TUE for a stimulant prescription for athletes in most elite sport settings must be requested and approved [83]. For convenience of use and prevention of misuse, long-acting formulations should be considered as first-line therapy [60, 61]. The slower fluctuation of medication blood levels in long-acting formulations may contribute to a decrease in the risk of drug misuse [84].

Nonstimulants may also be considered when an athlete requires medication for ADHD [29, 61, 75]. Nonstimulants include atomoxetine, bupropion, clonidine, and guanfacine.

Atomoxetine is the first-line medication for ADHD treatment among sports psychiatrists, presumably because of fewer regulations and safety concerns compared to stimulants [29]. Atomoxetine selectively inhibits norepinephrine transporters to increase the concentration of norepinephrine and dopamine in synapses within the prefrontal cortex [85]. As with stimulants, atomoxetine can cause side effects, specifically for this medication including increase in blood pressure and heart rate, nausea, decreased appetite, weight loss, sedation, acute liver injury, and increased suicidality [86]. In addition, atomoxetine takes a significantly longer time before providing a clinical effect compared to stimulants [29].

Bupropion is an antidepressant that works via dopamine and norepinephrine reuptake inhibition and is occasionally used off-label for ADHD [21, 87]. Limited evidence is available regarding the effectiveness of bupropion in improving ADHD symptoms [87]. The alpha-2 agonists clonidine and guanfacine have shown superiority over placebo in the treatment of ADHD [88]. Monotherapy with both drugs improved hyperactivity, impulsivity, inattention, and comorbid oppositional defiant disorder symptoms in individuals with ADHD [89]. However, possible side effects include sedation and cardiac side effects such as hypotension, bradycardia, and QTc prolongation [89, 90].

Conclusion

ADHD is a common neurodevelopmental disorder in elite athletes, with few studies reporting the precise prevalence in athletes. ADHD symptoms may negatively affect sports performance, and the condition may play a salient role in the choice of both a career in sports and competition at elite levels. The management of ADHD should focus on psychosocial interventions with or without medication to optimize short- and long-term outcomes for elite athletes in sports and in life.

References

1. Thomas R, Sanders S, Doust J, et al. Prevalence of attention-deficit/hyperactivity disorder: a systematic review and meta-analysis. Pediatrics. 2015;135(4):e994–1001. https://doi.org/10.1542/peds.2014-3482.
2. MacLean L, Prabhakar D. Attention-deficit/hyperactivity disorder and sports: a lifespan perspective. Psychiatr Clin N Am. 2021;44:419–30.
3. American Psychiatry Association. Diagnostic statistical manual of mental disorders. 5th ed. Arlington, VA: American Psychiatric Association; 2013.
4. Willcutt EG, Doyle AE, Nigg JT, et al. Validity of the executive function theory of attention-deficit/hyperactivity disorder: a meta-analytic review. Biol Psychiatry. 2005;57(11):1336–46.
5. Moulahoum H, Zihnioglu F, Timur S, et al. Novel technologies in detection, treatment and prevention of substance use disorders. J Food Drug Anal. 2019;27(1):22–31.
6. Aylward EH, Reiss AL, Reader MJ, et al. Basal ganglia volumes in children with attention-deficit hyperactivity disorder. J Child Neurol. 1996;11(2):112–5.
7. Wyciszkiewicz A, Pawlak MA, Krawiec K. Cerebellar volume in children with attention-deficit hyperactivity disorder (ADHD). J Child Neurol. 2017;32(2):215–21.
8. Mahone EM, Crocetti D, Ranta ME, et al. A preliminary neuroimaging study of preschool children with ADHD. Clin Neuropsychol. 2011;25(6):1009–28.
9. Castellanos FX, Aoki Y. Intrinsic functional connectivity in attention-deficit/hyperactivity disorder: a science in development. Biol Psychiatry Cogn Neurosci Neuroimaging. 2016;1:253–61.
10. Kelly C, Biswal BB, Craddock RC, Castellanos FX, Milham MP. Characterizing variation in the functional connectome: promise and pitfalls. Trends Cogn Sci. 2012;16:181–8.
11. Shaw P, Eckstrand K, Sharp W, et al. Attention-deficit/hyperactivity disorder is characterized by a delay in cortical maturation. Proc Natl Acad Sci U S A. 2007;104(49):19649–54.
12. Polanczyk G, de Lima MS, Horta BL, Biederman J, Rohde LA. The worldwide prevalence of ADHD: a systematic review and meta regression analysis. Am J Psychiatry. 2007;164(6):942–8. https://doi.org/10.1176/ajp.2007.164.6.942.
13. Doernberg E, Hollander E. Neurodevelopmental disorders (ASD and ADHD): DSM-5, ICD-10, and ICD-11. CNS Spectr. 2016;21(4):295–9. https://doi.org/10.1017/s1092852916000262.
14. Agnew-Blais JC, Polanczyk GV, Danese A, Wertz J, Moffitt TE, Arseneault L. Evaluation of the persistence, remission, and emergence of attention-deficit/hyperactivity disorder in young adulthood. JAMA Psychiatry. 2016;73(7):713–20. https://doi.org/10.1001/jamapsychiatry.2016.0465.
15. Faraone SV, Biederman J, Mick E. The age-dependent decline of attention deficit hyperactivity disorder: a meta-analysis of follow-up studies. Psychol Med. 2006;36(2):159–65. https://doi.org/10.1017/s003329170500471x.
16. Agnew-Blais JC, Polanczyk GV, Danese A, Wertz J, Moffitt TE, Arseneault L. Are changes in ADHD course reflected in differences in IQ and executive functioning from childhood to young adulthood? Psychol Med. 2019;50:2799–808. https://doi.org/10.1017/s0033291719003015.
17. Poysophon P, Rao AL. Neurocognitive deficits associated with ADHD in athletes: a systematic review. Sports Health. 2018;10(4):317–26.
18. Martin T. Public report of major league baseball's joint drug prevention and treatment program. 2018. http://www.mlb.com/documents/3/8/2/301315382/IPA_2018_Public_Report_113018.pdf.
19. USA Today. Exemptions for ADHD drugs in MLB drop to lowest in decade. USA Today. 2019. (National Ed.). https://www.usatoday.

com/story/sports/mlb/2019/11/29/exemptions-for-adhd-drugs-in-mlb-drop-to-lowest-in-decade/40727985/.

20. Plessow F, Pascual-Leone A, McCracken CM, Baker J, Krishnan S, Baggish A, Connor A, Courtney TK, Nadler LM, Speizer FE, Taylor HA, Weisskopf MG, Zafonte RD, Meehan WP III. Self-reported cognitive function and mental health diagnoses among former professional american-style football players. J Neurotrauma. 2020;37(8):1021–8. https://doi.org/10.1089/neu.2019.6661.

21. Putukian M, Kreher JB, Coppel DB, Glazer JL, McKeag DB, White RD. Attention deficit hyperactivity disorder and the athlete: an American Medical Society for Sports Medicine position statement. Clin J Sport Med. 2011;2:392–400.

22. Kowatch R, Monroe E, Delgado S. Not all mood swings are bipolar disorder. Curr Psychiatry. 2011;10(2):38–52.

23. Geller B, Williams M, Zimerman B, et al. Prepubertal and early adolescent bipolarity differentiate from ADHD by manic symptoms, grandiose delusions, ultra–rapid or ultradian cycling. J Affect Disord. 1998;51(2):81–91. https://doi.org/10.1016/S0165-0327(98)00175-X.

24. Harmon KG, Drezner JA, Gammons M, et al. American Medical Society for Sports Medicine position statement: concussion in sport. Br J Sports Med. 2013;47(1):15–26.

25. Nelson LD, Guskiewicz KM, Marshall SW, et al. Multiple self-reported concussions are more prevalent in athletes with ADHD and learning disability. Clin J Sport Med. 2016;26(2):120–7.

26. Williams WH, Potter S, Ryland H. Mild traumatic brain injury and post-concussion Syndrome: a neuropsychological perspective. J Neurol Neurosurg Psychiatry. 2010;81(10):1116–22.

27. McCrory P, Meeuwisse W, Johnston K, et al. Consensus statement on Concussion in Sport 3rd International Conference on Concussion in Sport held in Zurich, November 2008. Clin J Sport Med. 2009;19(3):185–200.

28. Esfandiari A, Broshek DK, Freeman JR. Psychiatric and neuropsychological issues in sports medicine. Clin Sports Med. 2011;30(3):611–27.

29. Reardon CL, Factor RM. Considerations in the use of stimulants in sport. Sports Med. 2016;46(5):611–7.

30. White RD, Harris GD, Gibson ME. Attention deficit hyperactivity disorder and athletes. Sports Health. 2014;6(2):149–56.

31. Pollak Y, Kahana-Vax G, Hoofien D. Retrieval processes in adults with ADHD: a RAVLT study. Dev Neuropsychol. 2008;33(1):62–73.

32. Pedersen A, Ohrmann P. Impaired behavioral inhibition in implicit sequence learning in adult ADHD. J Atten Disord. 2018;22(3):250–60.

33. Han DH, Kim BN, Cheong JH, et al. Anxiety and attention shifting in professional baseball players. Int J Sports Med. 2014;35(8):708–13.

34. Ginsberg Y, Hirvikoski T, Lindefors N. Attention Deficit Hyperactivity Disorder (ADHD) among longer-term prison inmates is a prevalent, persistent and disabling disorder. BMC Psychiatry. 2010;10:112.

35. Spencer T, Biederman J, Wilens T, et al. A large, double-blind, randomized clinical trial of methylphenidate in the treatment of adults with attention-deficit/hyperactivity disorder. Biol Psychiatry. 2005;57(5):456–63.

36. Regnart J, Truter I, Meyer A. Critical exploration of co-occurring attention-deficit/hyperactivity disorder, mood disorder and substance use disorder. Exp Rev Pharmacoecon Outc Res. 2017;17(3):275–82.

37. Barkley RA, Brown TE. Unrecognized attention-deficit/hyperactivity disorder in adults presenting with other psychiatric disorders. CNS Spectr. 2008;13(11):977–8.

38. Schiweck C, et al. Comorbidity of ADHD and adult bipolar disorder: a systematic review and meta-analysis. Neurosci Biobehav Rev. 2021;124:100. PMID: 33515607.

39. McIntosh D, Kutcher S, Binder C, et al. Adult ADHD and comorbid depression: a consensus-derived diagnostic algorithm for ADHD. Neuropsychiatr Dis Treat. 2009;5:137–50.

40. Caye A, Rocha TB, Anselmi L, et al. Attention-deficit/hyperactivity disorder trajectories from childhood to young adulthood: evidence from a birth cohort supporting a late-onset syndrome. JAMA Psychiatry. 2016;73(7):705–12.

41. Alexander SJ, Harrison AG. Cognitive responses to stress, depression, and anxiety and their relationship to ADHD symptoms in first year psychology students. J Atten Disord. 2013;17(1):29–37.

42. Barkley RA, Murphy KR, Dupaul GI, et al. Driving in young adults with attention deficit hyperactivity disorder: knowledge, performance, adverse outcomes, and the role of executive functioning. J Int Neuropsychol Soc. 2002;8(5):655–72.

43. Zamani Sani SH, Fathirezaie Z, Sadeghi-Bazargani H, Badicu G, Ebrahimi S, Grosz RW, Sadeghi Bahmani D, Brand S. Driving accidents, driving violations, symptoms of attention-deficit-hyperactivity (ADHD) and attentional network tasks. Int J Environ Res Public Health. 2020;17(14):5238. https://doi.org/10.3390/ijerph17145238.

44. Kirino E, Imagawa H, Goto T, et al. Comorbidities, healthcare utilization and work productivity in Japanese patients with adult ADHD. PLoS One. 2015;10(7):e0132233.

45. Parr JW. Attention-deficit hyperactivity disorder and the athlete: new advances and understanding. Clin Sports Med. 2011;30(3):591–610.

46. Brown TE. Attention deficit disorder: the unfocused mind in children and adults. New Haven, CT: Yale University Press; 2005.

47. Conner ML. Attention deficit disorder in children and adults: strategies for experiential educators. In: Experiential Education: A Critical Resource for the 21st Century, Proceedings Manual of the Annual International Conference of the Association for Experiential Education. Austin, TX, USA, 3–6 November 1994, vol. 22; 1994. p. 177–82. https://files.eric.ed.gov/fulltext/ED377013.pdf. Accessed 5 Feb 2021.

48. Hupfeld KE, Abagis TR, Shah P. Living "in the zone": hyperfocus in adult ADHD. Atten Defic Hyperac Disord. 2019;11:209.

49. Hartmann T. Attention deficit disorder: a different perception. Grass Valley, CA: Underwood Books; 1993.

50. Takacs A, Shilon Y, Janacsek K, et al. Procedural learning in Tourette syndrome, ADHD, and comorbid Tourette-ADHD: evidence from a probabilistic sequence learning task. Brain Cogn. 2017;117:33–40.

51. Vierkant T. Self-knowledge and knowing other minds: the implicit/explicit distinction as a tool in understanding theory of mind. Br J Dev Psychol. 2012;30(Pt 1):141–55.

52. Perroud N, Hasler R, Golay N, et al. Personality profiles in adults with attention deficit hyperactivity disorder (ADHD). BMC Psychiatry. 2016;16:199.

53. Kang KD, Han DH, Hannon JC, et al. Temperamental predictive factors for success in Korean professional baseball players. Psychiatry Investig. 2015;12(4):459–65.

54. Cloninger CR. A systematic method for clinical description and classification of personality variants. A proposal. Arch Gen Psychiatry. 1987;44(6):573–88.

55. Nazeer A, Mansour M, Gross KA. ADHD and adolescent athletes. Front Public Health. 2014;2:1–7.

56. Kiluk BD, Weden S, Culotta VP. Sport participation and anxiety in children with ADHD. J Atten Disord. 2009;12(6):499–506.

57. McKune AJ, Pautz J, Lombard J. Behavioural response to exercise in children with attention-deficit/hyperactivity disorder. S Afr J Sports Med. 2003;15(3):17–21.

58. Choi JW, Han DH, Kang KD, Jung HY, Renshaw PF. Aerobic exercise and attention deficit hyperactivity disorder: brain research. Med Sci Sports Exerc. 2015;47(1):33–9.

59. Seixas M, Weiss M, Muller U. Systematic review of national and international guidelines on attention-deficit hyperactivity disorder. J Psychopharmacol. 2012;26(6):753–65.
60. Reardon CL, Creado S. Psychiatric medication preferences of sports psychiatrists. Phys Sportsmed. 2016;44(4):397–402.
61. Perrin AE, Jotwani VM. Addressing the unique issues of student athletes with ADHD. J Fam Pract. 2014;63(5):E1–9.
62. Stewman CG, Liebman C, Fink L, et al. Attention deficit hyperactivity disorder: unique considerations in athletes. Sports Health. 2018;10(1):40–6.
63. Pelham WE, Burrows-Maclean L, Gnagy EM, et al. Transdermal methylphenidate, behavioral, and combined treatment for children with ADHD. Exp Clin Psychopharmacol. 2005;13(2):111–26.
64. Wolraich M, Brown L, Brown RT, et al. ADHD: clinical practice guideline for the diagnosis, evaluation, and treatment of attention-deficit/hyperactivity disorder in children and adolescents. Pediatrics. 2011;128(5):1007–22.
65. Wiggins D, Singh K, Getz HG, et al. Effects of brief group intervention for adults with attention deficit/hyperactivity disorder. J Ment Health Couns. 1999;21(1):82–93.
66. Solanto MV, Marks DJ, Mitchell KJ, Wasserstein J, Kofman MD. Development of a new psychosocial treatment for adult ADHD. J Atten Disord. 2008;11(6):728–36.
67. Virta M, Vedenpaa A, Gronroos N, Chydenius E, Partinen M, Vataja R, et al. Adults with ADHD benefit from cognitive-behaviorally oriented group rehabilitation: a study of 29 participants. J Atten Disord. 2008;12(3):218–26.
68. Hesslinger B, Tebartz van Elst L, Nyberg E, et al. Psychotherapy of attention deficit hyperactivity disorder in adults-a pilot study using a structured skills training program. Eur Arch Psychiatry Clin Neurosci. 2002;252(4):177–84.
69. Razoki B. Neurofeedback versus psychostimulants in the treatment of children and adolescents with attention–deficit/hyperactivity disorder: a systematic review. Neuropsychiatr Dis Treat. 2018;14:2905–13.
70. Bezchlibnyk-Butler KZ, Jeffries JJ, Procyshyn RM. Clinical handbook of psychotropic drugs. Göttingen: Hogrefe Publishing; 2012.
71. Hamilton RM, Rosenthal E, Hulpke-Wette M, et al. Cardiovascular considerations of attention deficit hyperactivity disorder medications: a report of the European Network on Hyperactivity Disorders work group, European Attention Deficit Hyperactivity Disorder Guidelines Group on attention deficit hyperactivity disorder drug safety meeting. Cardiol Young. 2012;22(1):63–70.
72. Drezner JA, O'Connor FG, Harmon KG, et al. AMSSM position statement on cardiovascular preparticipation screening in athletes: current evidence, knowledge gaps, recommendations, and future directions. Clin J Sport Med. 2016;26(5):347–61.
73. Howe AS, Boden BP. Heat-related illness in athletes. Am J Sports Med. 2007;35(8):1384–95.
74. May DE, Kratochvil CJ. Attention-deficit hyperactivity disorder: recent advances in paediatric pharmacotherapy. Drugs. 2010;70(1):15–40.
75. Conant-Norville DO, Tofler IR. Attention deficit/hyperactivity disorder and psychopharmacologic treatments in the athlete. Clin Sports Med. 2005;24(4):829–43, viii.
76. Becker SP, Froehlich TE, Epstein JN. Effects of methylphenidate on sleep functioning in children with attention-deficit/hyperactivity disorder. J Dev Behav Pediatr. 2016;37(5):395–404.
77. Fullagar HHK, Skorski S, Duffield R, et al. Sleep and athletic performance: the effects of sleep loss on exercise performance, and psychological and cognitive response to exercise. Sports Med. 2015;45:161–86.
78. Veliz P, Boyd C, McCabe SE. Adolescent athletic participation and nonmedical Adderall use: an exploratory analysis of a performance-enhancing drug. J Stud Alcohol Drugs. 2013;74(5):714–9.
79. Greydanus DE, Patel DR. Sports doping in the adolescent athlete the hope, hype, and hyperbole. Pediatr Clin N Am. 2002;49(4):829–55.
80. Jacobs I, Bell DG. Effects of acute modafinil ingestion on exercise time to exhaustion. Med Sci Sports Exerc. 2004;36(6):1078–82.
81. Benson K, Flory K, Humphreys KL, et al. Misuse of stimulant medication among college students: a comprehensive review and meta-analysis. Clin Child Fam Psychol Rev. 2015;18:50–76.
82. Lakhan SE, Kirchgessner A. Prescription stimulants in individuals with and without attention deficit hyperactivity disorder: misuse, cognitive impact, and adverse effects. Brain Behav. 2012;2(5):661–77.
83. World Anti-Doping Agency (WADA). World anti-doping agency prohibited list. Montreal, QC: WADA; 2019. https://www.usada.org/substances/prohibited-list.
84. Swanson J, Gupta S, Lam A, et al. Development of a new once-a-day formulation of methylphenidate for the treatment of attention-deficit/hyperactivity disorder: proof-of-concept and proof-of-product studies. Arch Gen Psychiatry. 2003;60(2):204–11.
85. Savill NC, Buitelaar JK, Anand E, et al. The efficacy of atomoxetine for the treatment of children and adolescents with attention-deficit/hyperactivity disorder: a comprehensive review of over a decade of clinical research. CNS Drugs. 2015;29:131–51.
86. Fredriksen M, Halmoy A, Faraone SV, et al. Long-term efficacy and safety of treatment with stimulants and atomoxetine in adult ADHD: a review of controlled and naturalistic studies. Eur Neuropsychopharmacol. 2013;23:508–27.
87. Verbeeck W, Bekkering GE, Van den Noortgate W, et al. Bupropion for attention deficit hyperactivity disorder (ADHD) in adults. Cochrane Database Syst Rev. 2017;10:CD009504.
88. Naguy A. Clonidine use in psychiatry: panacea or panache. Pharmacology. 2016;98(1–2):87–92.
89. Hirota T, Schwartz S, Correll CU. Alpha-2 agonists for attention-deficit/hyperactivity disorder in youth: a systematic review and meta-analysis of monotherapy and add-on trials to stimulant therapy. J Am Acad Child Adolesc Psychiatry. 2014;53(2):153–73.
90. Joo SW, Kim HW. Treatment of children and adolescents with attention deficit hyperactivity disorder and/or Tourette's disorder with clonidine extended release. Psychiatry Investig. 2018;15(1):90–3.

Personality Disorders

11

Carla Edwards

Introduction

Many elements related to personality have been extensively described in psychological, psychiatric, and sports performance literature. Personality theory has been explored through writings by historical philosophers such as Hippocrates (460–370 BCE) and Galen (129–199 CE) as well as by modern researchers and clinicians [1]. While most concepts of personality describe consistent and stable elements spanning cognitive, affective, and behavioral domains, there are subtle differences that distinguish them. Several of these concepts will be briefly explored as this chapter delves deeper into the dimension of personality disorders in sports.

It is helpful to have an understanding of the definitions of and salient points regarding several relevant terms before proceeding through the rest of this chapter:

- **Personality:** defined by the American Psychiatric Association (APA) as the way of thinking, feeling, and behaving that makes a person different from another person. It is influenced by the individual's genetic factors, environment, and experiences [2].
- **Personality traits:** reflect a person's characteristic pattern of thoughts, feelings, and behaviors. The Five-Factor Model of personality traits is a widely used system that implies where a person stands on a basic set of trait dimensions persisting over time and across situations. It identifies five broad categories that capture most character traits, including openness, conscientiousness, extraversion, agreeableness, and neuroticism (referred to as the acronym OCEAN). Each dimension also encompasses a number of more specific facets [3]. Other models describe additional main personality traits (including the HEXACO model, which adds honesty-humility as a sixth dimension). Critics of personality trait models argue that individuals do not act consistently from one situation to the next and are influenced by external factors [4].
- **Personality construct:** an important concept in understanding and defining the influence of an individual's core character, temperament, belief systems, and experiences on their interpretations, reactions, and relationships. It is further defined as an abstraction that is inferred through observations regarding cognitive, affective, and behavioral responses in various settings [5, 6].
- **Personality disorder:** a persistent way of thinking, feeling, and behaving that deviates from the expectations of an individual's culture and causes distress or functional impairment [7].

A deeper understanding of how personality elements impact an athlete's development, relationships, interactions, and performance can potentially allow the athlete, coach, or athlete support personnel to optimize supports and approaches to training.

A Diagnostic Challenge

Due to the abstract nature of personality, historical debate has challenged methods of measurement, characterization of pathology, and thresholds for establishing diagnoses. Major organizations involved with defining and classifying diseases have disagreed on nomenclature and thresholds for identification of disorders. The American Psychiatric Association's Diagnostic and Statistical Manual of Mental Disorders 5th edition (DSM-5) describes the general concept of personality disorders and further defines criteria for ten specific personality disorders (grouped according to similar features) [7].

Additional categories capture personality change due to another medical condition and other situations in which symptoms are impairing but do not fully satisfy the criteria of a specific disorder. The DSM-5 criteria for General Personality Disorder are listed in Fig. 11.1, while the clusters and specific personality disorders are listed in Fig. 11.2.

C. Edwards (✉)
Department of Psychiatry and Behavioral Neurosciences,
McMaster University, Hamilton, ON, Canada
e-mail: edwardcd@mcmaster.ca

A. An enduring pattern of inner experience and behavior that deviates markedly from the expectations of the individual's culture. This pattern is manifested in two (or more) of the following areas:

    1. Cognition (i.e., ways of perceiving and interpreting self, other people, and events)

    2. Affectivity (i.e., the range, intensity, liability, and appropriateness of emotional response)

    3. Interpersonal functioning

    4. Impulse control

B. The enduring pattern is inflexible and pervasive across a broad range of personal and social situations.

C. The enduring pattern leads to clinically significant distress or impairment in social, occupational, or other important areas of functioning.

D. The pattern is stable and of long duration, and its onset can be traced back at least to adolescence or early adulthood.

E. The enduring pattern is not better accounted for as a manifestation or consequence of another mental disorder.

F. The enduring pattern is not due to the direct physiological effects of a substance (e.g., a drug of abuse, a medication) or a general medical condition (e.g., head trauma).

Fig. 11.1 Diagnostic and Statistical Manual of Mental Disorders 5th edition diagnostic criteria for general personality disorder [7]

The International Statistical Classification of Diseases and Related Health Problems (11th edition; ICD-11; World Health Organization, 2019) approaches identification and classification of personality disorders according to dimensions of severity applied to a general description of a personality disorder. According to the ICD-11, to satisfy diagnostic criteria for a personality disorder, an individual must demonstrate problems in interpersonal relationships and functional impairment, which is further specified as "mild," "moderate," or "severe" based on descriptions of degrees of severity [8]. The ICD-11 criteria for General Personality Disorder and its related specifiers are listed in Fig. 11.3 [9]. The ICD-11 also introduced a new descriptive concept called "personality difficulty," which captures problems associated with interpersonal interactions but does not surpass the impairment severity threshold to be considered a disorder. Personality difficulty is manifested in "cognitive and emotional experience and expression only intermittently or at low intensity" and is not considered a diagnosis. The defined threshold for personality difficulty is one criterion less than the cut-off for personality disorder as measured on the Structural Clinical Interview for DSM-IV Avis II (SCID II). Although personality difficulty is conceptualized as less impairing than a personality disorder, it is not a benign state. In the UK National Morbidity study, which assessed 8400 individuals for personality pathology and mental health, nearly half of the respondents (48.3%) fulfilled criteria for personality difficulty [10]. According to study results, this population was more likely to seek visits with their general practitioners and mental health workers, attend a community medical center, or be admitted to a mental hospital. Although the study did not focus on the athlete population, findings suggest that a significant percentage of individuals experience intermittent or low-intensity difficulties related to features of their personalities. The global incidence of personality disorders has been reported as 5–12% [11, 12].

While personality features are expressed by the individual, they are experienced by everyone in the environment. As individual as one's own personality construct is, so is the interpretation of the expression of those personality features by others who are, in turn, influenced by their own personality constructs. These social transactions can be experienced positively or negatively, potentially influenced by whether the personality constructs of the individuals are concordant ("agreeable") or discordant ("disagreeable"). With the multitude of personality features, styles, and constructs that are

Fig. 11.2 Diagnostic and Statistical Manual of Mental Disorders 5th edition personality disorder clusters and specific personality disorders with brief descriptions [7]

Cluster A: the "odd, eccentric" cluster

Paranoid Personality Disorder: a pervasive distrust and suspiciousness of others such that their motives are interpreted as malevolent, beginning by early adulthood and present in a variety of contexts.

Schizoid Personality Disorder: a pervasive pattern of detachment from social relationships and a restricted range of expressions of emotions in interpersonal settings, beginning by early adulthood and present in a variety of contexts.

Schizotypal Personality Disorder: a pervasive pattern of social and interpersonal deficits marked by acute discomfort with, and reduced capacity for, close relationships as well as by cognitive or perceptual distortions and eccentricities of behavior, beginning by early adulthood and present in a variety of contexts.

Cluster B: the "dramatic, emotional, erratic" cluster

Antisocial Personality Disorder: a pervasive pattern of disregard for and violation of the rights of others, occurring since the age of 15 years, and further defined with additional elements of behavior, affect, and cognitive elements that reflect deviation from societal norms and expectations. An individual must be at least 18 years of age to receive this diagnosis.

Borderline Personality Disorder: a pervasive pattern of instability of interpersonal relationships, self-image, and affects, and marked impulsivity, beginning by early adulthood and present in a variety of contexts. Additional criteria further define specific challenges with cognition, affect, and behaviour that significantly impact interpersonal relationships and function.

Histrionic Personality Disorder: a pervasive pattern of excessive emotionality and attention-seeking, beginning by early adulthood and present in a variety of contexts.

Narcissistic Personality Disorder: a pervasive pattern of grandiosity (in fantasy or behavior), need for admiration, and lack of empathy, beginning by early adulthood and present in a variety of contexts.

Cluster C: the "anxious, fearful" cluster

Avoidant Personality Disorder: a pervasive pattern of social inhibition, feelings of inadequacy, and hypersensitivity to negative evaluation, beginning by early adulthood and present in a variety of contexts.

Dependent Personality Disorder: a pervasive and excessive need to be taken care of that leads to submissive and clinging behavior and fears of separation, beginning by early adulthood and present in a variety of contexts.

Obsessive-Compulsive Personality Disorder: a pervasive pattern of preoccupation with orderliness, perfection, and mental and interpersonal control, at the expense of flexibility, openness, and efficiency, beginning by early adulthood and present in a variety of contexts.

present within the sports world, there are many opportunities for personality differences or challenges to cause disruption.

Personality disorders are specific diagnoses that are made following clinical evaluation and consideration of multiple facets of an individual's internal and interpersonal experience, while exploring historic and current cognitive, affective (emotional), behavioral, and relational aspects of perception and function. Specific screening instruments exist for elucidation of diagnostic criteria for the ICD-11/DSM-5 Personality disorders (aligned with the DSM-5 Alternative Model for Personality Disorders), and other versions exist for specific DSM-IV personality disorders [13, 14]. While several high-profile athletes have openly disclosed their diagnoses, most challenges in personality are inferred based on patterns of interaction or behavior either observed or experienced.

Fig. 11.3 International Classification of Diseases for Mortality and Morbidity Statistics (11th revision) personality disorder description, specifiers, and personality trait domain qualifiers [9]

Personality disorder is characterised by problems in functioning of aspects of the self (e.g., identity, self-worth, accuracy of self-view, self-direction), and/or interpersonal dysfunction (e.g., ability to develop and maintain close and mutually satisfying relationships, ability to understand others' perspectives and to manage conflict in relationships) that have persisted over an extended period of time (e.g., 2 years or more). The disturbance is manifest in patterns of cognition, emotional experience, emotional expression, and behaviour that are maladaptive (e.g., inflexible or poorly regulated) and is manifest across a range of personal and social situations (i.e., is not limited to specific relationships or social roles). The patterns of behaviour characterizing the disturbance are not developmentally appropriate and cannot be explained primarily by social or cultural factors, including socio-political conflict. The disturbance is associated with substantial distress or significant impairment in personal, family, social, educational, occupational or other important areas of functioning.

Mild: Specific manifestations of personality disturbances are generally of mild severity. Mild Personality Disorder is typically not associated with substantial harm to self or others, but may be associated with substantial distress or with impairment in personal, family, social, educational, occupational or other important areas of functioning that is either limited to circumscribed areas (e.g., romantic relationships; employment) or present in more areas but milder.

Moderate: Specific manifestations of personality disturbance are generally of moderate severity. Moderate Personality Disorder is sometimes associated with harm to self or others, and is associated with marked impairment in personal, family, social, educational, occupational or other important areas of functioning, although functioning in circumscribed areas may be maintained.

Severe: There are severe disturbances in functioning of the self (e.g., sense of self may be so unstable that individuals report not having a sense of who they are or so rigid that they refuse to participate in any but an extremely narrow range of situations; self view may be characterised by self-contempt or be grandiose or highly eccentric). Problems in interpersonal functioning seriously affect virtually all relationships and the ability and willingness to perform expected social and occupational roles is absent or severely compromised. Specific manifestations of personality disturbance are severe and affect most, if not all, areas of personality functioning. Severe Personality Disorder is often associated with harm to self or others and is associated with severe impairment in all or nearly all areas of life, including personal, family, social, educational, occupational, and other important areas of functioning.

Personality Trait qualifiers:

Negative affectivity
Detachment
Disinhibition
Dissociality
Anankastia
Borderline pattern

Personality Applications in Sports

At the core of the effort and skill they bring to their sports, athletes, and coaches are human beings. They enter their sports journey with the genetic influences with which they were born and a history of life experiences outside of sports, including family, relationships, losses, hardships, triumphs, and various sources of adversity. Personality development is informed by these experiences, and sports can have an influential role if the individual is actively involved in sports during their formative years, when the child experiences rapid cognitive, social, emotional, and physical development.

Longitudinal studies have explored the influence of genetic and environmental factors on personality development and stability. While genetic factors have been identified as important for maintaining personality stability throughout the lifespan, unique environmental factors act to promote personality change [15]. Research suggests that personality is more variable throughout childhood and adolescence, and

personality continuity may plateau in early adulthood [16, 17]. These elements are important in application to sports if sport participation is considered an environmental influence on personality development or conversely if personality influences sport participation.

In addition to the influence of sports on the development and consolidation of an athlete's personality features, research has explored the personality traits that are found most frequently in successful athletes. Information gathered from such research may inform the "type" of athlete that is selected to a team or may guide coaching and mental performance strategies applied to training and competition. A sample of elite male athletes from Poland suggested that athletes who had attained the highest levels of success demonstrated lower levels of neuroticism, higher levels of extraversion, and higher levels of openness to experiences and conscientiousness according to the Five-Factor Model [18, 19]. Professional athletes have been found to have higher levels of self-esteem, sensation-seeking, and mental health as compared to amateur athletes, and differences have been reported in the personality characteristics of athletes who compete in individual and team sports [20]. One study demonstrated that athletes from individual sports scored significantly higher on measures of conscientiousness and autonomy, while team sports athletes scored higher on measures of agreeableness and sociotropy (defined as the tendency to place an inordinate value on relationships over personal independence) [21, 22].

Factors contributing to "positive personality" in Olympic athletes, which is conceptually related to resilience, are potentially protective against the exceptional stressors that this population faces [23, 24].

These factors include motivation, confidence, focus, perceived social support, and subsequent ability to positively adapt within the context of significant adversity [25]. Further relationships between resilience and personality are suggested with the recognized differences in individual responses to stress and adversity, and the conceptualization that the capacity for resilience develops over time in the context of interactions between the person and their environment [23, 26, 27].

Personality Disorders in Sports

While the Psychology literature has explored the influence of personality traits on athletic performance, success, and relationships, research exploring personality *disorders* in sport is considerably more sparse [28]. One study exploring the presence of personality disorders in a sample of 101 actively competing Egyptian athletes across different sports (as identified by the SCID II) demonstrated that 42/101 athletes (41.5%) fulfilled criteria for one personality disorder, while 13/101 athletes (12.9%) satisfied criteria for more than one personality disorder [29]. These rates are significantly higher than those measured in the general population and are likely not representative of the true incidence of personality disorders in all athlete populations.

Personality disorders can cause disruptions in the sport setting if the manifestations of the individual's challenges negatively influence their interpersonal relationships (i.e., via conflict, dependence, or clinginess), emotional regulation (i.e., via mood volatility, irritability, anger, tearfulness), interpretations of others' intentions, and behavior (i.e., via yelling, accusations, spitefulness, self-harm behaviors or suicidal threats). The external presentation of a personality disorder disturbance is often characterized as disruptive behavior.

Most sport personnel and settings are not equipped to manage disruptive behaviors, particularly those that are intense and present safety concerns. It is important to have qualified mental health personnel on the integrated/multidisciplinary support team to help the athlete and team personnel understand the behaviors and create support plans for de-

escalation and safety. Mental Health Action Plans and Emergency Action Plans should be created and made available to the athlete and all athlete support personnel to assist in response and ongoing management.

Case Illustrations

Negative impacts of personality disorder manifestations are experienced by many people in the sport environment regardless of the role of the individual who has the personality disorder. These anonymized, composite case illustrations demonstrate disruptions related to an athlete as well as a coach.

Case 1: Athlete

Allison was a 21-year-old female Olympic basketball player who was referred for Sports Psychiatry consultation after several episodes of behavioral disturbances and outbursts in the team environment.

Behaviors of concern included extreme negative reaction to criticism, yelling, hitting the wall with her fist, threatening to kill herself, and impulsively leaving practice on multiple occasions. She had a lengthy history of self-harm behavior (including cutting her wrists, hitting herself in the head, and minor intentional medication over-ingestions), which typically occurred when she was "in a negative headspace." Impulsive behavior undertaken in response to intense negative feelings about herself included excessive drinking, bingeing and purging, and sexual promiscuity (after which she always experienced intense guilt). Sexual promiscuity also occurred in the context of desperate attempts to avoid being alone. Several of these outbursts occurred while the team was traveling and training in different countries. Psychiatric consultation revealed that reactive mood lability began in her early adolescence and persisted as she left home to train in various high-performance sport settings. She repeatedly experienced volatility in her relationships, including with teammates, coaches, team personnel, and friends. Distress intolerance led to the described behavioral outbursts. She had numerous visits to the local emergency department while in crisis, and she described three previous suicide attempts. Allison had previous diagnoses of depression and attention-deficit/hyperactivity disorder (ADHD), and fulfilled diagnostic criteria for borderline personality disorder.

Although Allison had previous psychiatric diagnoses, the primary diagnosis contributing to her challenges was borderline personality disorder. Although there is frequently negative stigma associated with this diagnosis, Allison expressed relief after receiving the diagnosis, as "something finally explained how I was thinking, feeling, and acting." She consented to a meeting with the coaches and athlete support personnel to explain the diagnosis and its manifestations. Allison participated in the development of a Mental Health Action Plan, and team personnel were educated about their roles in support of the athlete. The athlete educated her teammates about her diagnosis and helped them understand her triggers, reactions, and responses that were helpful or harmful.

Comment Behavioral disturbances are often interpreted as "bad behavior," which can result in an athlete being released from a team or expelled from a program. When these disturbances occur in the context of a mental health disorder, the involvement of qualified mental health personnel can assist in proper identification of the problem and activation of appropriate education, treatment, and support pathways.

Case 2: Coach

James was a swim coach at a high-performance center who coached dozens of athletes at the Olympic Games over his 40 years of coaching. He was well known for his "temper tantrums" and resistance to having any "external" personnel or clinicians involved with his athletes, as "his way was the only way."

During training camps, he demanded the best vehicles and training times, often at the expense of his colleagues and other athletes in the program. He frequently teased his athletes and called them derogatory names or highlighted their disabilities. He regularly told integrated/multidisciplinary support team members that they were stupid, their roles were worthless, and that they were not needed. He considered every Olympic medal won by his athletes as "his." Athletes were told that they had no skill, that he was the only one who could make them "good," and that if they attempted to train anywhere else, they would not make the Olympic team. Some athletes in his group were reluctant to socialize with athletes from other high-performance centers (even when the groups merged for major competitions) due to fear of his anger and vexatious behavior. Others emulated his behavior by berating clinicians, being rude and dismissive to staff and other athletes, and throwing things around the team preparation area when they did not get what they wanted. While organizational personnel recognized the problems created in the environment based on the coach's (and athletes') behavior, it was predominantly tolerated since the coach "produced results."

Comment The patterns of beliefs, interpersonal relationships, and behavior exhibited by this coach were consistent with narcissistic personality disorder. Many of his actions can also be considered maltreatment and abuse of athletes and staff. Individuals demonstrating this personality profile are often entitled, difficult to engage in negotiation or com-

promise, and negatively impact the environment in multiple ways. Due to the value placed on success and results, it is unsurprising that this type of behavior is tolerated in elite or professional sports settings when it is perpetrated by an individual who is identified as a key contributor to those results. For the overall health and functioning of the sport environment, codes of conduct and standards of behavior should be established and enforced. A safe mechanism for reporting maltreatment should also be clearly communicated.

Summary

Dimensions of personality can potentially be useful in identifying desirable traits in athletes that are linked to success. However, personality disorders can lead to significant functional impairment and disturbances in the sport setting. Behavioral disturbances related to personality disorders can significantly impact the sport environment and affect everyone in that setting. Disruptive behavior is sometimes tolerated if it is perpetrated by an individual who is deemed to be integral to the team's success. Most sport personnel and settings are not equipped to manage intense behavioral disturbances that may involve threats to safety. The involvement of qualified mental health personnel can assist in proper identification of the problem and activation of appropriate education, treatment, and support pathways. Mental Health Action Plans and Emergency Action Plans can proactively assist athletes, coaches, and support personnel by identifying roles and protocols for management, support, and safety.

References

1. Clark LA, Watson D. Temperament: an organizing paradigm for trait psychology. In: John OP, Robins RW, Pervin LA, editors. Handbook of personality: theory and research. 3rd ed. New York, NY: Guilford Press; 2008. p. 265–86.
2. American Psychiatric Association. What are personality disorders? Washington, DC: American Psychiatric Association; n.d.. https://www.psychiatry.org/patients-families/personality-disorders/what-are-personality-disorders. Accessed 8 Nov 2021.
3. Costa PT, McCrae RR. Revised NEO personality inventory and NEO five-factor inventory: professional manual. Odessa, FL: Psychological Assessment Resources; 1992.
4. Diener E, Lucas RE, Cummings JA. Personality traits. In: Cummings JA, Sanders L, editors. Introduction to psychology. Saskatoon, SK: University of Saskatchewan Open Press; 2019. https://openpress.usask.ca/introductiontopsychology/. Licensed under a Creative Commons Attribution-NonCommercial-ShareAlike 4.0 International License, except where otherwise noted. https://openpress.usask.ca/introductiontopsychology/chapter/personality-traits/. Accessed 24 Oct 2021.
5. Teglasi H, Simcox AG, Kim N-Y. Personality constructs and measures. Psychol Sch. 2007;44(3):215–28.

6. Smith GT. On construct validity: issues of method and measurement. Psychol Assess. 2005;17(4):396–408. https://doi-org.libaccess.lib.mcmaster.ca/10.1037/1040-3590.17.4.396. Accessed 8 Nov 2021.

7. American Psychiatric Association. Personality disorders. In: Diagnostic and statistical manual of mental disorders. 5th ed. Washington, DC: American Psychiatric Association; 2013. https://doi.org/10.1176/appi.books.9780890425596.dsm18. Accessed 8 Nov 2021.

8. Mulder RT. ICD-11 Personality disorders: utility and implications of the new model. Fron Psychiatry. 2021;12:655548. https://doi.org/10.3389/fpsyt.2021.655548. Accessed 8 Nov 2021.

9. World Health Organization. International classification of diseases for mortality and morbidity statistics (11th Revision). Geneva: WHO; 2018. https://icd.who.int/browse11/l-m/en. Accessed 8 Nov 2021.

10. Yang M, Coid J, Tyrer P. Personality pathology recorded by severity: national survey. Br J Psychiatry. 2010;197(3):193–9. https://doi.org/10.1192/bjp.bp.110.078956.

11. Volkert J, Gablonski TC, Rabung S. Prevalence of personality disorders in the general adult population in Western countries: systematic review and meta-analysis. Br J Psychiatry. 2018;213(6):709–15. https://doi.org/10.1192/bjp.2018.202. PMID: 30261937.

12. Winsper C, Bilgin A, Thompson A, et al. The prevalence of personality disorders in the community: a global systematic review and meta-analysis. Br J Psychiatry. 2020;216(2):69–78. https://doi.org/10.1192/bjp.2019.166. PMID: 31298170.

13. Bach B, First MB. Application of the ICD-11 classification of personality disorders. BMC Psychiatry. 2018;18:351. https://doi.org/10.1186/s12888-018-1908-3.

14. Skodol AE, First MB, Bender DS, et al. Module II. Structured clinical interview for personality traits. In: First MB, Skodol AE, Bender DS, Oldham JM, editors. Structured clinical interview for the DSM-5 alternative model for personality disorders (SCID-AMPD). Arlington, VI: American Psychiatric Association; 2018.

15. Krueger RF, Johnson W. Behavioral genetics and personality: a new look at the integration of nature and nurture. In: John OP, Robins RW, Pervin LA, editors. Handbook of personality: theory and research. 3rd ed. New York, NY: Guilford Press; 2008. p. 287–310.

16. Roberts BW, DelVecchio WF. The rank-order consistency of personality traits from childhood to old age. Psychol Bull. 2000;126:325. https://doi.org/10.1037/0033-2909.126.1.3.

17. Terracciano A, McCrae RR, Costa PT. Intra-individual change in personality stability and age. J Res Pers. 2010;44(1):3137. https://doi.org/10.1016/j.jrp.2009.09.006.

18. Piepiora P. Assessment of personality traits influencing the performance of men in team sports in terms of the big five. Front Psychol. 2021;12:679724. https://doi.org/10.3389/fpsyg.2021.679724.

19. Piepiora P. Personality profile of individual sports champions. Brain Behav. 2021;11(6):e02145. https://doi.org/10.1002/brb3.2145. PMID: 33951345; PMCID: PMC8213921.

20. Samadzadeh M, Abbasi M, Shahbazzadegan B. Comparison of sensation seeking and self-esteem with mental health in professional and amateur athletes, and non- athletes. Procedia Soc Behav Sci. 2011;15:1942–50. https://doi.org/10.1016/j.sbspro.2011.04.032.

21. Nia M, Besharat MA. Comparison of athletes' personality characteristics in individual and team sports. Procedia Soc Behav Sci. 2010;5:808–12. https://doi.org/10.1016/j.sbspro.2010.07.189.

22. American Psychological Association. Dictionary of psychology. "Sociotropy". Washington, DC: American Psychological Association; n.d.. https://dictionary.apa.org/sociotropy. Accessed 16 Nov 2021.

23. Cnen T-W, Chiu Y-C, Hsu Y. Perception of social support provided by coaches, optimism/pessimism, and psychological well-being: gender differences and mediating effect models. Int J Sports Sci Coach. 2021;16(2):272–80. https://doi.org/10.1177/1747954120968649.

24. Fletcher D, Sarkar M. A grounded theory of psychological resilience in Olympic champions. Psychol Sport Exerc. 2012;13:669–78.

25. Luthar SS, Cicchetti D, Becker B. The construct of resilience: a critical evaluation and guidelines for future work. Child Dev. 2000;71:543e562. https://doi.org/10.1111/1467-8624.00164.

26. Rutter M. Psychosocial resilience and protective mechanisms. Am J Orthopsychiatry. 1987;57:316e331. https://doi.org/10.1111/j.1939-0025.1987.tb03541.x.

27. Egeland B, Carlson E, Sroufe LA. Resilience as process. Dev Psychopathol. 1993;5:517e528. https://doi.org/10.1017/S0954579400006131.

28. Allen MS, Greenlees I, Jones M. Personality in sport: a comprehensive review. Int Rev Sport Exerc Psychol. 2013;6:184–208. https://doi.org/10.1080/1750984X.2013.769614.

29. Hendawy HMFM, Awad EAA. Personality and personality disorders in athletes. In: Baron DA, Reardon CL, Baron SH, editors. Clinical sports psychiatry. London: Wiley-Blackwell; 2013. p. 58–60. https://doi.org/10.1002/9781118404904.ch6.

Bipolar and Psychotic Disorders

Alan Currie ⓘ and R. Hamish McAllister-Williams ⓘ

Introduction

Late adolescence and early adulthood are the peak ages of performance in most sports [1]. They are also the peak periods for the onset and first presentation of bipolar and psychotic disorders [2, 3]. Thus, whilst the prevalence in elite sport of these common and serious conditions is not known with any certainty, they are undoubtedly likely to appear in that environment [4]. These disorders will have a significant impact on both the health and performance of an athlete and have a worse outcome if diagnosis and treatment are delayed [5, 6]. In addition, they are likely to require treatment with medication, possibly in the long term. Therefore, all those who work in sport would benefit from a basic understanding of the features of these disorders, how they might present, and the importance of ready access to expert assessment, diagnosis, and treatment.

Diagnosis: Bipolar Disorder

Bipolar disorder is a recurrent condition where the central feature is episodic mood disturbance [7]. At one pole, episodes of elevated mood are described and called mania (or hypomania if less severe). At the other are episodes of low mood or depression, which have similar features to those seen in a depressive disorder. In general, in bipolar disorder, depressive episodes are more common than manic or hypomanic ones, though there is a great deal of variation between individuals. Mixed episodes are also occasionally seen where there are symptoms of both depression and mania in the same episode. Usually one mood state predominates, with some depressive features seen in a predominantly manic state or vice versa. Mixed episodes tend to be particularly unpleasant and distressing for the individual. Several subtypes of bipolar disorder are described with episodes of mood disturbance as the common feature. The characteristics of each subtype are summarised in Table 12.1.

In bipolar I disorder, a manic episode must have been present at least once in a person's life, although hypomanic episodes may also occur. In bipolar II disorder, there are

A. Currie (✉)
Regional Affective Disorders Service, Cumbria, Northumberland, Tyne and Wear NHS Foundation Trust, Newcastle, UK

Department of Sport and Exercise Science, University of Sunderland, Sunderland, UK
e-mail: alan.currie@cntw.nhs.uk

R. H. McAllister-Williams
Regional Affective Disorders Service, Cumbria, Northumberland, Tyne and Wear NHS Foundation Trust, Newcastle, UK

Affective Disorders, Northern Centre for Mood Disorders, Translational and Clinical Research Institute, Newcastle University, Newcastle upon Tyne, UK
e-mail: Hamish.mcallister-williams@newcastle.ac.uk

Table 12.1 Subclassification of bipolar disorder [7]

Disorder	Distinguishing characteristics
Bipolar I disorder	At least one manic episode
	Likely also to have had depressive episodes
Bipolar II disorder	At least one depressive episode
	At least one hypomanic episode
Cyclothymic disorder	At least 2 years of episodes of hypomanic and depressive symptoms
	Episodes do not meet full criteria for mania, hypomania or depression
Substance/medication-induced bipolar and related disorder	Symptoms relate to exposure to, intoxication by, or withdrawal from a substance or medication capable of producing mood disturbance
Bipolar and related disorder due to another medical condition	Mood disturbance is a direct physiological consequence of another medical condition
Other specified bipolar and related disorder	Symptoms do not meet full criteria for more specific bipolar spectrum disorder, e.g.: • Short duration hypomania • Hypomania with subsyndromal depressive episodes • Hypomania without depressive episodes • Short duration cyclothymia
Unspecified bipolar and related disorder	Symptoms do not meet full criteria and the reason is not, or cannot, be specified

hypomanic but not manic episodes. Cyclothymia is a form of bipolar disorder in which there are recurrent episodes of both hypomanic and depressive symptoms (not meeting full criteria for hypomanic and depressive episodes) over a period of 2 years or more.

When episodes are attributable to substance use, medication, or another medical condition, then a separate diagnosis is given. Medical conditions associated with mood disturbance are usually more of a consideration in older populations, where they are more common. Examples of these conditions include thyroid disease, multiple sclerosis, and cortical or subcortical brain lesions. Presentation of hypomania or mania for the first time in later life is unusual and a careful history and examination are essential with further investigations including imaging studies often required. Note, however, that a careful history (with corroboration) may occasionally identify earlier and subclinical episodes. A full medication history is also needed, with an awareness of which medications are especially associated with mood changes, e.g. corticosteroids and thyroid replacement therapy. Some performance enhancing drugs (PEDs) used by athletes and others may produce mood and/or psychotic symptoms, and the assessment of an athlete presenting with these symptoms should include a careful enquiry about their use and further investigations as indicated [4, 8–12]. Occasionally, symptoms of mania or hypomania emerge during antidepressant treatment, and in these circumstances an episode is only diagnosed if symptoms persist beyond the expected physiological effect of that treatment.

Mania and Hypomania

The main feature of a manic episode is elevated mood with increased activity or energy. The abnormality of mood is quite distinct from that usually experienced by the patient and is persistent. This is associated with a persistent increase in activity or energy. An irritable, rather than elated, mood is sometimes seen. Psychotic symptoms (e.g. grandiose delusions) may be present, and, if so, are consistent with the patient's elevated mood (mood congruent) and indicative of illness/episode severity.

Associated Symptoms

Seven associated symptoms are described, and at least three need to be present to meet the criteria for mania (four or more if the mood state is one of irritability rather than elation). These are:

- Grandiosity and increased self esteem
- Diminished need for sleep where the individual may not experience tiredness and awakens subjectively refreshed and energetic after only a few hours

- More talkative with pressure to keep talking
- The subjective experience of racing thoughts, which might be evident to others too and described as flight of ideas
- Easily distracted by unimportant or irrelevant stimuli and events
- Increased activity, which may be goal directed towards usual activities or restless agitation, which is less purposeful
- Activities with harmful consequences such as spending sprees or sexual indiscretions

Impairment of Functioning

Symptoms lead to a marked impairment in social or occupational functioning. This criterion is also met if hospitalisation is necessary to prevent harm or if psychotic symptoms (delusions or hallucinations) are present.

All of these features need to be present most of the time, on most days for at least 1 week, to constitute a manic episode.

The features of a hypomanic episode are similar except that the episode is not severe enough to cause marked impairment in functioning, psychotic features are absent, and symptoms need only be present for 4 days.

Depression

The depressive episodes seen in bipolar disorder are like those seen in depressive disorders. The Diagnostic and Statistical Manual of Mental Disorders 5th edition (DSM-5) describes the following nine symptoms or groups of symptoms that constitute a major depressive episode:

- Depressed mood such as sadness, emptiness, hopelessness, or appearing tearful
- Marked reduction in interest or pleasure for almost all activities
- Weight change, which might be weight loss or weight gain (5% or more) or a sustained increase or decrease in appetite
- Reduced or increased sleep
- Psychomotor changes such as retardation and feeling slowed down or alternatively agitation
- Loss of energy and fatigue
- Feeling worthless or with thoughts of excessive or inappropriate guilt. These thoughts might reach the intensity of a delusion, where they are fixed and held with strong conviction even when alternative evidence is presented
- Reduced concentration, indecision, and a diminished ability to think clearly

- Recurrent thoughts of death or suicidal ideation or a suicide attempt or specific plan

At least five of the nine symptoms listed must be present. In addition, there will be clinically significant distress or impairment in functioning, and the symptoms should not be attributable to another medical condition. Symptoms must be present for at least 2 weeks and include at least one of the first two symptoms of depressed mood or loss of interest.

Mixed States

Mixed states may occur when features of mania/hypomania and depression are seen during the same episode. A manic or hypomanic episode with mixed features is characterised by a full manic or hypomanic syndrome and at least three depressive symptoms present on most days during the episode. A depressive episode with mixed features is characterised by a full depressive syndrome and at least three manic or hypomanic symptoms.

Illness Course

Although bipolar disorder is an episodic illness, many patients spend extended periods in a symptomatic state, and subsyndromal symptoms are common. Patients with bipolar I disorder are reported to experience symptoms 47.3% of the time (53.9% in bipolar II), with depressive symptoms the most common, especially in bipolar II disorder [13, 14].

Rapid Cycling

Patients may also cycle rapidly from episode to episode. This is defined as four episodes or more within 12 months. To make this subtype diagnosis, there should be at least partial remission for a minimum of 2 months between episodes of the same polarity, although episodes can occur in any order or combination. The presence of rapid cycling is an indicator of poor outcome and/or poor prognosis.

Diagnostic Issues

Hypomanic episodes are typically shorter than episodes of mania and are, by definition, associated with less functional impairment. One consequence of this is that an individual with a hypomanic episode may not present for medical attention and indeed may welcome the experience of mood elevation and increased energy [15]. Subsequent depressive episodes may, however, be more unpleasant, unwanted, and

lead to seeking medical advice. If there is no inquiry about previous hypomanic episodes at this presentation, then the diagnosis of bipolar disorder will be missed, and the patient misclassified as having major depressive disorder. A good practice point in the assessment of presentation of a new episode of depression is to always inquire about previous hypomanic symptoms.

In a very physically active individual such as an athlete, it may be harder to spot 'excessive' energy or activity levels, and indeed over-activity may be normalised or obscured in the context of athletic training [16]. Anabolic androgenic steroids (AAS) and stimulants are also occasionally misused by athletes [8, 12]. Stimulants may produce transient mood changes and are associated with a broad range of mental health symptoms [17], and AAS are associated with subsyndromal mood disturbance towards either pole of hypomania or depression [9–11]. Their use should be considered in the assessment of any athlete presenting with mood disturbance [4].

Differential Diagnosis

Substance Use Disorders

Many substances can promote changes in mood, and symptoms may be relatively short-lived, self-limiting, and not meet full criteria for either depression or hypomania [4]. There is frequently a close temporal relationship between substance use and mood disturbance. The use of substances may be acknowledged during a sensitive inquiry, and corroborative reports from family or friends may be helpful [12].

Personality Disorder

Impulsive behaviours and marked changes in mood can be a feature of borderline personality disorder. However, the observed changes in mood are frequently towards anger or irritability and are usually triggered abruptly by an interpersonal cue. These changes also tend to be less sustained and can disappear just as quickly as they emerge [7]. The DSM-5 specifies that the intense emotions of borderline and other personality disorders should typically last only a few hours at most. Other features of borderline personality disorder will also be apparent such as efforts to avoid real or imagined abandonment, an unstable self-image and chronic feelings of emptiness.

Other distinctions have also been suggested [18]. Notably, borderline personality disorder 'evolves', e.g. with some emotional dysregulation present in childhood and adolescence, whilst bipolar II has an 'onset episode' and discontinuity in presentation, from absence of symptoms to their clear presence. The nature of mood episodes may also be different. In borderline personality disorder, the dysregulated mood state is unpleasant, even painful. In contrast, whilst anger and irritability can be prominent in the elevated mood state of bipolar disorder, the shift is usually to a more care-free state where anxiety and worry disappear and euphoria, grandiosity, and creativity are accompanied by feelings of invincibility. Another helpful distinction may be the response after a 'high' episode. In borderline personality disorder, the patient justifies their actions taken whilst they were in an elevated mood or blames them on others, whilst in bipolar disorder, they are more likely to be regretted with feelings of guilt or even shame.

A complication is that individuals with borderline personality disorder are at increased risk of developing depressive episodes, and it has been reported that bipolar and borderline personality disorders commonly co-exist [19].

Attention-Deficit/Hyperactivity Disorder (ADHD)

In ADHD, there may be features similar to mania or hypomania such as increased energy, distractibility, and over-talkativeness with a tendency to interrupt others. However, the primary disturbance is in behaviour and attention, in contrast to the primary disturbances in mood seen in bipolar disorder. In ADHD, symptoms are also persistent rather than episodic.

It is important to note that bipolar disorder and ADHD frequently occur together [20], and it has been reported that 5% of adolescents and young adults presenting with ADHD go on to receive a diagnosis of bipolar disorder [21].

Diagnosis: Psychosis

Psychotic disorders are characterised by symptoms such as delusions, hallucinations, and disorganised speech. In schizophrenia, additional symptoms are required to make the diagnosis, and there are a broad range of symptoms for an extended period of 6 months or more. Other psychotic disorders share similar features, albeit over a narrower range of symptoms or for a shorter duration or both [7].

For a diagnosis of schizophrenia, at least two of the five features listed in Table 12.2 must be present, and one of these must be delusions, hallucinations, or disorganised speech. A hallucination is a perception without a stimulus, e.g. hearing a voice when there is no one present. Hallucinations can occur in any sensory modality, e.g. auditory, visual, or tactile hallucinations. In schizophrenia, the voice that is heard may speak in the third person or as a running commentary on one's actions. Other auditory hallucinations include multiple voices conversing with each other or hearing one's thoughts spoken out loud. A delusion is a fixed belief that is usually false and held against evidence to the contrary. It is not in keeping with one's cultural background, e.g. a religious belief. Examples include paranoid delusions such as believing that one is under surveillance or being followed. In schizophrenia, there may be

Table 12.2 Schizophrenia and other psychotic disorders [7]

Schizophrenia	Two of five features must be present (at least one of: delusions, hallucinations, or disorganized speech):
	• Delusions
	• Hallucinations
	• Disorganized speech (at least one of these first three must be present)
	• Marked behavioural disturbance
	• Negative symptoms (e.g. diminished emotional expression or avolition)
	Marked deterioration in functioning
	Continuous disturbance for 6 months
	Associated features that may support the diagnosis:
	• Inappropriate affect such as laughing in the absence of an appropriate stimulus
	• Dysphoric mood with anxiety, anger, or depression
	• Cognitive deficits (e.g. in memory, language, and executive functions)
	• Deficits in social cognition, e.g. inability to infer the intentions of others
Schizophreniform disorder	Two of five features of schizophrenia (at least one of: delusions, hallucinations, or disorganized speech)
	Shorter duration (1–6 months)
	May be a provisional diagnosis, i.e. when the patient still has ongoing symptoms but not (yet) for 6 months
Brief psychotic disorder	At least one of delusions, hallucinations, disorganised speech
	Disorganized behaviour may also be present
	Symptoms for between 1 day and 1 month but eventual return to full functioning
	Can occur in response to a severe stressor (and then sometimes called *brief reactive psychosis*)
Delusional disorder	At least one delusion for at least 1 month
	Hallucinations not prominent
	Functioning and behaviour are not markedly impaired or bizarre
Schizoaffective disorder	Episode of depression or mania concurrent with at least two of the five features of schizophrenia
	Delusions or hallucinations for at least 2 weeks outside mood episode
	Mood symptoms are present for the majority of the illness
Psychotic disorder due to another medical condition	Delusions or hallucinations with significant distress or functional impairment
	History, examination, or laboratory findings suggest symptoms are the direct pathophysiological consequence of the medical condition
	Not better explained by another mental disorder or by delirium

(continued)

Table 12.2 (continued)

Substance- or medication-induced psychotic disorder	Delusions and/or hallucinations with significant distress or functional impairment
	Symptoms during or soon after substance intoxication or withdrawal
	Does not occur exclusively during the course of a delirium
	Substance is capable of producing delusions and/or hallucinations
	Not better explained by another psychotic disorder or by delirium
Attenuated psychosis syndrome (a 'condition for further study')	At least one of (present at least once per week for 1 month) delusions, hallucinations, disorganized speech
	Symptoms are distressing and disabling
	Symptoms below threshold for diagnosis of any other psychotic disorder (e.g. less severe and/or more transient)

more bizarre delusions such as experiencing thoughts or actions as being controlled by an outside agent (passivity); that thoughts are removed by an external force (thought withdrawal); that others can access one's thoughts (thought broadcasting); or that thoughts are being put into one's mind (thought insertion). Disorganised speech may manifest as jumping from one topic to another (sometimes called derailment or loosening of associations), an inability to answer questions directly (tangential speech), and in severe cases, speech that is incomplete, incomprehensible, and incoherent. This is sometimes called a word salad because the words appear as a mixture without the usual grammatical structure. Disorganised behaviours may also be seen, e.g. catatonic behaviour, where the individual shows a marked reduction in reactivity to their surroundings. Examples include negativism (resistance to instructions), catatonic excitement (markedly excessive and purposeless activity), and mutism or stupor (complete lack of verbal or motor responses). Occasionally, there may be grimacing, stereotyped repetitive movements, or echoing of the speech of others.

In schizophreniform disorder, there may be the same range of symptoms but for a shorter duration (1–6 months). In consequence, this is often a provisional diagnosis as the patient may have on-going symptoms and may in time go on to fulfill the diagnostic criteria for schizophrenia. A brief psychotic disorder is diagnosed when psychotic symptoms have been present for a still shorter duration of up to 1 month. In addition, there are usually a narrower range of symptoms, without the associated features seen in schizophrenia and a full return to functioning after the episode. A delusional disorder is diagnosed when delusions occur in the absence of hallucinations, functional impairment, or bizarre behaviours. A diagnosis of schizoaffective disorder is considered when there are features of schizophrenia concurrent with an epi-

sode of depression or mania. There must, however, be psychotic symptoms for at least 2 weeks outside the episode of mood disturbance (to distinguish this condition from bipolar disorder), although symptoms of mood disturbance are present for the majority of the illness.

Psychotic symptoms can also emerge secondary to a medical condition or its treatment, or as a result of substance intoxication or withdrawal. As with bipolar disorder, substances used by athletes such as AAS may be associated with mental health symptoms or disorders, including psychosis. The attenuated psychosis syndrome is not a diagnosis as such but is described as a 'condition for further study'. It is described as 'psychosis-like' with symptoms that are less severe and below the threshold for a psychotic diagnosis. Symptoms are more transient, and insight is relatively maintained, though there may be noticeable functional impairment whilst symptomatic. It is relevant in sport as many of those in sporting populations will be in late adolescence or early adulthood, which is the period when attenuated psychotic symptoms are most likely to emerge. More knowledge is needed on the course and prognosis of attenuated psychotic symptoms including the likelihood of resolution or progression to a full psychotic syndrome and which if any interventions are helpful.

Diagnostic Issues in Sport

An important issue to consider for all those who work with athletes is that the peak age of sporting performance shows significant overlap with the onset of many serious mental health disorders such as bipolar and psychotic disorders [1]. These conditions may arise co-incidentally in this population and require expert assessment, diagnostic clarification (especially if the presentation appears to be with attenuated symptoms), and further management. A second issue is that mood disturbance and psychotic symptoms can emerge in the context of misuse of substances by athletes for performance or other reasons [9–11]. The use of AAS is an example of how substance use can mimic the episodic mood disturbance of bipolar disorder. Hypomanic symptoms can emerge with AAS use and especially with high doses and/or multiple drugs, whilst depressive symptoms are associated with more chronic use and during withdrawal [9, 11]. Thus, both 'poles' may be seen. Substance use disorders are also found comorbid with bipolar disorder, and a positive drug screen or history of use does not exclude a diagnosis of bipolar disorder. Other substances that have been used by athletes and that are associated with psychotic symptoms and mood disturbance include stimulants, cannabis, and glucocorticoids [8, 22].

Prevalence

The general population lifetime prevalence of bipolar disorder is around 0.4% for type I, 0.6% for type II, and 1.4% for subthreshold symptoms [2]. There is regional variation in the lifetime prevalence of schizophrenia and related psychotic conditions, but the figure in most areas is around 0.5% [23]. Psychotic *symptoms* are a much commoner experience, especially in adolescence, reported in 7.5% of 13- to 18-year old where they do not necessarily indicate a psychotic disorder [24]. However, careful assessment and, if necessary, follow-up, are advised.

There are no reliable data on the prevalence of bipolar and psychotic disorders in populations of elite athletes [4, 25–27] although there are case reports of high-profile athletes who have been able to achieve sporting success in spite of their illness. Athlete Suzy Favor Hamilton has written and published her experiences of bipolar disorder [28]. She has described the history of bipolar disorder in her family, the stigma attached to this, and her own experiences of depression. She has offered a graphic account of a manic episode in association with being prescribed antidepressant medication, which includes her report of uncharacteristic and disinhibited sexual behaviour driven by her elevated mood state.

> *My doctor put me on another anti-depressant. The effects were immediate. I felt great. I felt beyond great. I felt alive. I wanted to live. Time for my fantasies to now become a reality. Our 20th wedding anniversary was coming up. A nice dinner date out on the town with flowers perhaps? Not for me. I wanted to go to Vegas, jump out of a plane, hire an escort, have a threesome. Bucket list stuff I never thought I would actually do. Never. I wanted it now.*

However, the functional impairments associated with schizophrenia may prove incompatible with a career in high-performance sport, and schizophrenia may be under-represented in populations of elite athletes for this reason [29].

Assessment

As with most other areas of clinical practise, the key to a good assessment is a comprehensive history and examination, supplemented by investigations. Early access to an expert assessment is strongly recommended. Delays in diagnosis and initiation of treatment are associated with poorer long-term outcomes [5, 6].

If bipolar disorder is being considered, then the assessment will need to include a detailed history of mood episodes including potential triggers and any symptoms that occur between episodes. A corroborative history from a family member or close acquaintance can be invaluable. The assessment should also consider the potential role of exercise in any mood disturbance. For example, is it a helpful way of managing symptoms, a symptom of elevated mood, or a contributory factor to mood instability and elevation [4]?

If a psychotic disorder or mania is being considered, then a specialist mental health assessment is indicated and may need to occur as a matter of urgency [4, 30]. The assessment should carefully evaluate all symptoms and include a risk assessment. Once again, a corroborative history can be invaluable.

The changes in mental status examination that are commonly found in mania and hypomania, and how they might be described in a written examination detailing a patient's presentation, are described below. Table 12.3 illustrates the features of symptoms commonly found in schizophrenia and other psychotic disorders.

Table 12.3 Symptoms in schizophrenia and other psychotic disorders [7]

Symptom	Features	Examples
Hallucination	A perception in the absence of an external stimulus. Can be in any sensory modality (e.g. auditory, visual, tactile).	Multiple voices conversing about the patient in the third person
		A running commentary of the patient's actions
		Hearing one's thoughts spoken aloud
Delusion	A fixed and strongly held belief that is almost always false, held against evidence that contradicts the belief, and is not in keeping with the patient's background or culture (e.g. religious belief)	A paranoid/persecutory belief of being followed or under surveillance
		Thoughts, actions, emotions are controlled by an external force or agent (passivity)
		Thoughts are removed from one's mind by an external agent (thought withdrawal); broadcast and read by others (thought broadcasting); put into one's mind by an external agent (thought insertion)
Disorganised speech	Spectrum from difficult to follow and hard to understand to complete incoherence	Questions are not directly answered (tangential speech)
		Jumps from topic to topic (loosening of associations or derailment)
		Jumbled incoherently and incomprehensible (word salad)
Disorganised behaviour	Catatonic symptoms	Bizarre postures, mutism, stupor
	Stereotypies	Repetitive rituals
	Echolalia or echopraxia	Echoing or copying speech/movement
	Grimacing	

(continued)

Table 12.3 (continued)

Symptom	Features	Examples
Negative symptoms	Social withdrawal	Absent from previous social activities
	Anhedonia	Reduced ability to experience activities as pleasurable
Emotional expression	Diminished or even absent range of emotions is expressed. Often called 'emotional blunting' or 'flattening of affect'	Reduced facial and vocal expressions and gestures in response to emotional stimuli
Avolition	Reduction of activities that are self-initiated	Deteriorating self-care and inattentive to personal hygiene. No longer participates in leisure activities
Deterioration in function	In at least one major area, e.g. work, relationships, self-care	Could include sporting performance in athletes
Incongruent affect	Mood is inconsistent (incongruent) with thoughts and actions. Mismatch between the emotion experienced and its expression	Appears happy and smiling (even giggling) when discussing a sad or unpleasant event or spontaneously for no reason
Dysphoric mood	Generalised unhappiness and dissatisfaction	May appear withdrawn and depressed. May display anxiety, frustration and restlessness
Cognitive deficits	Deficits in attention; working memory; verbal learning; executive functions	Impaired ability to sustain attention on a task; difficulty remembering a phone number before dialling it; difficulty learning a list; difficulties with problem solving, goal directed behaviour, flexibility in response to change, and planning
	Often presents subtly and before psychotic symptoms are apparent	
	May persist even when psychotic symptoms have responded to treatment	
Difficulties in social cognition	Impairments in social processing	Difficulty in perceiving and interpreting facial expression of others. Problems with mentalising (attending to mental states of self and others)

Mental Status Examination in Mania and Hypomania

Note that the interviewer is trying to build an overall picture, and one specific detail is insufficient to make a diagnosis.

Appearance

Comment on the clothing type, which might be brightly coloured, even garish or untidy. The subject may be inattentive to personal hygiene and, in severe cases, might look exhausted (whilst denying this). Be alert also for evidence of factors that may complicate the presentation such as alcohol or stimulant use.

Behaviour

Aim to describe what can be seen in a manner that would allow a non-observer to easily conjure an image of the patient. Try to be specific, e.g. if the patient is overfamiliar or hostile, then say how and give examples. Arousal may be increased, with increased vigilance or distractibility. Restlessness may be evident, and eye contact may not be sustained. Facial expressions reflect the underlying mood state, with excessive smiling or laughing. Disinhibition may be reflected in disregard for the usual social conventions and manners.

Mood

This should be rated both subjectively and objectively. Subjectively, there may be feelings such as being full of energy and excitement or 'on top of the world', which are usually described as welcome and pleasant experiences. Objectively, the patient may appear elated or irritable, and the latter may be a consequence of frustration when others do not share their ideas and plans. There may be fleeting mood swings (lability) towards low mood or even tearfulness.

Speech

The rate of speech production is typically increased. The patient may be hard to interrupt and seek out others to listen to their ideas. Greater degrees of pressured speech merge into flight of ideas where there are still connections between each element of the conversation, but they can be hard to follow and the connections may be weak (e.g. rhymes or puns). This is to be distinguished from the thought disordered speech of schizophrenia, where there are no connections and conversation jumps from one topic to another unconnected topic (e.g. knight's move thinking). Recording verbatim examples of speech to illustrate these features is difficult but invaluable.

Thinking

Abnormalities of thinking can be present in both form and content. The rate or flow (form) of thoughts is often increased, and this can feel unpleasant. The content will likely reflect their elevated mood state (mood congruence) such as ambitious plans or schemes and an exaggerated estimation of abilities and status. Ideas may reach the intensity of delusions, e.g. becoming convinced of special powers or abilities or believing to have been chosen for a special mission or purpose. If delusions are clearly incongruent with the observed mood state, then a diagnosis of schizoaffective or other psychotic disorder should be considered.

Perceptions

Psychotic symptoms such as delusions or hallucinations are usually a marker of illness severity and therefore seen only in more severe manic states. Mood congruence is the norm, e.g. a voice telling of special powers, and could be perceived as the voice of God or a person of high status.

Cognitive Abilities

If these are disturbed, this is most usually seen as deficits in sustaining attention with easy distractibility from external noise or other minor intrusions. This can extend to increased vigilance and even suspiciousness. The patient usually remains fully orientated.

Around 40% of people with bipolar disorder have some associated cognitive impairment [31], and there may be problems with executive function and memory even when mood symptoms are relatively absent [32]. Deficits are more pronounced in bipolar I disorder and in those with psychotic symptoms [33] but are generally not as problematic as in schizophrenia [34].

Insight

Insight is usually significantly impaired in mania, but often less so in hypomania. Patients may not recognise that they are ill or that their behaviour is unusual. However, they may recognise it as a change from their previous functioning, e.g. acknowledging increased energy, reduced need for sleep, and the novelty of their plans. Regaining insight during recovery can be a source of significant embarrassment for patients.

Physical Examination

The manic patient may show signs of exhaustion and sleep deprivation even though still physically overactive. The clinician should look for signs of self-neglect, even malnutrition, especially in patients with negative or depressive symptoms. Soft neurological signs may be seen in schizophrenia, including impairments in motor coordination and sequencing of complex movements. Examination may also reveal the increased arousal, dilated pupils, and motor tics that can be seen with stimulant use, or signs of AAS use such as acne, needle marks, testicular atrophy, or gynecomastia in men and hirsutism, breast atrophy, and clitoromegaly in women.

Investigations

Initial investigations are helpful in several respects. They will exclude or identify alternative causes of a disturbed mood; identify other conditions, e.g. poor nutrition or substance misuse that may exacerbate symptoms and complicate the illness course; and provide a baseline that will inform the choice of medications and future medication management [16, 35, 36].

Evaluation of Co-morbid Conditions and Complications

Laboratory studies may include:

- Complete blood count (CBC) to screen for anaemia and infections. Raised mean cell volume (MCV) can reveal harmful use of alcohol.
- Comprehensive metabolic panel (CMP) including electrolytes and kidney function, particularly if there is a state of under-nutrition and poor hydration through neglect or if there is co-morbid disordered eating.
- Glucose and/or HbA1c to screen for diabetes.
- Proteins, which may be lowered by poor nutrition.
- Thyroid function, as disturbances may cause depression or mania. Lithium treatment may also result in hypothyroidism.
- Liver function tests, especially if there are concerns about alcohol use.
- C-reactive protein (CRP) to screen for underlying inflammatory processes, e.g. lupus.

Other tests may be indicated depending on the patient's presentation and may include urinary drug screen for cannabinoids and amphetamines, structural brain imaging, electroencephalogram (EEG), and autoimmune screen.

Baseline Investigations When Antipsychotic or Mood Stabilising Medications Are Indicated

Depending on the particular medication chosen, these may include:

- CBC: Some mood stabilisers (e.g. valproate) are known to suppress bone marrow, and a baseline count is helpful.
- CMP: Lithium treatment will need adjusting if there is any impairment of renal function, and renal function must be monitored whenever lithium is prescribed.
- Glucose and lipids (ideally fasting): Antipsychotic medication is associated with the later development of metabolic syndrome.
- Prolactin: A baseline is helpful as many antipsychotic medications will elevate levels via dopamine blockade.

ECG: This is done to screen for prolonged QTc interval and the associated risk of arrhythmias with some antipsychotic medications.

Management

A delay in diagnosis of either bipolar or psychotic disorders is associated with a worse longer-term outcome. Confirmation of the diagnosis is an essential prerequisite to treatment and especially to use of mood stabilising or antipsychotic medications, which are often prescribed for long periods and can have side effects that impact athletic performance [4, 35, 37, 38].

Psychological Interventions

Psychotherapy can be used in the depressive phase of bipolar disorder, although much of the evidence is extrapolated from interventions used in depressive disorders and, in addition, is not sports specific. Cognitive behavioural therapy (CBT), interpersonal psychotherapy (IPT), and family interventions may be used [39, 40]. For longer-term prophylaxis in bipolar disorder, psychoeducation is frequently recommended and includes information on the nature and likely course of the illness; factors that can trigger destabilisation; strategies to address early warning signs of relapse; and appropriate use of short-term and long-term medication [41]. Interpersonal social rhythms therapy has also been recommended and reported to help maintain functioning [42, 43]. Central to this therapy is the development of regular daily routines and avoiding disruption to circadian rhythms and the sleep wake cycle. CBT and family interventions are also recommended alongside antipsychotic medication in the management of psychotic disorders [44, 45].

Exercise

Exercise may bring benefits for those who experience either bipolar or psychotic disorders, but evaluating and recommending exercise requires attention to some specific issues in athletic populations [46]. In some cases, the increased activity seen in mania or hypomania may be missed in the context of intense athletic training [16]. In bipolar disorder, rhythmic types of exercise such as running or swimming may aid mood regulation for some [47]. However, others report that exercise can contribute to symptoms of mood elevation [47], and exercise may have similar antidepressant and mood elevating properties as antidepressant medication [48] in those with an underlying propensity to bipolar disorders. In prospective studies, the incidence of bipolar disorders is also slightly higher in those who are regular exercisers at baseline [49]. Participants in high-risk sports such as mountain biking or rock climbing also report worsened bipolar symptoms [50].

An important consideration, therefore, when evaluating an athlete with bipolar disorder is to consider the nature of their physical activity and its potential role in their illness. This includes considering whether exercise is a manifestation of the disorder; a helpful way of managing symptoms; or a factor contributing to increased instability of mood (especially hypomanic or manic symptoms) [4]. Adjustments to the nature and intensity of exercise may need to be incorporated into short-term management of the condition, e.g. substituting higher intensity and higher risk activities with lower intensity and more soothing exercise patterns. In the longer term, it can also be helpful to refrain from training late in the evening and thus avoid the potentially activating effects of exercise [46].

There are many potential benefits from exercise and sports participation [51, 52]. Functional impairments and longer-term disability seen in psychotic disorders are correlated with cognitive symptoms and especially impairments in executive functions, and exercise may offer some protection via improved cognitive function [53, 54]. Physical activity may help to protect against the significant longer-term morbidity and mortality that is primarily related to metabolic syndrome associated with more chronic psychotic disorders and their treatment [55]. Sports participation can help those with psychotic conditions to experience recovery and a fulfilling and purposeful life in spite of their illness [56] and may also be a means to address the multiple social exclusions experienced by many of those with more long-term psychotic disorders [55]. Therefore, although the functional impairments of psychotic disorders such as schizophrenia may prove incompatible with a sustained career in high-performance sport [4, 29], athletes in this position should be supported with an 'exit-strategy' to a more recreational level of sports participation rather than being lost entirely to the world of sport [4].

Medication in Bipolar and Psychotic Disorders

Athlete-specific guidance is limited, but general population guidance along with athlete-specific guidance is summarised in Table 12.4. Prescribing in bipolar disorder is directed at both the episodes of mood disorder (depression and hypomania/mania) and, most importantly, long-term prophylaxis (preventing relapse and sustaining functional capacity) [39, 40, 57]. When recommending medication to an athlete, it is necessary for the prescriber to take careful consideration of not only the health benefits of treatment but also the impact on health and performance of side effects [37]. In addition, prescribing for athletes may need to account for unusual pharmacodynamics (e.g. the physiological stresses of the athlete's training and competition) and pharmacokinetics (e.g. how an athlete's body handles prescribed medication) [35, 46]. One issue that does not usually arise when prescribing for

Table 12.4 Medication guidance for the general population and the athlete population in bipolar and psychotic disorders [35, 37, 38, 44, 45, 57, 58]

	Bipolar mania	Bipolar depression	Bipolar prophylaxis	Psychosis
General guidance	Haloperidol, Olanzapine, Risperidone, Quetiapine; Lithium (slow effect); Valproate (slow effect)	Quetiapine, Lurasidone, Olanzapine/fluoxetine, Lamotrigine (very slow effect), Lithium (slow effect)	Both poles: Lithium, Quetiapine; Primarily mania: Valproate, Olanzapine, Risperidone; Primarily depression: Lurasidone, Lamotrigine	Any FGA or SGA depending on tolerability. Some guidance recommends SGA unless previous good response to FGA. Clozapine recommended for treatment-resistant cases.
Athlete guidance	Quetiapine; Lurasidone; Lamotrigine	Aripiprazole; Quetiapine; Lurasidone	Lithium; Aripiprazole; Quetiapine; Lurasidone; Lamotrigine	Aripiprazole; Lurasidone; Quetiapine

FGA first-generation antipsychotic, *SGA* second-generation antipsychotic

athletes with bipolar or psychotic disorders is the need to apply for a Therapeutic Use Exemption (TUE), as none of the commonly prescribed medications are associated with enhancement of sporting performance beyond simple restoration of health.

Acute Mania/Hypomania

In acute mania, there is a rapid onset of antimanic effect with antipsychotic medication, usually within hours or days. In addition, benzodiazepines, whilst not specifically antimanic, may have a role in reducing acute behavioural disturbance in the first few days of treatment [39, 40, 57]. Whilst both first- (FGA) and second-generation antipsychotics (SGA) can be used, SGA are generally preferred in adolescents and in athletes since individuals with bipolar disorder appear to be more prone to extrapyramidal side effects compared with individuals with schizophrenia [35, 37, 39]. Guidance recommends aripiprazole for adolescents because of its favourable metabolic profile [40], and athlete specific recommendations are summarised in Table 12.4. For less severe mania and hypomania, both lithium and valproate can be used, but have a slower onset of antimanic effect, and valproate should not be used in women of child-bearing age (which includes most female athletes) [39]. Occasionally, relapse occurs in those already taking prophylactic medication. In these circumstances, the first steps are to check adherence (e.g. by careful inquiry of patient and family supplemented if necessary by checking serum levels of lithium or valproate) and to adjust and optimise treatment accordingly [39, 40, 57]. This is supplemented by acute treatment as necessary and as described above. For those who develop manic or hypomanic symptoms whilst taking conventional antidepressant medication, this should be reviewed as soon as possible by an experienced mental health clinician (ideally the clinician with on-going and longer-term prescribing responsibilities) and may need to be stopped abruptly. The extent of acute behavioural disturbance and associated risks in acute mania are such that inpatient care is often indicated and may need to be undertaken by statutory or enforced means if insight is lacking and/or risks are high (see Chap. 20).

Depression

Conventional antidepressant medications have not been generally proven to be effective in bipolar depression, and in addition may precipitate switching into mania or hypomania [59, 60]. Guidance is to avoid them if possible and to only use them cautiously and usually only in combination with longer-term antimanic treatment, especially in bipolar I disorder. Selective serotonin reuptake inhibitors (SSRIs) and bupropion seem relatively less likely than other antidepressants to cause a switch into mania and are often preferred for this reason [60]. There is better evidence for recommending quetiapine, lurasidone, or olanzapine/fluoxetine in combination (OFC) [57]. Lamotrigine can also be used but is effective more slowly and requires careful titration [61]. Lithium has more equivocal evidence but can be recommended if shown to be previously effective [57].

Prophylaxis

For longer-term prophylaxis and prevention of future episodes in bipolar disorder, the best evidence is for lithium [39, 40, 57]. It is the usual first-line recommendation in guidelines and is effective at preventing relapse into either depression or hypomania/mania. Quetiapine may also prevent both depressive and hypomanic/manic episodes [62], but lamotrigine shows better prophylactic efficacy for depression than for hypomania/mania [40, 57]. Valproate and a range of antipsychotic medications including aripiprazole, lurasidone, olanzapine, and risperidone are more effective in the prophylaxis of hypomania/mania than depression [40, 57].

Psychosis

Long-term medication is usually recommended even after a single psychotic episode and reduces the risk of relapse [36, 44, 45]. Side effect profile influences the choice of drug, and although first-generation antipsychotic (FGA) and second-generation antipsychotic (SGA) medications show similar efficacy, some guidance preferentially recommends SGAs unless there is a documented good previous response to an FGA [45]. As in bipolar disorder, athletes may find side effects such as weight gain, sedation, and motor symptoms especially problematic, and thermoregulation may also be an issue for some [35, 37]. These concerns will influence both the choice of drug and the dosing regimen.

Athlete Prescribing Considerations

Athlete-specific evidence to guide treatment choice is limited and largely restricted to expert opinion that extrapolates from general guidance accounting for the specific needs of athletes in terms of health (and therefore indirectly performance) benefits and safety/tolerability [35, 37, 38].

Whilst lithium offers many advantages in terms of efficacy, it is associated with side effects such as tremor, which can impair motor performance, and careful monitoring of serum levels is required [35]. This is especially important in those who exercise intensely, as dehydration may raise levels towards toxicity [37], whilst sweat loss may theoretically lower serum lithium to below therapeutic levels [63, 64]. FGAs may be more likely to impair motor performance through the development of extrapyramidal symptoms, whilst some SGAs are associated with sedation and weight gain, which can be particularly undesirable for many athletes [4, 35, 37]. Although quetiapine may cause both weight gain and tremor (and therefore negatively impact performance), it is reported to have a lesser impact on thermoregulation and resting heart rate than other SGAs [46]. However, some antipsychotics (including quetiapine) can promote QTc prolongation, which may influence choice of medication for elite athletes [4, 37, 65]. When antipsychotics are prescribed for acute mania, they are typically used for weeks or a few months, whilst for bipolar prophylaxis and management of psychosis, they are likely to be prescribed for much longer durations (many months or more likely years) and this is a factor to be considered when evaluating tolerability. Some side effects might be bearable for a few weeks but would be much harder to tolerate over several years [4]. The timing of medication dosing throughout a daily cycle can also be manipulated to incorporate training and competition needs, e.g. not training in the few hours after taking medication that is even mildly sedating [46].

Conclusions

Bipolar and psychotic disorders are common and potentially serious conditions, but effective treatments are available. However, there are some important issues for sport to address to ensure the health and support the performance of athletes with these conditions.

Early identification is important, and delays in diagnosis and treatment are associated with poorer long-term outcomes. There may be some additional diagnostic issues to consider in sport, e.g. the difficulty in assessing over-activity in mania in those who are in intense physical training and the emergence of psychotic and mood symptoms in those who are using performance-enhancing substances such as AAS or stimulants.

Sport must also consider the importance of access to good mental health care. This extends beyond overcoming the stigma and barriers to care to include access to the specific and specialist expertise required to support and treat athletes with bipolar and psychotic disorders in the short, medium, and long term. The mental health expertise required to do this necessitates not just knowledge and skills in the management of the disorders themselves but an ability to apply this in the unusual environment of elite sport and accounting for the unique needs of the individual athlete. This might include modifications to a training programme to help manage the disorder and adjustments to medication regimens to accommodate training and competition. Sadly, it may also include supporting a small number of athletes with an exit strategy from elite sport if their illness proves incompatible with continued performance at that level but where continued sports participation will bring long-term health benefits.

References

1. Moesch K, Kenttä G, Kleinert J, Quignon-Fleuret C, Cecil S, Bertollo M. FEPSAC position statement: mental health disorders in elite athletes and models of service provision. Psychol Sport Exerc. 2018;38:61–71.
2. Merikangas KR, Jin R, He J-P, Kessler RC, Lee S, Sampson NA, et al. Prevalence and correlates of bipolar spectrum disorder in the world mental health survey initiative. Arch Gen Psychiatry. 2011;68(3):241–51.
3. Kessler RC, Amminger GP, Aguilar-Gaxiola S, Alonso J, Lee S, Üstün TB. Age of onset of mental disorders: a review of recent literature. Curr Opin Psychiatry. 2007;20(4):359–64.
4. Currie A, Gorczynski P, Rice SM, Purcell R, McAllister-Williams RH, Hitchcock ME, et al. Bipolar and psychotic disorders in elite athletes: a narrative review. Br J Sports Med. 2019;53(12):746–53.
5. Post RM, Leverich GS, Kupka RW, Keck PE, McElroy SL, Altshuler LL, et al. Early-onset bipolar disorder and treatment delay are risk factors for poor outcome in adulthood. J Clin Psychiatry. 2010;71(7):864–72.
6. Nordentoft M, Rasmussen JØ, Melau M, Hjorthøj CR, Thorup AAE. How successful are first episode programs? A review of the evidence for specialized assertive early intervention. Curr Opin Psychiatry. 2014;27(3):167–72.
7. American Psychiatric Association. Diagnostic and Statistical Manual of Mental Disorders (DSM-5). 5th ed. Washington, DC: American Psychiatric Publishing; 2013. p. 1–947.
8. Baron DA, Reardon CL, Baron SH. Doping in sport. In: Baron DA, Reardon CL, Baron SH, editors. Clinical sports psychiatry: an international perspective. 1st ed. Oxford: John Wiley & Sons; 2013. p. 21–32.
9. Bahrke MS. Psychological and behavioral effects of anabolic -androgenic steroids. Int J Sport Exerc Psychol. 2005;3(4):428–45.

10. Trenton AJ, Currier GW. Behavioural manifestations of anabolic steroid use. CNS Drugs. 2005;19(7):571–95.

11. Piacentino D, Kotzalidis G, Casale A, Aromatario M, Pomara C, Girardi P, et al. Anabolic-androgenic Steroid use and Psychopathology in Athletes. A systematic review. Curr Neuropharmacol. 2015;13(1):101–21.

12. Morse ED. Substance use in athletes. In: Baron DA, Reardon CL, Baron SH, editors. Clinical sports psychiatry. Oxford: John Wiley & Sons; 2013. p. 1–12.

13. Judd LL, Akiskal HS, Schettler PJ, Endicott J, Maser J, Solomon DA, et al. The long-term natural history of the weekly symptomatic status of bipolar I disorder. Arch Gen Psychiatry. 2002;59(6):530–7.

14. Judd LL, Akiskal HS, Schettler PJ, Coryell W, Endicott J, Maser JD, et al. A prospective investigation of the natural history of the long-term weekly symptomatic status of bipolar II disorder. Arch Gen Psychiatry. 2003;60(3):261–9.

15. Hantouche EG, Akiskal HS, Lancrenon S, Allilaire JF, Sechter D, Azorin JM, et al. Systematic clinical methodology for validating bipolar-II disorder: data in mid-stream from a French national multi-site study (EPIDEP). J Affect Disord. 1998;50(2–3):163–73.

16. Markser V, Currie A, McAllister-Williams RH. Mood disorders. In: Currie A, Owen B, editors. Sports psychiatry. 1st ed. Oxford: Oxford University Press; 2016. p. 31–51.

17. McKetin R, Leung J, Stockings E, Huo Y, Foulds J, Lappin JM, et al. Mental health outcomes associated with the use of amphetamines: a systematic review and meta-analysis. EClinicalMedicine. 2019;16:81–97.

18. Parker G. Is borderline personality disorder a mood disorder? Br J Psychiatry. 2014;204(4):252–3.

19. Frías Á, Baltasar I, Birmaher B. Comorbidity between bipolar disorder and borderline personality disorder: prevalence, explanatory theories, and clinical impact. J Affect Disord. 2016;202:210–9.

20. Schiweck C, Arteaga-Henriquez G, Aichholzer M, Edwin Thanarajah S, Vargas-Cáceres S, Matura S, et al. Comorbidity of ADHD and adult bipolar disorder: a systematic review and meta-analysis. Neurosci Biobehav Rev. 2021;124:100–23.

21. Chu CS, Tsai SJ, Hsu JW, Huang KL, Cheng CM, Su TP, et al. Diagnostic progression to bipolar disorder in 17,285 adolescents and young adults with attention deficit hyperactivity disorder: a longitudinal follow-up study. J Affect Disord. 2021;295:1072–8.

22. Creado S, Reardon C. The sports psychiatrist and performance-enhancing drugs. Int Rev Psychiatry. 2016;28(6):564–71.

23. Goldner EM, Hsu L, Waraich P, Somers JM. Prevalence and incidence studies of schizophrenic disorders: a systematic review of the literature. Can J Psychiatr. 2002;47(9):833–43.

24. Kelleher I, Connor D, Clarke MC, Devlin N, Harley M, Cannon M. Prevalence of psychotic symptoms in childhood and adolescence: a systematic review and meta-analysis of population-based studies. Psychol Med. 2012;42(9):1857–63.

25. Rice SM, Purcell R, De Silva S, Mawren D, McGorry PD, Parker AG. The mental health of elite athletes: a narrative systematic review. Sports Med. 2016;46(9):1333–53.

26. Reardon CL. Psychiatric comorbidities in sports. Neurol Clin. 2017;35(3):537–46.

27. Reardon CL, Factor RM. Sport psychiatry: a systematic review of diagnosis and medical treatment of mental illness in athletes. Sports Med. 2010;40(11):961–80.

28. Favor Hamilton S, Tomlinson S. Fast girl: a life spent running from madness. 1st ed. New York, NY: Harper Collins; 2016. 304 p.

29. Ströhle A. Sports psychiatry: mental health and mental disorders in athletes and exercise treatment of mental disorders. Eur Arch Psychiatry Clin Neurosci. 2019;269(5):485–98.

30. Currie A, McDuff D, Johnston A, Hopley P, Hitchcock ME, Reardon CL, et al. Management of mental health emergencies in elite athletes: a narrative review. Br J Sports Med. 2019;53(12):772–8.

31. Iverson GL, Brooks BL, Langenecker SA, Young AH. Identifying a cognitive impairment subgroup in adults with mood disorders. J Affect Disord. 2011;132(3):360–7.

32. Robinson LJ, Thompson JM, Gallagher P, Goswami U, Young AH, Ferrier IN, et al. A meta-analysis of cognitive deficits in euthymic patients with bipolar disorder. J Affect Disord. 2006;93(1–3):105–15.

33. Bora E. Neurocognitive features in clinical subgroups of bipolar disorder: a meta-analysis. J Affect Disord. 2018;229:125–34.

34. Carvalho AF, Bortolato B, Miskowiak K, Vieta E, Köhler C. Cognitive dysfunction in bipolar disorder and schizophrenia: a systematic review of meta-analyses. Neuropsychiatr Dis Treat. 2015;11:3111.

35. Johnston A, McAllister-Williams RH. Psychotropic drug prescribing. In: Currie A, Owen B, editors. Sports psychiatry. 1st ed. Oxford: Oxford University Press; 2016. p. 133–43.

36. Barnes TRE, Drake R, Paton C, Cooper SJ, Deakin B, Ferrier IN, et al. Evidence-based guidelines for the pharmacological treatment of schizophrenia: updated recommendations from the British Association for Psychopharmacology. J Psychopharmacol. 2020;34(1):3–78.

37. Reardon CL. The sports psychiatrist and psychiatric medication. Int Rev Psychiatry. 2016;28(6):606–13.

38. Reardon CL, Creado S. Psychiatric medication preferences of sports psychiatrists. Physician Sport Med. 2016;44(4):397–402.

39. Hirschfield RMA, Bowden CL, Gitlin MJ, Keck PE, Suppes T, Thase ME, et al. Treatment of patients with bipolar disorder. American Psychiatric Association Practice Guidelines. 2nd ed. Washington, DC: American Psychiatric Association; 2010. p. 1–82.

40. National Institute for Health and Care Excellence. Bipolar Disorder (update): the assessment and management of bipolar disorder in adults, children and young people in primary and secondary care. London: NIHCE; 2014.

41. Colom F, Vieta E, Reinares M, Martínez-Arán A, Torrent C, Goikolea JM, et al. Psychoeducation efficacy in bipolar disorders: beyond compliance enhancement. J Clin Psychiatry. 2003;64(9):1101–5.

42. Frank E, Swartz HA, Kupfer DJ. Interpersonal and social rhythm therapy: managing the chaos of bipolar disorder. Biol Psychiatry. 2000;48(6):593–604.

43. Frank E, Soreca I, Schwartz H, Fagiolini A, Mallinger AG, Thase ME, et al. The role of interpersonal and social rhythm therapy in improving occupational functioning in patients with bipolar I disorder. Am J Psychiatry. 2008;165(12):1559–65.

44. National Institute for Health and Care Excellence. Psychosis and schizophrenia in adults: prevention and management. London: NIHCE; 2014.

45. Lehman AF, Lieberman JA, Dixon LB, McGlashan TH, Miller AL, Perkins DO, et al. Practice guideline for the treatment of patients with schizophrenia. 2nd ed. Washington, DC: American Psychiatric Association; 2010. p. 1–184.

46. Bradley SL, Reardon CL. Bipolar disorder and eating disorders in sport: a case of comorbidity and review of treatment principles in an elite athlete. Phys Sportsmed. 2021;50:84–92.

47. Wright K, Armstrong T, Taylor A, Dean S. 'It's a double edged sword': a qualitative analysis of the experiences of exercise amongst people with bipolar disorder. J Affect Disord. 2012;136(3): 634–42.

48. Duman CH, Schlesinger L, Russell DS, Duman RS. Voluntary exercise produces antidepressant and anxiolytic behavioral effects in mice. Brain Res. 2008;1199:148–58.

49. Strohle A, Hofler M, Pfister H, Muller A-G, Hoyer J, Wittchen H-U, et al. Physical activity and prevalence and incidence of mental disorders in adolescents and young adults. Psychol Med. 2007;37(11):1657–66.

50. Dudek D, Siwek M, Jaeschke R, Drozdowicz K, Styczeń K, Arciszewska A, et al. A web-based study of bipolarity and impul-

sivity in athletes engaging in extreme and high-risk sports. Acta Neuropsychiatr. 2016;28(03):179–83.

51. Firth J, Cotter J, Elliott R, French P, Yung AR. A systematic review and meta-analysis of exercise interventions in schizophrenia patients. Psychol Med. 2015;45(7):1343–61.

52. Dauwan M, Begemann MJH, Heringa SM, Sommer IE. Exercise improves clinical symptoms, quality of life, global functioning, and depression in schizophrenia: a systematic review and meta-analysis. Schizophr Bull. 2016;42(3):588–99.

53. Pajonk F-G, Wobrock T, Gruber O, Scherk H, Berner D, Kaizl I, et al. Hippocampal plasticity in response to exercise in schizophrenia. Arch Gen Psychiatry. 2010;67(2):133–43.

54. Scheewe TW, van Haren NE, Sarkisyan G, Schnack HG, Brouwer RM, de Glint M, et al. Exercise therapy, cardiorespiratory fitness and their effect on brain volumes: a randomised controlled trial in patients with schizophrenia and healthy controls. Eur Neuropsychopharmacol. 2013;23:675–85.

55. Currie A, Malik R. Exercise participation and mental health. In: Currie A, Owen B, editors. Sports psychiatry. 1st ed. Oxford: Oxford University Press; 2016. p. 107–16.

56. Carless D. Narrative, identity, and recovery from serious mental illness: a life history of a runner. Qual Res Psychol. 2008;5(4):233–48.

57. Goodwin GM, Haddad PM, Ferrier IN, Aronson JK, Barnes TRH, Cipriani A, et al. Evidence-based guidelines for treating bipolar disorder: revised third edition recommendations from the British Association for Psychopharmacology. J Psychopharmacol. 2016;30(6):495–553.

58. Barnes T. Schizophrenia Consensus Group of British Association of Psychopharmacology. Evidence-based guidelines for the pharmacological treatment of schizophrenia: recommendations from the British Association for Psychopharmacology. J Pharmacol. 2011;25(5):567–620.

59. Sidor MM, MacQueen GM. Antidepressants for the acute treatment of bipolar depression. J Clin Psychiatry. 2011;72(2):156–67.

60. Post RM, Altshuler LL, Leverich GS, Frye MA, Nolen WA, Kupka RW, et al. Mood switch in bipolar depression: comparison of adjunctive venlafaxine, bupropion and sertraline. Br J Psychiatry. 2006;189(2):124–31.

61. Geddes JR, Calabrese JR, Goodwin GM. Lamotrigine for treatment of bipolar depression: independent meta-analysis and meta-regression of individual patient data from five randomised trials. Br J Psychiatry. 2009;194(01):4–9.

62. Weisler RH, Nolen WA, Neijber A, Hellqvist Å, Paulsson B. Trial 144 Study Investigators. Continuation of quetiapine versus switching to placebo or lithium for maintenance treatment of bipolar I disorder. J Clin Psychiatry. 2011;72(11):1452–64.

63. Jefferson JW, Greist JH, Clagnaz PJ, Eischens RR, Marten WC, Evenson MA. Effect of strenuous exercise on serum lithium level in man. Am J Psychiatry. 1982;139(12):1593–5.

64. Miller EB, Pain RW, Skripal PJ. Sweat lithium in manic-depression. Br J Psychiatry. 1978;133(5):477–8.

65. Beach SR, Celano CM, Noseworthy PA, Januzzi JL, Huffman JC. QTc Prolongation, Torsades de Pointes, and Psychotropic Medications. Psychosomatics. 2013;54(1):1–13.

Mental Health and Sport-Related Concussion

13

Vuong Vu and Aaron Jeckell

Introduction

Our understanding and appreciation of concussions has undergone a tremendous evolution in the past several decades. Far from the moderate to severe brain injuries with which concussions used to be conflated, the past several decades have brought us a new and more nuanced appreciation of this type of injury. Increased knowledge of sport-related concussions (SRCs) has enabled us to allow athletes to compete more safely and receive more effective treatment when injured. However, there is a paucity of data specific to SRCs in the elite athlete (EA). Most current studies examine youth and amateur athletes (AAs), as they make up a greater share of those injured. Although still an extremely heterogeneous group, it is important to consider some of the factors that distinguish EAs from other athletes. EAs tend to be larger, stronger, and compete at a higher level of speed and intensity as compared to AAs. EAs have generally been competing for longer, exposing them to a greater potential for injury. EAs are more likely to be late adolescents or young adults. They are also more likely to have access to immediate and advanced medical interventions as needed. Keeping these important differences in mind, we will explore how an SRC presents and can be managed in the EA, while making note of the limitations of current data and where generalizing available information is appropriate.

Background

Definition

An SRC describes a collection of symptoms that can appear after a transmission of force to the brain is experienced during participation in a sport activity. These indicators can vary but include a cluster of neuropsychiatric symptoms that appear within hours of injury and typically resolve over a matter of days to weeks. An SRC does not necessitate an impact to the head, only that the force be transmitted to the brain. An SRC may lead to neuropathological/neurochemical changes, but the impairment is said to be a functional disturbance rather than a structural injury. Loss of consciousness (LOC), once believed to be synonymous with SRC, is not required and is relatively uncommon in this type of injury [1].

An SRC leads to a complex neurochemical disruption in the brain and, in some cases, diffuse axonal injury [2]. After experiencing a concussive injury, a neurochemical cascade is set off in which ionic balances in the cerebral neurons are disrupted. To regain homeostasis, the brain requires additional oxygen and glucose supplied by cerebral blood flow to fuel sodium–potassium pumps. This occurs in the context of a relative energy disparity as blood flow to the brain is decreased in the aftermath of an SRC. These physiological changes are linked to the clinical symptoms seen in concussions [3]. Specifically, this energy imbalance can lead to a disturbance of functional networks that can cause impaired cognition, mood disturbance, vestibulo-ocular dysfunction, sleep disturbance, and a range of other symptoms [4].

In addition, an SRC can result in diffuse and multifocal damage to the axons within the white matter of the brain. This can account for impaired interactions between a variety of brain regions, exacerbating the range of symptoms described above. While macroscopic injury can occur with concussive impacts, SRC symptoms are not due to focal macroscopic brain injury [5].

It is important to distinguish an SRC from a mild traumatic brain injury (mTBI) that is experienced by the general

V. Vu (✉)
Northwest Permanente Physicians and Surgeons, PC, Portland, OR, USA

A. Jeckell
Vanderbilt University Medical Center, Broward Health, Coral Springs, FL, USA

population. Athletes who experience SRC may undergo baseline neurocognitive testing and physical examinations, as they are required by many athletic governing bodies. Athletes are likely to be helmeted or wearing protective equipment at the time of impact. EAs often have immediate and follow-up medical support available by specialists with specific training in the management of SRC. In addition, EAs may experience unique psychosocial factors that can contribute to injury and recovery including eagerness to return to sport, financial or scholarship incentives, and pressure from media and fans. Individuals who experience mTBI outside of the sport setting are unlikely to have baseline measures and are less likely to be wearing safety equipment when injured. In these cases, medical care may be delayed or never take place. While the impacts that EAs experience can be extremely forceful, a nonathlete mTBI often involves extreme impacts via vehicle collision, falls from height, or assault. LOC is less common in an SRC than in a non-SRC, which may lead to SRC being underreported [6].

Biomechanics

The physics of concussion has been studied extensively since the mid-twentieth century using animals, humans, machinery, and computational models. Ommaya and Gennarelli established that a rotational force component was more likely to lead to developing a concussion [7]. Efforts to identify a precise gravitational force at which a concussion occurs have been unyielding. Studying the dynamics of a human brain during an impact is extremely difficult and is limited by medical, ethical, and technological constraints. Animal models that focus primarily on small mammals are inadequate in their generalizability to humans. Cadaveric studies cannot reveal active biochemical changes or post-impact symptom development. The heterogeneity of elite athletes compounds these difficulties. A contemporary review of the literature does indicate several crucial findings. Although there is no specific threshold, a concussion can and does occur at lower impacts than previously believed. Conversely, athletes can experience multiple high-impact collisions (e.g., more than 80 times the force of gravity) in a season and not manifest concussion symptoms. Both linear and rotational impacts are important when considering the risk of concussion. Relying on the impact magnitude alone cannot predict clinical outcomes such as symptom severity, neuropsychological function, and time course [8].

Epidemiology

An estimated 1.6–3.8 million SRCs occur annually in the United States across all levels of play, a figure that factors unreported or unrecognized cases [9]. Up to 50% of concussed athletes do not immediately report the presence of

concussion-related symptoms [10]. Although SRCs account for a relatively small percentage of overall sport injuries, they are highly visible with the potential for significant repercussions. Additionally, SRCs have been covered extensively in the sports media over the past several decades with high-profile EAs publicly reporting short- and long-term effects of this injury. Data specific to the rates of concussion in EAs have been limited as present studies have tended to focus on youth/amateur athletes. Data regarding the frequency of SRCs in competition as compared to those in practice have been mixed.

The rates of concussion can be measured in terms of athlete exposure (AE), defined as a single athlete participating in a sport (practice or competition) in a way that exposes them to potential injury. A 2018 meta-analysis examining men's and women's elite-level rugby, ice hockey, European football, and men's American football found that the highest density of SRCs was in rugby (3.89 and 3.00 SRCs per 1000 h and AEs, respectively) and the lowest was in men's American football (0.01 and 0.08 per 1000 h and AEs, respectively). The authors found that in EAs, an SRC was rare in practice compared to competition, and women participating in ice hockey and European football were at an increased risk when compared to their male counterparts [11].

Among National Collegiate Athletic Association (NCAA) athletes, one study analyzing data from 2009 to 2014 found that SRCs in EAs represented 6.2% of all injuries reported. SRCs were reported at a greater rate in competition versus practice, though this varies by sport. The sports with the highest rates of SRCs were men's wrestling, men's and women's ice hockey, and men's (American) football. The sport with the greatest number of reported SRCs was men's football followed by men's ice hockey and women's soccer. A majority of SRCs occurred from player contact, and 9% were recurrent on average across the 25 sports included. Across the 5-year span, the national incidence of SRCs did not appear to increase linearly; however, year-to-year increases were seen in men's football, women's ice hockey, and men's lacrosse. The increases could be explained by a greater number of sport participants, a greater sensitivity to recognition of SRC among players, clinicians, and staff, or a more unsafe style of play [12].

Caution should be exercised when interpreting SRC rates for men's wrestling and men's/women's ice hockey, as the total sample reported was far less than that of men's football. One may hypothesize that these specific sports have higher rates due to being full-contact; however, women's ice hockey is not as there is no checking allowed. One may also take into consideration that an SRC may be misdiagnosed as it can present similarly to other common ailments, such as dehydration, seen in these specific sports [13].

There were a greater number of concussions during practice in men's football and in men's and women's basketball.

This could be due to factors such as a greater number of AEs in practices versus competition and the varying levels of protective equipment worn during practices [12].

A study looking at data among NCAA athletes from 2018 to 2019 did show a greater number of concussions observed during practice over competitions and that men's football had the highest total number of concussions followed by women's soccer. The data also showed similar rates between men and women with regard to symptom severity or recovery time [14].

Risk Factors

Identifying specific medical, including psychiatric, risk factors for experiencing an SRC and prolonged recovery is complicated by the fact that athletes are an extremely heterogeneous group participating in a wide range of activities that each confer their own set of risk factors. Any activity in which athletes travel at a high velocity or interact with moving objects of substantial mass confers a risk of experiencing an SRC. Sports that involve incidental collisions have additional risk, and sports where collisions are routine tend to have the highest risk. Other factors that have been studied and detailed in this section include the type of sport being played, the age of the athletes involved, the gender of the athlete, a history of previous concussion or mental health issue, and the level of play.

Legarreta et al. found that both a personal and a family history of psychiatric disorders, independently, are risk factors for prolonged recovery [15]. Those with preinjury mood or anxiety symptoms are more likely to experience them after an SRC [16]. Careful assessment of preinjury mental health issues can help a clinician predict and target interventions.

Data on age as a risk factor for prolonged recovery from an SRC have been mixed. Youth athletes are more likely to experience a concussion, and recovery may be expected to take longer [17–19]. Many studies support a gradient effect with older athletes recovering faster than youths. Other studies posit that teenage and high school athletes may be the highest-risk age group for a prolonged recovery. This can possibly be explained by teens being more developmentally advanced with an improved ability to express their feelings and symptoms verbally along with other psychosocial factors more relevant to that age range [20].

The role of gender and the risk of an SRC has been mixed, but many studies report that women have higher rates of SRCs within a given sport [21, 22]. Iverson et al. found that females have longer recovery periods, greater likelihood of symptoms persisting beyond 1 month, and higher reporting of symptoms before and after an injury when compared to males [20]. A 2020 scoping review analyzing female soccer players of all ages found specific sex disparities that may account for the higher rates of SRCs in females, including greater linear and rotational head acceleration, reduced neck strength (in addition to narrower and longer necks), greater injury rate with contact with the ball or ground, hormonal influences (specifically the late luteal phase with low progesterone and estrogen, both of which have been shown to be neuroprotective), and more sensitive effects on the brain structure (i.e., faster acceleration led to more jarring of the brain) [23]. Another article demonstrated how neurons in the female brain have narrower microtubules and may be more vulnerable to axonal shearing forces that typically occur in an SRC [24].

Many studies have found that a prior history of SRC increases the likelihood of experiencing a future SRC, presumably by lowering the impact threshold necessary to develop SRC symptoms [20]. In 2018, Putukian et al. replicated findings that a history of concussion increases the risk of future concussion in athletes [25]. A prior SRC is also associated with symptoms persisting for more than 1 month. Athletes with premorbid learning disorder and/or attention-deficit/hyperactivity disorder (ADHD) may be at a higher risk of experiencing concussion but not necessarily a prolonged recovery. There were mixed results on how specific clinical symptoms such as LOC or amnesia accounted for the severity of an SRC or the length of recovery. There were consistent findings that greater acute and subacute symptoms were associated with lengthier recovery [20]. Putukian et al. reinforced how higher symptom severity and more total symptoms, especially headaches, steadiness on one's feet, and worse concentration, could lead to longer recovery time frames [25].

Studies from 2014 and 2015 demonstrated that having experienced an SRC is a risk factor for lower extremity (LE) injury in EAs, but it is not yet known whether the converse is true [26, 27]. It would be intuitive to surmise that a nonconcussive injury that significantly alters an athlete's typical style of play, especially if participating in a contact sport, might increase their susceptibility to experiencing an SRC.

Early Age of Exposure to Sports

Evidence supports that an earlier estimated age of first exposure (eAFE) to high-risk sports incurs a higher risk of experiencing an SRC. Data addressing whether earlier eAFE reliably leads to late-life cognitive impairment and mental health disorders have thus far been mixed. Studies have predominantly focused on those who have participated in tackle football, limiting the generalizability to other sports.

One 2021 study aimed to evaluate how an earlier age of first exposure (less than 12 years of age) to amateur football contributed to long-term brain health outcomes in middle-aged men. Those who began playing football at a younger age did expectedly report more years of playing football and a greater number of lifetime concussions compared to the group of men who began playing football at age 12 or later; the former group also reported experiencing their first concussion at a younger age compared to the latter group. The two groups demonstrated similar rates of physical, cognitive, and mental health concerns at their current ages [28]. This particular study was a high-powered replication of two older studies (2016 and 2019 publications) that also showed no major association of long-term consequences of early exposure to football in retired National Football League (NFL) players [29, 30]. There are two other former studies (2015 and 2017 publications) that reflect opposing results, with indications that an earlier age of exposure to football is associated with a greater impairment of self-reported cognitive and neuropsychiatric symptoms in older men [31, 32]; notably, these specific studies showed mixed results and had different recruitment/inclusion criteria.

Caccese et al. authored papers from 2019 to 2021 that also explored the risks of an earlier age of first exposure to SRCs in females and males, though primarily focusing on symptoms experienced by college-age athletes and not later in life. The authors replicated findings that an earlier age of first exposure was associated with a higher total number of lifetime concussions in males and females but was not associated with significant neurocognitive deficits in college-age athletes [33–35].

There is a need for future longitudinal studies that examine this question applied to a larger and more diverse sample with matched controls and careful consideration of other factors that can lead to similar outcomes (substance use, socioeconomic factors, etc.). The results thus far may help provide more data for families who have fears about their children participating in certain sports at younger ages.

Early Injury Evaluation

Time to evaluation in younger athletes may be important considering a developing brain that is susceptible to injury and is experiencing a high rate of neurodevelopment. A prolonged recovery can lead to persistent symptoms of concussion that impact mood regulation, sleep, general physical health, and cognitive performance, and it is important to know whether time to evaluation can impact this trajectory in youth and older elite athletes alike.

A 2021 study evaluated the importance of early injury evaluation after concussion in pediatric populations and found that youths seen by a treatment team within 28 days after injury had shorter recovery times when compared to youths who had evaluations later than 28 days after injury. This study had male and female participants and concussions

that involved sporting and nonsporting (e.g., falls and non-sport recreation) activities. There were no significant differences between early (less than 14 days to evaluation after injury) and mid (14–28 days to evaluation after injury) evaluations with regard to recovery time [36]. A 2020 study supported findings of benefits from earlier clinic evaluations after concussion for improved recovery times, but the time frames were shorter (within 7 days versus 8–20 days) and the population studied was all athletes [37]. The 2021 study suggested that there may not be an increased risk of prolonged recovery with time to evaluation within 28 days, which can be important for athletes with limited access to care such as those in rural settings, where there may be some feasibility around telehealth services for concussion evaluation. Another critical point of the 2021 study was the incorporation of individualized and early exercise therapy, which will be addressed further in the Preventative and Treatment Strategies section of this chapter.

Other Specific Populations

In a 2021 study of elite para-athletes, results showed the rates of SRC comparable to other athletes. Despite multiple unique intrinsic and extrinsic risk factors that the para-athlete population sometimes faces, including impaired bodily senses (e.g., vision, balance, or executive functioning) and dependence on assistive devices (e.g., wheelchairs or a specific guide), the data only highlighted that female para-athletes and those with vision impairment had higher SRC rates, SRCs generally occurred during training, and the usual mechanism of injury was collision with an apparatus or another person [38]. This study referenced how nearly half of the SRCs could have been prevented and provided suggestions on how to modify systems to better protect the athletes.

Wallace et al. reviewed racial differences in youth athletes and found that Black athletes reported less knowledge about concussion symptoms and were also less likely to receive a diagnosis in the emergency department (ED) when compared to White athletes. The study also showed that White athletes were more likely to have a history of concussion diagnosis. Although not statistically significant, there was a trend toward White athletes receiving more ED orders and more head imaging. The presence of an athletic trainer helped reduce disparities of access to care and follow-up [39]. A separate study focusing on SRCs in youth and college-age athletes found that Black athletes reached symptom resolution faster and had a quicker return to school when compared to White athletes. The authors surmised that lower concussion symptom knowledge and a less serious attitude toward SRCs among Black athletes contributed to less reporting of concussion symptoms [40]. A third study analyzing NCAA Division 1 college athletes showed that Black college athletes were less likely to disclose experiencing concussion symptoms when compared to White college athletes, though it was not a significant difference. There were significant differences in the reasons cited for nondisclosure, as the Black athletes reported not thinking it was a concussion at the time and being fearful of being seen as weak by their peers. There were findings that White athletes and their parents had greater knowledge of concussion symptoms. Others found that females as well as any athlete with a history of concussion or greater concussion knowledge had higher odds of disclosing concussion symptoms [41].

Clinical Presentation

SRC symptoms typically develop within minutes to hours but can also manifest immediately after impact. Common initial symptoms include headache, dizziness, coordination impairment, nausea/vomiting, disorientation, confusion, or emotionality. In the immediate aftermath of an impact suspected to cause an SRC, a general medical and neurological examination needs to be performed in conjunction with standardized assessment tools such as the Sport Concussion Assessment Tool 5 (SCAT-5). These objective measures are crucial. An EA may be motivated to suppress or mask symptoms due to eagerness to support their teammates, intrinsic pressure to perform, fear of appearing weak, or extrinsic motivators such as financial or scholarship incentives. An athlete may not know how serious a concussion can be or may simply be unaware of what their symptoms mean to their health or long-term ability to participate in sport [42, 43].

Mental Health and Other Physical Symptoms

SRC symptoms are frequently clustered into four categories: somatic, sleep, cognitive, and emotional. It is not uncommon to see a symptom in one cluster evolve into or directly influence other symptoms. An EA who experiences significant sleep impairment after an SRC may subsequently feel a decline in their mood or mental fogginess. Large-scale meta-analyses have identified an association between SRC in athletes and the development of depressive symptoms, though causation cannot be established [44]. Many of these studies are limited by methodological issues and have concerns of potential bias. Other studies have demonstrated that the risk of experiencing depression after an injury is not unique to SRC [45]. Evidence linking SRC to anxiety is mixed, with insufficient data to draw definitive conclusions.

A 2021 study comprised of college athletes compared symptomatically and asymptomatically concussed athletes with control athletes and found that the symptomatic athletes had worse depressive symptoms and more cognitive disturbance, specifically slower reaction time and worse response accuracy [46]. A 2021 review study of youth and elite-level athletes analyzed ball heading in European football and found no clear evidence of short-term harmful cognitive effects; however, a few of the studies replicated negative effects on reaction time and memory capability [47].

Studies have reviewed the risk of lower extremity (LE) injury after an SRC. There are hypotheses and evidence that neurocognitive impairment (e.g., decreased reaction time and diminished working memory as alluded to above) from concussion can lead to mechanical compensatory strategies that ultimately put the athlete at a greater risk of injury, specifically anterior cruciate ligament strains and sprains [48, 49]. A separate study looking specifically at players in the NFL found no increased risk of LE injury after an SRC but also pointed out how NFL players have different levels of contact and playing/rest time in comparison to other sports with greater rates of LE injury including soccer and basketball [50].

There are emerging data surrounding concussion effects on autonomic function (e.g., blood pressure, heart rate, respiratory rate), but no clear conclusions can be drawn. In an examination of youth male EAs, Harrison et al. found that concussed athletes had increased heart rate variability only during exertional activities (cognitive or physical exercises), pointing to the importance of recognizing post-SRC deficits during functional activities and not just at rest [51].

When considering the development of mood or other physical symptoms in EAs after an SRC, one must consider the psychosocial factors in addition to those regarded as purely more "biological." An EA may be unfamiliar with mental health struggles prior to experiencing an SRC. The predominant culture in elite sport is such that any displays of perceived weakness are discouraged. As such, an athlete may struggle to relate their mental health symptoms or may even be ashamed of experiencing them. Fear and lack of understanding of the short- and long-term risks associated with an SRC may be another limiting factor that impacts symptom disclosure [52].

Recovery

Recovery from an SRC can vary depending on the level of play, age, or gender. A typical recovery time frame has been defined as 10–14 days for adults and approximately 4 weeks for children [1]. A 2018 study among Air Force cadets found differences in these time frames among athletes, specifically significant differences in the recovery time of men versus women (24.7 days versus 35.5 days, respectively) and also elite versus nonelite (25.4 days versus 34.7 days, respectively). The study referenced that EAs may recover faster given their superior fitness, more incentive to return to sport, and access to greater medical care as compared to nonelites [53].

A 2021 study analyzing collegiate athlete data consisting of males and females from 22 different sports spanning 2014–2018 agreed that 1 month was the appropriate estimation of a "normal" recovery timeline for return to play (RTP) across all athletes. Resetting the normalized time frame to 1 month may help reduce the stigma associated with needing a longer recovery. The same study also demonstrated that athletes who experienced concussions during competition had quicker recovery than during practice; the authors hypothesized that there was greater medical attentiveness for potentially faster recognition and evaluation of a concussion during competition. Concussions occurring during practice tend to be in the off-season, and medical staff may be more conservative with RTP timelines. This study also replicated results from other referenced studies that both greater initial injury severity and a history of three or more concussions had longer recovery time frames [54]. When considering recovery from an SRC, a provider must not rigidly adhere to a recovery timetable and instead focus on how the athlete presents.

Return-to-learn (RTL) protocols are a crucial element in recovery for youth athletes or those who are still in school. McCrory et al. summarized RTL and RTP as stepwise strategies starting with light activities that do not exacerbate symptoms and gradually progressing with eventual return to school or play full time [1]. For those struggling to advance through the RTL protocol, Herring et al. provided suggestions of accommodations including extra time for homework and exams, avoidance of noisy environments, and allowance of frequent breaks during learning and testing activities to name a few [55]. The Concussion in Para-Sport group released a thorough position statement in 2021 with specific guidelines on how to adjust RTP and RTL protocols, given the particular impairments that para-athletes have [56].

Newer evidence has refuted the once-held belief that an athlete must adhere to a certain window of inactivity, sometimes lasting weeks. Rather, mild cardiovascular activity that does not exacerbate any symptoms and is started after 1–2 days of physical and cognitive rest may speed up recovery [55, 57].

Haider et al. examined a population of predominantly SRC data in male and female youth from 2016 to 2019 and found specific criteria that were able to predict with high accuracy the future development of persistent post-concussive symptoms. The criteria examined included a history of multiple concussions, days since injury, severity of injury, and deficits in gait, orthostatic balance, and vestibulo-ocular system. As most youth athletes with SRC can wait 1 month before being concerned about prolonged symptoms,

this examination can help with early implementation of the recovery protocol for children at a greater risk [58].

Kirkwood et al. made suggestions about how to lessen or even eliminate nocebo effects caused by unnecessary interventions, inappropriate diagnostic examinations, or general confusion relating to SRCs. These include using milder language regarding injury, maintaining a positive framework of recovery rather than deficits, providing education and reassurance of expected symptoms and timelines, and sticking to evidence-based recommendations and treatments [59]. Accordingly, "overparenting" of youth after SRC was found to prolong recovery, and emotional distress worsened clinical outcomes [60].

A clinician must take all factors (not limited to age, gender, general medical/psychiatric history, sport played, symptoms experienced, or level of play) of each unique athlete into consideration when developing a treatment and recovery plan. When cumulative data suggest that an athlete is at a heightened risk of a prolonged recovery, it is worthwhile to consider early interventions and treatment in anticipation of experiencing extended symptomatology.

Preventative and Treatment Strategies

Screening

Athletes benefit from receiving a pre-participation evaluation during the off-season that should include a thorough history and nature of previous head injuries, migraines, and mental health disorders [1, 55]. It may also be beneficial to obtain baseline assessments of neurological and cognitive functions such as via the Sport Concussion Assessment Tool 5 (SCAT-5) or Immediate Post-Concussion Assessment and Cognitive Testing (ImPACT) [14, 55].

It is important to be able to recognize an SRC when it occurs, paying close attention to the mechanism of injury and the perceptible signs of change from baseline behavior such as having a blank stare and/or a decrease in mobility or balance. When suspicion is high enough to pull an athlete from play, the athlete should be taken to a quiet setting for a more thorough physical and cognitive evaluation. With the advancement of technology usage, there may be access to video footage and time to hear from independent spotters present to provide additional information of the presence and severity of a potential SRC [55, 61].

Targeted Education

There has been an increased focus on improving SRC knowledge with the intention of refining SRC recognition, greater adherence to recovery protocols, and a more measured understanding of injury severity. Efforts have been made to involve healthcare providers, athletes, coaches, staff, referees, and parents in the education process. A 2021 survey of professional team physicians revealed that support for routine educational meetings on SRC catered toward athletes and team staff [62]. Coaches can play a large role in creating an atmosphere in a team that promotes education, careseeking, and decreasing stigma of SRC [63].

A 2021 study evaluated an online training program (HEADS UP from the Centers for Disease Control and Prevention) designed for healthcare providers and found that it increased concussion knowledge as well as improved the ability to execute the learned guidelines, including reducing unnecessary neuroimaging and no longer prescribing strict rest for extended periods of time [64]. Other studies examined how online training programs can be used for parents and youth coaches. One found that online education programs, which can be easily disseminated to large audiences, can improve concussion knowledge; however, there is evidence that in-person training actually decreases concussion events and improves implementation of concussion guidelines [65].

Other studies showed that parent education around concussion has been lacking and would be important to target, given how symptoms can present hours or days post injury. Education can be catered toward populations for which there are barriers (e.g., cultural, language, age, or socioeconomic) to knowledge and create more equitable opportunities to learn factual risks and preventative strategies [66–68].

A survey of youth sports referees found that a majority believed that they could play a larger role in player safety, specifically with regard to concussion identification during competition. Many officials are not required to receive any formal training about SRC through their respective governing bodies but would be open to it, potentially improving SRC detection [69].

Nonpharmacological Interventions

Although data have been mixed, when worn properly, helmets and headgear in their respective sports may provide protection against SRCs and other kinds of head injuries. The usage of mouth guards can prevent oral injuries, but the data are inconclusive with regard to protection against SRCs [55, 70]. However, there is a trade-off that occurs with the use of protective equipment that may attenuate the risk of an SRC. Adding protective gear adds weight and size, leading to larger and heavier individuals capable of delivering a more forceful impact [71]. Athletes wearing protective equipment may feel emboldened to engage in a higher-risk style of play, something termed "risk compensation," thereby increasing

their risk of experiencing an SRC [72]. Although the evidence supporting the use of helmets to prevent an SRC may be limited, there is good evidence that they can prevent more severe injuries such as fractures and contusions, and, as such, their use should be promoted.

A small study in professional hockey players examined the potential of a head and neck cooling device to be worn shortly after an SRC injury. The results demonstrated a shorter RTP time frame when compared to that of controls, though this needs to be replicated in a larger and more diverse population. The device purportedly works via neuroprotective potential from hypothermia induction, with slowing of the neuroinflammatory cascade that likely occurs after an SRC [73].

Although not immediately applicable and generalizable to EAs, two studies examining mixed athlete populations (adolescent and university levels) explored how incorporation of neck exercises to strengthen neck muscles and lessen neck muscle fatigue could play a role in reducing SRCs. Neck exercises may be able to facilitate greater stabilization of one's head during impact and lower the likelihood of neck acceleration [74, 75].

Many rules have been instituted in different sports to promote athlete safety, with some specifically aimed at reduction of SRC incidents. For example, American football has rules prohibiting hitting a defenseless receiver in the head or neck region or leading a tackle with the top of one's helmet. A study comparing statistics in high school football before and after implementation of the targeting rule showed a lower trend in SRCs. Coaching staff should prioritize teaching appropriate playing techniques that protect athletes from injury [55, 76]. In adolescent and nonelite hockey, there has been enactment of policies disallowing body checking, which has resulted in lower concussion rates and even decreases in medical costs [77, 78].

In the first days to weeks after an SRC injury, most EAs return to baseline with limited need for medical intervention. In addition to strict adherence to an RTP/RTL protocol, participation in nonexertional team activities can mitigate feelings of isolation, a common factor in those who develop post-injury depressive symptoms. Ongoing attention from the athlete's support system, avoidance or lessened usage of illicit and other mind-altering substances, and psychotherapy can be applicable for some athletes at any point in recovery [79–81].

Medications and Supplements

Symptoms that persist beyond 1 month may warrant pharmacological interventions. No medications are approved by the US Food and Drug Administration (FDA) to treat SRC, though treatments can be considered to target specific symptoms. Variable symptom presentations are common in EAs, and it is important to evaluate and consider each individual thoroughly [82].

Sleep deficits have been demonstrated to delay recovery from an SRC, particularly due to compounding effects on mood and cognition. Initial recommendations may include limiting screen time, teaching sleep hygiene techniques, and implementing cognitive behavioral therapy for insomnia (CBT-I). If medications are warranted, then melatonin is a safe choice and incurs relatively low concern for potential oversedative effects. There is some evidence that melatonin may have a neuroprotective effect after a TBI [83], though this has not specifically been studied in EAs. Medications that can cause sedation or cognitive impairment should be avoided, as they can mask or mirror symptoms during recovery. Trazodone can be considered as a second-line option. Sedative-hypnotic agents such as benzodiazepines and zolpidem are to be avoided, given the concerns surrounding their habit-forming nature and negative effects on cognition and arousal [79, 82, 84, 85].

Headaches are a common somatic symptom after an SRC. For headaches that do not resolve with short-term use of nonsteroidal anti-inflammatory drugs (NSAIDs) or acetaminophen, some may recommend tricyclic antidepressants (TCAs) such as amitriptyline. TCAs can provide dual benefits in athletes with comorbid insomnia symptoms as they can be sedating. TCAs should be used with caution for certain athletes due to their sedating effect as well as possible weight gain and cardiac side effects [79, 82, 84, 85].

Emotional symptoms such as depression and anxiety may be experienced after an SRC. Aside from recommending ongoing emotional support from those close to the athlete and maintenance of social/team activities, medications such as selective serotonin reuptake inhibitors (SSRIs) or TCAs can be considered. This is especially true for athletes who have a preinjury history of depression and/or anxiety or for those with a strong history of these conditions [79, 84]. In particular, sertraline has been shown to potentially benefit both mood and cognitive symptoms in those with nonsport TBI [86].

Post-SRC cognitive deficits may include problems with attention, fatigue, and mental fogginess. Stimulants such as methylphenidate and amphetamines have shown efficacy to help resolve cognitive deficits [87–89]. Athletes and healthcare providers must be cognizant of their respective sports' regulations on the usage of stimulants, as their use is often prohibited by sports governing bodies without prior use authorization. For nonelite youth athletes with ADHD, a large cohort study showed that the usage of stimulants reduced SRC incidence [90]. Amantadine has been studied with mixed results pertaining to resolution of cognitive symptoms [91, 92].

There is ongoing research around the efficacy of using vitamins and supplements that may be neuroprotective and may help treat and/or prevent symptomatic head injury sequelae. Riboflavin, magnesium, and feverfew are frequently recommended for SRC-related headache or migraine, and fish oil is often recommended for potential neuroprotective effects [93, 94]. Recommending supplements can be complicated, as these substances face limited regulatory scrutiny, dosing can be variable, and research is needed to verify their safety and efficacy.

Diagnostic Testing

Neuroimaging

An SRC often yields negative findings on conventional neuroimaging (e.g., X-ray, magnetic resonance imaging (MRI), computed tomography (CT)) and is typically discouraged. Neuroimaging can be considered in circumstances where there is greater than 30 s of LOC, prolonged altered mental status, severe headache, focal neurological deficits, or seizure [1, 4, 95]. MRI, positron emission tomography (PET) scans, and other neuroimaging techniques are mostly reserved for research purposes [55]. Current neuroimaging research focuses on the neuropathological changes due to recurring head injury. There is much consideration around whether these anatomical changes have clinical relevance or predictability of other neurodegenerative disease processes such as chronic traumatic encephalopathy (CTE), but no major conclusions have been drawn thus far [96, 97].

Biomarkers

Efforts to identify a biomarker that can clearly and quickly diagnose and track recovery from an SRC have been unyielding. Current avenues of research include analyzing urine, blood, and even saliva. Potential biomarkers include calcium-binding protein S100β, glial fibrillary acidic protein (GFAP), serum neurofilament light chain protein (NFL), and various Tau proteins [98–100].

Case Example

Dolores is a 23-year-old female ice hockey player representing her nation at an elite level. During practice a month before a qualifying game, she was looking over her shoulder when she collided with a teammate. She struck the side of her head against the teammate's shoulder, leading to a rapid and forceful rotation of her head. She immediately fell to the ice and attempted to stand up but felt dizzy and light-headed. After her licensed athletic trainer helped her off the ice, she began experiencing a headache, photophobia, and felt nauseated with an episode of emesis. Due to the severity of her symptoms, she was taken to the nearest emergency department for evaluation. A physical exam revealed an athletic female with no overt signs of trauma. Except for the appearance of fatigue and a headache, her neurological exam was normal. Her head MRI was negative. She struggled to remember the collision, and her concentration was impaired. She was diagnosed with a concussion and instructed to rest for several days. This was her third lifetime concussion. She has a history of ADHD and had been on stimulants in the past. Her mother was diagnosed with depression that was successfully managed using an SSRI.

After 1 week, she was still symptomatic but eager to return to play in anticipation of the important game. Without telling her trainer, she attempted to skate with some teammates at full exertion. This led to an immediate exacerbation of her symptoms, most notably dizziness, headache, and photophobia. She confided in her trainer, who explained the severity of her injury and the importance of a full recovery. Together, they made an appointment to see a sports psychiatrist to discuss her symptoms.

At 20 days post injury, she continued to struggle with daily headaches, insomnia, and mild depression. She was able to walk at a light pace, but mild exertion continued to lead to symptom exacerbation. She expressed guilt and disappointment regarding her injury and was placing a great deal of pressure on herself to recover rapidly. After careful discussion with her mental health providers, trainers, and coaching staff, she decided that she would forgo the upcoming competition, recognizing that attempting to compete while still recovering from an SRC could be disastrous. Instead, she elected to focus on recovery and to be available for future competitions. Due to several risk factors for a prolonged recovery, a decision was made to initiate pharmacotherapy in conjunction with physical therapy and strict adherence to a regimented RTP protocol. Her psychiatrist started her on duloxetine to target her mood symptoms and headache. She started taking melatonin at bedtime for sleep as well as magnesium and riboflavin to target her headache.

At 6 weeks post injury, her symptoms had fully subsided, and she was able to complete the RTP protocol with a full return to activity. She remained on the nutritional supplements for several more months and tapered off duloxetine after 6 months as per evidence-based recommendations for the duration of the treatment for major depressive disorder [101].

References

1. McCrory P, Meeuwisse W, Dvorak J, Aubry M, Bailes J, Broglio S, et al. Consensus statement on concussion in sport—the 5th international conference on concussion in sport held in Berlin, October 2016. Br J Sports Med. 2017;51(11):838.
2. Hutchinson EB, Schwerin SC, Avram AV, Juliano SL, Pierpaoli C. Diffusion MRI and the detection of alterations following traumatic brain injury. J Neurosci Res. 2018;96(4):612–25.
3. Giza CC, Hovda DA. The new neurometabolic cascade of concussion. Neurosurgery. 2014;75(Suppl 4):S24–33.
4. Harmon KG, Clugston JR, Dec K, Hainline B, Herring S, Kane SF, et al. American Medical Society for Sports Medicine position statement on concussion in sport. Br J Sports Med. 2019;53(4):213–25.
5. Bailes JE, Hudson V. Classification of sport-related head trauma: a spectrum of mild to severe injury. J Athl Train. 2001;36(3):236–43.
6. Sojka P. "Sport" and "non-sport" concussions. CMAJ. 2011;183(8):887–8.
7. Ommaya AK, Gennarelli TA. Cerebral concussion and traumatic unconsciousness. Correlation of experimental and clinical observations of blunt head injuries. Brain. 1974;97(4):633–54.
8. Guskiewicz KM, Mihalik JP. Biomechanics of sport concussion: quest for the elusive injury threshold. Exerc Sport Sci Rev. 2011;39(1):4–11.
9. Langlois JA, Rutland-Brown W, Wald MM. The epidemiology and impact of traumatic brain injury: a brief overview. J Head Trauma Rehabil. 2006;21(5):375–8.
10. Coronado V, McGuire L, Faul M, Sugerman D, Pearson W. Traumatic brain injury epidemiology and public health issues. In: Brain injury medicine: principles and practice. New York, NY: Demos Medical Publishing; 2012. p. 84–100.
11. Prien A, Grafe A, Rössler R, Junge A, Verhagen E. Epidemiology of head injuries focusing on concussions in team contact sports: a systematic review. Sports Med. 2018;48(4):953–69.
12. Zuckerman SL, Kerr ZY, Yengo-Kahn A, Wasserman E, Covassin T, Solomon GS. Epidemiology of sports-related concussion in NCAA athletes from 2009-2010 to 2013-2014: incidence, recurrence, and mechanisms. Am J Sports Med. 2015;43(11):2654–62.
13. Weber AF, Mihalik JP, Register-Mihalik JK, Mays S, Prentice WE, Guskiewicz KM. Dehydration and performance on clinical concussion measures in collegiate wrestlers. J Athl Train. 2013;48(2):153–60.
14. Bohr AD, Aukerman DF, Harmon KG, Romano R, Hernández TD, Konstantinides N, et al. Pac-12 CARE-Affiliated Program: structure, methods and initial results. BMJ Open Sport Exerc Med. 2021;7(2):e001055.
15. Legarreta AD, Brett BL, Solomon GS, Zuckerman SL. The role of family and personal psychiatric history in postconcussion syndrome following sport-related concussion: a story of compounding risk. J Neurosurg Pediatr. 2018;22(3):238–43.
16. Zemek R, Barrowman N, Freedman SB, Gravel J, Gagnon I, McGahern C, et al. Clinical risk score for persistent postconcussion symptoms among children with acute concussion in the ED. JAMA. 2016;315(10):1014–25.
17. Gessel LM, Fields SK, Collins CL, Dick RW, Comstock RD. Concussions among United States high school and collegiate athletes. J Athl Train. 2007;42(4):495–503.
18. Guskiewicz KM, Weaver NL, Padua DA, Garrett WE Jr. Epidemiology of concussion in collegiate and high school football players. Am J Sports Med. 2000;28(5):643–50.
19. Halstead ME, Walter KD, Moffatt K. Sport-related concussion in children and adolescents. Pediatrics. 2018;142(6):e20183074.

20. Iverson GL, Gardner AJ, Terry DP, Ponsford JL, Sills AK, Broshek DK, et al. Predictors of clinical recovery from concussion: a systematic review. Br J Sports Med. 2017;51(12):941–8.

21. Baldwin GT, Breiding MJ, Dawn CR. Epidemiology of sports concussion in the United States. Handb Clin Neurol. 2018;158:63–74.

22. Kerr ZY, Chandran A, Nedimyer AK, Arakkal A, Pierpoint LA, Zuckerman SL. Concussion incidence and trends in 20 high school sports. Pediatrics. 2019;144(5):e20192180.

23. Blyth RJ, Alcock M, Tumilty DS. Why are female soccer players experiencing a concussion more often than their male counterparts? A scoping review. Phys Ther Sport. 2021;52:54–68.

24. Sanderson K. Why sports concussions are worse for women. Nature. 2021;596(7870):26–8.

25. Putukian M, Riegler K, Amalfe S, Bruce J, Echemendia R. Preinjury and postinjury factors that predict sports-related concussion and clinical recovery time. Clin J Sport Med. 2021;31(1):15–22.

26. Nordström A, Nordström P, Ekstrand J. Sports-related concussion increases the risk of subsequent injury by about 50% in elite male football players. Br J Sports Med. 2014;48(19):1447–50.

27. Pietrosimone B, Golightly YM, Mihalik JP, Guskiewicz KM. Concussion frequency associates with musculoskeletal injury in retired NFL players. Med Sci Sports Exerc. 2015;47(11):2366–72.

28. Iverson GL, Caccese JB, Merz ZC, Büttner F, Terry DP. Age of first exposure to football is not associated with later-in-life cognitive or mental health problems. Front Neurol. 2021;12:647314.

29. Solomon GS, Kuhn AW, Zuckerman SL, Casson IR, Viano DC, Lovell MR, et al. Participation in pre-high school football and neurological, neuroradiological, and neuropsychological findings in later life: a study of 45 retired national football league players. Am J Sports Med. 2016;44(5):1106–15.

30. Roberts AL, Pascual-Leone A, Speizer FE, Zafonte RD, Baggish AL, Taylor H Jr, et al. Exposure to American Football and Neuropsychiatric Health in former national football league players: findings from the football players health study. Am J Sports Med. 2019;47(12):2871–80.

31. Alosco ML, Kasimis AB, Stamm JM, Chua AS, Baugh CM, Daneshvar DH, et al. Age of first exposure to American football and long-term neuropsychiatric and cognitive outcomes. Transl Psychiatry. 2017;7(9):e1236.

32. Stamm JM, Bourlas AP, Baugh CM, Fritts NG, Daneshvar DH, Martin BM, et al. Age of first exposure to football and later-life cognitive impairment in former NFL players. Neurology. 2015;84(11):1114–20.

33. Caccese J, Schmidt J, Moody J, Broglio S, McAllister T, McCrea M, et al. Association between sports participation history and age of first exposure to high-risk sports with concussion history. Res Sports Med. 2021:1–13.

34. Caccese JB, DeWolf RM, Kaminski TW, Broglio SP, McAllister TW, McCrea M, et al. Estimated age of first exposure to American Football and Neurocognitive Performance Amongst NCAA male student-athletes: a cohort study. Sports Med. 2019;49(3):477–87.

35. Caccese JB, Iverson GL, Cameron KL, Houston MN, McGinty GT, Jackson JC, et al. Estimated age of first exposure to contact sports is not associated with greater symptoms or worse cognitive functioning in male U.S. Service Academy Athletes. J Neurotrauma. 2020;37(2):334–9.

36. Cassimatis M, Orr R, Fyffe A, Browne G. Early injury evaluation following concussion is associated with improved recovery time in children and adolescents. J Sci Med Sport. 2021;24(12):1235–9.

37. Kontos AP, Jorgensen-Wagers K, Trbovich AM, Ernst N, Emami K, Gillie B, et al. Association of time since injury to the first clinic visit with recovery following concussion. JAMA Neurol. 2020;77(4):435–40.

38. Lexell J, Lovén G, Fagher K. Incidence of sports-related concussion in elite para athletes - a 52-week prospective study. Brain Inj. 2021;35(8):971–7.

39. Wallace J, Hou BQ, Hajdu K, Tang AR, Grusky AZ, Lee T, et al. Healthcare navigation of black and white adolescents following sport-related concussion: a path towards achieving health equity. J Athl Train. 2021;

40. Yengo-Kahn AM, Wallace J, Jimenez V, Totten DJ, Bonfield CM, Zuckerman SL. Exploring the outcomes and experiences of Black and White athletes following a sport-related concussion: a retrospective cohort study. J Neurosurg Pediatr. 2021;28:516–25.

41. Wallace J, Beidler E, Register-Mihalik JK, Hibbler T, Bretzin A, DeMedal S, et al. Evaluating concussion nondisclosure in college athletes using a health disparities framework and appreciation for social determinants of health. J Athl Train. 2021;

42. Tjong VK, Baker HP, Cogan CJ, Montoya M, Lindley TR, Terry MA. Concussions in NCAA varsity football athletes: a qualitative investigation of player perception and return to sport. J Am Acad Orthop Surg Glob Res Rev. 2017;1(8):e070.

43. Caron JG, Benson AJ, Steins R, McKenzie L, Bruner MW. The social dynamics involved in recovery and return to sport following a sport-related concussion: a study of three athlete-teammate-coach triads. Psychol Sport Exerc. 2021;52:101824.

44. Rice SM, Parker AG, Rosenbaum S, Bailey A, Mawren D, Purcell R. Sport-related concussion and mental health outcomes in elite athletes: a systematic review. Sports Med. 2018;48(2):447–65.

45. Mainwaring LM, Hutchison M, Bisschop SM, Comper P, Richards DW. Emotional response to sport concussion compared to ACL injury. Brain Inj. 2010;24(4):589–97.

46. Sicard V, Harrison AT, Moore RD. Psycho-affective health, cognition, and neurophysiological functioning following sports-related concussion in symptomatic and asymptomatic athletes, and control athletes. Sci Rep. 2021;11(1):13838.

47. McCunn R, Beaudouin F, Stewart K, Meyer T, MacLean J. Heading in football: incidence, biomechanical characteristics and the association with acute cognitive function-a three-part systematic review. Sports Med. 2021;51(10):2147–63.

48. Kakavas G, Malliaropoulos N, Blach W, Bikos G, Migliorini F, Maffulli N. Ball heading and subclinical concussion in soccer as a risk factor for anterior cruciate ligament injury. J Orthop Surg Res. 2021;16(1):566.

49. Avedesian JM, Covassin T, Baez S, Nash J, Nagelhout E, Dufek JS. Relationship between cognitive performance and lower extremity biomechanics: implications for sports-related concussion. Orthop J Sports Med. 2021;9(8):23259671211032246.

50. Jildeh TR, Meta F, Young J, Page B, Okoroha KR. Concussion in national football league athletes is not associated with increased risk of acute, noncontact lower extremity musculoskeletal injury. Orthop J Sports Med. 2021;9(5):23259671211003491.

51. Harrison AT, Lane-Cordova A, La Fountaine MF, Moore RD. Impact of concussion history on heart rate variability during bouts of acute stress. J Athl Train. 2021;

52. Jeckell AS, Fontana RS. Psychosocial aspects of sport-related concussion in youth. Psychiatr Clin N Am. 2021;44:469.

53. D'Lauro C, Johnson BR, McGinty G, Allred CD, Campbell DE, Jackson JC. Reconsidering return-to-play times: a broader perspective on concussion recovery. Orthop J Sports Med. 2018;6(3):2325967118760854.

54. Broglio SP, McAllister T, Katz BP, LaPradd M, Zhou W, McCrea MA. The natural history of sport-related concussion in collegiate athletes: findings from the NCAA-DoD CARE Consortium. Sports Med. 2022;52:403.

55. Herring S, Kibler WB, Putukian M, Solomon GS, Boyajian O, Neill L, et al. Selected issues in sport-related concussion (SRC mild traumatic brain injury) for the team physician: a consensus statement. Br J Sports Med. 2021;55(22):1251.

56. Weiler R, Blauwet C, Clarke D, Dalton K, Derman W, Fagher K, et al. Infographic. The first position statement of the Concussion in Para Sport Group. Br J Sports Med. 2022;56:417.

57. Lawrence DW, Richards D, Comper P, Hutchison MG. Earlier time to aerobic exercise is associated with faster recovery following acute sport concussion. PLoS One. 2018;13(4):e0196062.

58. Haider MN, Cunningham A, Darling S, Suffoletto HN, Freitas MS, Jain RK, et al. Derivation of the Buffalo Concussion Physical Examination risk of delayed recovery (RDR) score to identify children at risk for persistent postconcussive symptoms. Br J Sports Med. 2021;55:1427.

59. Kirkwood MW, Howell DR, Brooks BL, Wilson JC, Meehan Iii WP. The Nocebo effect and pediatric concussion. J Sport Rehabil. 2021;30:837–43.

60. Trbovich AM, Preszler J, Emami K, Cohen P, Eagle S, Collins MW, et al. Is overparenting associated with adolescent/young adult emotional functioning and clinical outcomes following concussion? Child Psychiatry Hum Dev. 2021;

61. Gouttebarge V, Goedhart EA, Orhant E, Patricios J. Avoiding a red card: recommendations for a consistent standard of concussion management in professional football (soccer). Br J Sports Med. 2022;56:308.

62. Gouttebarge V, Ahmad I, Iqbal Z, Orhant E, Rosenbloom C, Sas K, et al. Concussion in European professional football: a view of team physicians. BMJ Open Sport Exerc Med. 2021;7(2):e001086-e.

63. Bissett JE, Kroshus E, Hebard S. Determining the role of sport coaches in promoting athlete mental health: a narrative review and Delphi approach. BMJ Open Sport Exerc Med. 2020;6(1):e000676-e.

64. Sarmiento K, Daugherty J, Waltzman D. Effectiveness of the CDC HEADS UP online training on healthcare providers' mTBI knowledge and self-efficacy. J Saf Res. 2021;78:221–8.

65. Feiss R, Lutz M, Reiche E, Moody J, Pangelinan M. A systematic review of the effectiveness of concussion education programs for coaches and parents of youth athletes. Int J Environ Res Public Health. 2020;17(8):2665.

66. Kerr ZY, Nedimyer AK, Kay MC, Chandran A, Gildner P, Byrd KH, et al. Factors associated with concussion-symptom knowledge and attitudes toward concussion care seeking in a national survey of parents of middle-school children in the US. J Sport Health Sci. 2021;10(2):113–21.

67. Haarbauer-Krupa JK, Register-Mihalik JK, Nedimyer AK, Chandran A, Kay MC, Gildner P, et al. Factors associated with concussion symptom knowledge and attitudes towards concussion care-seeking among parents of children aged 5-10 years. J Saf Res. 2021;78:203–9.

68. Kim S, Connaughton DP. Youth soccer parents' attitudes and perceptions about concussions. J Adolesc Health. 2021;68(1):184–90.

69. King C, Coughlan E. Blowing the whistle on concussion knowledge and education in youth sport referees. Open Access J Sports Med. 2021;12:109–17.

70. Tjønndal A, Austmo WF. Athletes' and coaches' attitudes toward protective headgear as concussion and head injury prevention: a scoping review. Front Sports Act Living. 2021;3:680773.

71. Youth CoS-RCi, Board on Children YaF, Medicine Io, Council NR. The National Academies collection: reports funded by National Institutes of Health. In: Graham R, Rivara FP, Ford MA, Spicer CM, editors. Sports-related concussions in youth: improving the science, changing the culture. Washington, DC: National Academies Press; 2014. p. 239–84.

72. Hedlund J. Risky business: safety regulations, risks compensation, and individual behavior. Inj Prev. 2000;6(2):82–90.

73. Gard A, Tegner Y, Bakhsheshi MF, Marklund N. Selective head-neck cooling after concussion shortens return-to-play in ice hockey players. Concussion. 2021;6(2):CNC90-CNC.

74. Elliott J, Heron N, Versteegh T, Gilchrist IA, Webb M, Archbold P, et al. Injury reduction programs for reducing the incidence of sport-related head and neck injuries including concussion: a systematic review. Sports Med. 2021;51:2373.

75. Peek K, Andersen J, McKay MJ, Versteegh T, Gilchrist IA, Meyer T, et al. The effect of the FIFA 11 + with added neck exercises on maximal isometric neck strength and peak head impact magnitude during heading: a pilot study. Sports Med. 2021;52:655–68.

76. Obana KK, Mueller JD, Saltzman BM, Bottiglieri TS, Ahmad CS, Parisien RL, et al. Targeting rule implementation decreases concussions in high school football: a national concussion surveillance study. Orthop J Sports Med. 2021;9(10):23259671211031191.

77. Emery CA, Eliason P, Warriyar V, Palacios-Derflingher L, Black AM, Krolikowski M, et al. Body checking in non-elite adolescent ice hockey leagues: it is never too late for policy change aiming to protect the health of adolescents. Br J Sports Med. 2021;56:12.

78. Currie GR, Lee R, Palacios-Derflingher L, Hagel B, Black AM, Babul S, et al. Reality check 2: the cost-effectiveness of policy disallowing body checking in non-elite 13- to 14-year-old ice hockey players. Int J Environ Res Public Health. 2021;18(12):6322.

79. Reardon CL. Psychiatric manifestations of sport-related concussion: careful diagnosis and management can help avoid unnecessary treatment or restrictions. Curr Psychiatry. 2020;19:22.

80. Silverberg ND, Hallam BJ, Rose A, Underwood H, Whitfield K, Thornton AE, et al. Cognitive-behavioral prevention of postconcussion syndrome in at-risk patients: a pilot randomized controlled trial. J Head Trauma Rehabil. 2013;28(4):313–22.

81. Tomfohr-Madsen L, Madsen JW, Bonneville D, Virani S, Plourde V, Barlow KM, et al. A pilot randomized controlled trial of cognitive-behavioral therapy for insomnia in adolescents with persistent postconcussion symptoms. J Head Trauma Rehabil. 2020;35(2):E103–e12.

82. Jeckell AS, Solomon GS. Pharmacological interventions in sport-related concussion. Pract Pain Manag. 2017;17(10):36–43.

83. Naseem M, Parvez S. Role of melatonin in traumatic brain injury and spinal cord injury. ScientificWorldJournal. 2014;2014:586270.

84. Meehan WP III. Medical therapies for concussion. Clin Sports Med. 2011;30(1):115–24, ix.

85. Halstead ME. Pharmacologic therapies for pediatric concussions. Sports Health. 2016;8(1):50–2.

86. Fann JR, Uomoto JM, Katon WJ. Cognitive improvement with treatment of depression following mild traumatic brain injury. Psychosomatics. 2001;42(1):48–54.

87. Tramontana MG, Cowan RL, Zald D, Prokop JW, Guillamondegui O. Traumatic brain injury-related attention deficits: treatment outcomes with lisdexamfetamine dimesylate (Vyvanse). Brain Inj. 2014;28(11):1461–72.

88. Kaelin DL, Cifu DX, Matthies B. Methylphenidate effect on attention deficit in the acutely brain-injured adult. Arch Phys Med Rehabil. 1996;77(1):6–9.

89. Whyte J, Hart T, Vaccaro M, Grieb-Neff P, Risser A, Polansky M, et al. Effects of methylphenidate on attention deficits after traumatic brain injury: a multidimensional, randomized, controlled trial. Am J Phys Med Rehabil. 2004;83(6):401–20.

90. Ali M, Dreher N, Hannah T, Li A, Asghar N, Spiera Z, et al. Concussion incidence and recovery among youth athletes with ADHD taking stimulant-based therapy. Orthop J Sports Med. 2021;9(10):23259671211032564.

91. Reddy CC, Collins M, Lovell M, Kontos AP. Efficacy of amantadine treatment on symptoms and neurocognitive performance among adolescents following sports-related concussion. J Head Trauma Rehabil. 2013;28(4):260–5.

92. Carabenciov ID, Bureau BL, Cutrer M, Savica R. Amantadine use for postconcussion syndrome. Mayo Clin Proc. 2019;94(2):275–7.

93. Vonder Haar C, Peterson TC, Martens KM, Hoane MR. Vitamins and nutrients as primary treatments in experimental brain injury: clinical implications for nutraceutical therapies. Brain Res. 2016;1640(Pt A):114–29.

94. Heileson J, Anzalone A, Carbuhn A, Askow A, Stone J, Turner S, et al. The effect of omega-3 fatty acids on a biomarker of head

trauma in NCAA football athletes: a multi-site, non-randomized study. J Int Soc Sports Nutr. 2021;18:65.

95. Giza CC, Kutcher JS, Ashwal S, Barth J, Getchius TS, Gioia GA, et al. Summary of evidence-based guideline update: evaluation and management of concussion in sports: report of the Guideline Development Subcommittee of the American Academy of Neurology. Neurology. 2013;80(24):2250–7.

96. Asken BM, Rabinovici GD. Identifying degenerative effects of repetitive head trauma with neuroimaging: a clinically-oriented review. Acta Neuropathol Commun. 2021;9(1):96.

97. McAllister D, Akers C, Boldt B, Mitchell LA, Tranvinh E, Douglas D, et al. Neuroradiologic evaluation of MRI in high-contact sports. Front Neurol. 2021;12:701948.

98. Wanner ZR, Southam CG, Sanghavi P, Boora NS, Paxman EJ, Dukelow SP, et al. Alterations in urine metabolomics following sport-related concussion: a (1)H NMR-based analysis. Front Neurol. 2021;12:645829.

99. Azizi S, Hier DB, Allen B, Obafemi-Ajayi T, Olbricht GR, Thimgan MS, et al. A kinetic model for blood biomarker levels after mild traumatic brain injury. Front Neurol. 2021;12:668606.

100. Hicks SD, Onks C, Kim RY, Zhen KJ, Loeffert J, Loeffert AC, et al. Refinement of saliva microRNA biomarkers for sports-related concussion. J Sport Health Sci. 2021;

101. Baldessarini RJ, Lau WK, Sim J, Sum MY, Sim K. Duration of initial antidepressant treatment and subsequent relapse of major depression. J Clin Psychopharmacol. 2015;35(1):75–6.

Substance Use and Substance Use Disorders

David R. McDuff, Michelle Garvin, and Donald L. Thompson

Introduction

The misuse of some substances is more common among elite athletes in certain sports than in the general population. These include the misuse of alcohol (binge drinking), cannabis, nicotine (oral tobacco), prescription stimulants (methylphenidate, amphetamine salts), and opioid pain medication [1–5]. Substance misuse is defined as illicit, risky, harmful, or heavy or problematic use and often indicates a shift to a more serious level of use. Sports medicine and mental health clinicians working with elite athletes or teams will routinely encounter cases of substance misuse, frequently associated with a mix of health, social, interpersonal, and legal/administrative problems. In addition, misuse is often associated with either general psychological distress or other mental health symptoms or disorders (e.g., anxiety, depression, insomnia). Routine screening (e.g., preseason, upon serious injury) using validated instruments such as the *Alcohol Use Disorders Identification Test-Consumption* (AUDIT-C) and the *Cut Down, Annoyed, Guilty, and Eye*-Opener modified for drugs (CAGE-drugs) is recommended [6].

The presence of substance use disorders is less commonly seen than substance misuse in active elite athletes because it can take many years for disorders to develop, and they typically reduce performance substantially. Use disorders are more likely to be seen, however, in transitioning or retired elite athletes or in active or retired coaches [7]. Substance use disorders are defined as a pattern of substance use that leads to significant distress and/or functional impairment and some of the following: (1) excessive or compulsive use; (2) failure to cut down or quit; (3) cravings or urges; (4) missing important obligations due to use or withdrawal; (5) use despite negative consequences; (6) physically hazardous use; and (7) tolerance and/or withdrawal symptoms [8]. The most common substance use disorders seen in active elite athletes or coaches are alcohol, nicotine, and cannabis. The most common use disorders seen in retired elite athletes are alcohol, nicotine, and opioids [1, 9].

When treating active or retired athletes or coaches with substance use disorders, it is important to collect a detailed history identifying the past and current patterns of substance use, routes of administration, and associated problems. In addition, any past treatment should be documented and reviewed for helpful components. Withdrawal symptoms and/or cravings must be managed immediately lest the athlete/coach resumes substance use. It is also important to look for co-occurring mental health symptoms or disorders as these often serve as recovery barriers or relapse triggers. One useful approach to conceptualizing the treatment plan is to use an Integrated Recovery Model (Fig. 14.1). This model identifies the substance use disorder itself (using the detailed history gathered), identifies stages of recovery over the first year (i.e., stop using, get comfortable, achieve life balance), and takes into consideration the key recovery barriers and/or relapse triggers [10, 11].

Integrating treatment of the use disorder with the major recovery barriers helps ensure that the treatment plan is comprehensive. Breaking down the recovery process in the first year into stages or phases that each have specific tasks can help athletes and providers focus on critical tasks and therefore make steady progress. For athletes and coaches, the best treatment plan creates a nonjudgmental support network and combines motivational interviewing (MI)/motivational enhancement therapy (MET) with medications that manage

D. R. McDuff (✉)
Psychiatry, University of Maryland School of Medicine, Baltimore, MD, USA

Baltimore Orioles (MLB), Maryland, MD, USA
e-mail: dmcduff@som.umaryland.edu

M. Garvin
Detroit Lions (NFL), Michigan, MI, USA

D. L. Thompson
Psychiatry, University of Maryland School of Medicine, Baltimore, MD, USA

Baltimore Orioles (MLB), Maryland, MD, USA

Detroit Lions (NFL), Michigan, MI, USA
e-mail: dthompso@som.umaryland.edu

© The Author(s), under exclusive license to Springer Nature Switzerland AG 2022
C. L. Reardon (ed.), *Mental Health Care for Elite Athletes*, https://doi.org/10.1007/978-3-031-08364-8_14

131

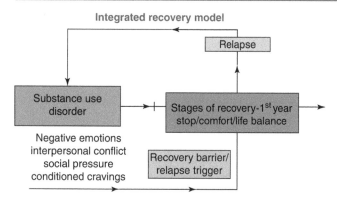

Fig. 14.1 Integrated Recovery Model of treatment for substance use disorders

acute and post-acute withdrawal symptoms, cravings, and common comorbid mental health symptoms (e.g., anxiety, anger, depression, insomnia, anergia) [12]. MI combined with group psychoeducation is also useful for athletes or coaches with substance misuse when their readiness to change may be low. Recent anonymized cases seen by the authors in both collegiate and professional sport settings in the United States have been presented to illustrate the key clinical points.

Common Substance Misuse and Use Disorders

Alcohol

Alcohol is a commonly used substance by athletes and nonathletes alike. Alcohol is used for its perceived relaxant effects, to reduce anxiety or tremors, and to improve confidence in performance. Additionally, outside of sport, alcohol is often used to reduce stress and enhance social connections. Despite its perceived benefits, there are many potential negative consequences of alcohol use on both performance and personal life. Although not a prohibited substance in most sports, many teams choose to impose limits on alcohol use in season to curb the negative impacts of alcohol on performance and health.

Alcohol use is common in athletes across genders at collegiate and professional levels. In US collegiate athletes, 76% of male and 79% of female athletes reported past-year alcohol use [13]. The combined gender past-year use rates were higher for division III athletes (81%) than those for either division II (74%) or division I (75%). The sports with the highest past-year use rates for men are ice hockey (93%), golf (88%), lacrosse (88%), and swimming (84%). For women, the highest use rates are in lacrosse (92%), ice hockey (91%), rowing (86%), and swimming

(84%) [13]. Another US study, using data from the National College Health Assessment II, showed that from 2011 to 2014, collegiate athletes were more likely than were nonathletes to be past or occasional users (1–19 days use) of alcohol in the past 30 days but not frequent users (20 or more using days) [4].

Binge drinking rates among US collegiate athletes are significant, with 44% of males reporting five or more drinks per drinking occasion in the past 2 weeks, whereas 39% of females reported drinking four or more drinks over the same period [13]. The binge drinking rates for male athletes in certain sports like lacrosse, ice hockey, rugby, and swimming are even higher, ranging from 50% to 70%. For women participating in lacrosse, ice hockey, and swimming, the binge drinking rates ranged from 49% to 57% [13]. Looking at more heavy consumption, 13% of male athletes reported having ten or more drinks per drinking occasion compared to only 1.4% of women. In a recently published survey of Brazilian collegiate athletes versus nonathletes from 2009, 67.6% have reported moderate to high-risk alcohol use as measured by the Alcohol, Smoking and Substance Involvement Screening Test (ASSIST). These elite collegiate athletes demonstrated greater odds of moderate to high-risk alcohol use compared to nonathletes (odds ratio (OR): 2.49, 95% confidence interval (CI): 1.36–4.54), but recreational athletes were no more likely than were nonathletes to report risky drinking [5].

Although use patterns are important to explore, the impact that use has on functioning is also critical. Studies show that student athletes experience negative impacts of alcohol use in the classroom, on the field, and in social life. For example, in a survey of collegiate athletes, the most common problems from alcohol misuse reported are: (1) hangover (52%); (2) forgot where you were or what you did (28.4%); (3) done something you later regretted (25.4%); (4) interrupted sleep (20.7%); (5) got into an argument/fight (16.8%); (6) missed a class (14.2%); (7) poor test or important project performance (7.1%); (8) performed poorly in practice or a game (7.4%); (9) got physically injured (6.8%); and (10) showed up late or missed a practice or game (2.3%) [13]. Alcohol also has significant negative impacts on performance including dehydration, insomnia, increased injury rates, decreased recovery from injury, reduced metabolic recovery, and weight gain [1].

Studies of professional athletes show rates of recent (past 30 days) adverse alcohol behaviors (i.e., regular, heavy, or binge drinking) using the AUDIT-C, ranging from 6% to 62.8% [7, 14–16]. In active professional male European football (soccer) players, the rates ranged from 6% to 17% depending on the country [14]. For professional male international rugby players from nine countries, the rate of new-onset adverse alcohol use was 22% [15]. The highest rates of adverse alcohol behaviors reported were seen in elite male rugby players from Australasia (68.6% preseason and 62.8% during the season) [16]. Rates in retired professional athletes appear to be higher than those in active players. In one study, former male and female Australian footballers reported significantly higher alcohol misuse rates (68.8%) compared with those in active male footballers (50.7%) and active female footballers (43.8%) [7]. There are no studies on the rates of alcohol misuse or use disorders in US professional athletes or collegiate or professional coaches; however, the experience of these writers suggests that the rates are clinically significant.

Case Study #1: Alcohol Misuse (Binge Drinking)

An 18-year-old female first-year college gymnast was referred by her therapist in the middle of the fall semester for evaluation of panic attacks. She had a history of generalized anxiety and inattention/distractibility dating back to elementary school. She was eventually diagnosed with attention-deficit/hyperactivity disorder (ADHD) in high school and successfully treated with lisdexamfetamine up to 70 mg. During her first semester in college, her anxiety symptoms increased due to academic/social stress and chronic injuries that prevented her from practicing. After a few therapy sessions and following a late-night emergency room visit after passing out in a bar after drinking many shots of distilled spirits with teammates, it became clear that she was engaging in regular binge drinking. Her blood alcohol level in the emergency room was more than twice the legal limit (0.19). The next day, she realized that she had multiple scratch marks on her breasts but had no recollection of how they got there. She did not think she was sexually assaulted. Her urine test for other substances, including cannabis, was negative.

Diagnoses (1) Attention-deficit/hyperactivity disorder, combined-type; (2) generalized anxiety disorder; (3) alcohol misuse (regular binge drinking); (4) foot and ankle ligament injury and Achilles tendon bone spurs, serious; (5) chronic asthma, controlled on an inhaler as needed.

Treatment For anxiety, she was started on low-dose venlafaxine extended-release (ER). The dosage was slowly increased over 6 weeks to 112.5 mg, and she was taught relaxation breathing and unwinding techniques with good results. For ADHD, she was continued on lisdexamfetamine 70 mg, but, over time, it was observed that her blood pressure and pulse were elevated, so her dosage was lowered to 50 mg. To address her alcohol misuse, she was referred to an alcohol and drug awareness class, which she attended weekly for 6 weeks.

Case Study #2: Severe Alcohol Use Disorder and Anxiety

A 38-year-old divorced father of two children and former college and professional football player was referred for evaluation by his head coach for drinking heavily prior to a practice, threatening his position as a collegiate offensive coordinator. He described a history of drinking 6–12 standard drinks of wine after practices and games dating back to late college. He used alcohol as a primary stress control strategy. After he retired from active play, his drinking increased to an all-day pattern, consuming 2–4 glasses of wine each morning and then 8–10 more, spaced throughout the day to prevent withdrawal symptoms. In addition to heavy drinking, he described stress-related anxiety and insomnia dating back to high school. He also struggled with chronic knee pain from loss of articular cartilage that prevented him from working out regularly. He reported a history of blackouts and passing out on multiple occasions with no arrests for driving under the influence even though he had driven intoxicated many times. There was no history of cannabis or other illicit substance use.

Diagnoses (1) Alcohol use disorder, severe; (2) generalized anxiety disorder; (3) sleep disorder (insomnia), alcohol-aggravated; (4) chronic left knee pain, recent unsuccessful arthroscopic surgery; (5) mildly elevated liver enzymes; (6) parent–child problem (special needs child); (7) recent death of a parent (mother).

His main recovery barriers were anxiety, insomnia, high-stress lifestyle, grief, and chronic knee pain (Fig. 14.2).

Treatment For alcohol use disorder, the following recommendations were made: (1) lorazepam 1 mg three to four times daily (with a plan for an eventual tapering protocol after detoxification); (2) disulfiram 250 mg daily; (3) oral

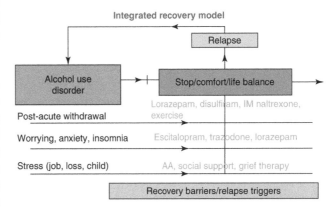

Fig. 14.2 Integrated Recovery Model of treatment for substance use disorder in Case Study #2

naltrexone 50 mg daily and then naltrexone intramuscularly monthly; (4) multivitamin, thiamine, and folic acid; (5) intensive outpatient care (12 weeks: 3 h/day, 5 days a week to start); (6) Alcoholics Anonymous meetings three times weekly; (7) group therapy and individual MET and grief therapy; (8) time off from work (8 weeks); and (9) regular exercise (swimming). For anxiety/stress control, the following were recommended: (1) escitalopram 15 mg daily; (2) lorazepam 1 mg three times daily as needed for post-acute withdrawal; and (3) regular exercise. For pain, the recommendations were: (1) improved nutrition and (2) regular exercise.

Case Discussions

Clinicians working with elite athletes will regularly encounter alcohol intoxication and associated problems as well as binge drinking. It is important, therefore, to educate athletes through prevention and intervention efforts and after an adverse alcohol event by informing them of the key factors influencing blood alcohol level. These are weight, percentage of body fat, sex, rate of drinking, alcohol concentration, natural sensitivity to alcohol's intoxicating effects, and tolerance if it has developed. It is also important to help athletes understand that alcohol is metabolized differently than are other substances (i.e., zero-order kinetics), resulting in slower elimination. It is estimated that most individuals metabolize about one drink an hour. For example, if an athlete consumes ten drinks in 4 h, then they will still have six drinks remaining to metabolize over the next 6 h. Athletes who take medications for anxiety or depression (e.g., selective serotonin or serotonin–norepinephrine reuptake inhibitors: SSRIs or SNRIs) or anxiety/insomnia (e.g., benzodiazepines, zolpidem) should be informed that these medications can boost alcohol's intoxicating effects by up to 50%. Identifying athletes who are engaging in frequent or risky alcohol use can help reduce its adverse effects and prevent advancement of misuse to a use disorder. Close monitoring of athletes for signs of frequent intoxication (e.g., hangover, lateness, arrests, arguments) or urine testing for alcohol in the morning are good ways to identify and intervene with frequent users [16]. Identifying periods of higher use within teams (e.g., off-season, post-game, bye weeks, etc.) can become a basis for psychoeducation sessions. Sessions combining psychoeducation and MI can be beneficial for athletes/coaches with low readiness to change levels.

Alcohol use disorders are more likely to be seen in older/retired athletes or coaches. If the athlete/coach has developed physiological dependence, then the management of withdrawal and cravings is the first step. This can be safely carried out in generally healthy persons in the outpatient setting using tapering dosages of benzodiazepines like chlordiazepoxide, lorazepam, or diazepam [2, 17, 18]. These can be administered in fixed reduction or symptom-triggered protocols. Sometimes it is helpful to continue low-dose benzodiazepines for a few weeks into the post-acute withdrawal period to reduce cravings. Other medications for cravings can be introduced during the acute and post-acute withdrawal periods. These include naltrexone, acamprosate, disulfiram, and gabapentin [19]. Several of these can be used concurrently (e.g., naltrexone and acamprosate, disulfiram and gabapentin). Since both naltrexone and disulfiram can cause a rise in liver enzymes, liver functioning should be systematically monitored during the first 6 months with use of either of these. In addition, naltrexone comes in the form of a depot injection that can be administered monthly. The effectiveness of any of these anti-craving medications is modest and not uncommonly associated with problems of poor adherence. Therefore, consideration should be given to the monitoring of their administration by an athletic trainer or a family member. Once withdrawal and cravings are managed, MI, behavioral strategies, and developing strong social support networks for recovery can be more effective.

Cannabis and Synthetic Cannabinoids

Cannabis is a flowering plant (e.g., *Cannabis sativa* and *Cannabis indica*) that is used to produce both medicinal and recreational marijuana. The cannabis plant contains more than 70 natural chemicals called cannabinoids, two of which are the primary components of most products on the market (legally or otherwise). These are delta-9-tetrahydrocannabinol (THC, the main high-producing chemical) and cannabidiol (CBD, which does not produce a high but may have medicinal properties). These natural cannabinoids as well as synthetically made ones exert their effects by interacting with endogenous cannabinoid receptors—cannabinoid receptor types 1 and 2 (CB1 and CB2)—in the brain, peripheral nerves, and other tissues (e.g., gastrointestinal tract, cardiovascular system) [20]. In the United States, cannabis is federally illegal and classified as a schedule 1-controlled substance [20]. Despite its illegality, cannabis is widely available, and its routes of administration (e.g., vaping, edibles, balms, tinctures) have expanded due to state-level medicalization and legalization. Additionally, THC content and THC:CBD ratios have risen substantially in both Europe and the United States since legalization began, increasing the likelihood of negative effects [21, 22].

There is a traditionally held view that marijuana is "safe or safer" than alcohol and is not addictive; however, about 9% of those who use it regularly will develop a substance use disorder. That number significantly rises (to 17%) among those who start using as teenagers and ranges from 25% to 50% among daily users [22]. The negative effects of short-term use include cough, impaired short-term memory (making learning and information retention harder), impaired motor coordination (impairing driving and making injury more likely), impaired judgment (increasing the risk of sexually transmitted diseases), and, in high doses, anxiety, panic attacks, and psychosis including paranoia [23]. The negative effects of long-term or heavy use, especially when starting during adolescence, include altered brain development, cognitive impairment, reduced life satisfaction and achievement, and increased risk of a psychotic disorder in persons with a predisposition to such disorders.

Synthetic cannabinoids are a class of chemicals that bind to the same receptors in the brain as THC, producing many of the same cannabis-like effects. Synthetic cannabinoids do not necessarily have the same chemical structure as THC, but their effects are usually much more intense, long-lasting, and unpredictable. Because of this, and their extremely high potency, even low doses of synthetic cannabinoids can produce toxic effects. The most common severe negative effects include irregular heartbeat, paranoia or other delusions, severe depression with suicidal thinking, hallucinations, inability to speak, anxiety or panic attacks, vomiting, confusion, poor coordination, kidney failure, and seizures [24]. Use can lead to hospitalizations or even death.

Cannabis use is prohibited by the National Collegiate Athletic Association (NCAA) and prohibited in competition by the World Anti-Doping Agency (WADA). Despite a lack of evidence to support cannabis use, its advancing legalization and medicalization in the United States and other countries has led many athletes to conclude that its use is not risky and may even be helpful for training/training recovery, performance, injury recovery, and relaxation [25]. In response to these changing perceptions, several US professional sports leagues, e.g., the National Football League (NFL) and Major League Baseball (MLB), have recently eliminated or reduced cannabis testing and sanctions in favor of the identification of daily or heavy users with the goal of providing treatment. Despite the perceived positive impacts on performance, cannabis use can have potentially negative impacts on performance including decreased reaction time, impaired coordination, and reduced motivation [26].

Most studies on cannabis use in sports are based on cross-sectional, self-report surveys, which, when compared to urine testing results, document widespread underreporting. Nevertheless, it appears that approximately one in four US collegiate athletes have used cannabis in the past year, with higher rates in division III versus division I (32.6% vs. 17.7%) and in those states where cannabis is recreationally/medically legal (38.7% vs. 26.1%) [13]. In addition, men and women in certain US collegiate sports such as ice hockey, lacrosse, wrestling, soccer, and swimming are more likely to use cannabis than are those in other sports. Finally, 2.5% of collegiate athletes report inhaling cannabis daily, potentially having a negative effect on mood, motivation, and learning [13]. There are no large studies on cannabis use among professional athletes, although reports from players indicate that its use is widespread and for many has replaced alcohol as a post-practice/game substance of choice.

Case Study #3: Synthetic Cannabis Withdrawal

A 23-year-old professional minor league baseball player with a prior history of cannabis misuse was being monitored by the league for compliance with treatment and continued abstinence through frequent, random urine drug screens. He was doing well in the program with more than 1 year of negative urine drug screens and full compliance with outpatient counseling. While the player was in the middle of a week-long road trip, the team psychiatrist received a phone call from the athletic trainer explaining that the player presented with onset of insomnia, anxiety, anorexia, abdominal pain with nausea and vomiting, diaphoresis, and tachycardia. During his medical assessment, he had admitted that during his time in the program, he had maintained abstinence from cannabis but had developed a daily habit of vaping CBD oil that he was purchasing from the Internet. He stated that he was using up to $80 a day worth of a specific CBD product. On this road trip, he had left his CBD oil at home and thus had abruptly stopped the CBD consumption 2 days prior to his presentation to the trainer. Cannabis withdrawal syndrome was considered, given his prior history, but, given the combination of his consistent denial of use coupled with the negative urine drug screens obtained through the extensive testing program in which he was participating, this was believed to be less likely. Although CBD withdrawal is not well-described in the literature, it was noted that the specific product that he was using had run afoul of the US Drug Enforcement Administration for adding synthetic cannabinoids into their advertised CBD products.

Diagnoses (1) Synthetic cannabis withdrawal, moderate; (2) cannabis use disorder, in full remission.

Treatment He was treated symptomatically with a 2-week tapering course of gabapentin in combination with anti-emetics and zolpidem 5 mg at night as needed for sleep. Upon return from the road trip, he also reintroduced himself to the CBD product with full resolution of his symptoms and agreed to gradually taper off the product over an 8-week period. He remained abstinent and without recurrent withdrawal symptoms while continuing in the outpatient treatment program.

Case Study #4: High-Potency Cannabis-Induced Paranoid Psychosis

A 22-year-old male, a previously healthy professional soccer player with no history of mental health disorders or substance misuse, was rehabilitating a hamstring injury during the season when the team psychiatrist received a late-night call from the head athletic trainer. The player had been apprehended by the police outside the home of an unknown family, who stated that he was trying to enter their home, calling for his mother to let him in. When the police arrived, they found his car, abandoned with the hazard lights flashing and a trail of clothing leading up to the house. Once at the home, the police found an incoherent, unclothed young man banging loudly on the front door, demanding to be let into the house. He was detained and transported to an emergency room for a medical evaluation under an emergency petition. His evaluation was notable for a profound thought disturbance of loosely associated, incoherent thought processes shrouded by extreme paranoia and agitation. His physical examination was unremarkable. His urine toxicology was positive for THC. He had no prior history of mental health disorders nor was there a family history of mental health or substance use disorders.

Diagnoses   (1) Cannabis-induced psychotic disorder, severe, with onset during intoxication; (2) no evidence of cannabis use disorder; (3) hamstring strain, moderate.

Treatment   He was voluntarily admitted to an acute psychiatric unit and stabilized on a low dose of risperidone over the course of 4 weeks. His thought disturbance persisted for several days, whereas his paranoia persisted for several weeks, with an eventual waning presence in his thought content. He subsequently admitted that over the course of 2 days prior to admission, he had consumed a large quantity of a highly potent form of THC, commonly referred to as "ear wax." The player denied previous cannabis use and estimated that he had smoked "over 50 hits" of the ear wax during those 2 days because he was bored during his rehabilitation. After discharge, he was maintained on risperidone for several months and then gradually weaned off under the care of a psychiatrist. Unfortunately, he was released by the team at the end of the season. In the months that followed, he became interested in yoga and mindfulness practices, ultimately utilizing these modalities to maintain his own mental health and launch a successful business career.

Case Study #5: Cannabis Use Disorder and Anxiety/Depression

A 19-year-old male collegiate football player was referred by his therapist to a psychiatrist in early spring for the evaluation of insomnia, anxiety, depression, inattention, cannabis use, and poor academic performance. He had been diagnosed with ADHD, inattentive-type, in late middle school and took methylphenidate reluctantly in high school for a few years. He eventually stopped it, saying that it increased his anxiety. In addition, he reported chronic anxiety, depression, and insomnia for which he self-medicated by smoking cannabis daily. He reported no prior treatment for anxiety or depression. During his second fall semester of college, his depression worsened to a moderately severe level, and he was unable to function optimally in school or sports. He spent much of his free time hanging out with friends and smoking cannabis. He was reluctant to take medications without consulting with his family.

Diagnoses   (1) ADHD, inattentive-type; (2) major depressive disorder, moderately severe; (3) generalized anxiety disorder; (4) insomnia disorder, stress-related; (5) poor medication adherence; (6) poor academic performance; (7) obesity.

His main recovery barriers were medication adherence, anxiety, insomnia, high-stress lifestyle, and friend group that promoted substance use.

Treatment   For ADHD, he was treated with behavioral therapy and academic accommodations, but he was reluctant to try even low-dose stimulant medication. He eventually agreed to try low-dose atomoxetine (25 mg) with some improvement and no side effects. For his depression and anxiety, he was started on 5 mg of escitalopram and the dosage was increased to 10 mg in 2 weeks with significant improvement. For insomnia, he was treated with trazodone 50–75 mg at bedtime, which was extremely helpful. With encouragement, he was able to stop cannabis use. He continued with twice monthly therapy. He did well until the end of the spring semester, when he slipped back into regular cannabis use and stopped taking his psychiatric medications. He was referred to a substance intensive outpatient program, and regular urine testing was started. In addition, he was restarted on escitalopram (10 mg), atomoxetine (increased to 40 mg), and trazodone (50–75 mg). Hydroxyzine 25–50 mg twice daily as needed for anxiety was added. He did well over the summer with significant reductions in symptoms and substance use but was injured during the fall season and stopped coming to treatment.

He resurfaced the following spring in crisis. Adjustment struggles to online learning and social isolation due to a global pandemic led to increased symptoms of anxiety, depression, suicidal ideation with a plan, insomnia, loss of motivation for schoolwork, and return to daily cannabis use. He had ceased taking depression and anxiety medications due to reported intolerance of side effects. He reported staying up most nights and simultaneously reported limited access to consistent, regular meals due to financial concerns and lack of team meals during the pandemic. Safety was the primary concern, and family support was engaged. The initial focus, after safety was ensured, was on regulating sleep and establishing food consistency. Daily support from the psychiatrist, psychologist, and/or team physician was

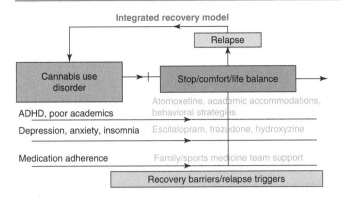

Fig. 14.3 Integrated Recovery Model of treatment for substance use disorder in Case Study #5

provided. Family members took on the role of assisting with medication management. Once sleep was regulated, safety concerns resolved. He eventually found a medication regimen with fewer side effects, and his adherence improved (Fig. 14.3).

Case Discussions

Clinical cases of cannabis intoxication, withdrawal, and use disorders have increased in sports medicine/mental health practices over the past decade as a result of US medicalization (at least 37 states) and legalization (at least 18 states) [27] and similar situations in other countries. The significant increase in cannabis THC levels and consumption methods as well as the widespread availability of more potent THC products (e.g., oils, concentrates, edibles) and synthetic cannabis (either purchased or as a contaminant) have resulted in more severe cases as demonstrated in the case studies.

Cannabis intoxication and withdrawal are the second most common reason for a substance-related emergency room visit in the United States, behind only cocaine [28]. Cannabis intoxication typically presents with anxiety/paranoia/panic, light-headedness/dizziness/vertigo, dysphoria, palpitations, and/or nausea/vomiting. The initial symptoms of cannabis withdrawal typically begin within 1–3 days after the last use, intensify over the first week, and remain for 1–2 weeks. The typical symptoms include irritability, aggression, anger, anxiety/nervousness, anorexia/weight loss, restlessness, depression, and a mix of physical symptoms including fever, chills, headache, abdominal pain, tremors, and sweats [28].

Studies have shown some modest benefits from a variety of medications in the management of cannabis withdrawal. Dronabinol, a CB1 agonist, which is US Food and Drug Administration (FDA)-approved for the treatment of acquired immunodeficiency syndrome (AIDS)-related anorexia and cancer chemotherapy vomiting, as well as gabapentin, a gamma-aminobutyric acid (GABA) modulator, are both helpful in reducing most withdrawal symptoms,

resulting in greater retention in treatment. Gabapentin is also helpful for reducing cravings and cannabis-related problems as well as improving cognitive dysfunction. Quetiapine and mirtazapine can be helpful for insomnia, anorexia, and reversing undesired weight loss, whereas zolpidem can also be used to improve sleep [29]. Unfortunately, most of these medications and other studies have shown little benefit in reducing the relapse rates of cannabis use disorder, except for perhaps topiramate, which has resulted in lowered use in adolescents [29]. Since none of these medications have been studied in athletes, they should be used with caution, starting with lower dosages and monitoring for side effects.

Opioids (Prescription Pain Medications)

Opioid analgesics are effective pain relievers for acute, severe athletic injuries requiring surgery and/or missed days from practice and competition. There are few long-term studies that support their use, however, in the treatment of chronic or subacute pain [30]. They are either naturally derived from the opium poppy (e.g., morphine, codeine), semi-synthetically made from morphine or similar compounds (e.g., oxycodone, hydrocodone), or synthesized independently (e.g., fentanyl, buprenorphine). They exert their effects by attaching to the opioid receptors in the cortex, mid-brain, brain stem, and spinal cord. The exact effects can vary across individuals, with some athletes reporting sedation and reduced mental quickness while others report stimulation (e.g., energy, motivation).

Opioid analgesic use in sports has decreased over the past decade in recognition of the negative consequences of the opioid epidemic over the last 20 years including rising rates of use disorders resulting in overdose and/or requiring treatment. For example, 18% of collegiate athletes reported using opioid analgesics with a prescription in 2013 compared to 11% in 2018. Use without a prescription dropped from 6% in 2013 to 3% in 2017 [13]. Most US collegiate and professional sports teams have removed opioid analgesics from training rooms and emergency travel kits.

Despite the risks associated with use and decreasing trends in use, opioid analgesic use without a prescription among collegiate athletes appears to be higher than that among collegiate nonathletes, especially among varsity male and female athletes with a current injury (17.9% versus 7.9% for males; 10.6% versus 6.7% for females) [3]. Retired US professional NFL athletes are even more likely to have used opioids during their playing careers (52%), and of these, 71% acknowledged misuse (no prescription or using differently than prescribed) [31]. A follow-up study of these same athletes 9 years later (2019) showed that almost 50% were still using opioids. This opioid use was also correlated with depressive symptoms, with retired players who reported continued opioid use being 5.93 times more likely to be experiencing current moderate to severe depressive symptoms than nonusing peers [9].

Case Study #6: Opioid and Muscle Relaxant Use Disorder

A 33-year-old married father of two children and recently retired professional football player (11 years in the NFL) was referred by his primary care physician and wife for the evaluation of chronic pain and overuse of pain medications and muscle relaxants. He presented with a 1-year history of escalating use of hydrocodone and carisoprodol. At the time of his initial evaluation, he was taking up to ten carisoprodol tablets and 20 hydrocodone tablets (200 morphine milligram equivalents) daily for chronic neck, shoulder, low back, and hip pain. He was obtaining some of his medication from physicians and buying some from friends. He reported poor pain relief, craving for the pills, and interdose withdrawal. He had previously been diagnosed with degenerative disc disease and traumatic arthritis and had two previous shoulder repairs (torn labrum). Psychiatric history revealed a long-term pattern of insomnia (difficulty falling and staying asleep) as well as untreated chronic anxiety. His stress level was extremely high due to his transition out of sport, financial strain from a failing business venture, and a need to establish a new career.

Diagnoses (1) Opioid and muscle relaxant use disorders, moderate; (2) generalized anxiety disorder; (3) insomnia disorder; (4) somatic symptom disorder with predominant pain.

His main recovery barriers/relapse triggers were chronic pain, anxiety, insomnia, and career uncertainty (Fig. 14.4).

Treatment For opioid use disorder and chronic pain, recommendations were: (1) buprenorphine 8 mg sublingually twice

daily; (2) massage therapy weekly; (3) stretching twice daily; and (4) trigger point injections. For anxiety, recommendations were: (1) sertraline up to 150 mg daily; (2) clonazepam 0.5 mg three times daily (while ensuring that concomitant opioid use was not occurring via urine testing); and (3) stress control therapy and career counseling. For insomnia, recommendations were: (1) trazodone 50–100 mg nightly; (2) unwinding routine; and (3) white noise at bedtime.

Case Discussions

Buprenorphine, a long-acting partial opioid agonist, is a highly effective medication that can be used to manage opioid withdrawal, reduce cravings, promote retention in treatment, and improve abstinence [32]. It is used sublingually, either as buprenorphine alone or as buprenorphine with naloxone. The latter formulation is typically used in those with a history of intravenous opioid use. An induction can be safely carried out in the outpatient setting with low starting dosages (i.e., 2–4 mg) to avoid precipitated withdrawal, which is more likely if the athlete or coach has been using fentanyl. A typical maintenance dosage of 8–24 mg in divided dosages two or three times a day is reached in 2–3 days. If buprenorphine is used to prevent relapse, then it should be continued for at least 6–12 months or longer. It is important to evaluate any athlete with an opioid use disorder for comorbid mental health symptoms and disorders (e.g., anxiety, depression) as these occur in 20–80% of these individuals in the general population, especially in adolescents and young adults [32].

Buprenorphine can also be used for the management of chronic pain that is common in transitioning or retired athletes or coaches [33]. In fact, a new formulation of buprenorphine with lower dosing was approved by the US FDA in 2016 for the treatment of chronic pain. The standard formulation can also be used and often results in lower pain levels with much less pain breakthrough. Unfortunately, buprenorphine (and methadone) are prohibited by the NCAA at all times and by WADA in competition; therefore, its use would necessitate a break in competition. Given the higher likelihood of long-term use of opioid analgesics by retired athletes with accompanying risks of overdose, tolerance/physiological dependence, poor pain control, and the development of a use disorder, buprenorphine should be strongly considered in this population.

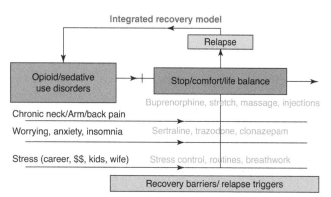

Fig. 14.4 Integrated Recovery Model of treatment for substance use disorder in Case Study #6

Stimulants (Caffeine, Nicotine, Cocaine, Over-the-Counter and Prescribed Stimulants)

Stimulants are a broad class of substances that stimulate the sympathetic nervous system via epinephrine or activation of brain circuits that use monoamines and other neurotransmitters (e.g., dopamine, norepinephrine, nicotine acetylcholine). This class includes many substances used regularly by athletes and coaches such as caffeine, nicotine, ephedrine, pseudoephedrine, synephrine, cocaine, methamphetamine, methylphenidate, amphetamine, modafinil, phentermine, and bupropion. They can be obtained legally, illicitly, over the counter, or with a prescription. Many members of this class are prohibited by WADA, professional sports leagues, and the NCAA because of their known performance-enhancing effects. For some prohibited substances, when prescribed clinically to treat ADHD, excessive daytime sleepiness, narcolepsy, depression, or obesity, they can be used by WADA or professional sport league-governed athletes and coaches after obtaining a therapeutic use exemption (TUE). The NCAA does not require TUEs per se but does have detailed requirements for diagnosis, management, and documentation for stimulant use to be considered justifiable.

Caffeine is the most widely used stimulant by elite athletes. It is attractive to some athletes during practice and competition because it increases alertness, muscle strength, endurance, and power [34]. Caffeine was prohibited by WADA until 2004, but its use has since been routinely monitored to track patterns through quantitative urine testing. Studies show that most (>70%) Olympic-level athletes use caffeine but that the levels for most sports are in the low to moderate ranges and therefore unlikely to enhance performance. Endurance sport athletes, however, such as those in cycling, rowing, and triathlon, use it at higher levels, warranting ongoing monitoring [35].

Nicotine obtained from oral tobacco is the second most widely used stimulant in sport, especially in US baseball, lacrosse, and ice hockey [13]. Sports clinicians will routinely encounter high-dose oral tobacco users who "dip" up to a can a day from awakening to bedtime. Efforts to quit among these individuals tend to be more successful in the off-season, with use patterns frequently returning as the playing season begins.

Prescribed stimulants, e.g., short- or long-acting methylphenidate or amphetamine, are the third most common category of stimulants used in sport. Approximately 8% of 40-person MLB rosters and 7% of NCAA student athletes have physician-prescribed stimulants (and a TUE in the case of the MLB) for ADHD [13, 36]. Importantly, an additional 5% of collegiate athletes use prescription stimulants without a prescription [13]. These stimulants are attractive to athletes because they increase alertness and sustained attention, boost energy, improve reaction time, and reduce hyperactivity and impulsivity [37]. Use of over-the-counter stimulants, e.g., ephedrine and synephrine, is also seen in sport. They are attractive to athletes as workout supplements or for weight loss. Athletes frequently use several stimulants together (stimulant stacking), especially caffeine, nicotine, ephedra, and/or prescribed stimulants. This practice of stimulant stacking can result in anxiety or insomnia due to synergistic stimulant effects.

Illicit stimulant use is seen in athletes just as in the general population. The most recent survey of collegiate athletes by the NCAA [13] has shown that past-year self-reported use of cocaine in 2013 compared to that in 2017 had increased from 2.6% to 5.2% for men and from 0.6% to 1.7% for women [13]. Substantially higher rates were seen in men's sports of lacrosse (22%), ice hockey (7%), and wrestling (7%) and in women's sports of lacrosse (6%) and ice hockey (4%). This is concerning since cocaine use has a moderate likelihood of developing into a use disorder and/or of being laced with fentanyl or other more potent synthetic opioids, making overdose a possibility.

Case Study #7: Stimulant Use Disorders and Insomnia

A 53-year-old married male and current professional baseball coach and former Major League Baseball (MLB) player was referred by his athletic trainer and team physician because of chronic insomnia and long-term high-dose caffeine and nicotine use. He routinely consumed 6–10 cups of brewed coffee (900–1500 mg) daily during the season and used a half-can of moist snuff every day. Reducing use led to rebound headaches. He had tried zolpidem 10 mg for insomnia in the past with positive results.

Diagnoses (1) Nicotine use disorder, moderate; (2) caffeine use disorder, moderate (3) chronic insomnia, severe, due to excessive use of stimulants and an active mind at night.

Treatment For his nicotine use disorder, he was prescribed varenicline 0.5 mg daily for 1 week while trying to reduce his intake by 25%. For the second week, the varenicline was increased to 0.5 mg twice daily with a goal of reducing his oral use by 50%. By the third week, his dosage was raised to 1 mg twice daily with few side effects and a substantial reduction in his cravings and use. He also utilized an oral tobacco substitute (gum) to satisfy his need to have something in his mouth. In addition to reducing his oral tobacco use, he switched to half-caffeinated/half-decaffeinated coffee and was able to reduce his daily intake to 4–6 cups.

For insomnia, he was educated about sleep hygiene including the importance of an unwinding routine and the use of white noise. He began to use melatonin 5 mg several hours before bedtime and was also given a prescription for trazodone 50–100 mg to be taken 90 min before bedtime. This regimen was only moderately effective, so he was given an additional prescription for zolpidem 5 mg as needed. He was instructed to take this nightly with the melatonin 5 mg

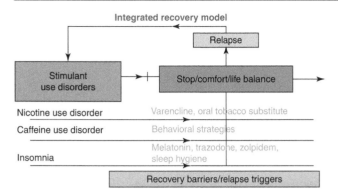

Fig. 14.5 Integrated Recovery Model of treatment for substance use disorder in Case Study #7

for a week to reset his sleep/awake cycle. Afterward, he used melatonin and trazodone or zolpidem as needed (Fig. 14.5).

Case Study #8: Severe Nicotine Use Disorder

A 42-year-old married professional football coach and former NFL player was referred by his team physician after a preseason dental exam revealed a precancerous buccal lesion due to heavy oral tobacco use. He had a long history of oral tobacco use dating back to high school. His use increased while in college and in his early years as a professional to one can of moist snuff daily. He would put in a dip immediately upon awakening and then dip regularly throughout the day, including one large dip just prior to bedtime. If he did not dip regularly, he would have intense cravings and mild withdrawal. In addition, he would frequently awaken during the night and need to put in a small dip to be able to fall back asleep. He was being pressurized by his wife and two children to quit and reported his readiness level to do so at 8/10, but his confidence was lower as he had tried to quit many times.

Diagnosis (1) Nicotine use disorder, severe; (2) oral leukoplakia; (3) chronic insomnia from nocturnal nicotine withdrawal.

Treatment For his nicotine use disorder, he was prescribed a 21 mg nicotine patch daily. Over the first 3 days of using the patch, he was instructed to supplement it with nicotine gum 4 mg hourly if needed. This would allow the patch nicotine level to reach a steady state, after which he would use the gum as needed for breakthrough cravings. After 2 weeks on the patch and gum, he switched to the nicotine patch and nasal spray. Bupropion sustained-release (SR) 100 mg daily was added during the day and increased to twice daily after 1 week. He also used a non-nicotine oral tobacco substitute for practices and games. Additionally, he was taught relaxation breathing and began to employ guided meditation exer-

cises during the day and at night. He successfully discontinued his oral tobacco after 1 month, his sleep improved, and his oral lesion resolved.

Case Study #9: Cocaine and Cannabis Use Disorders

A 21-year-old male collegiate baseball player was referred by his athletic trainer and sports psychologist for the evaluation of anxiety, depression, poor academic performance, and substance misuse (cannabis). He described a long history of regular stimulant (cocaine), opioid (pain pills), alcohol, and cannabis use dating back to high school. Additionally, he reported a traumatic developmental history of unstable housing and ongoing physical and emotional abuse by his father for which he carried much resentment. Urine testing was positive for cannabis and cocaine. He acknowledged this use as well as binge drinking, saying that substances were the only thing that reduced his anxiety and depression. In class, he reported difficulty concentrating, taking notes, and organizing his work.

Diagnoses (1) Generalized anxiety disorder; (2) major depressive disorder, moderately severe, substance-aggravated; (3) ADHD, combined-type; (4) intermittent explosive disorder; (5) cannabis and cocaine use disorders.

Treatment For anxiety and depression, he was started on sertraline 25 mg daily, increasing the dosage slowly to 150 mg daily over the first month. He also began to learn stress control strategies to manage his emotional activation, especially his anger. For ADHD, he was started on methylphenidate ER 18 mg. This dosage was increased to 54 mg daily without much improvement, so it was changed to lisdexamfetamine 40 mg daily with better results. He was prescribed an as-needed evening dosage of immediate-release amphetamine salts 10 mg for an extended duration of action when needed for academic purposes. For his substance use disorders, he was regularly urine tested and was enrolled in a low-intensity outpatient program. When this proved insufficient, he enrolled in an off-campus intensive outpatient program. He improved in many areas over the next few months but continued to struggle with his anger/resentment and alcohol and cannabis use.

Case Discussions

Nicotine (oral tobacco or vaping) use disorder, anecdotally, is the most commonly encountered stimulant use disorder in sports medicine practice. Withdrawal and cravings can be effectively managed with nicotine replacement therapy (NRT). NRT comes in various formulations including the patch, gum, lozenge, nasal spray, or inhaler. The patch takes 3 days or more to reach a steady state, so supplementation with short-acting products, e.g., nicotine gum or nasal spray, is typically necessary [1]. The 6-month meta-analytic abstinence rate for NRT is 16.9% versus 10.5% for placebo [38].

For the ongoing treatment of nicotine use disorder, other US FDA-approved medications with demonstrated effectiveness should be considered, including bupropion, varenicline, or the two in combination. Bupropion is an antidepressant medication that impacts brain dopamine and norepinephrine circuits. Varenicline is a partial nicotine acetylcholine receptor agonist that manages withdrawal, suppresses cravings, and supports abstinence. The typical maintenance dosage of bupropion is either the SR formulation 100 mg twice daily or the XL formulation at 150 mg daily. The 6-month meta-analytic abstinence rate for bupropion is 19.0% versus 11% for placebo. For varenicline, the typical maintenance dosage is 1 mg twice a day, but it can be started at lower dosages (i.e., 0.5 mg once or twice a day) while the athlete/coach is still using. The 6-month meta-analytic abstinence rate for varenicline is 25.6% versus 11.1% for placebo. The combination of bupropion and varenicline together along with psychosocial support and behavioral counseling has the highest abstinence rate [38]. Perhaps the most effective identification strategy for oral tobacco use disorder, which is common is US baseball, lacrosse, and ice hockey, is counseling following an annual dental screening looking for gum irritation or oral lesions [1].

Other stimulant use disorders (e.g., cocaine, nonprescription amphetamines) are not commonly seen in sport, presumably due to the detrimental effects on health and performance. However, the misuse (e.g., excessive dosages taken at night to study) of prescribed stimulants and the concurrent use of several stimulants (i.e., caffeine, nicotine, prescribed stimulants) even in low dosages can lead to increased anxiety, irritability, insomnia, gastrointestinal distress, and, paradoxically, poor concentration [1].

Summary and Conclusions

While substance use disorders are not common among actively participating collegiate and professional athletes due to the negative impacts on performance and daily functioning, substance misuse is common and, in some cases, is more prevalent among athletes than the general population. Providers working with this population will encounter misuse of many substances, particularly alcohol, cannabis, opioids, and stimulants. Additionally, substance use disorders are more commonly seen among retired athletes and coaches. The case examples presented above highlight misuse and use disorder cases along with comorbidities, barriers to treatment, and combined psychopharmacological and psychotherapeutic approaches to treating athletes and coaches.

Early identification is critical in curbing misuse and preventing the progression to a use disorder. Integrating regular screenings for substance misuse at yearly pre-participation examinations and training sports medicine staff along with organizational staff on the signs and symptoms of misuse are strategies that should be employed by teams and organizations to help with identification. For some substances (specifically nicotine), annual physical examinations can help identify individuals who may be struggling with misuse or a use disorder. Collaboration among all members of the sports medicine team (e.g., athletic trainers, physicians, other mental health providers) is critical.

Once an individual is referred to treatment, utilizing an Integrated Recovery Model can help with conceptualization of the problem and development of an appropriate treatment plan. A thorough assessment including pattern of use, previous quit attempts, comorbid conditions (mental health disorders and other physical health disorders), and barriers to treatment should be conducted. Treatment planning should then address goals for the first year of treatment including stopping use and finding comfort and life balance. In stopping use, the focus is on addressing withdrawal symptoms, suppressing cravings, ceasing use, and maintaining abstinence. MI, group psychoeducation, and behavioral and social support interventions paired with an appropriate medication regimen will be the most beneficial. Addressing comorbid conditions that may be underlying or maintaining use patterns is critical. Depression, anxiety, and insomnia are common comorbid presentations in athletes/coaches seeking treatment for substance misuse/use disorders. Appropriate treatment of these symptoms will help remove barriers to recovery and enhance success in maintaining abstinence.

While data on substance use patterns in the NCAA student athlete population are available, there are limited data for coaches and professional athletes. More robust research will help gain an understanding of the breadth of misuse and use disorders among these populations, which can help inform the need to allocate resources for prevention, early identification, and treatment.

References

1. McDuff D, Stull T, Castaldelli-Maia JM, Hitchcock ME, Hainline B, Reardon CL. Recreational and ergogenic substance use and substance use disorders in elite athletes: a narrative review. Br J Sports Med. 2019;53(12):754–60. https://doi.org/10.1136/bjsports-2019-100669.

2. Stull T, Morse E, McDuff DR. Substance use and its impact on athlete health and performance. Psychiatr Clin North Am. 2021;44(3):405–17. https://doi.org/10.1016/j.psc.2021.04.006.

3. Ford JA, Pomykacz C, Veliz P, McCabe SE, Boyd CJ. Sports involvement, injury history, and non-medical use of prescription opioids among college students: an analysis with a national sample. Am J Addict. 2018;27(1):15–22. https://doi.org/10.1111/ajad.12657.

4. Clarest J, Grandner M, Athey A, McDuff D, Turner R. Substance use among collegiate athletes versus non-athletes. Athl Train Sports Health Care. 2021;13:e443.

5. Mannes Z, Hasin D, Martins S, Goncalves P, Livne O, de Oliviera L, de Andrade A, McReynolds L, Hainline B, Castedelli-Maia J. Do elite college athletes have a higher likelihood of moderate to high risk alcohol and cannabis use compared to non-athletes? Results from a national survey in Brazil. Braz J Psychiatry. 2022;44:289.

6. Gouttebarge V, Bindra A, Blauwet C, et al. International Olympic Committee (IOC) Sport Mental Health Assessment Tool 1 (SMHAT-1) and Sport Mental Health Recognition Tool 1 (SMHRT-1): towards better support of athletes' mental health. Br J Sports Med. 2021;55(1):30–7. https://doi.org/10.1136/bjsports-2020-102411.

7. Kilic O, Carmody S, Upmeijer J, Kerkhoffs G, Purcell R, Rice S, Gouttegarge V. Prevalence of mental health symptoms among male and female Australian professional footballers. BMJ Open Sport Exerc Med. 2021;7:e001043. https://doi.org/10.1136/bmjsem-2021-001043.

8. American Psychiatric Association. Diagnostic and statistical manual of mental disorders. 5th ed. Washington DC: American Psychiatric Association; 2013.

9. Mannes ZL, Dunne EM, Ferguson EG, Cottler LB, Ennis N. History of opioid use as a risk factor for current use and mental health consequences among retired National Football League athletes: a 9-year follow-up investigation. Drug Alcohol Depend. 2020;215:108251. https://doi.org/10.1016/j.drugalcdep.2020.108251.

10. McDuff DR, Solounias BL, RachBeisel J, Johnson JL. Psychiatric consultation with substance abusers in early recovery. Am J Drug Alcohol Abuse. 1994;20(3):287–99. https://doi.org/10.3109/00952999409106015.

11. McDuff DR, Muneses TI. In: White R, Wright D, editors. Mental health strategy: addictions interventions with the dually diagnosed in addiction intervention: strategies to motivate treatment-seeking behavior. New York: The Haworth Press; 1998.

12. Substance Abuse Mental Health Services Administration Advisory. Using motivational interviewing in substance use disorder treatment. Rockville, MD: SAMHSA; 2021. https://store.samhsa.gov/product/advisory-using-motivational-interviewing-substance-use-disorder-treatment/pep20-02-02-014?referer=from_search_result.

13. NCAA. National study on substance use habits of collegiate student athletes. Indianapolis, IN: NCAA; 2018. http://www.ncaa.org/sites/default/files/2018RES_Substance_Use_Final_Report_FINAL_20180611.pdf

14. Gouttebarge V, Backx FJ, Aoki H, Kerkhoffs GM. Symptoms of common mental disorders in professional football (soccer) across five European countries. J Sports Sci Med. 2015;14(4):811–8. PMID: 26664278; PMCID: PMC4657424.

15. Gouttebarge V, Hopley P, Kerkhoffs G, et al. A 12-month prospective cohort study of symptoms of common mental disorders among professional rugby players. Eur J Sport Sci. 2018;18(7):1004–12. https://doi.org/10.1080/17461391.2018.1466914.

16. Du Preez EJ, Graham KS, Gan TY, Moses B, Ball C, Kuah DE. Depression, anxiety, and alcohol use in elite rugby league players over a competitive season. Clin J Sport Med. 2017;27(6):530–5. https://doi.org/10.1097/JSM.0000000000000411. PMID: 28107218.

17. Walters P, Hillier B, Passetti F, et al. Diagnosis and management of substance use disorders in athletes. Adv Psychiatry Behav Health. 2021;1:135–43. https://doi.org/10.1016/j.ypsc.2021.06.001.

18. Reardon CL, Bindra A, Blauwet C, et al. Mental health management of elite athletes during COVID-19: a narrative review and recommendations. Br J Sports Med. 2020;55:608. https://doi.org/10.1136/bjsports-2020-102884.

19. Reus VI, Fochtmann LJ, Bukstein O, et al. The American Psychiatric Association Practice Guideline for the Pharmacological Treatment of Patients With Alcohol Use Disorder. Am J Psychiatry. 2018;175(1):86–90. https://doi.org/10.1176/appi.ajp.2017.1750101.

20. Zou S, Kumar U. Cannabinoid receptors and the endocannabinoid system: signaling and function in the central nervous system. Int J Mol Sci. 2018;19(3):833. https://doi.org/10.3390/ijms19030833.

21. ElSohly MA, Chandra S, Radwan M, Majumdar CG, Church JC. A comprehensive review of cannabis potency in the United States in the last decade. Biol Psychiatry Cogn Neurosci Neuroimaging. 2021;6(6):603–6. https://doi.org/10.1016/j.bpsc.2020.12.016.

22. Chandra S, Radwan MM, Majumdar CG, Church JC, Freeman TP, ElSohly MA. New trends in cannabis potency in USA and Europe during the last decade (2008-2017). Eur Arch Psychiatry Clin Neurosci. 2019;269(1):5–15. https://doi.org/10.1007/s00406-019-00983-5. Published correction appears in Eur Arch Psychiatry Clin Neurosci. 2019 May 23.

23. Volkow ND, Baler RD, Compton WM, Weiss SR. Adverse health effects of marijuana use. N Engl J Med. 2014;370(23):2219–27. https://doi.org/10.1056/NEJMra1402309.

24. Castaneto MS, Gorelick DA, Desrosiers NA, et al. Synthetic cannabinoids: epidemiology, pharmacodynamics, and clinical implications. Drug Alcohol Depend. 2014;144:12–41.

25. Docter S, Khan M, Gohal C, Ravi B, Bhandari M, Gandhi R, Leroux T. Cannabis use and sport: a systematic review. Sports Health. 2020;12(2):189–99. https://doi.org/10.1177/1941738120901670. PMID: 32023171; PMCID: PMC7040945.

26. Ware MA, Jensen D, Barrette A, Vernec A, Derman W. Cannabis and the health and performance of the elite athlete. Clin J Sport Med. 2018;28:480–4.

27. National Conference of State Legislatures. State Medical Marijuana Laws. Washington, DC: NCSL; n.d.. https://www.ncsl.org/research/health/state-medical-marijuana-laws.aspx. Accessed 9 Sep 2021.

28. Takakuwa KM, Schears RM. The emergency department care of the cannabis and synthetic cannabinoid patient: a narrative review. Int J Emerg Med. 2021;14(1):10. https://doi.org/10.1186/s12245-021-00330-3.

29. Brezing CA, Levin FR. The current state of pharmacological treatments for cannabis use disorder and withdrawal. Neuropsychopharmacology. 2018;43(1):173–94. https://doi.org/10.1038/npp.2017.21233.

30. Tucker HR, Scaff K, McCloud T, et al. Harms and benefits of opioids for management of non-surgical acute and chronic low back pain: a systematic review. Br J Sports Med. 2020;54(11):664. https://doi.org/10.1136/bjsports-2018-099805.

31. Cottler LB, Ben Abdallah A, Cummings SM, Barr J, Banks R, Forchheimer R. Injury, pain, and prescription opioid use among former National Football League (NFL) players. Drug Alcohol Depend. 2011;116(1–3):188–94. https://doi.org/10.1016/j.drugalcdep.2010.12.003.

32. Borodovsky JT, Levy S, Fishman M, Marsch LA. Buprenorphine treatment for adolescents and young adults with opioid use disorders: a narrative review. J Addict Med. 2018;12(3):170–83. https://doi.org/10.1097/ADM.0000000000000388.

33. Rudolf GD. Buprenorphine in the treatment of chronic pain. Phys Med Rehabil Clin N Am. 2020;31(2):195–204. https://doi.org/10.1016/j.pmr.2020.02.001.

34. Grgic J, Grgic I, Pickering C, Schoenfeld BJ, Bishop DJ, Pedisic Z. Wake up and smell the coffee: caffeine supplementation and exercise performance-an umbrella review of 21 published meta-analyses. Br J Sports Med. 2020;54(11):681–8. https://doi.org/10.1136/bjsports-2018-100278. PMID: 30926628.

35. Aguilar-Navarro M, Muñoz G, Salinero JJ, Muñoz-Guerra J, Fernández-Álvarez M, Plata MDM, Del Coso J. Urine caffeine concentration in doping control samples from 2004 to 2015. Nutrients. 2019;11(2):286. https://doi.org/10.3390/nu11020286. PMID: 30699902; PMCID: PMC6412495.

36. Martin T. Report of major league baseball's joint drug prevention and treatment program. 2018. http://www.mlb.com/documents/3/8/2/301315382/IPA_2018_Public_Report_113018.pdf.

37. Han DH, McDuff D, Thompson D, Hitchcock ME, Reardon CL, Hainline B. Attention-deficit/hyperactivity disorder in elite athletes: a narrative review. Br J Sports Med. 2019;53(12):741–5. https://doi.org/10.1136/bjsports-2019-100713. PMID: 31097459.

38. Patnode CD, Henderson JT, Coppola EL, Melnikow J, Durbin S, Thomas RG. Interventions for tobacco cessation in adults, including pregnant persons: updated evidence report and systematic review for the US Preventive Services Task Force. JAMA. 2021;325(3):280–98. https://doi.org/10.1001/jama.2020.23541.

Behavioral Addictions: Excessive Gambling and Gaming

15

Jeffrey Derevensky

Behavioral Addictions

Behavioral addiction is a relatively new concept in psychiatry and was first introduced in the Diagnostic and Statistical Manual of Mental Disorders 5th edition (DSM-5) by the American Psychiatric Association in 2013 [1]. This is not to suggest that many of the disorders believed to be subsumed under behavioral disorders have recently evolved; rather, it has become a new way to classify certain disorders. While this chapter will touch upon gambling and gaming disorders (GDs), other behavioral disorders including Internet addiction, social networking addiction, food addiction, hypersexual disorders, love addiction, exercise addiction, excessive use of smartphones, and compulsive buying disorders have become associated with behavioral addictions and can negatively impact the elite athlete's mental health and performance. Based upon strong empirical and clinical evidence, a growing number of risky behaviors have been found to result in short-term rewards but can become persistent problems over time. If these behaviors are engaged in too frequently, then they are often accompanied by adverse consequences to the individual. Such behaviors share many similarities with other forms of addictive behaviors (e.g., substance addictions) [2]. The American Psychiatric Association, the World Health Organization (WHO), the American Society for Addiction Medicine, the International Society for Addiction Medicine, and the Canadian Society for Addiction Medicine have all acknowledged behavioral addictions, using somewhat similar clinical criteria. However, those disorders subsumed under the framework of behavioral addictions have often varied.

The commonalities found among all behavioral addictions include six core components: (a) salience (the activity becomes extremely important in the individual's life and dominates the person's thinking and behavior); (b) mood modification (this refers to the emotional impact that the behavior has upon the individual, with many individuals using the behavior as a form of psychological escape or as a means of arousal or avoidance of unpleasant events); (c) tolerance (the need to increase the time spent or the frequency of the behavior to achieve the desired mood modifications); (d) withdrawal (unpleasant symptoms when an individual reduces or stops the behavior); (e) conflict (interpersonal conflicts, conflicts with work, socialization, hobbies, or interests); and (f) relapse (the tendency to return to earlier patterns of excessive behavior after the original behavior has been stopped or periods of control) [3].

Although there is a growing body of neuroscience, neurobiological, and behavioral research supporting behavioral addictions, much of the current thinking relies upon using a biopsychosocial model to explain both the acquisition and maintenance of a wide number of behavioral disorders. In essence, to best understand the phenomenon, one must look at the interplay between a number of factors: biological (genetic predispositions impacting the brain), psychological (emotional, behavioral, and cognitive factors), and sociocultural influences (the influence of friends, peer group, family, importance of winning, and broader culture) [4, 5].

Elite Athletes Are Not Immune to a Wide Variety of Mental Health Symptoms and Disorders

Throughout this book, it is evident that elite athletes are not immune to a large number of mental health symptoms and disorders. In many cases, they are believed to be at an even higher risk compared to their peers. They train hard, are highly competitive, and have great athletic aspirations. Whether engaged in traditional sports or in newer virtual sports, the desire to be the best in one's sport is of paramount importance to an athlete. Within the "athletic world," there has always been an emphasis on physical fitness and mental well-being. This has never been more apparent as when

J. Derevensky (✉)
International Centre for Youth Gambling Problems and High Risk Behaviors, McGill University, Montreal, QC, Canada
e-mail: jeffrey.derevensky@mcgill.ca

Simone Biles, an Olympic icon gymnast with multiple Olympic gold medals and world championship titles, withdrew from several competitions in the 2021 Tokyo Olympics to address her mental health needs. Elite athletes are first and foremost individuals with the same frailties as others. They may train excessively, have inordinate pressures placed upon them (often self-imposed), which can result in a number of adverse consequences, and may only be active in their respective sport for a limited amount of time. When examining behavioral addictions associated with elite athletes, it is important to note that there are significant gender, age, and other cultural factors that impact the athlete.

Gambling Behaviors and Disordered Gambling Among Elite Athletes

The expansion of gambling internationally has been unprecedented during the past decade and continues to be one of the fastest growing industries worldwide. Alongside the growth of traditional forms of gambling (e.g., casinos, poker, horse racing, lottery, etc.), newer forms of gambling have emerged (e.g., local slot machine parlors, gambling via the Internet, mobile device wagering, sports wagering, e-sports gambling), and gambling has become a socially accepted recreational form of entertainment. In most jurisdictions, gambling is typically believed to be an adult activity, yet there is abundant international research suggesting that children and adolescents are actively participating in multiple forms of both regulated and unregulated gambling activities in spite of governmental age restrictions and prohibitions [6]. The age to gamble, in general, and the types of gambling permitted are often age-restricted and are dependent upon governmental regulations. Most recently, sports wagering (including propositional wagering – prop bets) and various forms of online wagering have been regulated in many US states, which has resulted in huge participation and revenues by gambling operators. Although the overall accessibility and availability have dramatically increased during the past decade, the prevalence rates of individuals with a gambling disorder have generally not risen among the general adult population. Typically, past-year self-reported prevalence rates of adults with gambling disorders generally range between 0.1% and 6%, with men reporting a higher incidence of problem gambling [7]. However, youth prevalence rates of problem gambling have been reported to be significantly higher, ranging from 0.2% to 12.3% in adolescents and young adults meeting the diagnostic criteria for problem/disordered gambling [8]. Variability in the rates of problem gambling has been attributable to accessibility and availability of multiple forms of gambling, instruments, and methodology used to assess gambling severity, cut-off scores on instruments, gender distributions, and time frames used

for assessing gambling problems. Nevertheless, it is important to note that irrespective of the study, youth problem gambling rates are typically higher than adult problem gambling rates. Still further, when looking at the prevalence of adult problem gambling, individuals aged 18–25 years report the highest prevalence of problem gambling. This is important to note as many elite athletes, depending upon their sport, fall in this age range where gambling problems seem to reach their peak and are the most pronounced.

Why Are Athletes Susceptible to Gambling and Gambling Disorders?

It is well acknowledged that a plethora of high-profile professional athletes, from all sports, have reportedly suffered from problematic gambling-related behaviors. Athletes including Pete Rose, Paul Horning, Art Schlichter, Rick Tocchet, Alex Rodriguez, Michael Jordan, Charles Barkley, John Daly, Wayne Rooney, and Evander Kane, along with a host of other international sports stars, have all had serious bouts of gambling-related problems. With significant fame and fortune, why would individuals risk losing everything? A number of reasons have been proposed as to why athletes tend to be more susceptible to gambling and gaming disorders. Curry and Jiobu [9] speculated that the socialization of athletes includes a continuous emphasis on competition, and this competitive nature has the potential to translate from the playing arena to the athletes' lives. As a result, gambling in its many forms provides the athlete with additional outlets in which they are able to compete. They suggest that athletes, like those who are dependent on alcohol or drugs, build a tolerance to the adrenaline rush associated with competition. This competitive approach may in fact be exacerbated when their professional careers hit a low or when faced with retirement. Given their knowledge of their particular sport, athletes may view gambling as a possible solution to financial difficulties. Yet, what we know is that in order to maintain the "high" associated with winning, they need to gamble for larger amounts of money and more frequently. This is especially true when their gambling losses mount (psychologists refer to this as "chasing behavior," a key characteristic of a gambling addiction). The continued losses typically result in more money gambled, guilt and shame complement financial losses, and there is a preoccupation with trying to regain control, ultimately ending in a cycle of escape, desperation, and hopelessness. The fact that gambling wagers can often be made anonymously via the Internet in many jurisdictions and gambling operators accept prop bets (where gamblers can bet on themselves) has plagued both collegiate and professional leagues who remain concerned about the integrity of the game. Younger collegiate athletes may also be susceptible to the potential to win money. It is also important to note that many athletes believe that their knowledge in one sport is generalizable to other sports and, as such, their gambling may well generalize across sporting events.

Prevalence of Gambling Problems/Disorders Among Athletes

Much of the available research comes from examination of the gambling behaviors of collegiate athletes. The National Collegiate Athletic Association (NCAA) in the United States has been monitoring gambling behaviors among college student athletes since 2004 in order to help meet the mental health demands of its students while simultaneously protecting the integrity of sporting events [10–15]. In a cross-sectional study, Richard et al. [16] looked at the gambling behaviors of four large samples of NCAA student athletes (2004, 2008, 2012, 2016). Across all the four cohorts, males consistently engaged in all forms of gambling activities more frequently than did female athletes (55% for males and 38% of females in the most recent study). While gambling participation rates decreased over the 12-year period and, in particular, problem gambling rates decreased for males (4% in 2004 and 1.8% in 2016), the prevalence rates are believed to be underestimated (players revealing a gambling problem are subject to losing their eligibility) and remain typically higher than those of their peers. Female problem/disordered gambling rates remained relatively the same (<1%) over the same time frame. The results from all four cohort studies confirm that collegiate student athletes typically start gambling for money before entering college. In spite of the NCAA regulations prohibiting gambling, there remains an appreciable number of college athletes experiencing a host of gambling-related problems. Håkansson et al. [17], using a much smaller Swedish sample of athletes engaged in a wide variety of sports, reported that 7% of athletes were identified as having gambling problems (14% of males; 1% of females). It should be noted that the NCAA studies have used a more detailed DSM screening measure than that used by Håkansson et al.'s study.

Although there remains some debate about whether or not fantasy sports wagering is a form of gambling, Marchica and Derevensky [14] reported that among collegiate student athletes, 48.1% of men and 25% of women who engaged in fantasy sports wagering could be identified as being at risk for a gambling disorder or have already met the clinical criteria for a gambling disorder.

In a study involving 1236 European professional athletes, Grall-Bronnec et al. [18] documented that 56.6% of athletes reported gambling at least once during the past year, with prevalence rates of problem gambling reaching 8.3%, and with betting on one's team, wagering online, and regular gambling being associated with gambling problems. Making bets on one's own team was specifically associated with past or current gambling problems. It should be noted that while legalized/government-related sports wagering in Europe has been available for many years, the introduction of prop bets is relatively new, thus affording athletes an ability to bet on themselves or against themselves. Weiss and Loubier [19], in comparing current, former, and nonathletes, reported that 13% of former athletes and 7% of current and professional athletes scored considerably higher on gambling severity screens and were more likely to be identified as problem gamblers compared to nonathletes. Professional and elite athletes were reported to be more likely to be engaged in gambling activities that were perceived to be "skill-based" forms of gambling (e.g., sports betting and poker) and were more likely to wager on the sport in which they participated.

Cultural and ethnic differences have also been found to impact one's gambling preferences [20]. A number of studies of nonathletes in the United States, Canada, and Australia [21–28] reported higher rates of disordered gambling among those identified as Native American [25, 28], Asian [22, 29], Black, and Hispanic [26] compared to Caucasian. While Nowak [30] reported that few studies have examined the ethnic and cultural differences among minority groups, those groups tend to have higher prevalence rates of problem gambling.

Understanding the Impacts of Disordered/Problem Gambling

While the vast majority of individuals gamble in a responsible, safe manner (setting and maintaining the amounts wagered and the frequency of gambling), disordered gamblers typically experience multiple negative outcomes, including risky behaviors, underperformance in athletic events, financial and social difficulties, and a host of concomitant mental health disorders. Problems associated with a gambling disorder are generally accompanied by decreased academic performance, difficulties in social relationships, depression, anxiety, feelings of hopelessness, heightened risk of suicide ideation and attempts, and substance use disorders [15, 31–40]. For an athlete, a gambling disorder becomes pervasive, interfering in all aspects, including athletic performance, of the individual's life.

Assessing for Disordered/Problem Gambling

Numerous screening instruments are used to assess both youth and adult problem gambling. It is important to note that these screens do not directly assess the amounts of money being wagered, as individual financial means differ dramatically. Rather, these gambling screens focus on gambling behaviors and their consequences. The DSM-5 (American Psychiatric Association) categorizes a gambling disorder as a Non-Substance-Related Disorder within the Substance-Related and Addictive Disorders section. Individuals meeting the diagnostic criteria are marked by a persistent and recurrent problematic gambling behavior, which leads to clinically significant impairment or distress, and endorse four or more of the following criteria in a 12-month period:

1. Needs to gamble with increasing amounts of money in order to achieve the same level of excitement and enjoyment
2. Is restless or irritable when attempting to cut down or stop gambling
3. Has made repeated unsuccessful efforts to control, cut back, or stop gambling
4. Is often preoccupied with gambling (e.g., having persistent thoughts of reliving past gambling experiences, handicapping or planning the next gambling venture, thinking of ways in which to get money to gamble)
5. Often gambles when feeling distressed (e.g., helpless, guilty, anxious, depressed)
6. After losing money gambling, often returns another day to get even (chasing one's losses)
7. Lies to conceal the extent of gambling involvement
8. Has jeopardized or lost a significant relation, job, or educational or career opportunity because of gambling
9. Relies on others to provide money to relieve desperate financial situations caused by gambling

A number of other clinical scales have been used for both adults and youth [6, 41]. Given these general diagnostic criteria, it is easy to see how applicable they would be for elite athletes.

Helping Athletes with a Gambling Problem/ Disorder

There currently exist no best practice guidelines for helping individuals with a severe gambling problem. Given that the gambling problem is often accompanied by other mental health problems and disorders, it is often recommended that comprehensive and expanded screening be used. Merely treating the gambling problem may mask some of the other underlying causes precipitating the gambling. The NCAA studies continue to reveal that athletic coaches and directors remain in a unique position to help deliver prevention programs and assist athletes with a gambling problem. In the

2016 survey among almost 20,000 NCAA college athletes, the three most effective ways to reduce problem gambling were to have coaches intervene, the use of imposed penalties, and discussions with teammates [42]. Accommodations for athletes to attend treatment facilities (as are often provided for substance use disorders) are warranted [15].

Mental health professionals treating individuals with a gambling disorder have employed a wide range of approaches: psychopharmacology, cognitive behavioral therapy (CBT), cognitive therapy, brief motivational interviewing, and the use of self-help groups (e.g., Gamblers Anonymous) [5, 6, 15]. The good news is that many individuals recover from a gambling disorder.

Gaming Disorders Among Elite Athletes

A gaming disorder (GD) has become an officially recognized mental health disorder by the World Health Organization (WHO) (International Classification of Diseases 11th Revision) [43], while being classified as a condition requiring further study prior to its formal inclusion in the DSM-5 (American Psychiatric Association) [1]. A GD is conceptualized to be a behavioral disorder and is broadly defined as a pattern of recurrent or persistent video gaming behavior over a period of at least 12 months. It is characterized by impaired control over gaming, increasing precedence of gaming over other life interests or activities, and a continuation or escalation of gaming despite negative consequences, psychological distress, or functional impairments [43]. Although individuals of all ages have been found to play video games, both online and via consoles, higher rates of GDs have been reported among children and adolescents compared to adults [44]. It is important to note that the gambling industry often refers to themselves as gaming to avoid any negative stigma associated with gambling. These two industries are different, yet there seems to be a migration of participants between the gaming and gambling industries.

Prevalence and Consequences of Gaming Disorders

Systematic reviews investigating the global prevalence rates of GDs have identified rates ranging from 1.0% to 19.9% among children and adolescents [45], with meta-analytic studies indicating pooled prevalence rates of approximately 4.6% [46]. Moreover, similar to gambling problems, males have been found to report greater rates of GDs compared to females [45, 46], with male adolescents being approximately four times more likely than females to report disordered gaming [46]. Comparing the prevalence rates across continents, Fam [46] identified that the rates of GDs among youth tend to be the highest in Asia (9.9%), followed by North America (9.4%), Australia (4.4%), and Europe (4.2%).

The study of problem gambling and GDs among elite athletes has been relatively sparse. The fact that elite athletes are engaged in gaming should not come as a great surprise given that many of the more popular games are sports-oriented (e.g., FIFA 22, NBA 2K22, Madden NFL 22, 18 Holes, Soccertastic, Superstar Football, etc.) The one study that directly addressed this issue reported that the general prevalence rates of problem gaming among elite athletes were comparable to the general population data, albeit on the lower end (2%) [17]. Although Håkansson et al.'s [17] findings suggest a relatively low prevalence rate for GDs among their elite athletes, they nevertheless concluded that there was a link between problematic video gaming and problem gaming for money. Finally, there is a growing body of evidence suggesting an association between gaming and general physical health including sleep and fatigue-related problems, a higher body mass index, and lower self-reported general health [47]. That said, it is important to note that the vast majority of individuals play games in a responsible manner with few gaming-related harms.

e-Sports Gaming

Electronic sports, or e-sports, refer to organized, competitive forms of video games that can be played individually or in a team. Such competitions are typically viewed by spectators either in person or via online streaming [48]. Advances in digital technologies have resulted in an exponential worldwide increase in the accessibility, engagement, and popularity of e-sports. Competitions have dramatically increased worldwide, with professional e-sports players having taken on the status of elite athletes, receiving high incomes through prize monies, sponsorship, and celebrity endorsements [49]. Professional e-sports players have been likened to athletes; they train, sweat, have aspirations of becoming world champion players, and strive to get into the Olympics (the International Olympic Committee is seriously considering making e-sports an Olympic event). Billionaires and gambling operators have invested heavily in e-sports organizations, with gambling operators building e-sports centers adjacent to their casinos and a growing number of colleges building e-sports arenas on their campuses. Not surprisingly, there are a growing number of studies suggesting that individuals wagering on e-sports tend to be younger, are more likely to be male, report wagering on a greater number of activities, regularly play video games, and are more frequently e-sports spectators [50, 51].

Consequences Associated with a Gaming Disorder

Individuals with a GD are reported to have increased difficulties with peers, poor parental relationships, academic difficulties, lower life satisfaction, greater levels of aggression, loneliness, depression, and anxiety [52]. Individuals with a GD have also been noted as having a significant health burden. It should be noted that youth that report gaming for excessive periods of time or exhibit greater symptoms of a GD have been found to report sleep difficulties (i.e., sleep deprivation, day–night reversal), dietary problems (i.e., malnutrition, dehydration), poorer general health, and increases in sedentary behavior [47, 53]. Not surprisingly, individuals with a GD are more likely to engage in novel forms of online gambling [54], with a number of studies noting the co-occurrence of problem video game playing and problem gambling [55]. Game developers are increasingly introducing gambling-like elements into video games [56], most often in the form of "loot boxes," which offer the player a chance to obtain rare items or in-game currency. Among a sample of 1348 adolescents, Marchica et al. [57] found that approximately 20% had wagered on e-sports during the past year. Wagering on e-sports was positively associated with gambling in general, problem gambling, and GD, as well as a number of externalizing behaviors. For athletes, gaming may represent a respite from the pressures associated with athletic competitions (sports games are among the most popular forms of gaming). It also may represent an alternative form of recreation, ultimately becoming a preoccupation, for injured athletes. There is new empirical evidence suggesting that athletes with a concussion would be best advised to reduce their screen time following their concussion. Macnow et al. [58], in a randomized controlled study, found that individuals with a concussion who engaged in screen time were less likely to recover quickly than were those who eliminated screen time. Interestingly, professional athletes like NBA star Kevin Durant turned to e-sports during the coronavirus lockdown of sporting events to play the NBA 2K20 video game on ESPN as a way of raising funds for charity [59], with other professional athletes investing in e-sports teams [60]. Cam Adair, who operates a website called GameQuitters. com, points to a number of elite international athletes with a gaming disorder [61].

Assessing for a Gaming Disorder

Due to the disproportional impact of GDs on youth, various measurement tools have been developed to assess for problem or disordered gaming. With regard to self-report measures, the most commonly utilized measurement tools include (a) the Game Addiction Scale [62], (b) the Pathological Gaming Scale [63], and (c) the Internet Gaming Disorder Scale—Short Form 9 [64]. These measures are typically derived from measures for gambling disorders. The items assess the severity of GD symptomatology over the past 6–12 months, with items including levels of (1) a preoccupation with gaming, (2) tolerance (i.e., the need for increasing amounts of time dedicated to gaming), (3) withdrawal symptoms when gaming is stopped, (4) loss of interest in activities other than gaming, (5) relapse/repeated unsuccessful attempts to stop gaming, (6) use of gaming for mood modification, (7) interpersonal conflicts, (8) lying/deception about gaming, and (9) jeopardizing academic/occupational success.

Helping Athletes with a Gaming Problem/Disorder

Similar to helping elite athletes with a gambling problem, there are currently no best practices developed for helping athletes with a gaming disorder. Examining other concomitant mental health issues that need to be addressed would represent a good beginning [65]. For some, gaming may be an alternative to grueling practices and training. For others, it may be a relief from boredom, and, for others, it may be one more form of competition, capitalizing on their competitive nature. Programs targeting emotional awareness and emotion regulation, self-care, and developing effective coping strategies may be useful [66]. Public health efforts and awareness campaigns differentiating healthy, recreational, or social gaming from problematic or disordered gaming will also be essential to develop greater societal awareness of this problem while not pathologizing all video game playing. For athletes unable to exhibit self-control, the use of self-blocking options (e.g., self-limiting time or night access), personalized feedback/alerts, and peer monitoring strategies can be helpful in reducing the consequences of problematic use. Other treatment strategies incorporate cognitive behavioral therapy (CBT), motivational interviewing, and mindfulness-based cognitive therapy [67]. Although a number of clinical studies have investigated the usefulness of pharmacological interventions for GDs, evidence as to their efficacy is limited.

Conclusions

Athletes appear to be particularly susceptible to a wide variety of mental health and behavioral addictions. While this chapter has only addressed gambling and gaming problems, because of the overrepresentation of young males, their high level of competitiveness, enhanced sensation-seeking behaviors, impulsivity, and increased risk-taking behaviors, there is little doubt that they may be more susceptible to engaging in these behaviors. With respect to gambling, the ability to wager online in isolation, the ability to try to alter the outcome of the game, and their knowledge of their sport may be contributing factors. Coaching staff and directors of athletics can play an important role in helping athletes with both gambling and gaming problems. Finally, although there is some preliminary research examining behavioral addictions among elite athletes, more research is necessary. Helping athletes overcome their mental health and behavioral difficulties needs to be prioritized.

References

1. American Psychiatric Association. Diagnostic and statistical manual of mental disorders (DSM–5): American Psychiatric Association; 2013.
2. Grant J, Potenza M, Weinstein A, Gorelick D. Introduction to behavioral addictions. Am J Drug Alcohol Abuse. 2010;36(5):233–41.
3. Griffiths M. A 'components' model of addiction within a biopsychosocial framework. J Subst Use. 2005;10(4):191–7.
4. Rosenberg K, Feder L. An introduction to behavioral addictions. In: Rosenberg K, Feder L, editors. Behavioral addictions: criteria, evidence, and treatment. London: Elsevier; 2014.
5. Derevensky J, Gilbeau L. Understanding youth gambling problems: prevention and treatment strategies. In: Grant J, Potenza M, editors. Pathological gambling: a clinical guide to treatment. 2nd ed. Washington, DC: American Psychiatric Association Publishing; 2021.
6. Derevensky J. Teen gambling: understanding a growing epidemic. New York: Rowman & Littlefield Publishers; 2012.
7. Calado F, Griffiths M. Problem gambling worldwide: an update and systematic review of empirical research (2000–2015). J Behav Addict. 2016;5(4):592–613.
8. Calado F, Alexandre J, Griffiths M. Prevalence of adolescent problem gambling: a systematic review of recent research. J Gambl Stud. 2017;33:397–424.
9. Curry T, Jiobu R. Do motives matter? Modeling gambling on sports among athletes. Sociol Sport J. 1995;12(1):21–35.
10. Ellenbogen S, Jacobs D, Derevensky J, Gupta R, Paskus T. Gambling behavior among college student-athletes. J Appl Sport Psychol. 2008;20(3):349–62.
11. Huang J, Jacobs D, Derevensky J. Sexual risk-taking behaviors, gambling, and heavy drinking among U.S. college athletes. Arch Sex Behav. 2010;39(3):706–13.
12. Huang J, Jacobs D, Derevensky J. DSM-based problem gambling: increasing the odds of heavy drinking in a national sample of U.S. college athletes. J Psych Res. 2011;45(3):302–8.
13. Huang J, Jacobs D, Derevensky J, Gupta R, Paskus T. Gambling and health risk behaviors among U.S. college student-athletes: findings from a national study. J Adol Health. 2007;40(5):390–7.
14. Marchica L, Derevensky J. Fantasy sports: a growing concern among college student-athletes. Int J Mentl Health Addict. 2016;14(5):635–45.
15. Derevensky J, McDuff D, Reardon C, Hainline B, Hitchcock M, Richard J. Problem gambling and associated mental health concerns in elite athletes: a narrative review. Br J Sports Med. 2019;53(12):761–6.

16. Richard J, Paskus T, Derevensky J. Trends in gambling behavior among college student-athletes: a comparison of 2004, 2008, 2012 and 2016 NCAA survey data. J Gambl Issues. 2019;41:73–100.

17. Håkansson A, Kenttä G, Åkesdotter C. Problem gambling and gaming in elite athletes. Addict Behav Rep. 2018;8:79–84.

18. Grall-Bronnec M, Caillon J, Humeau E, Perrot B, Remaud M, Guilleux A, et al. Gambling among European professional athletes: prevalence and associated factors. J Addict Dis. 2016;35(4):278–90.

19. Weiss S, Loubier S. Gambling behaviors of former athletes: the delayed competitive effect. UNLV Gam Res Rev. 2008;12(1):53–60.

20. Okuda M, Liu W, Cisewski J, Segura L, Storr C, Martins S. Gambling disorder and minority populations: prevalence and risk factors. Curr Addict Rep. 2016;3(3):280–92.

21. Alegría A, Petry N, Hasin D, Liu S, Grant B, Blanco C. Disordered gambling among racial and ethnic groups in the US: results from the National Epidemiologic Survey on Alcohol and Related Conditions. CNS Spectr. 2009;14(3):132–43.

22. Blaszczynski A, Huynh S, Dumlao V, Farrell E. Problem gambling within a Chinese speaking community. J Gambl Stud. 1998;14(4):359–80.

23. Petry N. A comparison of treatment-seeking pathological gamblers based on preferred gambling activity. Addiction. 2003;98(5):645–55.

24. Shaffer H, Hall M, Vander Bilt J. Estimating the prevalence of disordered gambling behavior in the United States and Canada: a research synthesis. Am J Public Health. 1999;89(9):1369–76.

25. Volberg R, Abbott M. Gambling and problem gambling among indigenous peoples. Subst Use Misuse. 1997;32(11):1525–38.

26. Welte J, Barnes G, Wieczorek W, Tidwell M, Parker J. Alcohol and gambling pathology among U.S. adults: prevalence, demographic patterns and comorbidity. J Stud Alcohol. 2001;62(5):706–12.

27. Westermeyer J, Canive J, Garrard J, Thuras P, Thompson J. Lifetime prevalence of pathological gambling among American Indian and Hispanic American veterans. Am J Public Health. 2005;95(5):860–6.

28. Zitzow D. Comparative study of problematic gambling behaviors between American Indian and non-Indian adolescents within and near a Northern Plains reservation. Am Indian Alsk Native Ment Health Res. 1996;7(2):14–26.

29. Rinker D, Rodriguez L, Krieger H, Tackett J, Neighbors C. Racial and ethnic differences in problem gambling among college students. J Gambl Stud. 2016;32(2):581–90.

30. Nowak D. College student-athlete gambling disorder: a review of research (1991-2017). J Psychiatr Ment Health. 2017;1:1–7.

31. Lorains F, Cowlishaw S, Thomas S. Prevalence of comorbid disorders in problem and pathological gambling: systematic review and meta-analysis of population surveys. Addiction. 2011;106(3):490–8.

32. Barnes G, Welte J, Tidwell M, Hoffman J. Gambling and substance use: co-occurrence among adults in a recent general population study in the United States. Int Gambl Stud. 2015;15(1):55–71.

33. Dowling N, Cowlishaw S, Jackson A, Merkouris S, Francis K, Christensen D. Prevalence of psychiatric co-morbidity in treatment-seeking problem gamblers: a systematic review and meta-analysis. Aust N Z J Psychiatry. 2015;49(6):519–39.

34. Bischof A, Meyer C, Bischof G, John U, Wurst F, Thon N, et al. Suicidal events among pathological gamblers: the role of comorbidity of axis I and axis II disorders. Psychiatry Res. 2015;225(3):413–9.

35. Black D, Coryell W, Crowe R, McCormick B, Shaw M, Allen J. Suicide ideations, suicide attempts, and completed suicide in persons with pathological gambling and their first-degree relatives. Suicide Life Threat Behav. 2015;45(6):700–9.

36. Stinchfield R, Hanson W, Olson D. Problem and pathological gambling among college students. New Dir Stud Serv. 2006;113:63–72.

37. Martin R, Usdan S, Cremeens J, Vail-Smith K. Disordered gambling and co-morbidity of psychiatric disorders among college students: an examination of problem drinking, anxiety and depression. J Gambl Stud. 2014;30(2):321–33.

38. Quigley L, Yakovenko I, Hodgins D, Dobson K, el-Guebaly N, Casey D, et al. Comorbid problem gambling and major depression in a community sample. J Gambl Stud. 2015;31(4):1135–52.

39. Brezing C, Derevensky J, Potenza M. Non–substance-addictive behaviors in youth: pathological gambling and problematic internet use. Child Adolesc Psychiatr Clin N Am. 2010;19(3):625–41.

40. Neighbors C, Rodriguez L, Rinker D, Gonzales R, Agana M, Tackett J, et al. Efficacy of personalized normative feedback as a brief intervention for college student gambling: a randomized controlled trial. J Consult Clin Psychol. 2015;83(3):500–11.

41. Stinchfield R. A review of problem gambling assessment instruments and brief screens. In: Richard D, Blaszczynski A, Nower L, editors. The Wiley-Blackwell handbook of disordered gambling. New York: Wiley Blackwell; 2013. p. 165–203.

42. Derevensky J, Gilbeau L. Preventing adolescent gambling problems. In: Heinz A, Romanczuk-Seiferth N, Potenza M, editors. Gambling disorder. Berlin: Springer International; 2019. p. 297–311.

43. World Health Organization. International classification of diseases 11th revision-ICD 11. World Health Organization; 2018.

44. Feng W, Ramo D, Chan S, Bourgeois J. Internet gaming disorder: Trends in prevalence 1998-2016. Addict Behav. 2017;75:17–24.

45. Stevens M, Dorstyn D, Delfabbro P, King D. Global prevalence of gaming disorder: a systematic review and meta-analysis. Aust N Z J Psychiatry. 2020;55(6):553–68.

46. Fam J. Prevalence of internet gaming disorder in adolescents: a meta-analysis across three decades. Scand J Psychol. 2018;59(5):524–31.

47. Huard Pelletier V, Lessard A, Piché F, Tétreau C, Descarreaux M. Video games and their associations with physical health: a scoping review. BMJ Open Sport Exerc Med. 2020;6(1):1–10.

48. Hamari J, Sjöblom M. What is eSports and why do people watch it? Int Res. 2017;27(2):211–32.

49. Funk D, Pizzo A, Baker B. eSport management: embracing eSport education and research opportunities. Sport Manag Rev. 2018;21(1):7–13.

50. Abarbanel B, Macey J, Hamari J, Melton R. Gamers who gamble: examining the relationship between eSports spectatorship and event wagering. J Emerg Sport Stud. 2020;3:1–23.

51. Macey J, Abarbanel B, Hamari J. What predicts eSports betting? A study on consumption of video games, eSports, gambling and demographic factors. New Media Soc. 2020;23(6):1481–505.

52. Richard J, Temcheff C, Derevensky J. Gaming disorder across the lifespan: a scoping review of longitudinal studies. Curr Addict Rep. 2020;7:1–27.

53. Saunders J, Hao W, Long J, King D, Mann K, Fauth-Bühler M, et al. Gaming disorder: its delineation as an important condition for diagnosis, management, and prevention. J Behav Addict. 2017;6(3):271–9.

54. Emond A, Griffiths M. Gambling in children and adolescents. Br Med Bull. 2020;136(1):21–9.

55. Derevensky J. Behavioral addictions: some developmental considerations. Curr Addict Rep. 2019;3(3):313–22.

56. Abarbanel B. Gambling vs. gaming: a commentary on the role of regulatory, industry, and community stakeholders in the loot box debate. Gaming Law Rev. 2018;22(4):231–4.

57. Marchica L, Richard J, Mills D, Ivoska W, Derevensky J. Between two worlds: exploring eSports betting in relation to problem gambling, gaming, and mental health problems. J Behav Addict. 2021;10(3):447–55.

58. Macnow T, Curran T, Tolliday C, Martin K, McCarthy M, Ayturk D, et al. Effect of screen time on recovery from concussion: a randomized clinical trial. JAMA Pediatr. 2021:1–8.

59. Russo D. 'Play ball!': Pro athletes like NBA star Kevin Durant turning to esports during coronavirus 2020. https://www.cnbc.com/2020/04/03/pro-athletes-turn-to-esports-to-stay-active-during-coronavirus.html.

60. Sayeed A. E-sports: top professional athletes who are involved in e-sports 2020. https://www.insidesport.co/esports-top-professional-athletes-who-are-involved-in-esports/.

61. Game Quitters. Are professional athletes addicted to video games? 2021. https://gamequitters.com/are-professional-athletes-addicted-to-video-games/.

62. Lemmens J, Valkenburg P, Gentile D. The internet gaming disorder scale. Psychol Assess. 2015;27(2):567–82.

63. Gentile D. Pathological video-game use among youth ages 8 to 18: a national study. Psychol Sci. 2009;20(5):594–602.

64. Pontes H, Griffiths M. Measuring DSM-5 internet gaming disorder: development and validation of a short psychometric scale. Comput Hum Behav. 2015;45:137–43.

65. González-Bueso V, Santamaría J, Fernández D, Merino L, Montero E, Ribas J. Association between internet gaming disorder or pathological video-game use and comorbid psychopathology: a comprehensive review. Int J Environ Res Public Health. 2018;15(4):668–88.

66. Greenberg M, Abenavoli R. Universal interventions: fully exploring their impacts and potential to produce population-level impacts. J Res Educ Eff. 2017;10(1):40–67.

67. King D, Delfabbro P, Wu A, Doh Y, Kuss D, Pallesen S, et al. Treatment of internet gaming disorder: an international systematic review and CONSORT evaluation. Clin Psychol Rev. 2017;54:123–33.

Athlete Mental Health Impacts of Harassment and Abuse in Sport

M. Mountjoy and C. Edwards

Introduction

As it turns out ... Dr Nassar was not a doctor, he in fact is, was, and forever shall be a child molester and a monster of a human being. End of story. He abused my trust; he abused my body and he left scars on my psyche that may never go away.
McKayla Maroney, Olympic Gold Medal Gymnast, London 2012 [1]

Sexual and psychological abuse in sport can profoundly impact the mental health of its victims, as described by the 2012 Olympic gold medalist McKayla Maroney in her victim impact statement at the criminal trial of the perpetrator of her abuse, Dr. Larry Nassar [1]. The impacts on the mental health of survivors can be devastating and long-lasting [2–4]. Reported mental health sequelae of sexual abuse within the sporting context include psychosomatic illnesses, eating disorders, substance misuse [5], and in adult survivors of abuse in sport, a reduction in self-reported quality of life as well as psychological distress [6]. Long-term post-traumatic stress disorder and dissociative symptoms in athletes are correlated with childhood psychological abuse in sport [3]. A study by Gervis and Dunn (2005) [7] identified other mental health sequelae from harassment and abuse in sport including substance use disorders, depression, anxiety, poor academic performance, loss of self-esteem, distorted body image, eating disorders, self-harm, and suicide.

Simone Biles (USA), during the summer Olympic Games in Tokyo 2021, withdrew from the gymnastics team event, citing the need to address her mental health [8]. As a survivor of sexual abuse from her former team physician, Dr. Larry Nasser, it became evident through the attention that Simone's revelation garnered from the media that sport needs to address harassment and abuse in sport to prevent mental health sequelae in athletes.

The International Olympic Committee (IOC) published a consensus statement on harassment and abuse in sport in 2016 [9]. In this document, the IOC consensus authors introduced a conceptual model that outlines the cultural context, the types of harassment and abuse, the mechanisms by which they are expressed in the sports environment, and the impacts of harassment and abuse on both the athletes and sports organizations (Fig. 16.1). In this model, mental health symptoms and disorders are suggested as potential indicative outcomes for athletes who have experienced harassment and abuse in sport.

Underpinning Statutory Documents Supporting Safe Sport

Many of the underpinning documents emphasizing the rights of individuals to an environment free from harassment and abuse are grounded in the United Nations Convention on the Rights of the Child (1989), specifically in articles 19 and 31 [10].

Article 19

1. *States Parties shall take all appropriate legislative, administrative, social and educational measures to protect the child from all forms of physical or mental violence, injury or abuse, neglect or negligent treatment, maltreatment or exploitation, including sexual abuse, while in the care of parent(s), legal guardian(s) or any other person who has the care of the child.*

Article 31

1. *States Parties recognize the right of the child to rest and leisure, to engage in play and recreational activities appropriate to the age of the child and to participate freely in cultural life and the arts.*

M. Mountjoy (✉)
Department of Family Medicine, McMaster University,
Kitchener, ON, Canada
e-mail: mmsportdoc@mcmaster.ca

C. Edwards
Department of Psychiatry, McMaster University,
Kitchener, ON, Canada
e-mail: edwardcd@mcmaster.ca

C. L. Reardon (ed.), *Mental Health Care for Elite Athletes*, https://doi.org/10.1007/978-3-031-08364-8_16

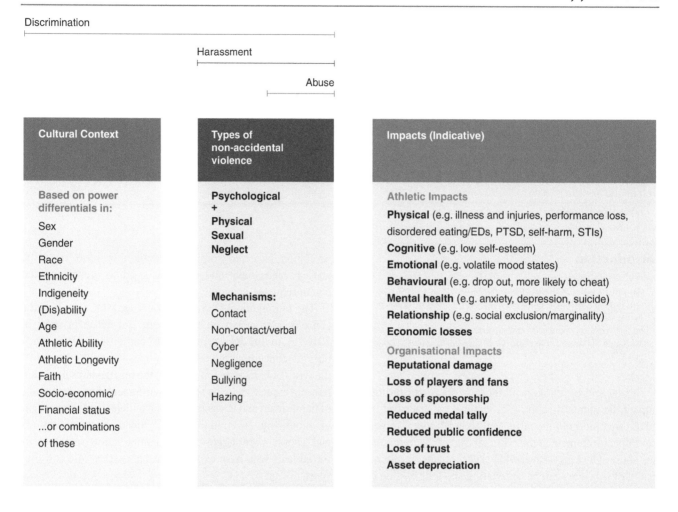

Discrimination

Harassment

Abuse

Cultural Context	Types of non-accidental violence	Impacts (Indicative)
Based on power differentials in: Sex Gender Race Ethnicity Indigeneity (Dis)ability Age Athletic Ability Athletic Longevity Faith Socio-economic/ Financial status ...or combinations of these	Psychological + Physical Sexual Neglect Mechanisms: Contact Non-contact/verbal Cyber Negligence Bullying Hazing	Athletic Impacts Physical (e.g. illness and injuries, performance loss, disordered eating/EDs, PTSD, self-harm, STIs) Cognitive (e.g. low self-esteem) Emotional (e.g. volatile mood states) Behavioural (e.g. drop out, more likely to cheat) Mental health (e.g. anxiety, depression, suicide) Relationship (e.g. social exclusion/marginality) Economic losses Organisational Impacts Reputational damage Loss of players and fans Loss of sponsorship Reduced medal tally Reduced public confidence Loss of trust Asset depreciation

Further details and examples of what can constitute harassment and abuse can be found in tha IOC Consensus Statement: Harassment and Abuse in Sport (2016).

Fig. 16.1 IOC conceptual model of harassment and abuse in sport [9]

Although this document is not sport-specific, it identifies the rights of children to be protected from harassment and abuse in all aspects of life, including recreational activities. The first publication demonstrating the importance of upholding human rights to prevent discrimination and violence in sport was published in 1998 [11] and 2004 [12] by Paolo David, the former secretary of the Committee on the Rights of the Child in the United Nations (UN) Office of the High Commission. The IOC published its first consensus statement on sexual harassment and abuse in sport in 2007 [13]. This seminal document highlighted the existing science in the field as well as identified prevention strategies and recommendations for sports organizations [13]. Another fundamental document was published by the United Nations Children's Fund (UNICEF) in 2010 [14], which reported the lack of child protection policies against harassment and abuse in sport from 119 countries surveyed, despite the pre-vious call to action in the 2006 publication of the UN World Report on Violence against Children [15].

In 2015, the IOC published a consensus statement on Youth Athlete Development, which underscored the importance of safeguarding this vulnerable population, and identified the concepts of medical mismanagement, abusive hazing rituals, and age-inappropriate training regimens [16]. Accompanying this publication was a supportive review paper that categorized the various forms of harassment and abuse threatening child athletes as being individual, relational, or organizational [17]. This document also outlined the principles of safeguarding the child athlete in sport and introduced a framework to facilitate the implementation of athlete safeguarding policies.

A second, more comprehensive IOC consensus statement was published in 2016, which extended the focus beyond sexual harassment and abuse to other forms including psychological, physical, and neglect. In addition to the conceptual model introduced above, athletes with particular vulnerability were identified, and the impacts of harassment and abuse on both athletes and sports organizations were discussed [9]. In addition, in 2016, the IOC implemented its first Games-Time Safeguarding Framework to safeguard athletes and other participants from harassment and abuse in sport during the Olympic Games in Rio de Janeiro, 2016 [18]. This Framework has been implemented at all subsequent editions of the Summer and Winter Olympic Games as well as the Youth Olympic Games [19].

The 2017 Kazan Action Plan is a consensus-based framework aimed at strengthening the connections between the United Nations' Sustainable Development Goals (SDGs) and sport policy developed by the United Nations Educational, Scientific and Cultural Organization (UNESCO) in consultation with the Intergovernmental Committee for Physical Education and Sport (CIGEPS) and more than 100 experts from the United Nations, sports organizations, academia, and nongovernmental organizations. The third action point addresses the integrity of sport and links safeguarding athletes to the Sustainable Development Goal (SDG) 16.2:

...the fundamental human rights of everyone affected by or involved in the delivery of physical education, physical activity and sport must be protected, respected and fulfilled in accordance with the United Nations Guiding Principles on Business and Human Rights.

The third action point also addresses the need to protect children, youth, and other vulnerable groups in sport (SDGs 5.2, 8.7, and 16.2, respectively) [20].

In addition, in 2017, the World Players Association, in collaboration with the Centre for Sport and Human Rights, developed a Universal Declaration of Player Rights. Right #3 states that all sport players have the right to participate in a sporting environment that is free from discrimination:

ENTITLED to equality of opportunity in the pursuit of sport without distinction of any kind and free of discrimination, harassment, and violence. A player's right to pursue sport cannot be limited because of his or her race, colour, birth, age, language, sexual orientation, gender, disability, pregnancy, religion, political or other opinion, responsibilities as a carer, property, or other status [21].

In 2018, the Children's Rights in Sport Principles was developed by the Japan Committee for UNICEF. This document was written to further develop the understanding of the child's rights and safeguarding within the sport context and purports 10 Sport Principles, four of which directly address safeguarding of children in sport:

- Principle (1) Commit to support the rights of children through non-discrimination (1c), and protection of children from all forms of violence (1d)

- Principle (3) Protection of children from violence and abuse in sport (3a), and protection of children from all forms of exploitation (3e)
- Principle (4) Protection of the physical and mental health of children (4a)
- Principle (5) Protection of the rights of children in sport through good governance encouraging the development of policies, procedures, guidelines, codes of conduct and reporting mechanisms (5a–e) [22]

A more recent IOC consensus statement that has directly linked athlete mental health to harassment and abuse in sport is the IOC consensus statement on the mental health of elite athletes (2019). Although this document largely focuses on the prevalence, diagnosis, and treatment of mental health disorders in elite athletes, it also identifies the intersection of harassment and abuse with adverse mental health outcomes [23]. For details on more underpinning IOC statutory documents related to safeguarding athletes in sport, please see Table 16.1.

Table 16.1 Underpinning statutes of the International Olympic Committee that serve to encourage the development and implementation of safeguarding initiatives, thereby promoting safe sport

Olympic Charter [24]	2.18 The mission of the IOC is to promote Olympism throughout the world and to lead the Olympic Movement. The IOC's role is … to promote safe sport and the protection of athletes from all forms of harassment and abuse
IOC Code of Ethics [25]	Article 1.4: Respect for international conventions on protecting human rights insofar as they apply to the Olympic games' activities, and which ensure in particular: • Rejection of discrimination of any kind on whatever grounds, be it race, colour, sex, sexual orientation, language, religion, political or other opinion, national or social origin, property, birth or other status • Rejection of all forms of harassment and abuse, be it physical, professional, or sexual, and any physical or mental injuries
Olympic Agenda 2020 + 5 [26]	Recommendation #3: Reinforce athletes' rights and responsibilities Recommendation #5: Further strengthen safe sport and the protection of clean athletes
Athletes' Declaration [27]	This declaration aspires to promote the ability and opportunity of athletes: 7. The protection of mental and physical health, including a safe competition and training environment and protection from abuse and harassment

(continued)

Table 16.1 (continued)

Recommendations for an IOC Human Rights Strategy [28]	IOC Human Rights Strategy over a 5-year timeline: • Deepen approach on prevention of harassment and abuse in sport (PHAS)
Basic Universal Principles of Good Governance of the Olympic and Sports Movement [29]	6.2 Protection of athletes It is the responsibility of each National Olympic Committee (NOC) to establish and govern safeguarding policies and to implement procedures and mechanisms to ensure a safe and supportive environment for athletes to practise their sport in the best conditions
Olympic Movement Medical Code [30]	1.1.1 Athletes enjoy the same fundamental rights as all patients in their relationships with physicians and health care providers, in particular, respect for: (a) Their human dignity (b) Their physical and psychological well-being (c) The protection of their health and safety
IOC Consensus Statements [13] [16] [9] [23]	2007 IOC Consensus Statement on sexual harassment and abuse in sport 2015 IOC Consensus Statement on youth athlete development 2016 IOC Consensus Statement on harassment and abuse (non-accidental violence) in sport 2019 IOC Consensus Statement on mental health in elite athletes
Safeguarding Frameworks for the Olympic Games and Youth Olympic Games [18, 19]	IOC Games-Time framework for safeguarding athletes and other participants from harassment and abuse in sport
Safeguarding athletes from harassment and abuse in sport: IOC Toolkit for IFs and NOCs [31]	A resource for International Federations and National Olympic Committees related to creating and implementing athlete safeguarding policies and procedures
IOC Certificate: Safeguarding Officer in Sport [32]	An online educational certificate program to equip those involved with safeguarding athletes of all ages from harassment and abuse in sport with knowledge, skills, and confidence
Athlete 365 Safe Sport for All [33]	Speak Up Reporting tool Safeguarding Officer contact information Consent in sport educational video IOC Athlete Safeguarding Course Sexual harassment and abuse in sport e-learning tool IOC safe sport webinar series for NOCs IOC athlete safeguarding webinar series for International Federations Athlete stories
IOC Safe Sport for Athletes Action Plan [34]	Action plan to strengthen safe sport/ safeguarding across the Olympic Movement to protect the physical and mental well-being of athletes
IOC Framework on Fairness, Inclusion and Non-Discrimination on the Basis of Gender Identity and Sex Variations [35]	1.4 Mechanisms to prevent harassment and abuse in sport should be further developed by taking into account the particular needs and vulnerabilities of transgender people and people with sex variations

Figure 16.2 outlines a timeline of pivotal global documents on the prevention of harassment and abuse in sport.

Science Base of Harassment and Abuse in Sport

Prevalence

The prevalence of harassment and abuse in sport is difficult to quantify in elite sport due to significant underreporting [6]; however, it is believed that it occurs at all levels of sport and in all sports [36–38]. There have been several studies published on the prevalence of sexual abuse in sport. One of the first prevalence studies conducted in Canadian elite athletes revealed that 1.9% of athletes under the age of 16 years reported sexual abuse [12]. A study conducted by Brackenridge et al. (2002) [39] identified a prevalence rate of 2–49% of sexual abuse in sport. A retrospective survey of elite Australian athletes identified a sexual abuse prevalence rate of 9.7% prior to the age of 18 years [11], and a large UK study of more than 60,000 youth athletes showed a prevalence rate of 3% for sexual harm and 29% for sexual harassment [40]. Another UK study also showed a prevalence of 75% for emotional harm and 24% for physical harm [41]. A 2015 Canadian study identified that 14% of a cohort of 359 youth athletes reported bullying while involved in sport [42]. A retrospective survey of 4000 adults in Belgium and The Netherlands revealed that almost half (44%) experienced at least one form of harassment and abuse while in sport: 14% sexual abuse (<18 years), 11% physical abuse, and 33% psychological abuse [6]. A study of elite athletics (track and field) athletes in Sweden identified a prevalence rate of 3% for sexual abuse and 18.3% for physical abuse, both of which were associated with an increased likelihood of sport-related injury in women [43].

Two international sports federations have also published prevalence studies: World Athletics (track and field) and FINA (Federation Internationale de Natation; aquatics). At the U20 World Athletics Championships, a survey of 380 athletes identified that 18% of males (M) and 15% of females (F) reported sexual abuse, 23%M/21%F verbal abuse, and 12%M/7%F physical abuse during sport [44]. In a survey at the FINA World Championships (2019), 15% of athlete participants reported having experienced harassment and abuse in sport and 9% had witnessed it. Almost half (40%) had experienced unwanted comments about their body shape or appearance. In all, 3% had experienced rewards in sport for sexual favors. Athletes who had experienced harassment and abuse had higher average scores for both depression and eating disorders and were more likely to express a need for psychotherapeutic support [45]. A recent review by World Athletics of more than 240,000 Twitter posts related to 161

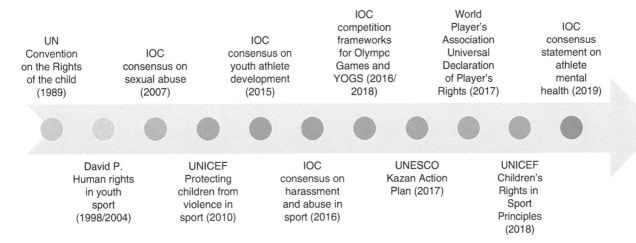

Fig. 16.2 A timeline of underpinning documents supporting safe sport

track and field athletes who competed in the Tokyo 2020 Olympic Games has revealed that nearly 15% of the athletes were targets of abusive posts (with 65% of the posts classified as "gravely abusive"). Nearly 70% of the targeted athletes were women [46].

While these studies have been in either a single sport, or a single geographic region, there are two studies on safeguarding of elite athletes representing multiple sports from around the world at the Summer (2018) [47] and Winter (2020) [48] Youth Olympic Games. Over half (52.5%) of the athletes surveyed in the Summer Youth Olympic Games (2018) reported that harassment and abuse was "likely,", "very likely," or "unsure" to occur in their sport [47]. In all, 61% of participating athletes in the Winter Youth Olympic Games responded similarly [48].

The scientific literature identifies four groups of athletes with a higher risk of harassment and abuse in sport: elite athletes [38, 49], child athletes [50], athletes with a disability [51, 52], and athletes who identify as LGBTQ (Lesbian, Gay, Bisexual, Transgender, Queer) [52, 53].

Evidence Base of Perpetrators of Harassment and Abuse in Sport

Perpetrators of sexual abuse in sport are more commonly reported to be male [54] and are in a position of power over the victim. Coaches are often identified as perpetrators of harassment and/or abuse within the sporting context [55, 56]. However, other members of the athlete entourage, such as the team physician, have also been identified as perpetrators in sport [57]. More recent evidence has demonstrated that athlete peers or teammates are also perpetrators of harassment and abuse in sport [56], especially male athletes in informal groups [58]. A study by Vertommen et al. (2021) identified the risk factors for sexual recidivism in sport, such

as deviant sexual behavior, the absence of an intimate relationship, and male victims [59]. A scoping review identified the risk factors for harassment and abuse in the coach–athlete relationship including closeness, power, blurred boundaries, and ambiguous roles [60].

Nonmental Health-Related Impacts of Harassment and Abuse

The impacts of harassment and abuse in sport can be devastating and long-lasting, beyond the period of abuse [61], and can affect peer athletes, friends, colleagues, and family members [9]. Athlete performance can be impaired, resulting in a loss of medal and sponsorship opportunities [62]. An impact of harassment and abuse is an increased risk of doping and/or willingness to cheat [63] and premature retirement from sport [3, 64].

Other impacts of sexual abuse may include local urogenital and anogenital trauma, sexually transmitted infections, and unwanted pregnancy [9]. The impacts of physical abuse may include injury, death, other medical problems, and developmental delays [65, 66]. Youth athletes are particularly vulnerable to physical abuse during the critical time of maturation and growth [67].

Mental Health Impacts of Harassment and Abuse

Mental health impacts of harassment and abuse (through direct and indirect mechanisms) have been extensively described in both athlete and nonathlete populations [2, 9, 68]. Athlete maltreatment can be experienced by any athlete during any stage of their sport journey, and youth who are sports prodigies may be at particular risk. The push to achieve extraordinary success places this special population at potential risk for a range of abuse, neglect, and boundary violations [69]. In addition to the risk of abuse and neglect, commodification of athletes, resulting from their inherent skills and sport potential, may lead to victimization of "by-proxy" ambitions. In this model, the athlete becomes an object onto which a perpetrator projects their own ambitions and is a tool used by the perpetrator to achieve what they perceive to be their own success. Potential perpetrators of "achievement by proxy" can include anyone in positions of authority or influence in the athlete's career, such as parents, coaches, mentors, agents, and sport systems. The specific effects on the mental health of athletes can include somatic manifestations of psychological disturbance, depression, avoidance, dependence, low self-esteem, anxiety, and substance misuse [69].

High-profile cases that thrust the topic of harassment and abuse in sport to the headlines provide windows into the experiences of the victims. A powerful army of 204 athletes who were abused by Larry Nassar provided impact statements during his sentencing hearing [70]. The long-standing effects on their mental health included depression, anxiety, substance use, post-traumatic stress disorder, difficulty with trust and intimacy, low self-worth, shame, and feeling "crushed, broken, and humiliated." At least three suicides have been attributed to the aftermath of Nassar's abuse, including gymnast Chelsea Markham and the fathers of gymnasts Melissa Imrie and Kyle Stephens. The constellation of mental health struggles described by these athletes is consistent with studies that have identified mental health sequelae such as substance use disorders, depression, anxiety, poor academic performance, loss of self-esteem, distorted body image, eating disorders, self-harm, and suicide [7].

Suicide has been identified as a mental health outcome of harassment and abuse in sport. In addition to Chelsea Markham, other youth athletes have ended their lives because of physical and sexual abuse experienced in sport [7]. *"Taibatsu,"* a Japanese term for corporal punishment, was found by Human Rights Watch researchers to be a common cultural practice in Japanese youth sports in 2020 [71]. Several Japanese athletes who had committed suicide cited physical and verbal abuse from their coach as the impetus for their suicide. A quantitative study of elite track and field athletes from Sweden identified an association between previous experience of physical or sexual abuse and suicidal ideation [72].

When long-standing abuse is finally exposed, it is common for reports to emerge that victims tried to report the abuse to teammates, coaches, parents, or sports administrators but were humiliated, threatened, bullied, and not believed. The psychological trauma experienced by the victims from the harassment and abuse is compounded if action is not taken to stop the abuse when an athlete reports the harassment or abuse to someone in a position of authority [73, 74].

Diagnosis of Mental Health Issues Resulting from Harassment and Abuse in Sport

Detection of mental health issues in athletes has been identified as a priority by the IOC and is supported by the IOC Consensus Statement on Mental Health in Elite Athletes (2019) [23]. Development of the Sport Mental Health Assessment Tool 1 (SMHAT-1) and the Sport Mental Health Recognition Tool 1 (SMHRT-1) has facilitated the ability to screen for general psychological well-being as well as a multitude of specific conditions (including trauma and abuse) [75]. Mental health screening should be regularly integrated in pre-participation questionnaires and implemented at identified check-in points during the year and as needed. Common presenting symptoms of athlete victims of abuse include psychosomatic illnesses, disordered eating, anxiety, depression, substance misuse, suicidal thoughts, self-harm, low self-esteem, poor body image, and sport drop out. All athletes who present with mental health symptoms should be screened for past or current experiences of harassment and abuse [9, 23]. Athletes who are suspected of having mental health challenges should be referred to a qualified mental health professional for further assessment and management [23, 75].

Treatment of Mental Health Disorders Related to Harassment and Abuse in Sport

Management of mental health disorders related to harassment and abuse in sport begins with the reporting mechanism. A safe, supportive process for athletes to report maltreatment, which includes protection from repercussions and retribution, may encourage higher rates of reporting. Investigation by a third party with no relationship with the organization is important for ensuring impartiality in the process. Passive attitudes, denial, nonintervention, and silence by authority figures may compound the initial trauma [76]. Connecting the victim of abuse with a qualified mental health professional is vital to begin the therapeutic process of exploration and support. Depending on the nature and severity of the symptoms, the affected individual may benefit from psychotherapy and/or medications. Psychotherapeutic modalities recommended for trauma include cognitive behavioral therapy (CBT), cognitive processing therapy, cognitive therapy, and prolonged exposure therapy [77]. If medications are warranted by symptom severity, then antidepressants from the selective serotonin reuptake inhibitor (SSRI) family, such as sertraline and fluoxetine, are considered reasonable choices for athletes [78, 79].

Prevention of Harassment and Abuse in Sport

Primary Prevention

Harassment and abuse in sport is an ethical and integrity issue, much like corruption, match fixing, and doping. As such, a "top-down" leadership commitment to prioritize safe sport and respect for athletes' rights within the sports organization is an essential component of prevention [9]. A cultural change for all within sport to avoid the commodification of athletes through a "win-at-all-costs" attitude is required [80].

Education of all members of sports organizations to raise awareness of the prevalence, risks, and impacts of harassment and abuse in sport is an important primary prevention strategy [9]. Importantly, all sports organizations should implement safeguarding policies and procedures as well as monitoring and evaluation systems. An example of a safeguarding framework developed by the UNICEF is the International Safeguards for Children in Sport [81]. To support the development and implementation of athlete safeguarding policies and procedures for the Olympic Movement, the IOC has published a guideline document with accompanying online webinars (Fig. 16.3) [82]. Sports organizations

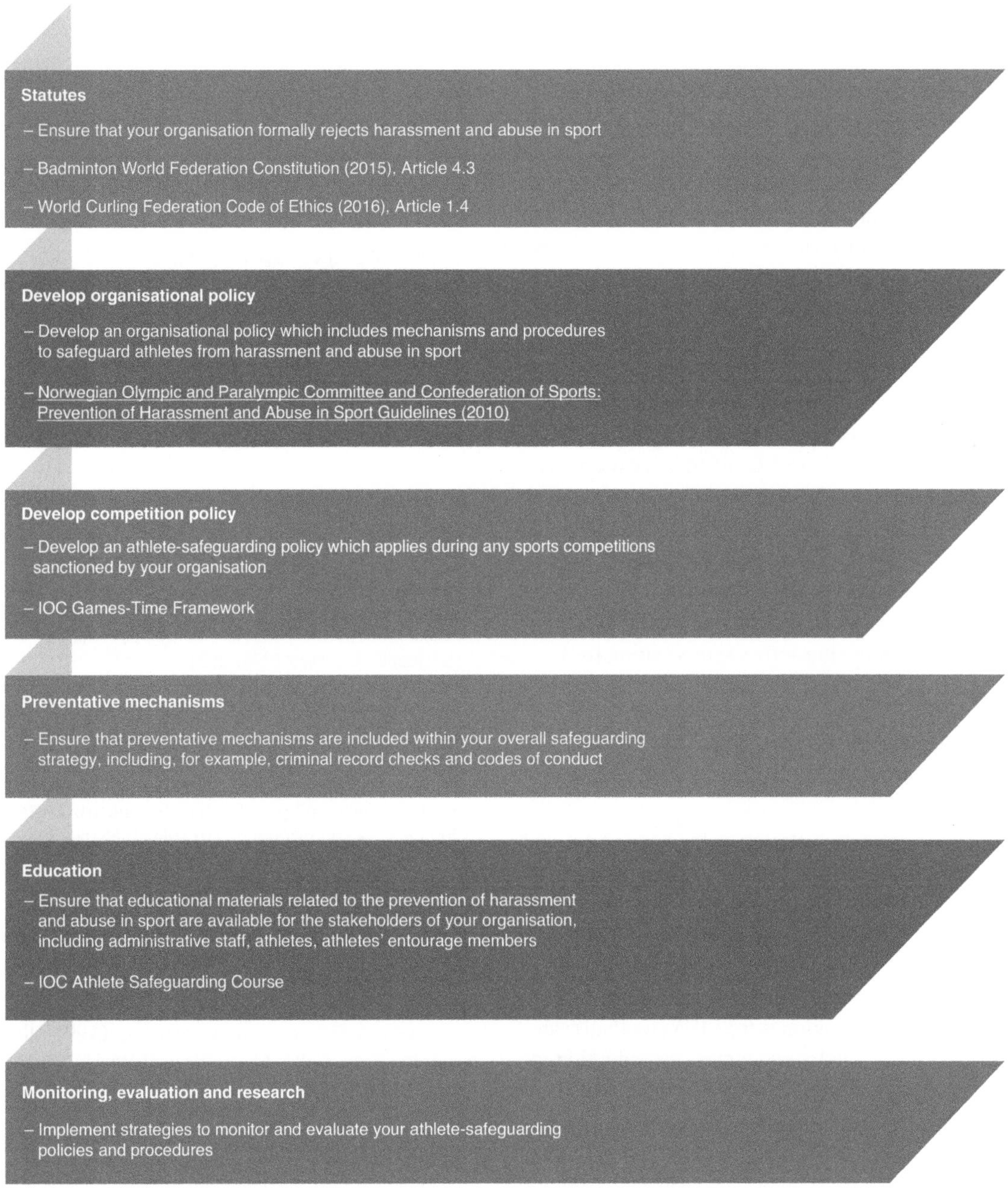

Statutes

– Ensure that your organisation formally rejects harassment and abuse in sport

– Badminton World Federation Constitution (2015), Article 4.3

– World Curling Federation Code of Ethics (2016), Article 1.4

Develop organisational policy

– Develop an organisational policy which includes mechanisms and procedures to safeguard athletes from harassment and abuse in sport

– Norwegian Olympic and Paralympic Committee and Confederation of Sports: Prevention of Harassment and Abuse in Sport Guidelines (2010)

Develop competition policy

– Develop an athlete-safeguarding policy which applies during any sports competitions sanctioned by your organisation

– IOC Games-Time Framework

Preventative mechanisms

– Ensure that preventative mechanisms are included within your overall safeguarding strategy, including, for example, criminal record checks and codes of conduct

Education

– Ensure that educational materials related to the prevention of harassment and abuse in sport are available for the stakeholders of your organisation, including administrative staff, athletes, athletes' entourage members

– IOC Athlete Safeguarding Course

Monitoring, evaluation and research

– Implement strategies to monitor and evaluate your athlete-safeguarding policies and procedures

Fig. 16.3 Safeguarding strategy flowchart overview [82]

should also implement competition safeguarding frameworks to protect the integrity of all participants [83, 84]. To mitigate physical abuse of athletes through medical mismanagement, all team physicians should abide by the ethical code of conduct as outlined in the Olympic Movement Medical Code [30]. Similarly, all elite sports organizations should implement the World Anti-Doping Code to protect athletes from the physical and psychological abuse caused by doping in sport [85]. Finally, supporting safeguarding research, specifically prevalence and intervention studies, is an indirect but important primary prevention strategy [9].

Secondary Prevention

An integral component of secondary prevention of harassment and abuse in sport is the education of all members of sports organizations on the recognition of harassment and abuse as well as the awareness of the reporting mechanisms. Robust safeguarding policies and procedures should include a detailed and appropriately resourced response system to manage athlete complaints and to provide referral pathways and neutral resolution mechanisms [9]. Team physicians should be knowledgeable of the subtle signs and symptoms of athlete presentations of harassment and abuse to facilitate early detection and to prevent prolonged abuse. In addition, team physicians should have the clinical competence to manage athlete disclosures of abuse and to provide appropriate medical and psychological support to the victim(s) [57, 66]. Sports organizations should have a certified and experienced safeguarding officer available both during sporting events and the training season [32]. All members of the safeguarding team should be trained in trauma-informed principles to mitigate unintentional secondary trauma [86]. Finally, the implementation of a global predator pipeline would prevent the recidivism of offenders in another sports setting [87].

Examples of Prevention Strategies for Harassment and Abuse in Sport

Many examples of prevention strategies for harassment and abuse in sport exist globally. With the objective of stopping abuse in sport, the Council of Europe developed an online platform to encourage dialogue, the reporting of abuse, the development of safeguarding initiatives, and the support of affected athletes [88]. Another example of a prevention strategy by an international federation is the FIFA (football) safeguarding toolkit, designed to encourage the adoption of athlete safeguarding strategies by its member federations [89]. In response to the exposure of systemic abuse in gymnastics, the United States Congress passed a law called "Empowering Olympic, Paralympic, and Amateur Athletes

Act of 2020" to establish safeguards to protect athletes from abuse in sport [90]. Another example of a multilayered approach to the prevention of harassment and abuse in sport is the IOC Safe Sport Action Plan (2020–2024), which provides a roadmap for a variety of safeguarding strategies targeting all members of the Olympic Movement including athletes, their entourage, sponsors, International Federations, National Olympic Committees, and Organizing Committees of the Olympic Games (OCOGS) [91].

Conclusions

By all stakeholders in sport working together with the common objective of preventing harassment and abuse in sport, many benefits can be realized. Importantly, given the significant mental health impacts on victims of harassment and abuse in sport, the implementation of prevention strategies should also result in the reduction of mental health symptoms and disorders in athletes. Thus, collectively, we can reach the objective of providing a sports environment that is safe and fulfilling for all [92].

Athletes of all ages have a right to engage in 'safe sport': an athletic environment that is respectful, equitable and free from all forms of non-accidental violence to athletes. Everyone involved in sport will benefit from a sporting environment that is free from fear or favour, and are just as entitled to express their human rights in the context of sport as they are in any other setting [9].

References

1. Maroney M. I thought I was going to die: read McKayla Maroney's statement in the Larry Nassar trial. Time Magazine. 2018. https://time.com/5109011/mckayla-maroney-larry-nassar-victim-impact-statement/. Accessed 1 Nov 2021.
2. Vertommen T, Kampen J, Schipper-van Veldhoven N, et al. Severe interpersonal violence against children in sport: associated mental health problems and quality of life in adulthood. Child Abuse Negl. 2018;76:459–68. https://doi.org/10.1016/j.chiabu.2017.12.013.
3. Fasting K, Brackenridge C, Walseth K. Consequences of sexual harassment in sport for female athletes. J Sexual Aggress. 2002;8:37–48. https://doi.org/10.1080/13552600208413338.
4. Tofler IR, Morse ED. The interface between sport psychiatry and sports medicine. Clin Sports Med. 2005;24(4):xv-i.
5. Sundgot-Borgen J, Fasting K, Brackenridge C, et al. Sexual harassment and eating disorders in female elite athletes—a controlled study. Scand J Med Sci Sports. 2003;13:330–5. https://doi.org/10.1034/j.1600-0838.2003.00295.
6. Vertommen T, Schipper-van Veldhoven N, Wouters K, et al. Interpersonal violence against children in sport in the Netherlands and Belgium. Child Abuse Negl. 2016;51:223–36. https://doi.org/10.1016/j.chiabu.2015.10.006.
7. Gervis M, Dunn N. The emotional abuse of elite child athletes by their coaches. Child Abuse Rev. 2004;13:215–23.
8. Killingal M. Simone Biles opens up about her mental health post Olympics: 'I'm still scared to do gymnastics'. CNN. https://www.

cnn.com/2021/10/22/sport/simone-biles-gymnastics-spt/index. html. Accessed 1 Nov 2021.

9. Mountjoy M, Brackenridge C, Arrington M, et al. The IOC consensus statement: harassment and abuse (nonaccidental violence) in sport. Br J Sports Med. 2016;50:1019–29. https://doi.org/10.1136/bjsports-2016-096121.

10. UNCRC. United Nations Convention on the Rights of the Child: resolution adopted by the general assembly. Geneva: United Nations; 1989. https://www.unicef.org/child-rights-convention/convention-text#. Accessed 1 Nov 2021.

11. David P. Children's rights and sport. In: Olympic review: Revue Olympique. 24. Lausanne: International Olympic Committee; 1998. p. 36–45.

12. David P. Human rights in youth sport: a critical review of children's rights in competitive sport. Taylor & Francis; 2004.

13. International Olympic Committee. Consensus Statement on "Sexual harassment and abuse in sport"; 2007. https://www.olympic.org/news/ioc-adopts-consensus-statement-on-sexual-harassment-and-abuse-in-sport. Accessed 1 Nov 2021.

14. Brackenridge C, Fasting K, Kirby S, et al. Protecting children from violence in sport: a review with a focus on industrialized countries. UNICEF Innocenti Research Centre; 2010. ISBN: 978-88-89129-96-8. https://www.unicef-irc.org/publications/pdf/violence_in_sport.pdf. Accessed 1 Nov 2021.

15. Pinheiro PS. United Nations Secretary-General's World report on violence against children. United Nations; 2006. http://www.violencestudy.org/IMG/pdf/English.pdf. Accessed 1 Nov 2021.

16. Bergeron M, Mountjoy M, Armstrong N, et al. International Olympic Committee consensus statement on youth athletic development. Br J Sport Med. 2015;49:843–51.

17. Mountjoy M, Rhind D, Tiivas A, et al. Safeguarding the child athlete in sport: a review, a framework, and recommendations for the IOC youth athlete development model. Br J Sport Med. 2015;49:883–6.

18. International Olympic Committee Safeguarding Framework: Rio de Janeiro Olympic Games; 2016. https://cdn.dosb.de/alter_Datenbestand/Bilder_allgemein/Veranstaltungen/Rio_2016/IOC_Framework_for_safeguarding_athletes.pdf. Accessed 1 Nov 2021.

19. International Olympic Committee. IOC Youth Olympic Games Framework for safeguarding athletes and other participants from harassment and abuse in sport. Hereinafter the "Framework". https://stillmed.olympic.org/media/Document%20Library/OlympicOrg/IOC/What-We-Do/Protecting-Clean-Athletes/Safeguarding/Lausanne-2020-YOG-framework-safeguarding-athletes.pdf#_ga52.56549032.2052076646.1599494602-1765704914.1497027285. Accessed 1 Nov 2021.

20. UNESCO. MINEPS VI Kazan Action Plan (KAP); 2017. https://en.unesco.org/mineps6/kazan-action-plan. Accessed 1 Nov 2021.

21. World Players Association. Universal declaration of players rights; 2017. https://sporthumanrights.org/library/universal-declaration-of-players-rights/. Accessed 1 Nov 2021.

22. United Nations. Centre for Sport and Human Rights. "The children's rights in sport principles"; 2018. https://www.sporthumanrights.org/library/childrens-rights-in-sport-principles. Accessed 1 Nov 2021.

23. Reardon C, Hainline B, Aron C, et al. International Olympic Committee consensus statement on mental health in elite athletes. Br J Sports Med. 2019;53(11):667–99. https://doi.org/10.1136/bjsports-2019-100715. Accessed 1 Nov 2021.

24. International Olympic Committee. Olympic Charter-In force as from 8 Aug 2021. https://stillmed.olympics.com/media/Document%20Library/OlympicOrg/General/EN-Olympic-Charter.pdf?_ga=2.161200373.959101447.1636944795-1451846925.1620655155. Accessed 1 Nov 2021.

25. International Olympic Committee. IOC Code of Ethics 2020. https://www.olympic.org/code-of-ethics. Accessed 1 Nov 2021.

26. International Olympic Committee. Olympic Agenda 2020+5: 15 recommendations. https://stillmedab.olympic.org/media/Document%20Library/OlympicOrg/IOC/What-We-Do/Olympic-agenda/Olympic-Agenda-2020-5-15-recommendations.pdf. Accessed 1 Nov 2021.

27. International Olympic Committee Athlete 365. Athlete's Declaration. https://olympics.com/athlete365/who-we-are/athletes-declaration/. Accessed 1 Nov 2021.

28. International Olympic Committee. Recommendations for an IOC Human Rights Strategy; 2020. https://stillmedab.olympic.org/media/Document%20Library/OlympicOrg/News/2020/12/Independent_Expert_Report_IOC_HumanRights.pdf. Accessed 1 Nov 2021.

29. International Olympic Committee. Basic universal principles of good governance of the Olympic and sports movement; 2008. https://stillmed.olympic.org/media/Document%20Library/OlympicOrg/IOC/Who-We-Are/Commissions/Ethics/Good-Governance/EN-Basic-Universal-Principles-of-Good-Governance-2011.pdf#_ga=2.183818085.277635013.1598965025-1765704914.1497027285. Accessed 1 Nov 2021.

30. International Olympic Committee. Olympic movement medical code; 2016. https://stillmed.olympic.org/media/Document%20Library/OlympicOrg/IOC/Who-We-Are/Commissions/Medical-andScientific-Commission/Olympic-Movement-Medical-Code-31-03-2016.Pdf. Accessed 1 Nov 2021.

31. International Olympic Committee. Safeguarding athletes from harassment and abuse in sport: IOC toolkit for IFs and NOCs. https://olympics.com/athlete365/app/uploads/2020/12/1428_Safeguarding_Toolkit_ENG_23d_screen_Full_2a-.pdf. Accessed 1 Nov 2021.

32. International Olympic Committee. IOC certificate: safeguarding officer in sport . https://www.sportsoracle.com/Safeguarding/Home/. Accessed 1 Nov 2021.

33. Athlete365 Safe Sport for all. https://olympics.com/athlete365/what-we-do/integrity/safe-sport/. Accessed 1 Nov 2021.

34. International Olympic Committee. Safe Sport Action Plan 2021–24. https://stillmed.olympics.com/media/Document%20Library/IOC/Athletes/Safe-Sport-Initiatives/2021-Safe-Sport-for-athletes-action-plan.pdf?_ga=2.10794996.1572138189.1637117182-1451846925.1620655155. Accessed 1 Nov 2021

35. IOC framework on fairness, inclusion, and non-discrimination on the basis of gender identity and sex variations. IOC-Framework-Fairness-Inclusion-Non-discrimination-2021.pdf (olympics.com). Accessed 16 Nov 2021.

36. Parent S, Fortier K. Prevalence of interpersonal violence against athletes in the sport context. Curr Opin Psychol. 2017;16:165–9.

37. Leahy T, Pretty G, Tenenbaum G. Prevalence of sexual abuse in organised competitive sport in Australia. J Sex Aggress. 2002;8(16–36):548.

38. Fasting K, Brackenridge C, Knorre N. Performance level and sexual harassment prevalence among female athletes in the Czech Republic. WSPAJ. 2010;19:26–32. 547

39. Brackenridge C, Fasting K. Sexual harassment and abuse in sport: the research context. J Sex Aggress. 2002;8:3–15.

40. Alexander K, Stafford A, Lewis R. The experiences of children participating in organised sport in the UK. London: NSPCC; 2011.

41. Stafford A, Alexander K, Fry D. 'There was something that wasn't right because that was the only place I ever got treated like that': children and young people's experiences of emotional harm in sport. Childhood. 2015;22:121–37.

42. Evans B, Adler A, Macdonald D, et al. Bullying victimization, and perpetration among adolescent sport teammates. Pediatr Exerc Sci. 2016;28(2):296–303. https://journals.humankinetics.com/view/journals/pes/28/2/article-p296.xml#:~:text=DOI%3A%20https%3A//doi.org/10.1123/pes.2015-0088.

43. Timpka T, Janson S, Jacobsson J, et al. Lifetime history of sexual and physical abuse among competitive athletics (track and field) athletes: cross sectional study of associations with sports and non-sports injury. Br J Sports Med. 2019;53(22):1412–7. https://doi.org/10.1136/bjsports-2018-099335.

44. Bermon S, Adami PE, Dahlström Ö, et al. Lifetime prevalence of verbal, physical, and sexual abuses in young elite athletics athletes. Front Sports Act Living. 2021;3:152–60. https://doi.org/10.3389/fspor.2021.657624.

45. Mountjoy M, Junge A, Magnusson C, et al. Beneath the surface: mental health and harassment & abuse of athletes participating in the FINA (aquatics) World Championships 2019. Clin J Sport Med. 2021;31(6):425–31. https://doi.org/10.1097/JSM.0000000000000814.

46. Pells E. Tokyo Olympians faced 'disturbing' level of abuse on social media, study shows. Associated Press. https://www.cbc.ca/sports/olympics/summer/trackandfield/world-athletics-social-media-1.6262375. Accessed 26 Nov 2021.

47. Mountjoy M, Vertommen T, Burrows K, Greinig S. #SafeSport: safeguarding initiatives at the Youth Olympic Games 2018. Br J Sports Med. 2020;54(3):176–82. https://doi.org/10.1136/bjsports-2019-101461.

48. Mountjoy M, Vertommen T, Tercier S, Greinig S, Burrows K. #SafeSport: perceptions of harassment and abuse from elite youth athletes at the Winter Youth Olympic Games, Lausanne 2020, Clin J Sports Med. 2022;32(3):297–305. https://doi.org/10.1097/JSM.0000000000000989. PMID: 34759180.

49. Vertommen T, Schipper-van Veldhoven NHMJ, Hartill MJ, et al. Sexual harassment and abuse in sport: the NOC*NSF helpline. Int Rev Sociol Sport. 2015;50:822–39.

50. LSEPS. European Union kids online report. London: Science LSoEaP; 2014.

51. Tuakli-Wosornu YA, Sun Q, Gentry M, et al. Non-accidental harms ('abuse') in athletes with impairment ('para athletes'): a state-of-the-art review. Br J Sports Med. 2020;54(3):129.

52. Kirby SL, Demers G, Parent S. Vulnerability/prevention: considering the needs of disabled and gay athletes in the context of sexual harassment and abuse. Int J Sport Exerc Psych. 2008;6(4):407–26.

53. Denison E, Kitchen A. Out on the fields. The first international study on homophobia in sport. Nielsen, Bingham Cup Sydney 2014, Australian Sports Commission, Federation of Gay Games; 2015. http://www.outonthefields.com/wp-content/uploads/2016/04/Out-on-the-Fields-Final-Report.pdf. Accessed 1 Nov 2021.

54. Fasting K, Brackenridge C, Sundgot-Borgen J. Prevalence of sexual harassment among Norwegian female elite athletes in relation to sport type. Int Rev Sociol Sport. 2004;39:373–86.

55. Sand TS, Fasting K, Chroni S, et al. Coaching behavior: any consequences for the prevalence of sexual harassment? Int J Sports Sci Coach. 2011;6:229–41.

56. Fasting K, Huffman D, Sand TS. Gender based violence in Zambian sport: prevalence and protection. Oslo: Norwegian Olympic and Paralympic Committee and Confederations of Sports; 2015.

57. Mountjoy M. 'Only by speaking out can we create lasting change': what can we learn from the Dr Larry Nassar tragedy? Br J Sports Med. 2019;53:57–60.

58. Vertommen T, Kampen J, Schipper-van Veldhoven N, et al. Profiling perpetrators of interpersonal violence against children in sport based on a victim survey. Child Abuse Negl. 2017;63:172–82. https://doi.org/10.1016/j.chiabu.2016.11.0.

59. Vertommen T, Verhelle H, Martijn FM, et al. Static and dynamic recidivism risk factors of people who have committed child sex offenses in sport. Front Sports Act Living. 2021;3:624548. https://doi.org/10.3389/fspor.2021.624548.

60. Gaedicke S, Schäfer A, Hoffmann B, et al. Sexual violence and the coach-athlete relationship—a scoping review from sport sociological and sport psychological perspectives. Front Sports Act Living.

2021;3:643707. https://doi.org/10.3389/fspor.2021.643707. PMID: 34056586; PMCID: PMC8155665.

61. Leahy T. Working with adult athlete survivors of sexual abuse. In: Hanrahan SJ, Andersen MB, editors. Routledge handbook of applied sport psychology: a comprehensive guide for students and practitioners. London: Routledge; 2010. p. 303–12.

62. Brackenridge CH. Spoilsports: understanding and preventing sexual exploitation in sport. London: Routledge; 2001.

63. Yukhymenko-Lescroart MA, Brown ME, Paskus TS. The relationship between ethical and abusive coaching behaviors and student-athlete well-being. Sport Exerc Perform Psychol. 2015;4:36–49.

64. Pinheiro MC, Pimenta N, Resende R, et al. Gymnastics and child abuse: an analysis of former international Portuguese female artistic gymnasts. Sport Educ Soc. 2014;19:435–50.

65. Burke M. Obeying until it hurts: coach-athlete relationships. J Philos Sport. 2001;28:227–40.

66. Marks S, Mountjoy M, Marcus M. Sexual harassment and abuse in sport: the role of the team doctor. Br J Sports Med. 2012;46:905–8.

67. DiFiori JP, Benjamin HJ, Brenner J, et al. Overuse injuries and burnout in youth sport: a position statement from the American Medical Society for Sports Medicine. Clin J Sport Med. 2014;24:3–20.

68. Schenk A, Fremouw WJ. Prevalence, psychological impact, and coping of cyberbully victims among college students. J School Violence. 2012;11:21–37.

69. Tofler IR, Knapp PK, Lardon MT. Achievement by proxy distortion in sports: a distorted mentoring of high-achieving youth. Historical perspectives and clinical intervention with children, adolescents and their families. Clin Sports Med. 2005;24:805–28.

70. Rahal S, Kozlowski K. 204 impact statements, 9 days, 2 counties, a life sentence for Larry Nassar. Detroit News; 2018. https://www.detroitnews.com/story/news/local/michigan/2018/02/08/204-impact-statements-9-days-2-counties-life-sentence-larry-nassar/1066335001/. Accessed 26 Nov 2021.

71. Human Rights Watch. I was hit so many times, I can't count. 2020. https://www.hrw.org/report/2020/07/20/i-was-hit-so-many-times-i-cant-count/abuse-child-athletes-japan. Accessed 1 Nov 2021.

72. Timpka T, Spreco A, Dahlstrom, et al. Suicidal thoughts (ideation) among elite athletics (track and field) athletes: cross-sectional study of associations with sexual and physical abuse victimization, aspects of sports participation, and psychological and behavioural resourcefulness. Br J Sports Med. 2021;55(4):198–205. https://doi.org/10.1136/bjsports-2019-101386.

73. Raakman E, Dorsch K, Rhind D. The development of a typology of abusive coaching behaviours within youth sport. Int J Sports Sci Coach. 2010;5:503–15.

74. Fasting K, Brackenridge C, Walseth K. Women athletes' personal responses to sexual harassment in sport. J Appl Sport Psychol. 2007;19:419–33.

75. Gouttebarge V, Bindra A, Blauwet, et al. International Olympic Committee (IOC) Sport Mental Health Assessment Tool 1 (SMHAT-1) and Sport Mental Health Recognition Tool 1 (SMHRT-1): towards better support of athletes' mental health. Br J Sports Med. 2021;55(1):30–7. https://doi.org/10.1136/bjsports-2020-102411.

76. Wenzel T, Zhu LJ. Posttraumatic stress in athletes. In: Baron DA, Reardon C, Baron SH, editors. Clinical sports psychiatry: an international perspective. New York: Wiley; 2013. p. 102–14.

77. American Psychological Association. Guideline development panel for the treatment of posttraumatic stress disorder in adults. Clinical practice guideline for the treatment of PTSD; 2017. https://www.apa.org/ptsd-guideline/ptsd.pdf. Accessed 26 Nov 202.

78. Department of Veterans Affairs, Department of Defense. VA/DOD clinical practice guideline for the management of posttraumatic stress disorder and acute stress disorder. Washington, DC: Department of Veterans Affairs; 2017.

79. Reardon CL, Creado S. Psychiatric medication preferences of sports psychiatrists. Phys Sportsmed. 2016;44:397–402.

80. Mountjoy M. #Time2Act: harassment and abuse in elite youth sport culture. Br J Sports Med. 2020;54:367–8.

81. Founders Group. International Safeguards for Children in Sport; 2014. International-Safeguards-for-Children-in-Sport-version-to-view-online.pdf (unicef.org.uk). Accessed 1 Nov 2021.

82. International Olympic Committee. Safeguarding athletes from harassment and abuse in sport: IOC Toolkit for IFs and NOCs. https://olympics.com/athlete365/app/uploads/2020/12/1428_Safeguarding_Toolkit_ENG_23d_screen_Full_2a-.pdf. Accessed 1 Nov 2021.

83. Mountjoy M, Moran J, Ahmed H, et al. Athlete health and safety at large sport events: the development of consensus-driven guidelines. Br J Sport Med. 2021;55(4):191–7. https://doi.org/10.1136/bjsports-2020-102771.

84. Mountjoy M. ASOIF guidelines for health care at International Federation events; 2020. https://library.olympic.org/Default/doc/SYRACUSE/354139/. Accessed 1 Nov 2021.

85. World Anti Doping Association. The World Anti Doping Code; 2021. https://www.wada-ama.org/en/what-we-do/the-code. Accessed 1 Nov 2021.

86. Mountjoy M, Vertommen T, Denhollander R, et al. Effective engagement of survivors of harassment and abuse in sport in athlete safeguarding initiatives: a review and a conceptual framework. Br J Sport Med. (accepted in publication).

87. Predator pipeline: NCAA looks the other way as athletes punished for sex offences play on, 2019. USA Today Network. https://gatehousenews.com/predatorpipeline. Accessed 1 Nov 2021.

88. Council of Europe. Start to talk, 2019. https://www.coe.int/en/web/sport/start-to-talk. Accessed 1 Nov 2021.

89. FIFA. FIFA Guardians—up to us: child safeguarding toolkit for member associations; 2019. https://resources.fifa.com/image/upload/toolkit-fifa-guardians.pdf?cloudid=nz1lyz3ykaioy7gwfmgs. Accessed 1 Nov 2021.

90. US Congress S.2330—Empowering Olympic, Paralympic, and Amateur Athletes Act of 2020. https://www.congress.gov/bill/116th-congress/senate-bill/2330. Accessed 1 Nov 2021.

91. International Olympic Committee. Safe Sport Action Plan 2021–24. https://stillmed.olympics.com/media/Document%20Library/IOC/Athletes/Safe-Sport-Initiatives/2021-Safe-Sport-for-athletes-action-plan.pdf?_ga=2.10794996.1572138189.1637117182-1451846925.1620655155. Accessed 1 Nov 2021.

92. Mountjoy M, Armstrong N, Bizzini L, et al. IOC Consensus Statement: training the elite child athlete. Br J Sports Med. 2008;42:163–4.

Psychological Response to Injury and Illness

Margot Putukian

Introduction

Participation in sport entails hours of training, practice, and competition with athletes spending time and energy working with coaches and other support staff to improve their skills and compete. Mental health (MH) is an important consideration in supporting the overall vigor and well-being of athletes. Several recent publications have focused on MH symptoms and disorders in athletes [1–5]. MH and well-being exist on a continuum, with resilience and thriving on one end and MH symptoms and disorders that significantly disrupt function and performance on the other. A systematic review and meta-analysis of 22 studies demonstrated a prevalence of MH symptoms and disorders in current and former elite athletes in males and females from team sports and combined Olympic sports that was significant, with the most common symptoms and disorders reported being anxiety, depression, sleep dysfunction, alcohol misuse, and general psychological distress [6].

Participation in sport includes the additional risk of injury and illness that may not necessarily be experienced by nonathletes. There is an interface between injury or illness and MH and performance that is quite complex, and understanding the risk factors for injury and/or illness is complicated [1–3, 5, 7, 8]. It is unclear whether participation in sport increases the risk of or potentially protects athletes from MH disorders. Sport entails unique stressors, and, accordingly, there are MH symptoms or disorders in athletes that are potentially seen more commonly than in their nonathlete peers. These stressors include sexual abuse, hazing and bullying, challenges related to retirement from or transition out of sport, and the psychological response to injury and illness [1, 2]. This chapter will focus on the psychological response to injury and illness.

Epidemiology

As mentioned previously, in a systematic review of elite sport athletes, several MH symptoms and disorders were reported in both current and former elite male and female athletes [6]. The prevalence ranged from 19% for alcohol misuse to 34% for anxiety/depression in current elite athletes and from 16% for distress to 26% for anxiety/depression in former elite athletes.

Specifically, for current athletes, in 11 studies of 3335 male and female athletes, 19.6% (95% confidence interval (CI): 16.0–23.0) reported symptoms of distress. In 10 studies of 4782 current athletes from various sports, 26.4% (95% CI: 21.6–31.2) reported symptoms of sleep disturbance. In 9 studies of 2895 current athletes from various sports, 33.6% (95% CI: 27.4–39.7) reported symptoms of anxiety/depression. In 11 studies of 5555 current athletes from various sports, 18.8% (95% CI: 11.1–26.5) reported symptoms of alcohol misuse. Cross-sectional studies demonstrated eating disorders (EDs)/disordered eating ($n = 7$ studies) in 1–28%, panic disorder ($n = 2$ studies) in 1–5%, and problem gambling ($n = 1$ study) in 2–7% [6].

Specifically, for former athletes, 15 studies were included, and prevalence data from 8 of them ($n = 1686$ male and female athletes from team sports and combined Olympic sports) demonstrated that 15.8% (95% CI: 16.0–23.3) reported symptoms of distress [6]. Sleep disturbance was reported in 20.9% (95% CI: 15.2–26.6) out of a total of 1579 former athletes ($n = 7$ studies) from various sports. Anxiety/depression was reported in 26.4% (95% CI: 21.4–31.4) out of a total of 1662 former athletes from various sports ($n = 8$ studies). Alcohol misuse was reported in 21.1% (95% CI: 14.7–27.4) out of a total of 1636 former athletes from various sports ($n = 8$ studies). Cross-sectional studies revealed eating disorders in 24–27% ($n = 2$ studies), dementia in 6% ($n = 1$ study), Alzheimer's disease in 12% ($n = 1$ study), and mild cognitive impairment in 23% ($n = 1$ study). This comprehensive review demonstrates the significant prevalence of MH symptoms and disorders in both current and former

M. Putukian (✉)
Major League Soccer, Princeton, NJ, USA

male and female elite athletes participating in a variety of sports [6].

The Context and Current Environment of Mental Health, Injury, and Illness in Elite Sport

The International Olympic Committee (IOC) has identified MH as a focus point, with the development of several new tools for athletes and several other stakeholders related to MH and wellness, including the Sports Mental Health Recognition Tool 1 and the Sports Mental Health Assessment Tool 1 as well as the IOC Mental Health Toolkit [9–11]. These tools have raised awareness, provided education to several stakeholders, and created a framework to understand important policies and procedures that can improve the delivery of MH care to athletes.

There are several barriers and facilitators to help-seeking behavior in athletes [11–13], and prevention programs should address these through education, policy development, mental health action plans, screening programs, and effective referral and treatment plans. The most important barriers to help-seeking behaviors in elite athletes are MH stigma, a lack of MH literacy, and the negative experience that some athletes had previously had when seeking help [11, 12]. Alternatively, facilitators to help-seeking behavior include encouragement from others, an established relationship with the health-care provider, positive previous interactions with the provider, support for help-seeking by others, especially coaches, and access to the Internet [11, 12].

Health-care providers can be instrumental in facilitating help-seeking behavior by providing educational programs, developing and implementing policies and programs, adding screenings for MH symptoms and disorders to sports physicals and office visits as indicated, and establishing MH plans and MH Emergency Action Plans. Given the relationship that many team physicians develop with athletes and teams, the ability to decrease the stigma surrounding MH is an important opportunity for improving the overall health and safety of athletes [1]. In addition, team physicians and other health-care providers that work with athletes are often involved throughout the injury/illness and are therefore in a position to recognize athletes that may be in distress related to their injury/illness [1–4].

Illness and Injury in Elite Athletes

Illness and injury have been associated with and identified as risk factors for several MH symptoms and disorders that occur commonly in athletes, including anxiety, depression, suicide, substance use, disordered gambling, trauma-related disorders, overtraining, and eating disorders (EDs) as well as issues related to transition/retirement from sport [5, 14–26]. Although controversial, there may, conversely, also be MH disorders and psychological stressors that an athlete experiences that can increase the risk of illness or injury [27–31]. Finally, there may be underlying MH disorders that are unmasked by the psychological response to injury or that complicate recovery from injury [27–29, 31–35].

The risk factors for injuries are multifactorial and often challenging to interpret. Injured athletes report a higher level of symptoms of both depression and anxiety compared to their noninjured peers [26, 36]. The risk factors for injury include both sociocultural and psychological factors [31, 37, 38]. The sociocultural risk factors include social pressures, limited social resources, a lifetime history of sexual or physical abuse, organizational stress (i.e., how the athlete feels about the structure and function of their team), stress related to a negative self-assessment of their academic or athletic performance, coaching quality (how they perceive their relationship with their coach), and the culture of their sport/team (e.g., the mindset of the team; win at all costs versus continued team growth) [3, 31, 39, 40]. The psychological risk factors include perfectionism, anxiety/worry, hypervigilance, poor body image or low self-esteem, limited coping resources, risk-taking behaviors, low mood state, or life event stress (e.g., stress associated with major life event stressors such as the death of a family member or starting at a new school). Life event stress can also include athlete-specific stressors such as injury or illness, fear of reinjury, failure in competitions, retirement from sport, or abuse related to sport (e.g., sexual abuse, hazing, bullying) [27–30, 33, 41].

Although there are limited prospective and/or conflicting results regarding the risk factors related to injury, life event stress and high stress response (e.g., negative emotional response after a sport injury or other stressful events) consistently demonstrate a relationship with injury risk [26, 29, 31, 37, 39, 40, 42–44]. Athletes with higher resiliency and "mental toughness" have lower rates of injury and lower rates of depression, stress, anxiety, and obsessive-compulsive symptoms [17, 21].

The psychological response to injury has been described previously as a model that suggested that the way an athlete appreciates their injury (cognitive appraisal) determines their emotional and behavioral responses [38]. This has formed the framework for much of the more recent literature. The cognitive, emotional, and behavioral responses can be influenced by several athlete-specific factors, can change over time, and can influence the rehabilitative process as well as an athlete's ability to return to sport. Understanding each of these responses is critical in understanding how they interact and what role the medical staff can play in providing additional support and improving outcome.

A cognitive response is how the athlete understands their injury or illness. It leads to an emotional response; both can be either "normal" or "problematic," [3] and both can affect behavioral responses such as goal setting, motivation, and compliance with treatment [37]. An emotional response is how the athlete feels about their injury or illness. This can include sadness, anger, frustration, changes in sleep or appetite, and lack of motivation [37].

Improved injury recovery has been shown in athletes that have more positive cognitive, emotional, and behavioral responses to injury [17, 27, 45–50]. Factors such as motivation [51], apprehension of reinjury [41, 52–54], and psychological readiness [55] are associated with a higher likelihood of return to the preinjury level of play and higher post-injury performances [50]. Higher levels of optimism and self-efficacy and lower levels of depression and stress are also associated with improved recovery from injury [17, 27, 46, 48–50, 54, 56–60].

Management of Injuries and Illnesses to Improve Outcomes

Strategies such as (1) using modeling techniques (e.g., videos, peer athletes) to decrease the fear of reinjury, (2) support of athlete autonomy (e.g., via explaining the purpose of rehabilitative exercises), (3) increasing confidence (e.g., via goal setting, functional tests), (4) providing social support, (5) finding a role for the athlete within their sport (e.g., monitoring statistics, helping the coach), and (6) stress inoculation training (e.g., to avoid the need for pain medication if the injury requires surgery) are all important for improving recovery [47, 60].

A recent publication has outlined a 24-week program via a randomized controlled trial (RCT) for athletes recovering from anterior cruciate ligament (ACL) surgical reconstruction. It plans to implement cognitive behavioral therapy modules targeting several psychological barriers to return to sport as an intervention [61]. The seven self-directed modules are provided using a smartphone application and address: (1) goal setting, (2) recovery, (3) return to sport, (4) return to performance, (5) staying injury-free, (6) handling thoughts and emotions, and (7) injury education [61]. The results of this RCT will be useful in determining whether a smartphone application that delivers cognitive behavioral therapy is effective in improving the number of athletes that return to various levels of sport after surgical treatment of their ACL injury.

Specific Situation: Sport-Related Concussion (SRC)

One of the most common injuries that is particularly challenging is a sport-related concussion (SRC) [62], which includes several nonspecific symptoms that are the same symptoms

endorsed by individuals with MH disorders. This overlap creates diagnostic challenges for health-care providers working to both diagnose and treat SRCs [63–65]. There are also data that suggest that athletes with SRC may develop MH symptoms and that athletes may use substances in order to cope with these emotions [66]. A prospective cohort study of male professional rugby players assessed at three time points (a baseline assessment and then follow-ups at 6 and 12 months) found that those players that sustained a concussion within 12 months of a baseline assessment were more likely to develop MH symptoms (odds ratio ranging from 1.5 (95% CI: 1.0–2.1) for distress to 2.0 (95% CI: 1.2–3.6) for adverse alcohol use). In this study, players who sustained a severe injury within 12 months of baseline were more likely to develop symptoms of anxiety/depression (odds ratio of 1.5 (95% CI: 1.1–2.0)) [67].

In male collegiate athletes who have been diagnosed with SRC, symptoms of depression, anxiety, and impulsivity are commonly noted [68]. In one study, 20% of collegiate athletes reported symptoms of depression after an SRC, with predictors including ethnicity (non-White), baseline reporting of symptoms of depression, the number of games missed after injury (the more the games, the more are the symptoms), and the number of years they had been involved in sport (more symptoms if fewer number of years in sport) [65]. A longer recovery time and/or persisting symptoms after an SRC, a preexisting history of mood or other MH disorders, a family history of MH disorders, and high-stress life events have been associated with the development of MH symptoms [16, 19, 69–72]. Individuals who have had an SRC report fear of reinjury [32, 67], an issue initially cited in athletes after ACL reconstruction [17, 46, 48, 49, 56, 73].

Other Injuries and Illnesses: Beyond Concussion

Whether the psychological response is different when in response to a musculoskeletal injury versus other types of injuries or illnesses such as concussion is unclear. The assumption might be that the response might be similar if the expectation (how severe the athlete appreciates the condition to be) is similar. A recent study has found that the response to a musculoskeletal injury and a concussion are similar when assessed using the Profile of Mood States (POMS) and the State-Trait Anxiety Inventory (STAI) [74]. The time to return to sport was similar, and this was an important consideration. In addition, there was improvement over time for both conditions, suggesting that psychological issues that occurred after an injury, whether musculoskeletal or a concussion, improved to baseline levels of function no matter the injury [74].

Another recent study has evaluated whether or not the premorbid psychological status of the athlete can predict how they handle a subsequent injury/illness and found that if the athlete had some previous experience with adversity, which was neither trivial nor overwhelming, then they did better than others with either nonexistent adversity or prior overwhelming adversity [75]. In this study, the authors prospectively evaluated preinjury adversity over a 5-year time period using a measure of adversity and then evaluated a measure of coping as well as psychological responses at the onset of injury, rehabilitation, and return to sport. They subsequently performed in-person interviews on a subset of the injured participants. They theorized that an explanation for their findings was that athletes with high preinjury adversities were excessively overwhelmed such that they were unable to cope with injury and those with low preinjury adversities had not developed coping abilities and lacked the resources needed to cope with injury [75]. More research is needed to further clarify future directions.

The human severe acute respiratory syndrome (SARS) coronavirus called COVID-19 [76] was first described in December 2019 and subsequently created a worldwide pandemic. It brought elite sports to a halt and postponed the Summer Olympic Games, moving them to Tokyo in the summer of 2021. The literature regarding the impacts of COVID-19 suggests the psychological effects of the pandemic on athletes [77–79]. At the collegiate level, a survey of >37,000 athletes demonstrated high rates of mental distress, with more than 25% reporting feeling sadness and a sense of loss and 8.3% reporting "feeling so depressed it has been hard to function" at least "constantly" or "most every day" [77]. Sleep dysfunction was reported in one in three (33%), and 80% reported having barriers to training including fear of exposure to COVID-19 (43%), lack of motivation (40%), feeling of stress or anxiety (21%), and sadness or depression (13%) [77]. It is clear that the mental health response to COVID-19 infection is significant not only for athletes but also for the general population at large, and ongoing efforts to recognize and identify athletes at risk for mental health symptoms and disorders are essential [78].

Future Directions

Over the past decade, more attention has been paid to the importance of psychological factors and how they relate to not only the risk of injury/illness but also how these factors may relate to recovery, rehabilitation, and return to sport [80]. MH issues are common in sport [1–6], and a better understanding of the importance of recovery [81], nutrition, and sleep [82] in supporting overall well-being and performance is expected [83].

More attention is being paid to the evaluation of psychological factors, unique stressors, and risk factors for injury—including psychological parameters—[84] and ultimately a better understanding of the psychological response to injury

and how to respond and support athletes that are injured or ill will be possible. Understanding the complexity that each individual athlete presents with their antecedent psychological factors, the social support network that they have in place, their prior adversity, and all the factors that can play a role in modifying their post-injury/illness response is an area of further research. Having a better understanding of the cognitive, emotional, and behavioral responses to injury, as well as the individual factors that can affect them, is also an area that merits additional attention.

References

1. Chang C, Putukian M, Aerni G, et al. Mental health issues and psychological factors in athletes: detection, management, effect on performance and prevention: American Medical Society for Sports Medicine Position Statement—executive summary. Br J Sports Med. 2020;54(4):216–20. https://doi.org/10.1136/bjsports-2019-101583.
2. Reardon C, Hainline B, Aron CM, et al. Mental health in elite athletes: International Olympic Committee consensus statement. Br J Sports Med. 2019;53(11):667–99.
3. Herring SA, Kibler WB, Putukian M, et al. Psychological issues related to illness and injury in the athletes and the team physician: a consensus statement—2016 update. Med Sci Sports Exerc. 2017;49(5):1043–54.
4. Inter-association Consensus Document: mental health best practices. Understanding and supporting student-athlete mental wellness. 2016. Updated 2020. https://ncaaorg.s3.amazonaws.com/ssi/mental/SSI_MentalHealthBestPractices.pdf. Accessed 1 Apr 2020.
5. Rice SM, Purcell R, De Silva S, et al. The mental health of elite athletes: a narrative systematic review. Sports Med. 2016;46:1333–53.
6. Gouttebarge V, Castaldelli-Maia JM, Gorczynski P, et al. Occurrence of mental health symptoms and disorders in current and former elite athletes: a systematic review and meta-analysis. Br J Sports Med. 2019;53(11):700–6. https://doi.org/10.1136/bjsports-2019-100671.
7. Putukian M. How being injured affects mental health. In: Brown GT, Hainline B, Kroshus E, Wilfert M, editors. Mind, body and sport: understanding and supporting student-athlete mental wellness. Indianapolis, IN: NCAA Press; 2014. p. 72–5.
8. Putukian M. The psychological response to injury in student athletes: a narrative review with a focus on mental health. Br J Sports Med. 2016;50:145–8.
9. Gouttebarge V, Abhinav B, Blauwet C, et al. The International Olympic Committee Sport Mental Health Assessment Tool 1 (SMHAT-1) and Sport Mental Health Recognition Tool 1 (SMHRT-1): towards better support of athletes' mental health. Br J Sports Med. 2021;55:30–7.
10. Rice S, Olive L, Gouttebarge V, et al. Mental health screening: severity and cut-off point sensitivity of the Athlete Psychological Strain Questionnaire in male and female elite athletes. BMJ Open Sport Exerc Med. 2020;6(1):e000712. . Published 2020 Mar 18. https://doi.org/10.1136/bmjsem-2019-000712.
11. IOC Toolkit. https://olympics.com/ioc/news/amp/ioc-launches-safe-sport-action-plan-and-mental-health-toolkit-for-elite-athletes.
12. Gulliver A, Griffiths KM, Christensen H. Barriers and facilitators to mental health help-seeking for young elite athletes: a qualitative study. BMC Psychiatry. 2012;12:157.
13. Confectioner K, Currie A, Gabana N, et al. Help-seeking behaviours related to mental health symptoms in professional football.

BMJ Open Sport Exerc Med. 2021;7(2):e001070. Published 2021 May 17.

14. Armstrong S, Omen-Early J. Social connectedness, self-esteem, and depression symptomatology among collegiate athletes versus non-athletes. J Am Coll Heal. 2009;57(5):521–6.

15. Beals KA, Manore MM. Disorders of the female athlete triad among collegiate athletes. Int J Sport Nutr Exerc Metab. 2002;12(3):281–93.

16. Guskiewicz KM, Marshall SW, Bailes J, et al. Recurrent concussion and risk of depression in retired professional football players. Med Sci Sports Exerc. 2007;39(6):903–9.

17. Hammond T, Gialloreto C, Kubas H, et al. The prevalence of failure-based depression among elite athletes. Clin J Sport Med. 2013;23:273–7.

18. Huang J-H, Jacobs DF, Deverensky JL, et al. Gambling and health risk behaviors among U.S. college student-athletes: findings from a national study. J Adolesc Health. 2007;10:390–7.

19. Kerr ZY, Thomas LC, Simon JE, et al. Association between history of multiple concussions and health outcomes among former college football players: 15-year follow-up from the NCAA Concussion Study (1999-2001). Am J Sports Med. 2018;46:1733–41.

20. Lindqvist AS, Moberg T, Ehmborg C, et al. Increased mortality rate and suicide in Swedish former elite male athletes in power sports. Scand J Med Sci Sports. 2013:1–6.

21. Proctor SL, Boan-Lenzo C. Prevalence of depressive symptoms in male intercollegiate student-athletes and nonathletes. J Clin Sport Psychol. 2010;4:204–20.

22. Weigand S, Cohen J, Merenstein D. Susceptibility for depression in current and retired student athletes. Sports Health. 2013;5(3):263–6.

23. Wolanin A, Gross M, Hong E. Depression in athletes: prevalence and risk factors. Curr Sports Med Rep. 2015;14(1):56–60.

24. Yang J, Peek-Asa C, Corlette JD, et al. Prevalence of and risk factors associated with symptoms of depression in competitive collegiate student athletes. Clin J Sport Med. 2007;17:481–7.

25. Kiliç Ö, Aoki H, Goedhart E, et al. Severe musculoskeletal time-loss injuries and symptoms of common mental disorders in professional soccer: a longitudinal analysis of 12-month follow-up data. Knee Surg Sports Traumatol Arthrosc. 2018;26(3):946–54. https://doi.org/10.1007/s00167-017-4644-1.

26. Rice SM, Gwyther K, Santesteban-Echarri O, et al. Determinants of anxiety in elite athletes: a systematic review and meta-analysis. Br J Sports Med. 2019;53(11):722–30. https://doi.org/10.1136/bjsports-2019-100620.

27. Ardern CL, Taylor NF, Feller JA, et al. A systematic review of the psychological factors associated with returning to sport following injury. Br J Sports Med. 2013;47:1120–6.

28. Ivarsson A, Johnson U. Psychological factors as predictors of injuries among senior soccer players. A prospective study. J Sports Sci Med. 2010;9:347–52.

29. Ivarsson A, Johnson U, Anderson MB, et al. Psychosocial factors and sport injuries: meta-analyses for prediction and prevention. Sports Med. 2017;47:353–65.

30. Ivarsson A, Johnson U, Lindwall M, et al. Psychosocial stress as a predictor of injury in elite junior soccer: a latent growth curve analysis. J Sci Med Sport. 2014;17(4):366–70.

31. Wiese-Bjornstal DM. Psychology and socioculture affect injury risk, response, and recovery in high-intensity athletes: a consensus statement. Scand J Med Sci Sports. 2010;20(Suppl 2):103–11.

32. Anderson MN, Womble MN, Mohler SA, et al. Preliminary study of fear of re-injury following sport-related concussion in high school sports. Dev Neuropsych. 2019;44(6):443–51.

33. Ivarsson A, Johnson U, Podlog L. Psychological predictors of injury occurrence: a prospective investigation of professional Swedish soccer players. J Sport Rehabil. 2013;22(1):19–26.

34. Iverson GL. Chronic traumatic encephalopathy and risk of suicide in former athletes. Br J Sports Med. 2014;48:162–4.

35. Nippert AH, Smith AM. Psychological stress related to injury and impact on sport performance. Phys Med Rehabil Clin N Am. 2008;19(2):399–418.

36. Gulliver A, Griffiths KM, Mackinnon A, et al. The mental health of Australian elite athletes. J Sci Med Sport. 2015;18:255–61.

37. Forsdyke D, Smith A, Jones M, et al. Psychosocial factors associated with outcomes of sports injury rehabilitation in competitive athletes: a mixed studies systematic review. Br J Sports Med. 2016;50:537–44.

38. Wiese-Bjornstal DM, Smith AM, Shaffer SM, et al. An integrated model of response to sport injury: psychological and sociological dynamics. J Appl Sport Psychol. 1998;10:46–69.

39. Johnson U, Ivarsson A. Psychological predictors of sport injuries among junior soccer players injury prediction in Swedish Soccer. Scand J Med Sci Sports. 2011;21:129–36.

40. Pensgaard AM, Ivarsson A, Nilstad A, et al. Psychosocial stress factors, including the relationship with the coach, and their influence on acute and overuse injury risk in elite female football players. BMJ Open Sport Exerc Med. 2018;4(1):e000317.

41. Ardern CL, Taylor NF, Feller JA, Webster KE. Fear of re-injury in people who have returned to sport following anterior cruciate ligament reconstruction surgery. J Sci Med Sport. 2012;15:488–95. https://doi.org/10.1016/j.jsams.2012.03.015.

42. van der Does HT, Brink MS, Otter RT, Visscher C, Lemmink KA. Injury risk is increased by changes in perceived recovery of team sport players. Clin J Sport Med. 2017;27(1):46–51. https://doi.org/10.1097/JSM.0000000000000306. PMID: 26945309.

43. Kellmann M, Bertollo M, Bosquet L, et al. Recovery and performance in sport: consensus statement. Int J Sports Physiol Perform. 2018;13(2):240–5. https://doi.org/10.1123/ijspp.2017-0759. Epub 2018 Feb 19. PMID: 29345524.

44. Staufenbiel SM, Penninx BW, Spijker AT, Elzinga BM, van Rossum EF. Hair cortisol, stress exposure, and mental health in humans: a systematic review. Psychoneuroendocrinology. 2013;38(8):1220–35. https://doi.org/10.1016/j.psyneuen.2012.11.015. Epub 2012 Dec 17. PMID: 23253896.

45. Burland JP, Toonstra J, Werner JL, et al. Decision to return to sport after anterior cruciate ligament reconstruction, part I: a qualitative investigation of psychosocial factors. J Athl Train. 2018;53(5):452–63.

46. Ardern CL. Anterior cruciate ligament reconstruction-not exactly a one-way ticket back to the preinjury level: a review of contextual factors affecting return to sport after surgery. Sports Health. 2015;7:224–30.

47. Podlog L, Banham SM, Wadey R, et al. Psychological readiness to return to competitive sport following injury: a qualitative study. Sport Psychol. 2015;29:1–14.

48. Gignac MA, Cao X, Ramanathan S, et al. Perceived personal importance of exercise and fears of re-injury: a longitudinal study of psychological factors related to activity after anterior cruciate ligament reconstruction. BMC Sports Sci Med Rehabil. 2015;7:4. http://www.biomedcentral.com/2052-1847/7/4.

49. Glazer DD. Development and preliminary validation of the Injury-Psychological Readiness to Return to Sport (I-PRRS) scale. J Athl Train. 2009;44:185–9.

50. Conti C, di Fronso S, Pivetti M, et al. Well-come back! Professional basketball players perceptions of psychosocial and behavioral factors influencing a return to pre-injury levels. Front Psychol. 2019;8(10):222. https://doi.org/10.3389/fpsyg.2019.00222. PMID: 30800089; PMCID: PMC6375854.

51. Podlog L, Eklund RC. Return to sport after serious injury: a retrospective examination of motivation and psychological outcomes. J Sport Rehabil. 2005;14:20–34. https://doi.org/10.1123/jsr.14.1.20podlog.

52. Ardern CL, Webster KE, Taylor NF, Feller JA. Return to sport following anterior cruciate ligament reconstruction surgery: a system-

atic review and meta-analysis of the state of play. Br J Sport Med. 2011;45:596–606. https://doi.org/10.1177/0363546513489284.

53. Ardern CL, Taylor NF, Feller JA, et al. Psychological responses matter in returning to preinjury level of sport after anterior cruciate ligament reconstruction surgery. Am J Sports Med. 2013;41:1549–58. https://doi.org/10.1177/0363546513489284.

54. Hsu C-J, Meierbachtol A, George SZ, et al. Fear of reinjury in athletes: implications for rehabilitation. 2016;9(2):162–7. https://doi.org/10.1177/1941738116666813.

55. Ardern CL, Österberg A, Tagesson S, et al. The impact of psychological readiness to return to sport and recreational activities after anterior cruciate ligament reconstruction. Br J Sport Med. 2014;48:1613–9. https://doi.org/10.1136/bjsports-2014-093842.

56. Czuppon S, Racette BA, Klein SE, et al. Variables associated with return to sport following anterior cruciate ligament reconstruction: a systematic review. Br J Sports Med. 2014;48:356–64.

57. Flanigan DC, Everhart JS, Glassman AH. Psychological factors affecting rehabilitation and outcomes following elective orthopaedic surgery. J Am Acad Orthop Surg. 2015;23(9):563–70. https://doi.org/10.5435/JAAOS-D-14-00225. Epub 2015 Jul 20. PMID: 26195567.

58. Everhart JS, Best TM, Flanigan DC. Psychological predictors of anterior cruciate ligament reconstruction outcomes: a systematic review. Knee Surg Sports Traumatol Arthrosc. 2015;23(3):752–62. https://doi.org/10.1007/s00167-013-2699-1. Epub 2013 Oct 15. PMID: 24126701.

59. Podlog L, Dimmock J, Miller J. A review of return to sport concerns following injury rehabilitation: practitioner strategies for enhancing recovery outcomes. Phys Ther Sport. 2011;12(1):36–42. https://doi.org/10.1016/j.ptsp.2010.07.005. Epub 2010 Aug 30. PMID: 21256448.

60. Hainline B, Turner JA, Caneiro JP, et al. Pain in elite athletes: neurophysiological, biomechanical and psychosocial considerations: a narrative review. Br J Sports Med. 2017;51:1259–64.

61. Ardern CL, Kvist J, BANG Trial Group. BAck iN the Game (BANG)—a smartphone application to help athletes return to sport following anterior cruciate ligament reconstruction: protocol for a multi-centre, randomised controlled trial. BMC Musculoskelet Disord. 2020;21(1):523 . Published 2020 Aug 8. https://doi.org/10.1186/s12891-020-03508-7.

62. McCrory P, Meeuwisse W, Dvořák J, et al. Consensus statement on concussion in sport-the 5th international conference on concussion in sport held in Berlin, October 2016. Br J Sports Med. 2017;51:838–47.

63. Echemendia RJ, Meeuwisse W, McCrory P, et al. The sport concussion assessment tool 5th edition (SCAT5): background and rationale. Br J Sports Med. 2017;51:848–50.

64. Kontos AP, Covassin T, Elbin RJ, et al. Depression and neurocognitive performance after concussion among male and female high school and collegiate athletes. Arch Phys Med Rehabil. 2012;93:1751–6.

65. Vargas G, Rabinowitz A, Meyer J, et al. Predictors and prevalence of postconcussion depression symptoms in collegiate athletes. J Athl Train. 2015;50:250–5.

66. McDuff DR, Baron D. Substance use in athletics: a sports psychiatry perspective. Clin Sports Med. 2005;24:885–97; Reardon C, Creado S. Drug abuse in athletes. Subst Abus Rehabil. 2014:95–105.

67. Kilic Ö, Hopley P, Kerkhoffs GMMJ, et al. Impact of concussion and severe musculoskeletal injuries on the onset of mental health symptoms in male professional rugby players: a 12-month study. BMJ Open Sport Exerc Med. 2019;5(1):e000693 . Published 2019 Dec 22. https://doi.org/10.1136/bmjsem-2019-000693.

68. Rice SM, Parker AG, Rosenbaum S, et al. Sport-related concussion and mental health outcomes in elite athletes: a systematic review. Sports Med. 2018;48:447–65.

69. Corwin DJ, Zonfrillo MR, Master CL, et al. Characteristics of prolonged concussion recovery in a pediatric subspecialty referral population. J Pediatr. 2014;165:1207–15.

70. Kerr ZY, Marshall SW, Harding HP, et al. Nine-year risk of depression diagnosis increases with increasing self-reported concussions in retired professional football players. Am J Sports Med. 2012;40(10):2206–12.

71. Lange RT, Iverson GL, Rose A. Depression strongly influences postconcussion symptom reporting following mild traumatic brain injury. J Head Trauma Rehabil. 2011;26.

72. Putukian M, Riegler K, Amalfe S, et al. Pre-injury and post-injury factors that predict sport-related concussion and clinical recovery. Clin J Sports Med. 2021;31(1):15–22. https://doi.org/10.1097/JSM.0000000000000705.

73. Garcia GH, Wu HH, Park MJ, et al. Depression symptomatology and anterior cruciate ligament injury: incidence and effect on functional outcome—a prospective cohort study. Am J Sports Med. 2016;44(3):572–9 . Published online Dec 1. https://doi.org/10.1177/0363546515612466.

74. Turner S, Langdon J, Shaver G, et al. Comparison of psychological response between concussion and musculoskeletal injury in collegiate athletes. Sport Exerc Perform Psychol. 2017;6(3):277–88. https://doi.org/10.1037/spy0000099.

75. Wadey R, Evans L, Hanton S, et al. Can preinjury adversity affect postinjury responses? A 5-year prospective, multi-study analysis. Front Psychol. 2019;10:1411. https://doi.org/10.3389/fpsyg.2019.01411.

76. World Health Organization. Novel Coronavirus 2019. https://www.who.int/emergencies/diseases/novel-coronavirus-2019. Accessed 31 May 2020.

77. NCAA: NCAA student-athlete COVID-19 well being study. http://www.ncaa.org/about/resources/research/ncaa-student-athlete-covid-19-well-being-study. Accessed 1 Jun 2020.

78. Reardon CL, Bindra A, Blauwet C, et al. Mental health management of elite athletes during COVID-19: a narrative review and recommendations. Br J Sports Med. 2020:bjsports-2020-102884. https://doi.org/10.1136/bjsports-2020-102884. PMID: 32967853.

79. McGuine TA, Biese KM, Petrovska L, et al. Mental health, physical activity, and quality of life of US adolescent athletes during COVID-19-related school closures and sport cancellations: a study of 13000 athletes. J Athl Train. 2021;56(1):11–9.

80. Truong LK, Mosewich AD, Holt CJ, et al. Psychological, social and contextual factors across recovery stages following a sport-related knee injury: a scoping review. Br J Sports Med. 2020;54:1149–56.

81. Herring SA, Kibler WB, Putukian M. Load, overload, and recovery in the athlete: select issues for the team physician—a consensus statement. Med Sci Sports Exerc. 2019;51(4):821–8. https://doi.org/10.1249/MSS.0000000000001910. PMID: 30882753.

82. Andrade A, Bevilacqua G, Casagrande P, Brandt R, Coimbra D. Sleep quality associated with mood in elite athletes. Phys Sportsmed. 2019;47(3):312–7.

83. Santi G, Pietrantoni L. Psychology of sport injury rehabilitation: a review of models and interventions. J Hum Sport Exerc. 2013;8(4):1029–44.

84. Li C, Ivarsson A, Lam LT, Sun J. Basic psychological needs satisfaction and frustration, stress and sports injury among university athletes: a four-wave prospective study. Front Psychol. 2019;10:665. https://doi.org/10.3389/psyg.2019.00665.

Overtraining Syndrome

Nekisa Haghighat and Todd Stull

Introduction

The elite athlete is no stranger to training volumes of high intensity and duration. The resulting injuries, fatigue, and mental strain are often accepted as part and parcel of the life of an athlete and perhaps even a necessary and expected sacrifice. However, overemphasis on training without adequate rest and recovery can quickly tip the scales toward overtraining at the expense of performance. When the balance between training and recovery remains disrupted over a prolonged period of time, a constellation of adverse health impacts emerges. These manifestations, which include both general medical and mental health symptoms, fall in the spectrum of varying severity and duration, ultimately progressing toward a disorder known as overtraining syndrome if left unchecked.

Historical Background

In 1936, the pioneering endocrinologist Hans Selye conceptualized a stress-driven process that he described as a "general adaptation syndrome," which is typically seen when an organism is damaged by a diverse array of nocuous agents [1]. This response develops over three stages: alarm, resistance, and exhaustion. In the first stage, the organism exhibits a "general alarm reaction" that manifests as a series of hormonal and physiological changes. If the initial insult is continued in relatively small doses or increments, then the organism will build up such resistance that the aforementioned changes are practically reversed by the end of the second stage. However, with continued stress, the organism exhausts this resistance and experiences a return of the initial physiological changes, often more severe and permanent.

N. Haghighat · T. Stull (✉)
Department of Psychiatry and Neuroscience,
University of California Riverside, Riverside, CA, USA
e-mail: nekisa.haghighat@medsch.ucr.edu; todd.stull@ucr.edu

Building upon these observations leads to the broader concepts of allostasis and allostatic load, which supplement the classic notion of homeostasis and stress. Allostasis refers to the process of maintaining stability, or homeostasis, by adapting to a stressor. Mediators of allostasis include stress hormones, such as glucocorticoids and catecholamines, the adrenocortical and autonomic nervous systems, proinflammatory cytokines, and metabolic hormones. Prolonged allostasis takes a toll on the human body, referred to as the allostatic load or the cumulative effect of chronic stress. Allostasis and allostatic load center around the brain as the interpreter of and the responder to environmental challenges and as the target of those challenges [2]. Allosteric changes in the brain—such as increased amygdala activation and atrophy of the hippocampus and prefrontal cortex—mimic the processes seen in depression and anxiety, indicating that maladaptive responses to stress may play a role in the development of these conditions.

Overview of Overtraining Syndrome

Overtraining syndrome (OTS) is a complex clinical disorder most prominent in the athletic population and is recognized in other occupations that demand intensive physical and emotional input in exchange for performance. OTS can be viewed as various outcomes falling in the spectrum or "well-being continuum," as described in the International Olympic Committee's (IOC) consensus statement on load in sport and risk of injury and is further illustrated and expanded upon in Fig. 18.1 [3]. On one end of the spectrum is the optimal state of homeostasis. The physical and psychological load exerted on an athlete can move their health along the continuum, progressing from homeostasis through a series of maladaptive changes that can ultimately lead to illness, injury, or even death on the other end of the spectrum. On the other hand, recovery works as a mutual counteragent that can shift the athlete's physical and psychological well-being back

Fig. 18.1 Overtraining
syndrome continuum

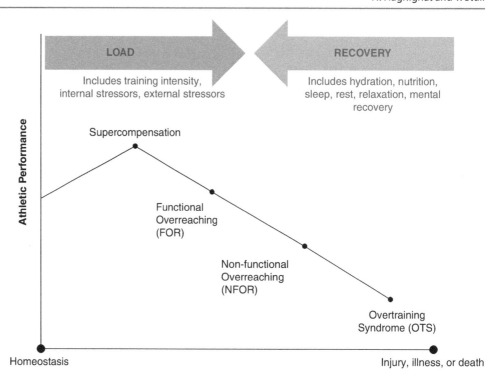

toward homeostasis. The constant push and pull between load and recovery thus determines the athlete's risk of developing one or many of the symptoms that fall under the umbrella of OTS.

Key Terminologies

Discussions revolving around OTS will inevitably utilize a range of different and often overlapping terminologies that vary from region to region. It is therefore important to clarify the key terms that are commonly used in research and clinical practice.

Load and Recovery

The IOC's consensus group broadly defines "load" as a sport and nonsport burden that functions as a stimulus applied to the human biological system, which can range from subcellular biological elements to the individual themselves. This burden encompasses physiological, psychological, and mechanical stressors [3]. Regarding OTS, it should be emphasized that this load includes stressors both within and outside of the sport that can affect the athlete's physical and psychological well-being.

As such, load can be further subdivided into external and internal stressors. "External load" refers to stimuli that are often measured independently of an athlete's internal characteristics. These include the frequency, type, and duration of training or competition, distance traveled, number of repetitions, power output, and other measurements unique to the sport. External load also includes factors outside of training or competition, such as life events and the impact of the sport on personal domains like relationships and academics.

In conjunction with biological and environmental factors, the external load will ultimately lead to physiological and psychological responses that are in turn referred to as the "internal load." Various aspects of the internal load can also be measured, often through objective and subjective tools. These include psychological inventories and scales and measurements of sleep, laboratory data, and vital signs [3].

"Recovery," on the other hand, works in direct opposition to load and can be divided into three essential components: hydration and nutrition, sleep and rest, and relaxation and mental recovery [4, 5]. An athlete who is provided adequate time for recovery and who incorporates these elements into that process lowers their risk for OTS and is more likely to see improvements in performance, rather than stagnation or even diminished performance.

Stages Along the Continuum

An athlete on the optimal end of the training spectrum is one whose training is adequately balanced by recovery, leading to an increase in athletic performance without compromising mental or other aspects of physical stability or homeostasis. Increasing the intensity of training past this point leads to overtraining.

Overtraining—usually undertaken to enhance performance—leads to an accumulation of training load, resulting in a short-term decrement in performance capacity. When provided with an appropriate recovery period, usually a matter of days, the athlete's physiological response can compensate for the training-related stress, leading to enhanced performance compared to baseline levels. This is referred to as "super-compensation." If the initial increase in the training load is not counteracted by an appropriate period of recovery, however, the short-term performance deficit will persist, leading to a state known as "functional overreaching (FOR)."

As overtraining intensity persists, the amount of time required to recover increases from days to weeks or months, as does the duration of the performance deficit. As a result, the athlete progresses from functional to "nonfunctional overreaching (NFOR)," a state of extreme overreaching that leads to stagnation or a decrease in performance that will not recover for several weeks or months. As the training load continues to increase without adequate rest and recovery, the athlete will enter a prolonged state of maladaptation with adverse changes in the markers of performance as well as in biological, neurochemical, and hormonal regulation mechanisms. This is known as overtraining syndrome.

The imbalance between training activity and recovery leads to chronic energy deprivation and inadequate mechanisms for repair and recovery. The body will initially make functional adaptations to restore homeostasis, but these will quickly be exhausted and replaced by maladaptive responses and further energy deprivation. Given the deprived state and low energy availability (EA), the central struggle will be balancing the continued desire to train hard with the reduced ability to do so. Overtraining can occur during all major forms of training, including resistance, anaerobic, aerobic, cognitive, and psychological training [6, 7].

Other Conditions Related to OTS

Overtraining syndrome and its related conditions have been described in athletic populations worldwide, with terminologies differing from region to region. "Unexplained underperformance syndrome (UUPS)" is often used interchangeably with OTS and refers to a persistent, unexplained performance deficit recognized by both the athlete and their trainer despite 2 weeks of relative rest. After a period of heavy training and competition, athletes who develop UUPS typically report fatigue and an unexpected sense of effort during continued training. In addition, they may experience frequent minor infections, stiff or sore muscles, disturbances in mood and sleep quality, and loss of energy, appetite, competitive drive, and libido [8].

"Burnout syndrome in athletes (BSA)" is a condition experienced by athletes who lose energy and the motivation to continue their training regimens. Athletes with BSA experience three central characteristics: emotional and physical exhaustion, a reduced sense of accomplishment, and sport devaluation. Psychological symptoms include negative self-talk, deterioration of interpersonal relationships, behavioral issues, and decreased performance. Physical symptoms often manifest as headaches, insomnia, fatigue, diminished appetite, and an increased rate of infections. The psychological and general physical impact of BSA unsurprisingly shares many commonalities and often overlaps with OTS.

Incidence and Prevalence of OTS

The lack of standardized diagnostic criteria for identifying OTS makes it challenging to assess the exact prevalence and incidence of the syndrome. Nevertheless, the current literature suggests that OTS is becoming more widely recognized and studied, with the prevalence estimated at 20–60% in elite athletes [6]. Earlier studies have evaluated the more general concept of training with insufficient rest, which was estimated to occur in 7–20% of athletes per training cycle with a higher risk among elite runners (60%) compared to lower-level runners (38%) [9]. The lifetime risk of OTS amongst runners is estimated to be 64% and 60% for males and females, respectively [10].

What is more, athletes who have previously experienced OTS are more likely to relapse. For example, one study found that 91% of college swimmers who experienced OTS during their freshman year had a repeat episode the following year, compared to an incidence of 34% among swimmers who had not experienced an initial episode of OTS as a freshman [11].

Even higher rates of OTS and related syndromes have been reported in other studies, but these are likely inflated due to the overlapping definitions of FOR, NFOR, and OTS/UUPS. Nevertheless, it is important to consider the widespread prevalence of these conditions, given the shared symptomatology and fluidity between these stages on the well-being continuum.

Theories Related to the Etiology of OTS

Multiple overlapping theories attempt to explain the etiology of OTS, ranging from classic theories focusing on neurochemical pathways to the more modern viewpoint of paradoxical deconditioning syndrome. The classic theories are based on an imbalance between training and recovery and can be confounded by variables such as inadequate nutrition, illness, psychosocial stressors, and sleep issues. These variables can lead to dysfunctions in immune response, inflammation, neurological function, hormone signaling, and metabolic systems. Despite the varied symptomatology and presentation of OTS, most theories seek to explain the etiology of the core features of OTS, including decreased physical performance, fatigue, and disrupted mood, sleep, and behavior.

Most classic theories postulate that different levels of amino acids and neurotransmitters play a role in OTS development. For example, the neurotransmitter serotonin (5-hydroxytryptamine, 5-HT) is a well-established regulator of mood, sleep, and behavior and is therefore implicated in the etiology of OTS as part of the "central fatigue hypothesis." In the brain, 5-HT is derived from tryptophan. Prolonged exercise increases the plasma levels of unbound or free tryptophan (F-TRP), leading to increased tryptophan uptake and 5-HT synthesis in the brain. Increased 5-HT, in turn, has been linked to feelings of lethargy and fatigue in humans [12, 13].

Meanwhile, exercise naturally leads to depletion of muscle glycogen stores, as glycogen is one of the primary sources of energy during prolonged exercise. Therefore, the "glycogen depletion hypothesis" proposes that diminished glycogen levels cause muscle fatigue and resulting impairments in athletic performance—one of the hallmarks of OTS. Furthermore, decreased glycogen stimulates the oxidation of branched-chain amino acids (BCAAs) to glucose in order to increase immediately available energy sources. The subsequent decrease in plasma BCAAs plays into the central fatigue hypothesis, as F-TRP and BCAAs use and compete for the same transport mechanism to cross the blood–brain barrier. In addition, an increased plasma F-TRP to BCAA ratio further increases tryptophan uptake into the brain and is an important determinant of the rate of 5-HT synthesis [6, 13, 14]. In addition, prolonged or high-intensity exercise has been shown to transiently decrease the levels of glutamine, which is integral for immune cell function. Therefore, the "glutamine hypothesis" theorizes that exercise-induced glutamine depletion may account for the increased rate of upper respiratory infections seen in OTS [15].

Other theories point to inflammation, cytokine release, and oxidative stress as the sources of muscle damage, fatigue, and increased susceptibility to infections seen in OTS. A baseline level of oxidative stress is expected during exercise, as the reactive oxygen species released by the damaged muscle cells facilitate cellular repair. The "oxidative stress hypothesis," however, postulates that excessive oxidative stress can become pathological. High levels of reactive oxygen species cause inflammation, muscle fatigue, and soreness, resulting in decreased athletic performance [16, 17]. In a similar vein, the "cytokine hypothesis" proposes that dam-

aged tissues elicit a local inflammatory response that involves the recruitment of cytokines. With adequate recovery, this inflammation can work to improve muscle strength and tissue healing. However, continued training in the absence of adequate recovery can amplify this response into a state of systemic inflammation. Persistent elevations in proinflammatory cytokines contribute to CNS and peripheral fatigue as well as negative changes in hormonal and metabolic functions [18–21].

Still other theories illustrate the role that different hormonal and nervous systems have in the dysregulation and maladaptive responses implicated in OTS. The "autonomic nervous system hypothesis" proposes that an imbalance in the autonomic nervous system accounts for some of the psychological and general physical symptoms of OTS, including fatigue, apathy, performance inhibitions, depression, and bradycardia [6, 22]. Various forms of negative feedback may cause this and sympathetic inhibition, resulting in surges of catecholamine release, increased metabolism, and elevated core temperatures during heavy exercise [23]. Similarly, the "hypothalamic hypothesis" attempts to elucidate the role of the hypothalamic–pituitary–adrenal (HPA) axis in the hormonal dysregulation seen in OTS, as evidenced by the alterations in key hormones such as cortisol, adrenocorticotropic hormone (ACTH), testosterone, growth hormone (GH), and prolactin in overtrained athletes [24, 25].

Evaluation and Diagnosis of OTS

Athletes affected by OTS will most often initially present with vague reports of unexplained underperformance. A thorough history will often reveal descriptions of persistently decreased athletic performance despite weeks to months of recovery and disturbances in mood. The athlete may express that they feel they need to exert considerably more effort during training or competition. They may also report a wide range of mood-related symptoms, including irritability, diminished motivation, depressed mood, and difficulty concentrating or cooperating with others. Athletes may notice changes in their sleep patterns with resulting feelings of persistent fatigue or daytime sleepiness. Finally, they may experience somatic complaints, including persistent muscle soreness or stiffness, recurrent overuse injuries, unexplained weight loss, or frequent illnesses such as upper respiratory infections.

General Medical and Psychiatric Evaluation

Athletes presenting with any of the symptoms mentioned above should undergo a thorough general medical and mental health evaluation, as OTS is often considered a diagnosis of exclusion. In particular, the clinician should gain a nuanced understanding of the athlete's training program, including any recent changes in frequency, duration, or intensity of training and the presence or absence of dedicated time for adequate sleep and recovery.

Initial laboratory tests should include a complete blood count, basic metabolic panel, ferritin level, and thyroid-stimulating hormone level. A monospot test may be indicated if the history suggests infectious mononucleosis, whereas an elevated resting heart rate warrants an electrocardiogram. Longitudinal screening tests or logs that assess changes in sleep, nutrition, weight, or mood are also helpful in evaluating symptoms over time. Any additional data obtained through the athlete's training program, such as training logs, reactive strength index, force plate data, counter jump data, or catapult data, could also provide more objective assessments.

Differential Diagnosis

The signs and symptoms of OTS span a wide range of mental and other physical symptoms that can mimic common or uncommon disorders seen in the typical sport population. The most immediate causes of general fatigue should be considered first, including insomnias and other sleep disturbances, nutritional deficiencies, anemia, and primary mental health disorders such as depression, generalized anxiety, and eating disorders. From a systems-based perspective, the differential diagnosis should include endocrine disorders such as hypothyroidism, diabetes mellitus, or adrenocortical insufficiency or excess, and cardiopulmonary conditions such as cardiomyopathies, congenital or acquired heart disease, and chronic pulmonary disease. Neurological conditions that should be considered include post-concussive syndromes as well as neuromuscular disorders. Infectious processes should also be included in the differential, such as post-viral syndromes, infectious mononucleosis, respiratory infections, hepatitis, and human immunodeficiency virus. A thorough psychosocial history must be conducted and should screen for drug-related conditions such as substance misuse and medication side effects and environmental and social stressors, such as interpersonal issues, major life events, and excessive cognitive demands like work or study hours.

Testing

At present, there is little evidence to support the use of biochemical, immunological, or hormonal testing to diagnose OTS. Laboratory tests help rule out other disorders on the differential, but OTS remains primarily a clinical diagnosis of exclusion. There is better evidence to support the use of questionnaires or other scales, especially to monitor progression and recovery during OTS. One commonly used scale is the Borg Rating of Perceived Exertion (RPE), which measures an individual's effort and exertion, breathlessness, and fatigue during a workout, indicating the intensity of a training activity [26]. An overtrained athlete may report higher RPE while simultaneously exhibiting decreased athletic performance.

Another more comprehensive tool to assess for the early indicators of OTS is the Profile of Mood States (POMS) questionnaire, a 65-item survey with six subscales that assess mood disturbances, including tension, depression, anger, vigor, fatigue, and confusion [27]. The Recovery-Stress Questionnaire for Athletes (RESTQ-Sport) is another useful scale that measures the frequency of current stress along with the frequency of recovery-associated activities. The 76-item scale also contains several subscales that explore general as well as sport-specific stress and recovery [28]. These various measures can help identify early OTS signs and monitor progression, but they are not specific to OTS. Nevertheless, they can be used in conjunction with one another and alongside a thorough history and diagnostic workup to gain a better understanding of OTS as well as an athlete's projected recovery.

Mental Health Diagnoses Associated with OTS

A complicated interplay exists between an athlete's mental health and other aspects of their physical health regardless of the presence or absence of OTS. These interactions between psychological and physiological factors account for the varied characteristics of OTS and related conditions. OTS and comorbid mental health disorders are not mutually exclusive. They can coexist, cause, exacerbate, or be mistaken for one another. Furthermore, many mental health disorders initially present during young adulthood, coinciding with the period when athletes are most likely to strive toward the peak of their athletic training. These considerations further emphasize the importance of a thorough mental health evaluation in athletes in general and in those suspected to be experiencing OTS in particular. The most common mental health diagnoses associated with OTS include mood disorders such as major depressive disorder (MDD) or chronic persistent depressive disorder, substance use disorders, disordered eating and sleep, anxiety, and trauma-related disorders.

Depressive Spectrum in Sport

Currie et al.'s view of the interplay between depression and sport presents depressive symptoms on a spectrum, with normal mood progressing toward a depressive illness [29].

Normal mood can be sustained by sporting activities, not just the physical activity itself but also additional elements that can improve mild depressive symptoms, such as interconnectedness, social support, and regular routines. As depressive symptoms increase, due to a primary depressive disorder or overtraining that can no longer be mitigated by the benefits of sport, the athlete may progress toward an overt depressive illness. Symptoms can manifest as major depressive disorder (MDD) or severe underrecovery and overtraining that mimics MDD.

Briefly, the signs and symptoms of MDD include depressed mood, anhedonia, changes in sleep, appetite, or weight, impaired concentration, fatigue or diminished energy, feelings of guilt, worthlessness, hopelessness, psychomotor changes, and suicidal thoughts or feelings. Most studies investigating depression among athletes have been conducted with collegiate-level athletes and have found the prevalence to range from 15.6% to 21%, with female athletes at a higher risk [30].

The association between physical activity and mood is widely acknowledged and studied. Current evidence indicates that, on average, moderate exercise improves mood, whereas intense exercise may lead to its deterioration. Mood disturbances are a valuable early indicator of OTS. More than 70% of athletes with NFOR and OTS reported emotional disturbances, indicating that athletes often detect early signs of overreaching by themselves before it is brought to the attention of trainers or health-care providers, making it all the more important to listen to the athlete when they begin to indicate that something is wrong [31]. One of the most meaningful comparisons of OTS and MDD is the athlete's avoidance and outright denial of each diagnosis. In both illnesses, the afflicted person tends to reject the implications of loss of control, diminished vitality, and inadequate coping skills. When in this state of denial, athletes tend to work harder to overcome their inadequacies, leading to more severe symptoms and dysfunction [32].

Other commonalities between OTS and depression include a lack of recovery from training, reduced performance, and chronic maladaptive responses. In addition to shared symptomatology, OTS and depression are characterized by remarkably similar changes in brain structures, neurotransmitters, endocrine pathways, and immune responses, suggesting similar origins. Perhaps the only apparent difference between the disorders is the manner in which dysfunction manifests and the athlete recuperates. The overtrained athlete will mostly suffer from deficits in athletic performance, which may recover with prolonged rest. The depressed athlete, however, will experience social, cognitive, and work-related dysfunction and will often feel worse with rest [32]. Similar to depressive disorders, anxiety and trauma-related disorders also overlap with OTS and should be screened for on initial history. Like OTS, anxiety and trauma disorders interfere with sleep, disrupt the autonomic nervous system, and cause impairments in energy, endurance, reaction time, and coordination, resulting in impaired athletic performances.

Disordered Eating: Female Athlete Triad Versus Relative Energy Deficiency in Sport

In 2005, the IOC released a since-updated consensus statement defining the female athlete triad as the widely recognized combination of disordered eating and irregular menstrual cycles among female athletes, leading to decreased endogenous estrogen and, in turn, low bone mineral density [33]. In 2007, the American College of Sports Medicine updated the definition of the triad to refer to the relationship between three interrelated components: energy availability (EA), menstrual function, and bone health [34]. Since then, a growing body of literature has further expanded our understanding of the triad and has reframed the condition as a relative energy deficiency resulting from an imbalance between dietary energy intake (EI) and the energy expenditure required to support homeostasis, health, and the activities of daily living, growth, and sporting activities. When viewed in this framework, it is clear that the triad can affect all genders, necessitating the introduction of a more comprehensive, broader term for the overall syndrome. As such, the IOC released an updated consensus statement in 2014 that goes beyond the female athlete triad to explore the newly coined relative energy deficiency in sport (RED-S). The statement defines RED-S as an impaired physiological function including, but not limited to, the metabolic rate, menstrual function, bone health, immunity, protein synthesis, and cardiovascular health caused by relative energy deficiency. Athletes affected by RED-S may experience impaired self-body image, low self-esteem, decreased muscle strength or endurance, impaired coordination, and a depleted fuel source—symptoms that overlap with OTS.

Sleep and Mental Health

The role of insomnia and other forms of disrupted sleep in OTS is complicated, as poor sleep can be a symptom, cause, or comorbidity of OTS. Inadequate or disrupted sleep is associated with many mental health disorders, including depressive and trauma-related disorders. Problems with sleep can lead to increased rates of injuries and infections, magnified perceived effort, reduced time to exhaustion and task failure, and impaired coordination and reaction time. Athletes with poor sleep often have hormonal imbalances, inflammation, immune dysfunction, and impaired emotional control and impulsivity, leading to problems on and off the field. Disentangling sleep disorders from OTS and related symptoms is inherently difficult and potentially unnecessary, as improving sleep should be a primary goal in improving an athlete's health, performance, and general well-being [35].

Substance Use Disorders

Substance use, misuse, and use disorders can also cause behavioral and physical disturbances that mimic OTS. It is important to note that this consideration is not just limited to illicit substances alone but also includes prescription medications, anabolic steroids, caffeine, supplements, or other substances that may otherwise be considered benign substances but can significantly impair athletic performance. A substance use disorder is a compulsive pattern of substance use that leads to loss of control, cravings, and negative consequences related to the personal and professional aspects of life. Regardless of the presence or absence of a substance use disorder, an athlete's addictive behavior—such as a relentless commitment to sustained and excessive training—can in and of itself cause OTS. Such behavior may be interpreted as a form of self-harm or a maladaptive attempt to communicate internal distress [36–38].

Treatment and Prevention of OTS

The most critical step in the treatment and management of OTS is to correctly identify the syndrome in the first place and the specific stressors that may be contributing to its etiology. A thorough history and diagnostic workup are critical to treating underlying disorders, including primary mental health disorders. Treatment of FOR is the most straightforward and involves balancing overload training with appropriate recovery, which typically amounts to a few days and minimal sacrifices in training. Rest and recovery are also the mainstays of treatment in NFO and OTS, though for prolonged periods that may require more disruptive sacrifices in training, such as missing competitions or delaying training cycles.

Given the significant role of mental health in the etiology, progression, and manifestation of OTS, referral to a mental health provider would be beneficial. First, however, it is vital to build a rapport with the athlete, listen to their concerns, and understand their perceptions. As previously mentioned, OTS and mental health disorders are commonly rejected diagnoses, so emphasis should be placed on reducing the stigma, accepting help, and referring to the appropriate mental health provider.

Recovery and prevention of OTS rely heavily on monitoring and adjusting the training load. Using scales such as the RPE, POMS, or REST-Q helps provide a more objective measure of the progress and assessment of interventions. Observation of the training load, effective use of performance measures, and utilization of mood questionnaires can interrupt the progression from FO to NFO and OTS [6, 7, 39]. Education also plays a crucial role in the prevention of OTS. Athletes and trainers alike should be aware that the initial signs of overreaching include feeling the need to increase training to compensate for decreased performance. Another warning sign is an increased rating of perceived exertion for a given workload, which can be screened early using the RPE.

Conclusions

Overtraining syndrome is a nebulous clinical diagnosis complicated by many overlapping syndromes, a multifactorial etiology, and an ever-changing terminology. The hallmarks of OTS include decreased athletic performance in the setting of increased training intensity without appropriate recovery, often accompanied by changes in mood, motivation, and general medical health. OTS represents a maladaptive response to an imbalance between exercise and recovery. It is mediated by complex neurohormonal processes and affects multiple domains of well-being, including mental health and other aspects of physical health. A thorough history is crucial in identifying OTS, as there are limited laboratory tests or diagnostic evaluations that can aid in its diagnosis—though these are important in ruling out other illnesses. Validated scales, such as the RPE, POMS, and REST-Q, can be utilized to screen for early signs of OTS and to adjust the training load and monitor recovery, which are the mainstays of the treatment of OTS. Finally, it is crucial to listen to the athlete, who is often the first to realize the warning signs of OTS. The apparently growing incidence of OTS and mental health disorders in athletes, coupled with the potentially irreversible psychological, professional, and social consequences, makes prevention, early identification, and effective management crucial in ensuring the health and well-being of the athlete.

References

1. Selye H. A syndrome produced by diverse nocuous agents. Nature. 1936;138(3479):32.
2. McEwen BS. Allostasis and allostatic load: implications for neuropsychopharmacology. Neuropsychopharmacology. 2000;22(2):108–24.
3. Soligard T, Schwellnus M, Alonso J-M, Bahr R, Clarsen B, Dijkstra HP, et al. How much is too much? (Part 1) International Olympic Committee consensus statement on load in sport and risk of injury. Br J Sports Med. 2016;50(17):1030–41.
4. Kenttä G, Hassmén P. Overtraining and recovery. Sports Med. 1998;26(1):1–16.

5. Chang C, Putukian M, Aerni G, Diamond A, Hong G, Ingram Y, et al. Mental health issues and psychological factors in athletes: detection, management, effect on performance and prevention: American Medical Society for Sports Medicine Position Statement—executive summary. Br J Sports Med. 2020;54(4):216–20.

6. Kreher JB, Schwartz JB. Overtraining syndrome: a practical guide. Sports Health. 2012;4(2):128–38.

7. Meeusen R, Duclos M, Gleeson M, Rietjens G, Steinacker J, Urhausen A. Prevention, diagnosis and treatment of the overtraining syndrome: ECSS position statement 'task force'. Eur J Sport Sci. 2006;6(01):1–14.

8. Budgett R, Newsholme E, Lehmann M, Sharp C, Jones D, Jones T, et al. Redefining the overtraining syndrome as the unexplained underperformance syndrome. Br J Sports Med. 2000;34(1):67–8.

9. Morgan WP, O'Connor P, Sparling P, Pate R. Psychological characterization of the elite female distance runner. Int J Sports Med. 1987;8(S 2):S124–S31.

10. Morgan WP, O'Connor PJ, Ellickson KA, Bradley PW. Personality structure, mood states, and performance in elite male distance runners. Int J Sport Psychol. 1988;19(4):247–63.

11. Raglin J. Overtraining and staleness-psychometric monitoring of endurance athletes. In: Handbook of research on sports psychology; 1993.

12. Young S. The clinical psychopharmacology of tryptophan. In: Nutrition and the brain (USA); 1986.

13. Mittleman KD, Ricci MR, Bailey SP. Branched-chain amino acids prolong exercise during heat stress in men and women. Med Sci Sports Exerc. 1998;30(1):83–91.

14. Fernstrom JD. Dietary precursors and brain neurotransmitter formation. Annu Rev Med. 1981;32(1):413–25.

15. Mackinnon LT, Hooper SL. Plasma glutamine and upper respiratory tract infection during intensified training in swimmers. Med Sci Sports Exerc. 1996;28(3):285–90.

16. Tanskanen M, Atalay M, Uusitalo A. Altered oxidative stress in overtrained athletes. J Sports Sci. 2010;28(3):309–17.

17. Tiidus PM. Radical species in inflammation and overtraining. Can J Physiol Pharmacol. 1998;76(5):533–8.

18. Carfagno DG, Hendrix JC. Overtraining syndrome in the athlete: current clinical practice. Curr Sports Med Rep. 2014;13(1):45–51.

19. Robson PJ. Elucidating the unexplained underperformance syndrome in endurance athletes. Sports Med. 2003;33(10):771–81.

20. Smith LL. Cytokine hypothesis of overtraining: a physiological adaptation to excessive stress? Med Sci Sports Exerc. 2000;32(2):317.

21. Smith LL. Overtraining, excessive exercise, and altered immunity. Sports Med. 2003;33(5):347–64.

22. Lehmann M, Foster C, Dickhuth H-H, Gastmann U. Autonomic imbalance hypothesis and overtraining syndrome. Med Sci Sports Exerc. 1998;30(7):1140–5.

23. Lehmann M, Foster C, Keul J. Overtraining in endurance athletes: a brief review. Med Sci Sports Exerc. 1993;25(7):854–62.

24. Cadegiani FA, Kater CE. Hormonal response to a non-exercise stress test in athletes with overtraining syndrome: results from the endocrine and metabolic responses on overtraining syndrome (EROS)—EROS-STRESS. J Sci Med Sport. 2018;21(7):648–53.

25. Kindermann W, Urhausen A. Diagnosis of overtraining what tools do we have. Rev Sports Med. 2002;32(2):95–102.

26. Williams N. The Borg rating of perceived exertion (RPE) scale. Occup Med. 2017;67(5):404–5.

27. Berger BG, Motl RW. Exercise and mood: a selective review and synthesis of research employing the profile of mood states. J Appl Sport Psychol. 2000;12(1):69–92.

28. Kellmann M, Kallus KW. Recovery-stress questionnaire for athletes: user manual. Human Kinetics; 2001.

29. Currie A, Arcelus J, Plateau C. Eating disorders. In: Currie A, Owen B, editors. Sports psychiatry. Oxford: OUP; 2016.

30. Wolanin A, Gross M, Hong E. Depression in athletes: prevalence and risk factors. Curr Sports Med Rep. 2015;14(1):56–60.

31. Birrer D, Lienhard D, Williams C, Röthlin P, Morgan G. Prevalence of non-functional overreaching and the overtraining syndrome in Swiss elite athletes. Schweizerische Zeitschrift für Sportmedizin und Sporttraumatologie. 2013;61(4):23–9.

32. Schwenk TL. The stigmatisation and denial of mental illness in athletes. Br J Sports Med. 2000;34(1):4–5.

33. Drinkwater B, Loucks A, Sherman R, Sundgot-Borgen J, Thompson R. International Olympic Committee (IOC) consensus statement on the female athlete triad. 2005.

34. Thomas DT, Erdman KA, Burke LM. American college of sports medicine joint position statement. Nutrition and athletic performance. Med Sci Sports Exerc. 2016;48(3):543–68.

35. Kroshus E, Wagner J, Wyrick D, Athey A, Bell L, Benjamin HJ, et al. Wake up call for collegiate athlete sleep: narrative review and consensus recommendations from the NCAA Interassociation Task Force on Sleep and Wellness. Br J Sports Med. 2019;53(12):731–6. https://doi.org/10.1136/bjsports-2019-100590.

36. Peluso MAM, Andrade LHSG. Physical activity and mental health: the association between exercise and mood. Clinics. 2005;60:61–70.

37. Souter G, Lewis R, Serrant L. Men, mental health and elite sport: a narrative review. Sports Med Open. 2018;4(1):1–8.

38. Ströhle A. Sports psychiatry: mental health and mental disorders in athletes and exercise treatment of mental disorders. Eur Arch Psychiatry Clin Neurosci. 2019;269(5):485–98.

39. Morgan W, Brown D, Raglin J, O'connor P, Ellickson K. Psychological monitoring of overtraining and staleness. Br J Sports Med. 1987;21(3):107–14.

Transitioning out of Elite Sport

Vincent Gouttebarge

Introduction

Mental health symptoms are commonly reported by elite athletes during their career, with prevalence rates ranging from 19% for alcohol misuse to 34% for anxiety/depression [1, 2]. The scientific literature as well as many anecdotal reports suggest that elite athletes are also likely to report mental health symptoms once they retire from their sport. Transitioning out of elite sport is indeed not easy as it is likely to have a behavioral and emotional impact on former elite athletes. During the transitioning process, elite athletes might face several challenges such as adjusting to a new life and lifestyle, being suddenly "like everyone else," or missing the sport atmosphere and competition. Depending on how well they cope with these challenges, former elite athletes might report mental health symptoms. This chapter focuses on these mental health symptoms (self-reported and not clinically diagnosed) that might occur after transitioning out of elite sport.

Occurrence of Mental Health Symptoms in Former Elite Athletes

Scientific information about the mental health symptoms occurring in the context of elite sports remains scarce. This is even more the case for the group of former athletes who might have struggled during transitioning out of elite sport. In the past two decades, a limited number of quantitative studies reporting the occurrence of mental health symptoms among former elite athletes were published, looking especially at symptoms of psychological distress, anxiety, depression, sleep disturbance, substance misuse, and disordered eating (Table 19.1). The available scientific evidence suggests that former elite athletes report mental health symptoms nearly as often as do active elite athletes or the general population [1, 2].

The prevalence of distress symptoms was shown to range between 9% and 39% among former elite athletes (mean age: 34–62 years; mostly male) from team sports (American football, cricket, football, ice hockey, rugby) and combined Olympic sports [3–10]. Recently, a cross-sectional study has found a 26% prevalence of distress symptoms among retired professional footballers, while a prospective cohort study showed that its 12-month incidence was 13% among Dutch former elite athletes (mean age: 50 years; various Olympic sports) [11, 12].

Symptoms of depression were reported by 15–42% of former American football players (mean age: 53–62 years), whereas symptoms of anxiety were experienced by 33% of former American ice hockey players (mean age: 57 years) [13–16]. The prevalence of anxiety/depression symptoms (not differentiated) ranged between 16% and 39% among

Table 19.1 Prevalence of mental health symptoms among former elite athletes from various sport disciplines

	Distress	Anxiety/depression	Sleep disturbance	Adverse alcohol use
Cricket	26	24	21	22
Football	9–18	19–39	11–28	8–32
Handball	16	16	12	7
Ice hockey	12	19	17	29
Olympic sports	18	29	22	27
Rugby	25	28	29	24

V. Gouttebarge (✉)
Department of Orthopedic Surgery and Sports Medicine, Amsterdam University Medical Centers, Amsterdam, The Netherlands
e-mail: v.gouttebarge@amsterdamumc.nl

former elite athletes (mean age: 34–51 years; mostly male) from team sports (American football, cricket, football, ice hockey, rugby) and combined Olympic sports [4, 6–10]. Recently, a cross-sectional study has found an 11% and 13% prevalence of anxiety and depression symptoms, respectively, among retired professional footballers, while a prospective cohort study showed that the 12-month incidence of anxiety/depression symptoms (not differentiated) was 28% among Dutch former elite athletes (mean age: 50 years; various Olympic sports) [11, 12].

The prevalence of sleep disturbance was shown to range between 11% and 29% among former elite athletes (mean age: 34–62 years; mostly male) from team sports (American football, cricket, football, ice hockey, rugby) and combined Olympic sports [4, 6–10]. Recently, a cross-sectional study has found a 33% prevalence of sleep disturbance among retired professional footballers, while a prospective cohort study showed that its 12-month incidence was 15% among Dutch former elite athletes (mean age: 50 years; various Olympic sports) [11, 12].

When it comes to substance misuse, the consumption of alcohol has been the most studied. The prevalence of alcohol misuse ranged from 6% to 32% among former elite athletes (mean age: 34–62 years; mostly male) from team sports (American football, cricket, football, ice hockey, rugby) and combined Olympic sports [4, 6–10]. Recently, a cross-sectional study conducted among retired professional footballers has found a 69% prevalence of alcohol misuse and a 10% prevalence of substance misuse [12]. A recent prospective cohort study has shown that the 12-month incidence of alcohol misuse was 7% among Dutch former elite athletes (mean age: 50 years; various Olympic sports) [11].

Disordered eating is commonly reported by former elite athletes from various Olympic sports, with prevalence rates reaching up to 27% [7]. Recently, a cross-sectional study has found a 40% prevalence of disordered eating among retired professional footballers, while a prospective cohort study showed that its 12-month incidence was 20% among Dutch former elite athletes (mean age: 50 years; various Olympic sports) [11, 12].

The Etiology of Mental Health Symptoms in Former Elite Athletes

The occurrence of mental health symptoms in elite sport is likely to be multifactorial and is the consequence of the interaction between psychosocial and sport-related stressors [2, 17, 18]. In former elite athletes, stressors related to an elite sport career might have long-term consequences, while transitioning out of elite sport might lead to mental health symp-

toms. In addition, former elite athletes are as any human being likely to report mental health symptoms as a consequence of psychosocial stressors.

Psychosocial Stressors

As indicated in the biopsychosocial model, biological (genetic, biochemical, etc.), psychological (mood, personality, behavior, etc.), and social (cultural, familial, socioeconomic, etc.) stressors, combined with adverse life events (e.g., death of a family member, relationship problem) and/or a particular vulnerability due to predisposition (e.g., genetic, personality, history), play a role in the occurrence of mental health symptoms (as well as other physical health problems) [17]. In former professional footballers, previous adverse life events were associated with a higher risk of mental health symptoms [3, 4]. A prospective cohort study showed that former professional footballers exposed to recent adverse life events were two to four times more likely to report mental health symptoms than were former players with no adverse life events [19]. Similar associations were found among former professional rugby players and former Dutch elite athletes [5, 7].

Stressors Related to an Elite Sport Career

Stressors related to a sports career might have long-term consequences on the mental health of former elite athletes. In former professional footballers, severe musculoskeletal injuries and subsequent surgeries occurring during a football career were associated with a higher risk of mental health symptoms [3, 4]. A similar association was found in Olympic sport disciplines: former Dutch elite athletes exposed to a higher number of severe injuries and/or surgeries were up to seven times more likely to report mental health symptoms by comparison to those less or unexposed [7]. Some scientific literature suggests that sports career-related concussions might lead, in the long term, to mental health symptoms among former elite athletes [20]. Retired professional American football players reporting three or more previous concussions were found to be three times more likely to be diagnosed with depression compared with those with no history of concussion [21]. Former professional athletes from football, ice hockey, and rugby who reported a history of six or more concussions were approximately up to five times more likely to report mental health symptoms [22]. Sport career dissatisfaction was shown to have long-term consequences as well: former Dutch elite athletes who were dissatisfied about their sports career were up to six times more likely to report mental health symptoms by comparison to those satisfied with their sports career [7]. A similar association was found among former professional rugby players [5].

Stressors Related to the Transition out of Elite Sport

Transitioning out of elite sport can be an impactful period for many athletes as they might be exposed to various stressors and challenges, among which include adjusting to a new life and lifestyle, being suddenly "like everyone else," or missing the sport atmosphere and competition [2]. This period is even more challenging for athletes forced to retire as they are more likely to report mental health symptoms by comparison to those who planned their time to transition out of sport. Former professional rugby players who were forced to retire (e.g., because of experiencing a career-ending injury) were more than twice as likely to report symptoms of distress in comparison to those who retired voluntarily [6]. In former professional footballers, employment status as well as a higher number of working hours were correlated with symptoms of distress and anxiety/depression (employment and more working hours associated with less distress) [23]. These findings confirm that combining an elite sport career with sustainable attention to education and career planning is important, while preparing for retirement from elite sport can ease athletes' transition and positively impact their well-being [2].

Duty of Care in Elite Sport

As stated by the World Health Organization (WHO) and the International Labour Organization (ILO), "protection, promotion, surveillance and maintenance of the highest degree of physical, mental and social well-being of workers in all occupations long after they enter their retirement years" is a fundamental human right that should be facilitated by social partners and stakeholders [24]. Therefore, stakeholders in elite sport have a duty to care, protect, and promote the long-term health of athletes. In professional football and rugby, an After Career Consultation was developed in order to empower the sustainable physical, mental, and social health and the quality of life of retired professional football and rugby players [25–27]. Analogously, an "exit health examination" focusing, among other things, on mental health should be developed and implemented in the context of elite sports. This could ease the process of transitioning out of elite sport, with clinicians playing a significant role in the

athletes' care and guidance. This role of clinicians might be even more relevant to former elite athletes at risk for mental health symptoms, especially those who were forced to transition out of their sport.

Clinicians' Role

Clinicians have an important role to play when elite athletes are transitioning out of sport, as they are likely to report mental health symptoms. Clinicians should screen elite athletes for mental health symptoms (and disorders) at the start of (and during) the transitioning process, as this will allow them to facilitate timely management and care for any identified mental health condition. Clinicians should also provide transitioning elite athletes with guidance toward the prevention of mental health symptoms.

The International Olympic Committee (IOC) Mental Health Working Group has developed the IOC Sport Mental Health Assessment Tool 1 (SMHAT-1) in order to assess elite athletes potentially at risk for or already experiencing mental health symptoms and disorders [28]. Relying on a three-step approach (step 1: triage; step 2: screening; and step 3: intervention and (re)assessment), the SMHAT-1 (Fig. 19.1) ideally should be used when any significant event for elite athletes occurs, including transitioning out of sport [28]. Subsequently, and if necessary, the management and care of elite athletes transitioning out of sport and reporting mental health symptoms should be facilitated in a timely manner. Generic approaches are available in order to manage mental health symptoms among former elite athletes, with such approaches including improvement in mental health literacy (through psychoeducation), physical activity, psychotherapy, and pharmacological treatment [2, 29]. It is worth mentioning that both mental health literacy (psychoeducation) and physical activity should be considered by clinicians as types of guidance for transitioning elite athletes that may prevent mental health symptoms.

Mental health literacy is defined as the cognitive and social skills that determine the motivation and ability of individuals to gain access to, understand, and use information in ways that promote and maintain good mental health [30]. This has come to include concepts related to the knowledge of effective self-management strategies, challenging the mental disorder stigma, awareness and use of mental health first aid to assist others, and the facilitation of help-seeking behaviors [30]. Such an organized process of disseminating balanced and evidence-based information about a medical condition to patients and their entourage (e.g., family, friends, colleagues) is an essential element of nearly all types

SMHAT-1

The Internationl Olympic Committee Sport Mental Health Assessment Tool 1

DEVELOPED BY THE IOC MENTAL HEALTH WORKING GROUP

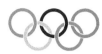

Athlete's name: _____   Athlete's ID number: _____

What is the SMHAT-1

The International Olympic Committee (IOC) Sport Mental Health Assessment Tool 1 (SMHAT-1) is a standardized assessment tool aiming to identify at an early stage elite athletes (defined as professional, Olympic, Paralympic and collegiate level; 16 and older) potentially at risk for or already experiencing mental health symptoms and disorders, in order to facilitate timely referral of those in need to adequate support and/or treatment.

Who should use the SMHAT-1

The SMHAT-1 can be used by sports medicine physicians and other licensed/registered health professionals, but the clinical assessment (and related management) within the SMHAT-1 (see step 3b) should be conducted by sports medicine physicians and/or licensed/registered mental health professionals. If you are not a sports medicine physician or other licensed/registered health professional, please use the IOC Sport Mental Health Recognition Tool 1 (SMHRT-1). Physical therapists or athletic trainers working with a sports medicine physician can use the SMHAT-1 but any guidance or intervention should remain the responsibility of their sports medicine physician.

To use this paper version of the SMHAT-1, please print it single-sided. The SMHAT-1 in its current form can be freely copied for distribution to individuals, teams, groups and organizations. Any revision requires the specific approval by the IOC MHWG while any translation should be reported to the IOC MHWG. The SMHAT-1 should not be re-branded or sold for commercial gain. Further information about the development of the SMHAT-1 and related screening tools (including psychometric properties) is presented in the corresponding publication of the British Journal of Sports Medicine.

Why use the SMHAT-1

Mental health symptoms and disorders are prevalent among active and former elite athletes. Mental health disorders are typically defined as conditions causing clinically significant distress or impairment that meet certain diagnostic criteria, such as in the Diagnostic and Statistical Manual of Mental Disorders 5th edition (DSM-5) or the International Classification of Diseases 10th revision (ICD-10), whereas mental health symptoms are self-reported, may be significant but do not occur in a pattern meeting specific diagnostic criteria and do not necessarily cause significant distress or functional impairment.

When to use the SMHAT-1

The SMHAT-1 should be ideally embedded within the pre-competition period (i.e., a few weeks after the start of sport training), as well as within the mid- and end-season period. The SMHAT-1 should also ideally be used when any significant event for athletes occurs such as injury, illness, surgery, unexplained performance concern, after a major competition, end of competitive cycle, suspected harassment/abuse, adverse life event and transitioning out of sport.

Step 1: Triage Tool — Athlete's form 1
Assessment with APSQ

| Score APSQ < 17 | Score APSQ ≥ 17 |

No further action needed

Step 2: Screening Tools — Athlete's form 2
Assessment with 6 screening instruments

Score ≥ 1
PHQ-9 item 9
= ACTION

| 6 screening instruments under threshold | 1 or more screening instruments at or above threshold |

Step 3a: Brief intervention and monitoring
- Single or combination of brief interventions
- Monitoring with APSQ (**Athlete's form 1**)

Step 3b: Clinical assessment
- Assessment (e.g., severity, complexity, diagnostic)
- Additional information (**Athlete's form 3**)
- Definition and application of treatment and support plan
- Referral to a mental health professional

Step 1. Triage tool for mental health symptoms and disorders

○ *ACTION: For this step, you need to refer to the Athlete's form 1. Complete the following.*

Calculate the total score by summing up the answers on the 10 items | Total Score

Total score 10 – 16 >>> No further action needed

Total score 17 – 50 >>> The athlete should complete the Athlete's form 2. Once the Athlete's form 2 is completed, proceed to step 2

Step 2. Screening tools for mental health symptoms and disorders

○ *ACTION: For this step, you need to refer to the Athlete's form 2. Complete the following.*

Screening 1 (anxiety)

Calculate the total score by summing up the answers on the 7 items | Total Score

Screening 2 (depression)

Calculate the total score by summing up the answers on the 9 items | Total Score

Note the score ('0', '1', '2' or '3') of the athlete on item 9 | Score

Screening 3 (sleep disturbance)

Calculate the total score by summing up the answers on the 5 items. | Total Score

Screening 4 (alcohol misuse)

Calculate the total score by summing up the answers on the 3 items | Total Score

Screening 5 (drug(s) use)

Calculate the total score by summing up the answers on the 4 items | Total Score

Note which drug(s) caused concerns or problems for the athlete | Drug(s)

Screening 6 (disordered eating)

Calculate the total score by summing up the answers on the first 6 items | Total Score

Fig. 19.1 The International Olympic Committee Sport Mental Health Assessment Tool 1 (SMHAT-1)

of health conditions and related treatment. Therefore, mental health literacy should be considered as a prerequisite to any subsequent approach applied to elite athletes transitioning out of sport.

Remaining physically active on a regular basis provides many health benefits, including improved sleep, stress relief, improved alertness, increased energy levels during the day, and healthy weight management. Research has shown that physical activity, including jogging, swimming, cycling, walking, gardening, and dancing, also has a significantly positive impact on mental health symptoms: it improves self-esteem and cognitive function and reduces anxiety and depression [2, 29]. This effect might be explained not only by physiological reactions (e.g., exercise-induced increase in blood circulation to the brain) but also by distraction, self-efficacy, and social interaction. The significance of physical activity for health in general and for mental health in particular should be acknowledged by clinicians with elite athletes transitioning out of sport.

By allowing patients to understand their feelings, and what makes them feel positive, anxious, or depressed, psychotherapy refers to a range of approaches that can help with mental health symptoms [2, 29]. One of the most commonly applied approaches to psychotherapy is cognitive behavioral therapy (CBT). Based on the relationship and dialogue between the patient and the clinician, this process can provide patients with the coping skills necessary to deal with difficult situations in a more adaptive and positive manner [2, 29]. When it comes to elite athletes transitioning out of sport, as performance-related matters are typically much less relevant, psychotherapy can provide the necessary safe and supportive environment that allows athletes to talk openly with someone who is objective, neutral, and nonjudgmental. As family members are likely to be substantially impacted by the process of transitioning out of elite sport and/or involved in the athletes' mental health symptoms, family therapy should be considered by clinicians.

Although mental health literacy, physical activity, and psychotherapy are typically the first-line treatments for mild to moderate mental health symptoms, medications may also be needed in some cases. When it comes to elite athletes transitioning out of sport, there are fewer particular considerations when prescribing psychiatric medications (in contrast to active athletes).

References

1. Gouttebarge V, Castaldelli-Maia JM, Gorczynski P, Hainline B, Hitchcock ME, Kerkhoffs G, et al. Occurrence of mental health symptoms and disorders in current and former elite athletes: a systematic review and meta-analysis. Br J Sports Med. 2019;53:700–6.
2. Reardon CL, Hainline B, Aron CM, Baron D, Baum AL, Bindra A, et al. Mental health in elite athletes: International Olympic Committee consensus statement (2019). Br J Sports Med. 2019;53:667–99.
3. Gouttebarge V, Frings-Dresen MH, Sluiter JK. Mental and psychosocial health among current and former professional footballers. Occup Med (Lond). 2015;65:190–6.
4. Gouttebarge V, Aoki H, Kerkhoffs G. Prevalence and determinants of symptoms related to mental disorders in retired male professional footballers. J Sports Med Phys Fitness. 2016;56:648–54.
5. Gouttebarge V, Kerkhoffs G, Lambert M. Prevalence and determinants of symptoms of common mental disorders in retired professional Rugby Union players. Eur J Sport Sci. 2016;16:595–602.
6. Brown JC, Kerkhoffs G, Lambert MI, Gouttebarge V. Forced retirement from professional Rugby Union is associated with symptoms of distress. Int J Sports Med. 2017;38:582–7.
7. Gouttebarge V, Jonkers R, Moen M, et al. The prevalence and risk indicators of symptoms of common mental disorders among current and former Dutch elite athletes. J Sports Sci. 2017;35:2148–56.
8. Gouttebarge V, Kerkhoffs G. A prospective cohort study on symptoms of common mental disorders among current and retired professional ice hockey players. Phys Sportsmed. 2017;45:252–8.
9. Kilic Ö, Aoki H, Haagensen R, Jensen C, Johnson U, Kerkhoffs G, et al. Symptoms of common mental disorders and related stressors in Danish professional football and handball. Eur J Sport Sci. 2017;17:1328–34.
10. Schuring N, Kerkhoffs G, Gray J, Gouttebarge V. The mental well-being of current and retired professional cricketers: an observational prospective cohort study. Phys Sportsmed. 2017;45:463–9.
11. Oltmans E, Confectioner K, Jonkers R, Kerkhoffs G, Moen M, Verhagen E, et al. A 12-month prospective cohort study on symptoms of mental health disorders among Dutch former elite athletes. Phys Sportsmed. 2022;50(2):123–31. https://doi.org/10.1080/0091 3847.2020.1868276.
12. Kiliç O, Carmody C, Upmeijer J, Kerkhoffs G, Purcell R, Rice R, et al. Prevalence of mental health symptoms among male and female Australian professional footballers. BMJ Open Sport Exerc Med. 2021;7:e001043.
13. Schwenk TL, Gorenflo DW, Dopp RR, Hipple E. Depression and pain in retired professional football players. Med Sci Sports Exerc. 2007;39:599–605.
14. Kerr ZY, Marshall SW, Harding HP Jr, Guskiewicz KM. Nine-year risk of depression diagnosis increases with increasing self-reported concussions in retired professional football players. Am J Sports Med. 2012;40:2206–12.
15. Hart J Jr, Kraut MA, Womack KB, Strain J, Didehbani N, Bartz E, et al. Neuroimaging of cognitive dysfunction and depression in aging retired National Football League players: a cross-sectional study. JAMA Neurol. 2013;70:326–35.
16. Willer BS, Tiso MR, Haider MN, Hinds AL, Baker JG, Miecznikowski JC, et al. Evaluation of executive function and mental health in retired contact sport athletes. J Head Trauma Rehabil. 2018;33:E9–E15.
17. Engel GL. The need for a new medical model: a challenge for biomedicine. Science. 1977;196:129–36.
18. Arnold R, Fletcher D. A research synthesis and taxonomic classification of the organizational stressors encountered by sport performers. J Sport Exerc Psychol. 2012;34:397–429.
19. van Ramele S, Aoki H, Kerkhoffs G, Gouttebarge V. Mental health in retired professional football players: 12-month incidence, adverse life events and support. Psychol Sport Exerc. 2017;28:85–90.
20. Gouttebarge V, Kerkhoffs GMMJ. Sports career-related concussion and mental health symptoms in former elite athletes. Neurochirurgie. 2021;67:280–2.
21. Guskiewicz KM, Marshall SW, Bailes J, McCrea M, Harding HP Jr, Matthews A, et al. Recurrent concussion and risk of depres-

sion in retired professional football players. Med Sci Sports Exerc. 2007;39:903–9.

22. Gouttebarge V, Aoki H, Lambert M, Stewart W, Kerkhoffs G. A history of concussions is associated with symptoms of common mental disorders in former male professional athletes across a range of sports. Phys Sportsmed. 2017;45:443–9.

23. Gouttebarge V, Aoki H, Verhagen E, Kerkhoffs G. Are level of education and employment related to symptoms of common mental disorders in current and retired professional footballers? Asian J Sports Med. 2016;7:e28447.

24. International Labour Organization. Health and life at work: a basic human right. Geneva: International Labour organization; 2009.

25. Carmody S, Jones C, Malhotra A, Gouttebarge V, Ahmad I. Put out to pasture: what is our duty of care to the retiring professional footballer? Promoting the concept of the 'exit health examination' (EHE). Br J Sports Med. 2019;53:788–9.

26. Gouttebarge V, Goedhart E, Kerkhoffs G. Empowering the health of retired professional footballers: the systematic development of an After Career Consultation and its feasibility. BMJ Open Sport Exerc Med. 2018;4:e000466.

27. Gouttebarge V, Janse van Rensburg DC, Kerkhoffs G. No time to waste: towards necessary health support for retired professional rugby players. South Afr J Sports Med. 2021;33:1–3.

28. Gouttebarge V, Bindra A, Blauwet C, Campriani N, Currie A, Engebretsen L, et al. International Olympic Committee (IOC) Sport Mental Health Assessment Tool 1 (SMHAT-1) and Sport Mental Health Recognition Tool 1 (SMHRT-1): towards better support of athletes' mental health. Br J Sports Med. 2021;55:30–7.

29. Reardon CL, Bindra A, Blauwet C, Budgett R, Campriani N, Currie A, et al. Mental health management of elite athletes during COVID-19: a narrative review and recommendations. Br J Sports Med. 2020:bjsports-2020-102884. https://doi.org/10.1136/bjsports-2020-102884.

30. Gorczynski P, Currie A, Gibson K, Gouttebarge V, Hainline B, Castaldelli-Maia JM, et al. Developing mental health literacy and cultural competence in elite sport. J Appl Sport Psychol. 2021;33(4):387–401. https://doi.org/10.1080/10413200.2020.1720045.

Mental Health Emergencies

Alan Currie [ID] and Allan Johnston [ID]

Introduction

What constitutes a mental health or psychiatric emergency might seem self-evident, but it is nonetheless important to be clear about how this situation is described and defined. To do so, it is helpful to draw parallels with other medical emergencies and, in addition, to consider the key components of a mental health emergency.

Examples of other medical emergencies in sport might include a compound fracture in a high-speed sport such as cycling or a player who collapses on the field of play as a consequence of a cardiac condition. In each case, a medical concern has presented itself suddenly, there is a high risk of an adverse outcome, and an immediate response is required. The latter two features in particular are the hallmarks of any medical emergency.

In psychiatric practice, the equivalent presentation would be an acute disturbance in an individual's mental state that poses a significant risk and that requires an urgent response (Table 20.1) [1]. Occasionally (and often with the benefit of hindsight), a mental state disturbance has a more insidious or subacute presentation but one that culminates in a scenario of high risk requiring an immediate response. A disturbance in mental state will be associated with either underlying mental health symptoms or disorders or with another medical disorder such as delirium. A disturbance can include features such as agitation, aggression, or violence [2, 3]. Other important characteristics of the mental state can include impairments in insight and judgment [3]. The risks posed by

Table 20.1 Features of a mental health emergency

Sudden (acute) presentation	The mental state disturbance appears without a prior warning. With hindsight, it may become apparent that there was a prodromal period or that early warning signs were present
High risk	The most obvious are the immediate risks to the safety of self and/or others. Other risks may emerge. For example, in mania, these can include significant financial risk or social embarrassment
Immediate response required	Immediate safety is of primary concern. Other concerns are: – Ready availability of clinical expertise – Knowledge of how to access this immediately

these mental state disturbances might be to the individuals themselves, to others in the vicinity, or to both [1, 3]. Risks to the individual might arise from suicidal thinking, intent, or behavior or from impaired judgment or recklessness (e.g., in mania, psychosis, or delirium), and risks to others may arise from disinhibited aggression or homicidal thoughts and behaviors. These situations require a rapid response, where safety is the primary consideration and where there should be ready availability of a clinical assessment [1]. Knowledge of the features of the emergency presentation can be invaluable later when planning preventative steps and early interventions for possible future episodes.

Prevalence

An important point about mental health emergencies in sport is that the entire range of mental health symptoms and disorders can present with acute disturbances and associated risks requiring urgent attention [1]. An emergency may result from delirium, substance use disorders, psychotic or bipolar disorders, depressive disorders, anxiety and related disorders, eating disorders, and personality disorders.

A. Currie (✉)
Regional Affective Disorders Service, Cumbria Northumberland Tyne and Wear NHS Foundation Trust, Newcastle, UK

Department of Sport and Exercise Sciences, University of Sunderland, Sunderland, UK
e-mail: alan.currie@cntw.nhs.uk

A. Johnston
Derbyshire Healthcare NHS Foundation Trust, Killamarsh, UK

English Institute of Sport, Sheffield, UK
e-mail: Allan.Johnston@nhs.net

Capturing data on mental health emergency presentations in elite sport is difficult, and the available data are likely to represent an underestimate. For example, at the 2012 Olympic Games in London, a dedicated mental health service for more than 10,000 athletes recorded only four mental health emergencies (International Olympic Committee (IOC)/cognacity data). Athletes may not present with emergency symptoms for the same reasons that they do not present with mental health symptoms generally, including stigma, low levels of mental health literacy, negative past experiences of seeking help, and busy schedules [4]. In addition, symptoms may resolve relatively quickly with supportive interventions, and the crisis may be short-lived. At a major games event, there may be "more pressing" issues such as injury or performance concerns, and mental health symptoms, despite their acuity, may not be addressed until later when the athlete returns home, or they may be managed in the moment without being systematically recorded. Initiatives to improve the availability of mental health services during major events were established around the delayed 2020 Olympic and Paralympic Games in Tokyo. The "Mentally Fit" campaign of the International Olympic Committee (IOC) provided all athletes access to a range of resources, educational materials, and a 24-hour helpline, accessible via a quick response (QR) code and publicized widely around the Games' sites and venues. The helpline was available in multiple languages and offered immediate triage and short-term therapeutic support if indicated. It was provided by Workplace Option LLC (a global well-being solutions provider) in partnership with the IOC and available in the immediate lead up to, during, and for an additional 3 months following the Games.

Types of Mental Health Emergencies

Delirium

Delirium may be a consequence of an underlying medical condition or its treatment, drug intoxication or withdrawal, or occasionally a toxin such as from an insect bite [5]. Because of its relationship with underlying medical conditions, delirium is often considered a disorder of old age. It is certainly more common in that age group and is less common in the age groups most represented in elite sport. However, some specific types of delirium have been reported in elite sport, e.g., after a concussion [6], secondary to hyperthermia, which may be exacerbated by stimulant use [7], or secondary to hyponatremia, which may be associated with overzealous hydration [8, 9].

Substance Use Disorders

Substance use disorders may lead to an emergency presentation as a consequence of either intoxication or withdrawal [1]. Athletes are known to misuse a range of substances that might lead to such a presentation. The pattern of alcohol use in elite sports indicates a prevalent binge pattern rather than regular heavy drinking, although both are seen [10–12]. This might make presentation during intoxication more likely than during withdrawal, although either is possible [1]. Perhaps the most important effect of alcohol is as a moderator of violent behavior and suicidal ideation via its disinhibiting effects. Cannabis is a common substance of misuse in certain sports [13], and the most common adverse effects are mild [14], although paranoid symptoms and severe acute anxiety have been reported, especially when high-potency preparations are used [15, 16]. Anabolic androgenic steroids (AAS) may be misused by elite athletes to improve performance [17]. Mood disturbances and psychotic symptoms can emerge. These are usually subsyndromal for either a hypomanic or psychotic episode, although higher doses and the use of multiple agents are associated with more severe disturbances of mental state [18–21]. AAS use may be associated with suicidality via at least two different mechanisms [22]. First, those who are current users may experience rapid mood changes associated with impulsive acts including the sudden emergence of suicidal thinking and behavior. Second, former users may develop more enduring mood disturbances including depression that is associated with sustained suicidal thoughts, intent, and plans. Stimulant drugs are also occasionally used by athletes either for recreational purposes or for performance enhancement [17]. They can promote significant agitation, aggression, and even psychotic symptoms [23, 24] and are associated with an increased risk of hyperthermia [7]. Opioids are an important class of drugs that can be misused by athletes [25, 26]. These are frequently taken by injured athletes either illicitly or as prescribed and are a commonly used substance in self-poisoning. In England, they account for 31% of self-poisoning fatalities (https://sites.manchester.ac.uk/ncish/reports/).

Bipolar and Psychotic Disorders

The incidence and prevalence of bipolar and psychotic disorders in elite sport are not known [27, 28]. What is known is that the age of onset of these disorders overlaps with the peak age of sporting performance [29] and that both of these conditions can lead to an emergency presentation [1]. For example, acute mania is associated with risky activities resulting from elevated mood, disinhibition, and impaired insight. Examples include excess spending, dangerous driving, or increased sexual activity [30]. The risks associated with an acute psychotic presentation might result from severe agitation, disorganized behavior, or behaviors associated with paranoid delusions or hallucinations [31].

Depression

Depressive symptoms are approximately as common in elite athletes as in the general population [32], and there are some sport-specific issues that may be associated with an emergency presentation. First, there is a relationship between depressive symptoms and sports injuries [33] and between sports injuries and complex emotional reactions including anger [34, 35]. Anger and depression in combination can serve to increase the risk of suicidal behavior. Second, depressive symptoms may be missed, at least in the early stages, with athletes reluctant to disclose symptoms [4, 36] or where symptoms are misattributed to overtraining [37]. A delay in symptom presentation or recognition increases the possibility of an emergency presentation if symptoms progress and the athlete reaches a crisis point [1].

Suicide

In a recent study of 402 elite athletes, the prevalence of suicidal thoughts was 15.6% (men, 17.4%; women, 14.2%). Despite one in six elite athletes reporting suicidal thoughts, 97% of those with such thoughts did not attempt suicide at any time. Among female athletes, a history of sexual abuse was the strongest determinant of both suicidal thoughts and actions, followed by the psychological sense of perceiving life as less-comprehensible, manageable, and meaningful. Among male participants, the main determinant of suicidal ideation was using an avoidant strategy for coping with life challenges [38].

Self-Harm

Self-harm can be defined as "any act of self-injury carried out by an individual irrespective of motivation." The exact rates are hard to discern, as most acts of self-harm do not result in presentation for medical attention. Self-harm is more common in women, and 16.7% of females will self-harm at some point in their lives compared to 4.8% of men [39]. Many people use self-harm, especially self-cutting, to

help manage distress and report that their actions do not have suicidal intent. Some report that their self-cutting is a way of preserving their life and is done to "reduce" suicidal thoughts, plans, or actions [40, 41].

Anxiety Disorders

Panic disorder, which is characterized by the abrupt onset of severe anxiety, is perhaps the most likely of the anxiety disorders to present as an emergency and is reported in 4.5% of elite athletes [42]. Phobias may also present suddenly, e.g., acute severe anxiety secondary to a flying phobia in an athlete who is traveling to an event and who may have been previously sensitized by an adverse flying experience [43].

Post-Traumatic Stress Disorder (PTSD)

This and related conditions may be more prevalent in elite athletes than in the general population, with reported rates of 13–25% in some studies. Contributory factors might include trauma directly experienced through sports participation, e.g., a severe sports injury or the traumatic consequences of abusive dynamics within sports teams [44].

Eating Disorders

Eating disorders are known to be prevalent in elite sports [45] but are more likely to require ongoing mental health treatment, support, and monitoring than to need an urgent mental health response. For an athlete with an eating disorder, the risks that require an urgent and immediate response are usually the result of general medical issues such as electrolyte disturbance, cardiac arrhythmias, or fractures [46]. However, these might lead to an athlete being deselected, which can result in significant emotional decompensation and an emergency mental health presentation [47].

Personality Disorders

Disorders of personality represent enduring patterns of inner experiences and outward behavior that are maladaptive, inflexible, and pervasive [5]. In consequence, management of these difficulties usually requires a long-term approach that can include extended psychotherapy. Nonetheless, emergency presentations can occur, and periods of significant emotional disturbance can be seen. For example, there are specific features of borderline personality disorder that are likely to promote a mental health emergency. Traits of this condition in the absence of the full syndrome can be similarly problematic. In this disorder, sufferers can be acutely sensitive to perceived rejection or abandonment and may respond with sudden and dramatic changes in mood with prominent and occasionally explosive anger. Behaviors in response to perceived rejection can also include impulsive acts such as self-harm or even suicidal behavior. In the context of elite sport, there are many potential triggers for this, most obviously if the athlete is deselected ("rejected"). Limited data also point to this being the most common subtype of personality disorder in competitive athletes [48]. Of particular note is the common comorbidity with borderline personality disorder of both eating disorders [49] and AAS use [18], and an athlete deselected for medical complications of an eating disorder or a doping violation may therefore be at an especially high risk.

Guidelines

An individual mental health emergency may in itself be unexpected, but for there to be "any" emergency is an expected occurrence at some point, and this requires advanced planning. Guidelines emphasize the helpfulness of a prepared written action plan detailing how to respond. Plans highlight the importance of, first, recognizing that it is an emergency, and second, clarity on the roles and responsibilities of staff and other team members. Safety is paramount, and good plans include the importance of knowing who to call and where the nearest facilities and expertise are located [50]. Plans that are consistent with other emergency situations and follow a similar template are valuable in this respect as general medical staff members will have greater awareness of the common elements of a response to a cardiac, musculoskeletal, or mental health emergency.

Planning Ahead

Those who work in sport recognize the value of planning ahead to mitigate or avoid adverse events, and advanced planning can lessen the impact of a mental health emergency presentation. Recurring crises of a similar nature or with the same individual should also be a signal to take a step back and evaluate what might need to be addressed in the organization or team's response or with the individual. Are there important gaps in service provision or response? Is it necessary to have a more detailed understanding of the athlete's underlying difficulties, perhaps via an expert mental health assessment by a sports psychiatrist?

Planning ahead will include developing familiarity with local mental health and emergency services. This applies to the services that are nearest to where the athlete or team is usually based. Importantly, it also extends to familiarity with the nearest and best services when traveling, especially with an athlete known to have a mental health disorder where an emergency presentation is possible.

Some sports organizations have created their own guidelines to assist support staff in planning for major events. Figure 20.1 is based on a template prepared by the Mental Health Expert Panel (MHEP) of the English Institute of Sport (EIS) and circulated to all sports in the UK and their respective support staff in preparation for a major international multisport event. The template includes simple points such as ensuring an adequate supply of medication, having more detailed information on the athlete's illness history, and the athlete's view of what is likely to be helpful in a crisis. It also includes a prompt to develop a more detailed mental health-care plan if this is necessary or desirable.

An example of a more detailed care plan is shown in Fig. 20.2. It is designed to be used by more specialist mental health staff such as a psychiatrist or clinical psychologist. It follows the biopsychosocial model that is familiar to most mental health practitioners and that allows for a comprehensive evaluation and subsequent interventions accounting for multiple relevant factors. The document also includes references to the principles of an individualized Wellness Recovery Action Plan (WRAP) such as daily health maintenance activities alongside identifying and responding to triggers and early warning signs [51]. Plans such as these are commonly used in many mental health services and have utility in avoiding or managing an emerging crisis [52].

Roles and Responsibilities

It is in the nature of emergencies that a rapid and decisive response is likely to be needed. For this reason, a clear and simple plan that describes the responsibilities of medical and support staff should be readily available and understood by all.

All staff should be aware of how to recognize an emergency, and whilst it is usually self-evident, it is nonetheless advisable to describe and define the scenarios that constitute an emergency. Examples of scenarios where there is a high level of risk that requires an immediate response include suicidal or homicidal ideation, highly agitated or threatening behavior, acute psychosis, delirium, confusion, intoxication, or overdose. All staff should also know who to contact for further help including the details of the local emergency services.

For most staff faced with an emergency, the first person to contact is likely to be a member of the medical team. This

As the event approaches, it is important to consider the mental health of those traveling as part of your team and to plan proactively.

It is recommended to consider the following during preparation:

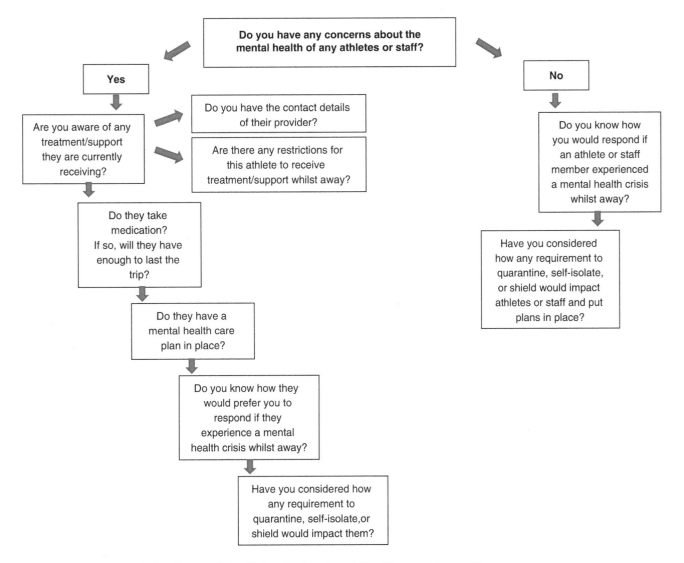

A more detailed guidance to help with the planning of mental health support for specific athletes and staff with known mental health problems is also available via the mental health clinicians (psychiatrists and clinical psychologists) working with your team.

Fig. 20.1 A template for mental health considerations in pre-event planning

might be the team doctor as there may not always be a trained mental health professional such as a psychiatrist or clinical psychologist readily available. Medical staff will be in a position to conduct an initial assessment, including assessing for any injuries or ingestion of harmful substances and deciding whether to call for emergency services or transport to the nearest emergency department. Medical staff will also be alert for signs of delirium on intoxication.

If there are trained mental health personnel nearby or readily accessible, they will also have a role in the initial assessment, de-escalation, arranging for further investigations, and prescribing of any necessary medications. The standard advice for mental health professionals is to try where possible to follow their usual emergency assessment processes even though the assessment may take place in unusual or suboptimal surroundings such as a

Template for mental healthcare

This document is intended to help with planning of mental health support in advance of a major event. The document can be used to support any athlete or staff member with a known mental health problem and would be developed in conjunction with their mental health practitioner.

The template uses the biopsychosocial model as its framework. This is a model that is a widely used and accepted way of understanding mental health concerns. It should provide a holistic and person-centred care plan to support mental health.

Biological	Psychological	Social
• Ensure optimum physical health (e.g., analgesia) and any health monitoring needed (e.g., blood tests).	• Develop a contact plan between the individual and their usual mental health clinician or mental health support team.	• Develop a contact plan with informal sources of support at home (friends and family, etc.).
• Review mood. Diarise or self-monitor using biological symptoms such as sleep, appetite and energy.	• Consider rating symptoms using tools such as PHQ9 for depression and GAD7 for anxiety. Ensure there are baseline ratings for comparison.	• Review the necessity for contact with team members, local practitioners, or services at the event. What is their availability and how will they be contacted?
• Optimise sleep. Attend to sleep hygiene. Implement interventions such as sleep CBT or medication as necessary.	• Risk assessment and safety planning when relevant.	• Anticipate any restrictions that might impede access to support, e.g., isolation requirements. Develop contingency plans to accommodate these.
• Ensure optimal nutrition. Consider specific dietary needs especially if there are concerns regarding energy availability, RED-S, or disordered eating.	• Consider if any specific resources or expertise may be needed, e.g., ready access to de-escalation exercise in a crisis.	• Plan for downtime and access to quiet spaces.
• Consider any alcohol or illicit substance use. Aim to stabilise well in advance (including safe withdrawal if needed).	• Consider using the Wellness Recovery Action Plan (WRAP) structure to plan self-care.	• Take one or two special home comforts with you.
• Medicines monitoring: ensure adequate supply. Adjust dosing schedule to accommodate time zone, climate, and competitive schedule.		• Reflect on usual routines and activity schedule. In particular, incorporate the little events during the day that help to sustain good health, including mental and other aspects of physical health. Ensure these are available and scheduled.
		• Pre-plan how you will use and access social media (if at all).

Fig. 20.2 Pre-event planning for mental health practitioners in sport including a Wellness Recovery Action Plan. *CBT* cognitive behavioral therapy, *RED-S* relative energy deficiency in sport, *PHQ9* Patient Health Questionnaire-9, *GAD7* General Anxiety Disorder-7

Wellness Recovery Action Plan (WRAP)

Consider writing out your own plan in each of the four areas below. It is a personal document, though others may help you develop it. Keep it safe and readily accessible. Share it with those you trust, including any mental health practitioners with whom you are working, if you wish.

---

1. How does 'well' feel? What are your signs of good mental health?
Describe yourself when you are well.

What feelings, actions, and behaviours are associated with this?

What does your 'inner voice' say when things are going well?

---

2. What keeps you well? What techniques or strategies have helped before?
Some people call this their 'wellness' toolbox. It might include:
- contacting friends, family and other supporters
- relaxation exercises and other stress reduction techniques
- focusing exercises
- affirming activities (take a moment to read or make a list of positive affirmations)
- diet
- light (e.g., time in daylight, low level lighting before sleep)
- good sleep quality

---

3. Triggers for stress? What factors might affect you?
What events or circumstances make you feel uncomfortable?

Recognising what might happen and dealing with the normal reaction to these events can prevent things from becoming worse.

---

4. Early warning signs? What symptoms might you notice when becoming stressed?
Debriefing after a previous crisis or significant health concern can be a helpful (albeit retrospective) way of identifying these early signs.

Consider reviewing a previous episode of distress/crisis with one of your supporters, perhaps including your mental health clinician.

Fig. 20.2 (continued)

hotel room or training facility [1, 53]. A collateral history from a close friend, teammate, or staff member who knows the athlete well can be helpful in determining the origins of the emergency presentation. Other staff may be trained in verbal de-escalation techniques, and this can be invaluable for the distressed, disturbed, or potentially aggressive athlete.

Management

General Management Issues

When there is an imminent risk of violence, the priority is safety. This means not only keeping the athlete safe but also considering the safety (general physical and psychological) of others in the vicinity [54]. If possible, bladed items and any poisons or toxins should be carefully removed from the athlete's possession. If there is no concern about imminent violence or need for immediate medical attention, then the priority is to connect with the athlete and help them manage their distress. Although it is an important principle to pursue the least-restrictive or coercive management option, it is nonetheless essential that the chosen option be safe.

Verbal De-escalation

Skills in verbal de-escalation are central and can reduce the need for medication to manage acute behavioral disturbances [55]. Medication can still be considered as an option to supplement verbal de-escalation or if verbal de-escalation is unsuccessful, with the safety of athletes and others in close proximity as the primary concern [1, 2].

Four stages of verbal de-escalation are described (Table 20.2.) The process begins with engagement, then moves onto establishing collaboration, the actual de-escalation, and ends with a debriefing. De-escalation requires some specialist training but can be an extremely helpful designated role within a support team.

Engagement includes simple measures such as polite, clear introductions. The athlete should be helped to orient to their surroundings and provided with reassurance. It is helpful to use short, simple sentences and phrases and to keep the personnel involved to a safe minimum, as multiple interactions can be overstimulating and confusing and can heighten agitation. There are techniques that will help foster a collaborative relationship even in an acute situation. These are based on active listening, which can be conveyed through speech and posture and will help identify thoughts, feelings, and immediate needs. Once the athlete is engaged and collaboration is established, the next stage is to de-escalate by coaching the athlete to calm themselves and regain control of

Table 20.2 De-escalation stages

1. Engagement	2. Establishing collaboration	3. De-escalation	4. Debriefing
Introduction Orientation Reassurance Concise, simple sentences One clinician (multiple interactions can be confusing and may escalate)	Active listening Conveyed through speech and body language Identify thoughts, feelings, and needs, e.g., "You seem troubled, would you like to say what's on your mind?" "You seem to be anxious/scared; would you like to talk about that?" "You seem troubled/scared; what would be helpful to you right now?"	Simple advice: "Let's sit somewhere quiet and talk." Use of grounding techniques, e.g., breathing, visualizing a favorite place Make an offer or gesture, e.g., warmth, food, drink	Later—When patient is calmed Patient and clinician each describe what happened Joint reflection on what might help next time

their emotions. Steps that can facilitate this include encouraging the athlete to find a quiet spot to sit and relay any of their concerns calmly. The athlete can be gently coached to use grounding techniques such as breathing or visualization, especially if they already have some familiarity with these exercises. Gestures such as offering something to eat or drink can be helpful too. The fourth stage is the debriefing, which can begin very quickly after the disturbance is diffused. Debriefing affords both parties an opportunity to describe and explain events from their perspectives and to reflect on what might be helpful in future situations.

Medication for Acute Behavioral Disturbances

Concerns that side effects of medication such as motor side effects, sedation, or weight gain may negatively impact performance [56–58] may be less relevant in an emergency where it may be riskier to withhold treatment and where treatment may only be needed for an extremely short period [1]. Two main groups of medications are used in the management of acute behavioral disturbances: benzodiazepines and antipsychotics [2] (Table 20.3). Benzodiazepines ought to be considered first unless there has been prior successful exposure to an antipsychotic and/or it is known that the athlete is presenting with symptoms of psychosis or mania, e.g., because of a known prior history of one of these conditions. The oral route is preferred, and if medication is indicated, then it can be used alongside verbal de-escalation, with each facilitating the other.

Table 20.3 Medication options in acute behavioral disturbance

	Benzodiazepines	Antipsychotics
Suggested use/ indications	If clinical information is limited	If history of bipolar or psychotic disorder
	No previous antipsychotic exposure	Especially if previous response to specific antipsychotic medication
	Known cardiovascular disease	Usually under the direction of a specialist (e.g., a psychiatrist)
Options	Lorazepam is preferred as it is short-acting: 1–2 mg Can be repeated after 4 h	*Drug (time of maximum plasma concentration):* Aripiprazole (3–5 h) Haloperidol (2–6 h) Olanzapine (5–8 h) Quetiapine (1.5 h) Risperidone (1–2 h) Others (specialist facility only): Loxapine can be inhaled The intramuscular route (e.g., haloperidol) is only for the most severe emergencies (often called "rapid tranquilization")
	Other oral benzodiazepines (e.g., diazepam with a half-life of 30–56 h) can be used depending on availability	
	Others: Midazolam can be administered via the buccal route Benzodiazepines may be co-administered with antipsychotics in severe cases (usually only under specialist supervision)	

Other routes of administration can be used but are generally only recommended if specialist supervision or facilities are available. Midazolam (a benzodiazepine) can be administered via the buccal route, and loxapine (an antipsychotic) can be taken by inhalation. Parenteral (e.g., intramuscular) administration can only be recommended in specialist facilities and if the level of acute disturbance warrants this, e.g., if de-escalation and oral pharmacological treatment methods are impossible or ineffective and a significant risk is present. Using the parental route is often termed "rapid tranquilization," and both benzodiazepine and antipsychotics can be administered intramuscularly. It should be noted, in addition, that parenteral diazepam is not recommended because of lack of evidence, and parental midazolam is not recommended because of the risk of respiratory depression.

Specific Management Issues

There are specific management issues that need to be considered for disorders or groups of disorders.

In delirium, the two priorities are, first, not to miss the diagnosis and, second, to identify and treat the underlying cause [59]. It is important not to misattribute symptoms to another disorder such as depression (diagnostic shadowing) as delays from misdiagnosis can have serious, even fatal consequences. In cases of substance use and intoxication, it is

important to know the features of common presentations. Immediate management priorities are the initial safety of the athlete and the need for monitoring. For intoxications that are not serious or may be self-limiting, such as many cases of alcohol intoxication, it may be sufficient to monitor the athlete (e.g., in a team hotel) without transferring them to the emergency department [60]. In other instances, transfer to the emergency department will be the only appropriate response, e.g., to administer naloxone in cases of opioid intoxication [1]. Once the intoxication is cleared, then, there is a need for a timely and comprehensive mental health assessment and development of a management plan to address any underlying difficulties [61].

For the athlete experiencing psychotic symptoms or mania (bipolar disorder), then the level of disturbance may warrant an inpatient mental health evaluation [62, 63]. If this is not required, then the athlete may still need to be prescribed a pharmacological agent in addition to the usual de-escalation measures. It is recommended to use benzodiazepines if the athlete is treatment-naive and/or their past history is unknown [2]. If the athlete has had previous exposure to antipsychotic medication or is in a specialist mental health facility, then antipsychotic medication can be used alone or alongside a benzodiazepine. If the athlete has a history of either psychosis or bipolar disorder, then advance planning in anticipation of an acute or emergency presentation can be especially valuable (Figs. 20.1 and 20.2).

For the athlete who may be experiencing suicidal thoughts with associated intent or behaviors, then it is essential to make a sensitive inquiry and crucial to listen to the athlete's response [64]. Immediate safety is the priority. Once the crisis is over, then it is recommended to begin developing a safety plan to deal with future eventualities during the post-event debriefing.

The management of acute, severe anxiety is largely carried out via behavioral means such as breathing or grounding techniques [43]. In some instances, benzodiazepines or beta-blockers may be offered, but there are concerns about their use in athletes as both may have a detrimental effect on athletic performance and are, in addition, prohibited substances in many sports [43, 57].

The emotional decompensation that can occur in athletes with underlying personality difficulties can be usually managed in the short term using techniques of psychological de-escalation. There are two important principles in the preventative management of this kind of difficulty. In the long term, this type of emotional decompensation is addressed by psychotherapy or other psychological interventions that help the athlete recognize and manage difficult emotions more effectively [65]. In addition, the hotspots for emotional decompensation can often be predictable and therefore, to a degree, preventable. For example, the decision to exclude an athlete who has an eating disorder from either training or competition is one that should occur as a last resort and at the end point of clear and agreed processes supported by policies [47].

Conclusions

The elements of a mental health emergency are the sudden presentation of a disturbance in mental state that is associated with a high level of risk and requires an immediate response. Features of the mental state disturbance might include severe agitation, aggression or violence, and/or impaired insight and judgment. Recognizing that an emergency is occurring is central to an appropriate and timely response and is supported by having clear and agreed upon definitions of what constitutes an emergency. Whilst data on the incidence of emergency presentations are sparse and difficult to collect, any mental health condition could result in an emergency presentation.

Safety is paramount when responding to an emergency, and this includes the safety of not only the affected individual but also those in the immediate vicinity. All support staff should be aware of what constitutes an emergency and their role in the immediate response, which may simply be knowing who to call. Selected staff, including medical staff, may have additional expertise in the initial response including a quick assessment of any injuries, detecting evidence of ingestion of any substances, and evaluating for the presence of delirium. Some staff may also have training in verbal de-escalation techniques or in prescribing calming or tranquilizing medication. Specialist mental health staff may additionally be available to assist with a more detailed assessment in the short term including understanding the nature of any underlying mental health disorder and initiating an appropriate immediate plan of care and treatment.

It is the duty of sports organizations and teams to develop and disseminate policies and processes for identifying and responding to mental health emergencies. Support staff should be appropriately trained and confident in their role and know where, when, and how to find additional expertise if needed.

References

1. Currie A, McDuff D, Johnston A, Hopley P, Hitchcock ME, Reardon CL, et al. Management of mental health emergencies in elite athletes: a narrative review. Br J Sports Med. 2019;53(12):772–8.
2. Patel MX, Sethi FN, Barnes TR, Dix R, Dratcu L, Fox B, et al. Joint BAP NAPICU evidence-based consensus guidelines for the clinical management of acute disturbance: De-escalation and rapid tranquillisation. J Psychopharmacol. 2018;32(6):601–40.
3. Newman BM, Ravindranath D. Managing a psychiatric emergency. Psychiatr Times. 2010;27(7):1–5.
4. Castaldelli-Maia JM, Gallinaro JGDME, Falcão RS, Gouttebarge V, Hitchcock ME, Hainline B, et al. Mental health symptoms and disorders in elite athletes: a systematic review on cultural influencers and barriers to athletes seeking treatment. Br J Sports Med. 2019;53(11):707–21.
5. American Psychiatric Association. Diagnostic and statistical manual of mental disorders (DSM-5). 5th ed. Washington, DC: American Psychiatric Publishing; 2013. p. 1–947.
6. Schuman G. Post concussion delirium in children: two cases. Neurology. 2014;82(10 Supplement):P5.309.
7. Macleod AD. Sport psychiatry. Aust N Z J Psychiatry. 1998;32(6):860–6.
8. Noakes TD, Norman RJ, Buck RH, Godlonton J, Stevenson K, Pittaway D. The incidence of hyponatremia during prolonged ultraendurance exercise. Med Sci Sports Exerc. 1990;22(2):165–70.
9. Hew-Butler T, Loi V, Pani A, Rosner MH. Exercise-associated hyponatremia: 2017 update. Front Med. 2017;4(21):1–10.
10. Green GA, Uryasz FD, Petr TA, Bray CD. NCAA study of substance use and abuse habits of college student-athletes. Clin J Sport Med. 2001 Jan;11(1):51–6.
11. Zhou J, Heim D. Sports and spirits: a systematic qualitative review of emergent theories for student-athlete drinking. Alcohol Alcohol. 2014;49(6):604–17.
12. Barry AE, Howell SM, Riplinger A, Piazza-Gardner AK. Alcohol use among college athletes: do intercollegiate, club, or intramural student athletes drink differently? Subst Use Misuse. 2015;50(3):302–7.
13. Brisola-Santos MB, Gallinaro JGM, Gil F, Sampaio-Junior B, Marin MCD, de Andrade AG, et al. Prevalence and correlates of cannabis use among athletes—a systematic review. Am J Addict. 2016;25(7):518–28.
14. Johns A. Psychiatric effects of cannabis. Br J Psychiatry. 2001;178(02):116–22.
15. Castaneto MS, Gorelick DA, Desrosiers NA, Hartman RL, Pirard S, Huestis MA. Synthetic cannabinoids: epidemiology, pharmacodynamics, and clinical implications. Drug Alcohol Depend. 2014;144:12–41.
16. Volkow ND, Baler RD, Compton WM, Weiss SRB. Adverse health effects of marijuana use. N Engl J Med. 2014;370(23):2219–27.
17. Reardon C, Creado S. Drug abuse in athletes. Subst Abus Rehabil. 2014;5:95–105.
18. van Amsterdam J, Opperhuizen A, Hartgens F. Adverse health effects of anabolic–androgenic steroids. Regul Toxicol Pharmacol. 2010;57(1):117–23.
19. Bahrke MS. Psychological and behavioral effects of anabolic—androgenic steroids. Int J Sport Exerc Psychol. 2005;3(4):428–45.
20. Piacentino D, Kotzalidis G, Casale A, Aromatario M, Pomara C, Girardi P, et al. Anabolic-androgenic steroid use and psychopathology in athletes. A systematic review. Curr Neuropharmacol. 2015;13(1):101–21.
21. Trenton AJ, Currier GW. Behavioural manifestations of anabolic steroid use. CNS Drugs. 2005;19(7):571–95.
22. Thiblin I, Runeson B, Rajs J. Anabolic androgenic steroids and suicide. Ann Clin Psychiatry. 1999;11(4):223–31.
23. McDuff DR, Baron D. Substance use in athletics: a sports psychiatry perspective. Clin Sports Med. 2005;24(4):885–97.
24. Baron DA, Reardon CL, Baron SH. Doping in sport. In: Baron DA, Reardon CL, Baron SH, editors. Clinical sports psychiatry: an international perspective. 1st ed. Oxford: Wiley; 2013. p. 21–32.
25. NCAA. NCAA national study on substance use habits of college student-athletes; 2018.
26. Ford JA, Pomykacz C, Veliz P, McCabe SE, Boyd CJ. Sports involvement, injury history, and non-medical use of prescription

opioids among college students: an analysis with a national sample. Am J Addict. 2018;27(1):15–22.

27. Reardon CL. Psychiatric comorbidities in sports. Neurol Clin. 2017;35(3):537–46.

28. Rice SM, Purcell R, De Silva S, Mawren D, McGorry PD, Parker AG. The mental health of elite athletes: a narrative systematic review. Sports Med. 2016;46(9):1333–53.

29. Moesch K, Kenttä G, Kleinert J, Quignon-Fleuret C, Cecil S, Bertollo M. FEPSAC position statement: mental health disorders in elite athletes and models of service provision. Psychol Sport Exerc. 2018;38:61–71.

30. Goodwin GM, Haddad PM, Ferrier IN, Aronson JK, Barnes TRH, Cipriani A, et al. Evidence-based guidelines for treating bipolar disorder: revised third edition recommendations from the British Association for Psychopharmacology. J Psychopharmacol. 2016;30(6):495–553.

31. Lehman AF, Lieberman JA, Dixon LB, McGlashan TH, Miller AL, Perkins DO, et al. Practice guideline for the treatment of patients with schizophrenia. 2nd ed. American Psychiatric Association; 2010. p. 1–184.

32. Gorczynski PF, Coyle M, Gibson K. Depressive symptoms in high-performance athletes and non-athletes: a comparative meta-analysis. Br J Sports Med. 2017;51(18):1348–54.

33. Putukian M. The psychological response to injury in student athletes: a narrative review with a focus on mental health. Br J Sports Med. 2016;50(3):145–8.

34. Baum AL. Suicide in athletes. In: Baron DA, Reardon CL, Baron SH, editors. Clinical sports psychiatry: an international perspective. 1st ed. Oxford: Wiley; 2013. p. 79–88.

35. Galambos SA, Terry PC, Moyle GM, Locke SA. Psychological predictors of injury among elite athletes. Br J Sports Med. 2005;39(6):351–4.

36. Markser VZ. Sport psychiatry and psychotherapy. Mental strains and disorders in professional sports. Challenge and answer to societal changes. Eur Arch Psychiatry Clin Neurosci. 2011;261:182–5.

37. Schwenk TL. The stigmatisation and denial of mental illness in athletes. Br J Sports Med. 2000;34(1):4–5.

38. Timpka T, Spreco A, Dahlstrom O, Jacobsson J, Kowalski J, Bargoria V, et al. Suicidal thoughts (ideation) among elite athletics (track and field) athletes: associations with sports participation, psychological resourcefulness and having been a victim of sexual and/or physical abuse. Br J Sports Med. 2021;55:198–205.

39. National Institute for Health and Clinical Excellence. Overview—self-harm in over 8s: long-term management. NICE; 2011.

40. Nock MK. Why do people hurt themselves? New insights into the nature and functions of self-injury. Curr Dir Psychol Sci. 2009;18(2):78–83.

41. Klonsky ED, Glenn CR. Assessing the functions of non-suicidal self-injury: psychometric properties of the Inventory of Statements about Self-injury (ISAS). J Psychopathol Behav Assess. 2009;31(3):215–9.

42. Gulliver A, Griffiths KM, Mackinnon A, Batterham PJ, Stanimirovic R. The mental health of Australian elite athletes. J Sci Med Sport. 2015;18(3):255–61.

43. McDuff DR. Adjustment and anxiety disorders. In: Currie A, Owen B, editors. Sports psychiatry. Oxford: Oxford University Press; 2016. p. 1–16.

44. Aron CM, Harvey S, Hainline B, Hitchcock ME, Reardon CL. Post-traumatic stress disorder (PTSD) and other trauma-related mental disorders in elite athletes: a narrative review. Br J Sports Med. 2019;53(12):779–84.

45. Sundgot-Borgen J, Torstveit MK. Prevalence of eating disorders in elite athletes is higher than in the general population. Clin J Sport Med. 2004;14:25–32.

46. Mountjoy M, Sundgot-Borgen J, Burke L, Carter S, Constantini N, Lebrun C, et al. The IOC consensus statement: beyond the Female Athlete Triad-Relative Energy Deficiency in Sport (RED-S). Br J Sports Med. 2014;48(7):491–7.

47. Currie A, Morse E. Eating disorders in athletes: managing the risks. Clin Sports Med. 2005;24(4):871–83.

48. Hendawy HM, Baron DA, Sei-Eldawla A, Fekry M, Hwidi D. Prevalence of psychiatric disorders and coping processes in a sample of Egyptian competitive athletes. Faculty of Medicine, Ain Shams University; 2012. p. 60–2.

49. Martinussen M, Friborg O, Schmierer P, Kaiser S, Øvergård KT, Neunhoeffer A-L, et al. The comorbidity of personality disorders in eating disorders: a meta-analysis. Eat Weight Disord. 2017;22(2):201–9.

50. National Collegiate Athletic Association Mental Health Task Force. Mental health best practices: understanding and supporting student athlete mental wellness; 2020. https://ncaaorg.s3.amazonaws.com/ssi/mental/SSI_MentalHealthBestPractices.pdf. Accessed 29 Dec 2021.

51. Copeland M. Wellness recovery action plan. Occup Ther Ment Health. 2002;17(3–4):127–50.

52. Copeland M. Overview of WRAP: wellness recovery action plan. Ment Health Recov Newslett. 2002;3:1–9.

53. Currie A, Johnston A. Psychiatric disorders: the psychiatrist's contribution to sport. Int Rev Psychiatry. 2016;28(6):587–94.

54. Substance Abuse and Mental Health Services Administration. Practice guidelines: core elements for responding to mental health crises. Rockville, MD: Center for Mental Health Services; 2009. p. 1–14.

55. Richmond JS, Berlin JS, Fishkind AB, Holloman GH, Zeller SL, Wilson MP, et al. Verbal de-escalation of the agitated patient: consensus statement of the American Association for Emergency Psychiatry Project BETA De-escalation Workgroup. West J Emerg Med. 2012;13(1):17–25.

56. Reardon CL, Creado S. Psychiatric medication preferences of sports psychiatrists. Phys Sportsmed. 2016;44(4):397–402.

57. Reardon CL. The sports psychiatrist and psychiatric medication. Int Rev Psychiatry. 2016;28(6):606–13.

58. Johnston A, McAllister-Williams RH. Psychotropic drug prescribing. In: Currie A, Owen B, editors. Sports psychiatry. 1st ed. Oxford: Oxford University Press; 2016. p. 133–43.

59. Garriga M, Pacchiarotti I, Kasper S, Zeller SL, Allen MH, Vázquez G, et al. Assessment and management of agitation in psychiatry: expert consensus. World J Biol Psychiatry. 2016;17(2):86–128.

60. McDuff D. Substance use and abuse. In: McDuff D, editor. Sports psychiatry: strategies for life balance and peak performance. 1st ed. Washington, DC: American Psychiatric Publishing; 2012. p. 85–128.

61. Donohue B, Loughran T, Pitts M, Gavrilova Y, Chow GM, Schubert K. Preliminary development of a brief intervention to prevent alcohol misuse and enhance sport performance in collegiate athletes. J Drug Abuse. 2016;2(3):1–9.

62. Hirschfield RMA, Bowden CL, Gitlin MJ, Keck PE, Suppes T, Thase Michael E, et al. Treatment of patients with bipolar disorder. 2nd ed. APA Practice Guidelines; 2010. p. 1–82.

63. Currie A, Gorczynski P, Rice SM, Purcell R, McAllister-Williams RH, Hitchcock ME, et al. Bipolar and psychotic disorders in elite athletes: a narrative review. Br J Sports Med. 2019;53(12):746–53.

64. Schreiber J, Culpepper L. Suicidal ideation and behavior in adults—UpToDate [Internet]. UpToDate; 2019. [cited 2019 Jan 29]. https://www.uptodate.com/contents/suicidal-ideation-and-behavior-in-adults.

65. National Institute for Health and Care Excellence. Borderline personality disorder: recognition and management. London; 2009.

Working with Diverse Athletes

Raphaela Shea Fontana, Aaron Jeckell, and Shane Creado

Introduction

Sport is a highly diverse activity that includes individuals from different cultural and racial backgrounds. "Diversity" can include different cultures, ethnicities, sexual orientations, and religious beliefs. An understanding of diversity moves us beyond our ethnocentric and egocentric viewpoints, allowing us to become better clinicians by strengthening the therapeutic alliance. "Culture" embodies layers of ethnicity, race, nationality, religion, regionalism, family, and group memberships [1]. Few things affect sport more profoundly than culture. The elite athlete (EA) is first a by-product of the culture in which they grow and develop. Culture may be considered as the blueprint for living—it provides the environmental forces that shape the morals, values, thoughts, feelings, and behaviors of our world's EAs.

As providers, it is critical that we work toward cultural humility as we enter the therapeutic arena with EAs and recognize that every EA has lived through their own unique experiences to get to where they are today. Culture, race, and ethnicity are tied to economic status and may affect an EA no differently than someone in the general population. While the Diagnostic and Statistical Manual of Mental Disorders 5th edition (DSM-5) has taken steps to consider cultural factors with the addition of the Cultural Formulation Interview, this metric is not specific to sports psychiatry and does not list specific cultural risk factors for which to assess. We will outline the utility of the biopsychosocial cultural spiritual

(BPSCS) model in approaching the cultural formulation of the EAs we encounter in treatment.

The Biopsychosocial Cultural Spiritual Model

The biopsychosocial model was first described in 1978 by George Engel, who believed that to understand and respond to a patient's suffering one must first understand the three core components of illness: biology, psychology, and social environment [2]. Although there has been controversy in recent years regarding this conceptual model [3], the majority of mental health professionals agree on the importance of seeing our patients as more than just an athlete or a mental health diagnosis. It remains pertinent to be mindful of the psychological sciences, neuroscience, and evolution of health care (including the presence of health inequities) among other factors when approaching the philosophical utility of the biopsychosocial model. In utilizing an expanded version of Engel's original model, the BPSCS formulation, we can now evolve and change our diagnostic assessment as the EA continues to grow and develop, providing new information along the way.

A BPSCS formulation consists of "4 P's": predisposing, precipitating, perpetuating, and protective factors [4]. Predisposing factors are areas of vulnerability that increase the risk of developing mental or other physical health conditions. Precipitating factors, also known as "stressors," are events that happen prior to the onset of symptoms. Perpetuating factors are conditions that continue to exacerbate or stress the problem. Protective factors offer protection and support to the patient, counteracting the other factors previously defined. These "4 P's" help outline the framework needed to understand the EAs with whom we are working at any given time (Table 21.1).

R. S. Fontana (✉)
Department of Psychiatry and Behavioral Medicine, Prisma Health—Upstate, Greenville, SC, USA

A. Jeckell
Department of Psychiatry and Behavioral Sciences, Vanderbilt University School of Medicine, Nashville, TN, USA

Broward Health Coral Springs, Coral Springs, FL, USA

S. Creado
Department of Psychiatry and Sleep Medicine, Amen Clinics, Inc.;
Shane Creado, LLC, Chicago, IL, USA

Table 21.1 The biopsychosocial cultural spiritual (BPSCS) model as a framework for working with diverse elite athletes. *EA* elite athlete

	Predisposing	Precipitating	Perpetuating	Protective
Biological	Genetics Substance use history Past psychiatric history and/ or symptoms Other medical illness Cognitive impairment Unresolved injury Demographics (age, sex, gender, race, ethnicity)	Medication nonadherence Other medical illness Relapse Cognitive impairment Injury Pregnancy/childbirth/ menopause	Medication nonadherence Substance use Cognitive impairment Other medical illness Debility Prolonged recovery from injury or illness	Medication adherence Responsiveness to treatment Exercise Abstinence from substance use
Psychological	Defense mechanisms/ego disruptions Adverse childhood events Schemas Low self-esteem Poor or tenuous interpersonal relationships Lack of support Weak nonathlete identity	Traumatic event Conflict/change in interpersonal relationships Identity conflict Lack of coping skills Distress intolerance Changes in cognition Grief/bereavement	Defense mechanisms Unstable interpersonal relationships Emotion dysregulation Lack of coping skills Athletic performance issues Trauma history	Mature defense mechanisms Positive and supportive interpersonal relationships Intrinsic motivation Resilience Mental toughness Good coping skills Exercise Balanced athletic identity
Social Cultural Spiritual	Low education level Adverse childhood events Health disparities Discrimination Social environment Cultural background Trauma	Legal stressors Housing instability Financial instability Inability to access health care Lack of a social support system Unemployment Identity crisis Media coverage Legal involvement	Inability to access health care Lack of a social support system Financial instability Unemployment Cultural/spiritual explanations of illness Media coverage	Experience navigating mental health treatment Health insurance Access to health care Spirituality and religious beliefs Adequate support system Employed Sport involvement

Predisposing Factors

Numerous factors can impact the likelihood of an EA developing mental health complications. While there is a paucity of high-quality research specific to this population, predisposing factors are critical to consider when developing a case formulation. Data support that EAs are vulnerable to a range of issues including mood disorders, trauma-related pathology, eating disorders, and substance use disorders [5]. The below two risk factors discussed are not the only predisposing risk factors to consider for an EA; the provider must remain mindful of the genetic factors, familial history, substance use, or other underlying medical etiologies to name a few.

Adverse Childhood Experiences (ACEs)

Adverse childhood experiences (ACEs) are traumatizing events that carry the potential to significantly change the psychological, emotional, and even neurobiological development of an individual. The Centers for Disease Control (CDC) groups ACEs into three categories—abuse, household challenges, and neglect. Abuse is comprised of physical, sexual, and/or emotional abuse. Household challenges can be varied and include household substance misuse, mental health symptoms and disorders, incarceration of a family member, family separation, and violence directed toward other family members at home. Neglect is typically considered to be emotional, physical, or resource-driven. Contemporary data have begun to emphasize community and larger systemic factors such as community violence, racism, and poverty as major contributors to ACEs.

Notably, ACEs can predispose any individual to health (including mental health) challenges later in life [6] and are unfortunately quite common. Several large-scale studies suggest that over half of the adults in the general population have experienced at least one ACE and a quarter of these adults have experienced two or more such events [7]. Data specific to athletes have been limited, though some studies suggest comparable statistics. A recent study of National Collegiate Athletic Association (NCAA) athletes has identified that 64.5% had experienced at least one ACE [8]. This is pertinent to EAs due to the propensity for ACEs to predispose an individual to worse general physical health and emotional flexibility as compared to someone without a trauma history, thereby possibly increasing the risk of injury or the development of poor coping strategies.

Systemic Discrimination

Socioeconomic status (SES) and financial factors can play a significant role in early sport participation and specialization. Unfortunately, systemic racism also plays a role in the disproportionate distribution of these resources and opportunities [9]. Access to different activities can vary considerably depending on the resources required for participation. For instance, ice hockey requires more equipment and specialized facilities that can be expensive to acquire and maintain as compared to soccer or basketball. As such, participation in these sports can stratify considerably based on the resources available to individuals and their communities.

Precipitating and Perpetuating Factors

Since both precipitating factors and perpetuating factors have a large amount of overlap and exist along a continuum,

they have been grouped together. The goal of this section is to provide a list of risk factors, in no particular order, for which to screen EAs within the framework of the DSM-5 Cultural Formulation Interview [10].

Perceived Identity

Our environment shapes our identity. As providers, it is crucial that we do not reject or support an EA's belief system or other proclivities. Our job is to understand their perceptions, thoughts, and feelings as a way to enhance our own understanding of their mental health symptoms to help bolster our treatment plan. It is important for the culturally aware provider to seek to understand an EA's sense of self in various domains (Table 21.2).

Table 21.2 The importance of recognizing the myriad of identities that may contribute to an elite athlete's emotional well-being

Domain	Clinical relevance	Examples
Religious/ spiritual identity	Certain religious or spiritual beliefs may help or hinder a clinician's ability to work with a given athlete. Treatment options may be limited based on an individual's religious background.	There are several religious groups that fear the presence of voodoo or "roots." In others, it is culturally acceptable for one to have visions of their recently deceased loved one. If the provider is unaware of these religious beliefs, then an EA could be wrongly diagnosed with psychosis or a primary thought disorder.
Political identity versus perceived political identity	Athletes from various sports leagues in the United States have been drawing focus on the systemic injustices experienced by minority groups. This is a charged sociopolitical issue. The mental health provider's role is to understand how the life experiences of their athletes impact them daily and how current events may be perceived differently by them relative to individuals from the same or a different background.	Kneeling during the national anthem or referencing social injustices on uniforms or equipment (e.g., representing the Black Lives Matter movement or LGBTQ+ equality). Any political statements made by athletes on the international stage at the 2020 Summer Olympics in Tokyo (held in 2021) were banned. There are instances of competition where athletes have refused to compete against athletes of another nation or cultural group with whom there is conflict.
National identity	Athletes from around the world come to certain countries to pursue collegiate and professional sports. There are several forces that shape an athlete's national identity in their formative years, such as the effects of mass migration, their country in turmoil, and millions of people settling in previously homogeneous countries.	A Japanese-Indian EA may want to represent Japan at the Olympics, but if the field is too competitive, then they may opt to represent India instead. On one hand, this can fulfill a lifelong dream of competing on the world stage, but on the other, it can lead to a feeling of betrayal of an athlete's own national identity.
Cultural identity	An athlete's cultural background can include many layers. An EA has the potential to be both impacted by and act as an impactful force on their culture. Their successes or failures can exert tremendous influence on the community that supports them or their team.	An EA immigrates from Colombia to the United States and feels a perceived inclination to change their culture to adapt to the environment around them. This can conflict with the EA's current belief system in the culture in which they grew up, and they may feel compelled to conform as opposed to upholding their cultural beliefs.
Racial identity	Racial identity is both externally imposed and internally constructed; when these two perceptions are at odds, it can create a significant amount of distress for the EA.	Biracial athletes may feel pressured to identify in a certain way by the media or teammates. An athlete may portray their racial identity publicly in a way that is divergent from how they internally identify. One cannot simply deny half of their heritage because of external pressure from social media without psychosocial consequences.
Athletic identity	Athletic identity is the degree to which an individual identifies with the athlete's role and looks to others for validation of that role [46]. Evidence has shown that a strong athletic identity can predispose EAs to adverse mental health outcomes when this identity is threatened by poor performance, retirement, injury, or mental health disorders.	Many in the athletic community adhere to the belief that it is admirable to play while hurt or injured. Axioms such as "pain is weakness leaving the body" are ubiquitous. This cultural practice may dissuade an athlete from acknowledging pain (including mental health suffering), predisposing them to a new or worse injury, and leaves room for bullying if an EA sits out an important competition due to an injury or illness.

(continued)

Table 21.2 (continued)

Domain	Clinical relevance	Examples
Societal identity	In some countries, sport is viewed as nonessential, whereas education is considered essential. Thus, a child's natural inclination toward sport may be curbed in favor of a more society-deemed appropriate future. In such environments, local governments, school districts, and other entities may direct resources away from sport, resulting in less-systematic and disciplined training for young athletes.	Japan can be considered as more of a collectivist society, whereas the United States is more of an individualistic society. For example, a vast majority of the Japanese public did not want the 2020 Olympic games to move forward, citing concerns about a global pandemic and the health implications on an international scale. Contrast this response with individuals exercising their personal liberties and attending packed sporting events in the United States. Neither culture is right or wrong, but this simply highlights the importance of the provider understanding societal impacts for the EA's participation in sport.
Ethnic identity	Ethnicity refers to a socially constructed identity based on one's self-concept and identification. An individual can identify as being part of multiple ethnic groups.	An athlete identifies as Muslim-American, stating that her parents are both from diverse ethnic backgrounds. She has felt torn about which sport to participate in because, although she loves gymnastics, her father is disapproving due to the uniform and what this symbolizes.
Gender identity	This is a complex discussion and a highly charged sociopolitical issue as it relates to participation in sport for LGBTQ+ EAs. There are several relevant issues, such as gender dysphoria, sports organizations' rules about transgender athletes, the debate about performance advantages based on the type of sport (e.g., gymnastics versus mixed martial arts), hormonal therapy and the age at which this was started by the EA, inherent biological differences among sexes, and other factors that are actively being discussed.	A transsexual male-to-female athlete dominates a volleyball match in the female category to such an extent that other competitors believe that there is an unfair advantage. The athlete provides appropriate documentation indicating that legally she is female and able to participate in sport. Many questions have come from similar scenarios. Is this fair? Should there be a specific blood hormone level to compete? Should a governing body restrict the right of transsexual athletes to compete in the gender category by which society and law accepts them as human beings?

EA elite athlete

Bullying/Hazing

Bullying, hazing, and sexual abuse in sport are ubiquitous. The underpinnings of each of these practices can vary considerably, with hazing being a type of "rite of passage," bullying being an exclusionary technique aimed at maintaining a social hierarchy, and sexual abuse serving the perpetrator and subjugating the victim [11, 12]. Unfortunately, many athletes have experienced some degree of maltreatment at some point in their sporting development. Studies have demonstrated that as many as 82% of NCAA athletes have experienced hazing, with 42% having experienced similar maltreatment during high school [13]. Despite the ubiquitous nature of hazing, there nonetheless exists a "code of silence" surrounding the practice that likely clouds the true incidence. Unfortunately, many athletes downplay the severity of these types of traumas due to fear of retaliation or belief that this maltreatment was for their improvement or the well-being of the team.

Media Coverage and Social Media Scrutiny

There has been no other time in modern history where athletes have been under greater media scrutiny. In addition to increased television coverage, we now have streaming and social media platforms where videos, clips, and memes of athletes can be disseminated to a limitless number of viewers with the click of a button. Material posted to Twitter, Facebook, and YouTube is often hyperbolic and inflammatory by design to increase exposure. As a result, a pseudo-journalistic industry has evolved where individuals work around the clock to develop an endless cycle of content focused on EAs and other high-profile individuals. This is all in addition to the preexisting social media scrutiny by fans and observers. An EA who is faced with a myriad of other stressors can be tipped into severe anxiety, depression, or suicidal thoughts and behaviors with the added burden of reading or seeing negative and hypercritical social media blasts. In extreme cases, EAs or even their loved ones have been the target of severe threats [14]. EAs who have any kind of online presence are subjected to an endless barrage of scrutiny or praise, which can dramatically contribute to stress or emotional distress.

Legal Stress/Regulations

Rules and regulations can be at the team, organizational, national, and international levels, and it can be extremely stressful for an EA to navigate these without support or guidance. Punishment for intended or unintended actions inside or outside the sports arena can range from simple fines to disqualification to being suspended or banned from sport. Rules are constantly evolving, and an EA may have little to no awareness or input when it comes to voicing their concerns regarding proposed regulations. This can be especially true when involving international competition or competition outside of one's regular league or organization and can lead to a sense of powerlessness, hopelessness, and defeat.

Athlete-Specific Cognitive Distortions

While cognitive distortions may not meet the criteria for a mental health disorder, they can certainly have a direct impact on an EA's performance and emotional well-being as well as a therapeutic relationship. An EA can begin to view their identity as a direct reflection of their own or their team's successes or failures if they start to become overly attached to the outcome in competition. Pressure can drive EAs to self-medicate with alcohol or other substances that can exacerbate or precipitate mental health disorders such as depression or anxiety. In the case of an EA, please see specific athlete-related cognitive distortions (Fig. 21.1).

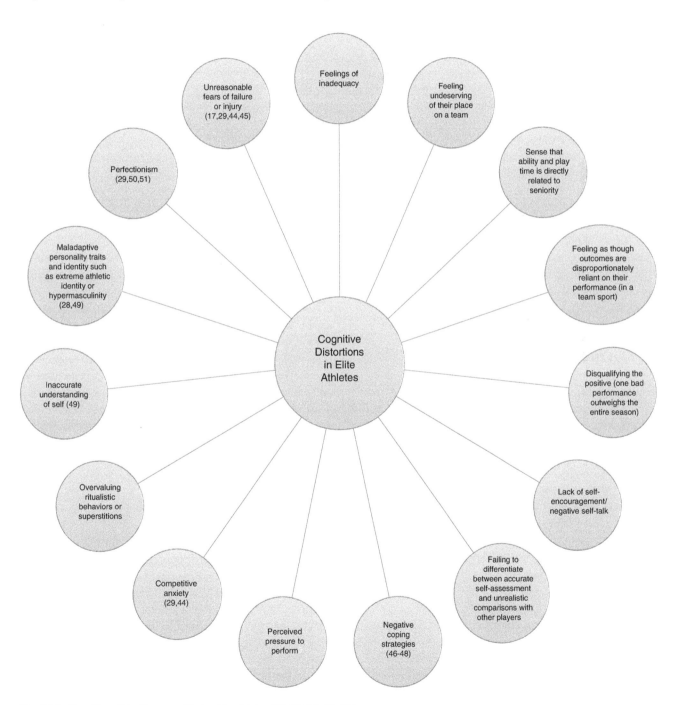

Fig. 21.1 Cognitive distortions specific to elite athletes [17, 29, 30, 47–54]

Financial Stress

Excelling in sport and achieving an elite status do not always correlate with financial success or stability. A recent study of Olympic athletes across 48 countries has found that 58% did not consider themselves to be financially stable; athletes responded that they frequently relied on family and donations to fund training and that financial instability negatively impacted performance [15]. Even athletes who participate in sports and are perceived to be living a life of profound wealth can face economic hardship after retirement. EAs may have unrealistic expectations about how long their careers or finances may last. The average athlete in any major league US sport (e.g., National Football League (NFL), National Basketball Association (NBA), Major League Baseball (MLB)) plays at that level for 5–7 years, which means that the average EA will retire around the age of 30 years old [16].

While athletes receive extensive training in their sport, they rarely receive financial education or advice. EAs may underestimate the taxes, agent fees, or other costs associated with their athletic status, whereas others may feel pressured to live a lavish and ostentatious lifestyle to conform to cultural expectations or to financially support family members. Some athletes acquire tremendous wealth with little to no understanding of how to manage their finances, making them vulnerable to predatory advisors during or after their careers. EAs who have experienced a sudden spike in wealth followed by financial hardship may encounter mental health issues later in life.

Barriers to Care

This can take many forms and is best summarized by Fig. 21.2. Stigma continues to be highlighted as a barrier to help-seeking behavior in athletes [17, 18]. The stigma against expressing anything that may be perceived as weakness is profound in the world of EAs. Just like how some may feel pressured to suppress the expression of physical pain, many athletes feel unable to safely disclose their mental health symptoms. There is a general view that athletes who seek help for psychological problems may be seen as weak by other athletes and coaches [19]. EAs are commonly upheld as a paragon of strength and, as such, any expression of weakness is often dissuaded.

Career Transition or Retirement from Sport

Career transitions are critical phases in an EA's career [20]. In all, 15–20% of athletes are expected to face serious adjustment difficulties, including a feeling of loss, identity crises, and distress, following athletic retirement [21]. Uncertainty about retirement [22] and retired status compared to active status [23] are significant risk factors for an EA to decompensate emotionally, especially if their identities are closely linked to sport and there is no set plan for retirement. Gouttebarge et al. showed that among current and former football (soccer) players, up to 39% of retired players faced mental health challenges including adverse nutritional and drinking behavior [23]. It is critical to identify an EA's sense of self both in and out of sport when developing a therapeutic rapport.

Travel Impacts

Professional sport often requires travel across time zones, and competitions cannot be adjusted to suit individual needs for each EA. Travel, regardless of distance, can disrupt normal routines and may lead to several downstream effects, such as mood fluctuations, changes in sleep patterns, higher cortisol levels, performance impairments, and lowered emotional resilience. Travel can further compound stressors when EAs are forced to be away from their support systems in times of joy (e.g., births of babies, weddings, birthdays, holidays) and sorrow (e.g., loss and bereavement).

Travel fatigue and jet lag can worsen sports performance, thereby compounding stress [24]. For example, the NBA season consists of 4–6 preseason games played across 3–4 weeks followed by an 82-game regular season played across 26 weeks (177 days). NBA players can fly up to 50,000 miles per season—roughly 20,000 more miles each season than NFL teams and far enough to circle the globe twice. Westward travel may also worsen performance as compared to eastward travel; NBA teams that traveled eastward scored more points per game and had a winning percentage of 45.4% compared with 36.2% for teams traveling westward [25]. Similar performance profiles have been reported in the NFL and the National Hockey League (NHL).

Injury

Serious injury, particularly a career-ending injury, is a significant risk factor for the development of mood disorders in athletes [26]. In addition, poor general health [27], such as chronic back pain [28], permanent disability [29, 30], osteoarthritis [31], overtraining syndrome, severe injury/surgery [32, 33], and low quality of sleep that can accompany injury [34, 35] are all significant stressors for an EA.

Sport-related concussions (SRCs) warrant special mention, in part, due to the potential harmful impact on mental health associated with this injury as well as the misinforma-

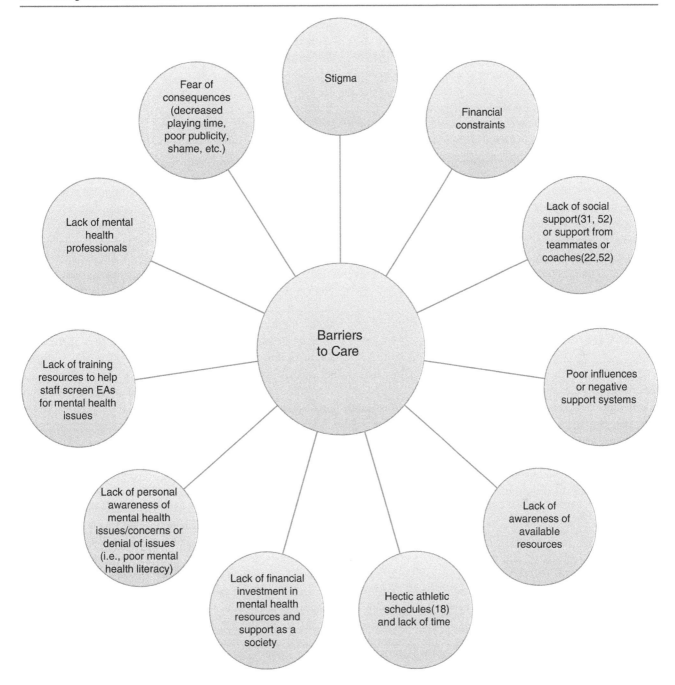

Fig. 21.2 Barriers to care for elite athletes [18, 23, 32, 55]. *EAs* elite athletes

tion and confusion surrounding this topic. SRCs can affect reaction time, resilience, and sleep patterns and lead to visual processing speed changes, tinnitus, pituitary dysfunction, dysautonomia, and many other conditions—each of which can present a unique challenge to an EA in recovery from this form of injury [36]. Immediate recognition and an appropriate response to an SRC is critical, as return to play pre-emptively can lead to poor outcomes. The number of prior concussions sustained, the severity of the sequelae, and other mental health and general medical comorbidities are all factors that can impact an EA's recovery. Each athlete will have

unique considerations when evaluating their treatment plan and future in sport after sustaining an SRC.

Protective Factors

Protective factors are features, experiences, or skills an individual possesses that promote resilience in the face of hardship or challenges. These are often extremely important in warding off or managing mental health symptoms and disorders, as the road to becoming an EA is filled with adversity.

Former Treatment

While the existence of a preexisting mental health disorder would be considered a predisposing risk factor for an EA, previous engagement in mental health treatment may serve as a protective factor. For the EA who is struggling, knowing how to seek out mental health resources can be protective and advantageous to their well-being. This is especially true if the EA has an established relationship with licensed mental health professionals or other resources. An EA who has had success navigating their mental health symptoms or disorders may also be more open to talking about their experiences with their family, friends, teammates, coaching staff, or even the media. Such an athlete may serve as an important example or role model to others who are struggling with their mental health. Having a support system in place has been shown to improve access to care and adherence to treatment.

Health Care

The EA may have access to numerous resources that would otherwise be more difficult to attain relative to the general population. Health care is no exception. Most professional teams employ medical staff, including trainers, nutritionists, physicians, and physical therapists. Elite-level professional organizations may even have expensive imaging machinery and other medical equipment on the premises of their stadium or training facility, thus greatly improving access to care.

Spirituality/Religious Beliefs

Despite some reports and visuals, there is a paucity of data specific to the rates of religiosity in the EA population. Several common visuals include seeing an EA make the sign of the cross on the sideline or seeing Bible scriptures or verses on an EA's body or equipment. It is also not uncommon to hear a prayer coming from the locker room or to read about teams relying on a clergy member to bless their performance on the field or to even curse the opponents. A recent study of EAs has found that high levels of religiosity were related to high levels of self-worth and low levels of shame when considering athletic failures [37]. Moreover, high levels of religiosity were correlated with greater levels of comfort in competition via higher levels of self-worth. However, there is also a documented association between the perceived perfection of God and the EA's personal performance being correlated with feelings of shame. Overall, this study sug-

gested that religiosity could be, but is not universally, a powerful resource in helping athletes deal with psychological difficulties and challenges [37].

Superstition

Many EAs adhere to superstitions or ritualistic behaviors as a technique to bring about a sense of familiarity to the unknown and unpredictable nature of competition. Paired with visualization and mindfulness techniques, rituals have the potential to provide an EA with a sense of control over difficult situations. These behaviors can range from a specific pregame activity or meal to touching or manipulating a piece of equipment in a certain manner. EAs are motivated to gain a competitive edge, so these superstitions and behaviors can evolve over time based on the results that they are perceived to bring about in competition or performance. At times, these can veer into maladaptive behaviors if adhering to them in any way interferes with the success of the individual or the team. As mental health providers, it is pertinent to identify whether these behaviors are pathological and a hindrance versus ritualistic and beneficial to the EA's performance.

Involvement in Sport

Involvement in sport can be expected to confer numerous protective benefits on the EA. An EA may enjoy a certain level of prestige and social benefit due to their involvement in sport. A membership in a team, organization, or community has been demonstrated to confer mental health benefits including an improved sense of self, greater feelings of interconnectedness, and lower levels of anxiety [38, 39]. This is prominent in circumstances where an EA is representing an organization to which they feel a strong emotional connection such as their national team or hometown organization.

Early data also suggest that among youths who have experienced ACEs, participation in a team sport is associated with improved mental health outcomes as an adult [40]. This is consistent with other data that demonstrated the significant mental health benefits associated with team sport participation [41, 42]. Researchers have found a correlation between ACEs and the resiliency seen in EAs that they link to a "motivational trigger," which fuels an intensity and passion for their chosen sport [43]. Although further studies are warranted, EAs are likely to benefit from involvement in sport as a method to build resilience after experiencing adversity and hardship.

Case 1

Anna is a bisexual, cis-gender, Asian-American, 18-year-old female figure skater who has been living away from home secondary to her desire to train for a national competition. Although she has been performing well, she has been distracted during practice—something that could put her personal safety at risk. When asked about this by the team psychiatrist, Anna confides that she has experienced sexual assault. She reports being taken advantage of by a medical staff member the previous weekend and later identifies as being raped. However, she also worries that by saying something she will get some of her teammates in trouble too since this occurred while a few of them were drinking alcohol together after a grueling practice week. She indicates that other teammates have told her about similar occurrences in recent months.

As more instances of abuse come to light, the practice rink, staff, and team come under close media scrutiny in their city. Anna, as well as other teammates, experience a high degree of publicity. She is bombarded with derogatory statements regarding her race and gender identity, and several journalists find information about her family history including allegations of physical abuse from a child protective services report when she was 7 years old. This further hampers her ability to perform in sport. She begins seeing a therapist and psychiatrist specifically to process her recent and past traumatic experiences. She identifies as having a high degree of anxiety and endorses symptoms consistent with post-traumatic stress disorder. She is started on a selective serotonin reuptake inhibitor (SSRI) due to the severity of her symptoms and begins trauma-focused cognitive behavioral therapy.

Anna responds well to treatment and feels empowered to continue competing in figure skating. However, she now feels conflicted and self-conscious about the traditional figure skating uniform that she has typically worn, one that she feels hypersexualizes athletes. After careful consideration and with the support of the coaching staff and administration, she makes the decision to wear a less-revealing leotard during competition. Even though the amount of clothing cover is not associated with an increased risk of sexual abuse in sport, she now feels able to shift her own focus from the exposure of her body to her athletic prowess and talent. She continues to perform extremely well and feels proud that she is serving as a positive role model to youth athletes everywhere.

Time for practice! The reader can create a biopsychosocial formulation for Anna's case presentation using the 4 P's outlined below (and you may think of more!):

- Predisposing factors: Systemic discrimination/racism, race and ethnicity, adverse childhood events, sex
- Precipitating factors: Sexual assault/trauma, substance use, heightened anxiety, living away from home, discrimination (racial, gender identity, sexual orientation)
- Perpetuating factors: Media scrutiny and undesired publicity, uniform, sexual orientation and gender identity, trauma history, discrimination, pandemic
- Protective factors: Seeking out general medical and mental health treatment, positive support system, supportive athletic administration, views self as a role model to youth athletes, involvement in sport/exercise, medication and treatment adherence, resilience

Importance of Cultural Humility

Providers must continually foster cultural humility while treating EAs. This means "admitting that *one does not know* and is willing to *learn from patients* about their experience, while being aware of one's own embeddedness in culture(s)," [44] and providing person-centered care through intrapersonal and interpersonal approaches. Differences in culture can possibly lead to misunderstanding the patient during treatment. Therefore, it is imperative that providers foster an understanding of cultural humility through self-assessment, appreciation of the patient's expertise, openness to balancing the power differential in the clinician–patient relationship, and dedication to lifelong learning to practice culturally and linguistically appropriate health-care services [44].

Cultural humility trainings are driven to be more "process-oriented" to enhance a provider's ability to provide patient-centered care, as compared to cultural competency training, which tends to be more "content-oriented" and aims to improve providers' knowledge and confidence in treating diverse patients [44]. Good patient–provider communication positively affects patient and provider satisfaction, patient adherence to therapy, and health outcomes [45]. Importantly, a willingness to "learn from patients" about their experiences does not mean that it is the athlete's job to educate the clinician. Providers should consider the recommendations in Table 21.3 when entering into a clinician–patient relationship with an EA who is culturally different from their own identification.

Table 21.3 Clinical pearls on how providers can foster cultural humility [44]

- Reflect on your own beliefs, values, and biases—both implicit and explicit—to see how your own culture may impact the care you provide to your patient.
- Adopt a person-centered stance where one is respectful of a patient's identity and their cultural background. Keep an open mind and invite the athlete to share any information about their background or current situation that they feel safe revealing.
- Humble oneself to counterbalance the authority that comes with being a provider, and equalize the physician–patient relationship.
- Gain knowledge and awareness both outside and inside the therapeutic alliance to help understand the practice and worldviews of different cultures.
- A technique that providers can implement in session is the Ask, Share, Compare, and Negotiate model (ASCN or "askin") as described by Kutob et al. [45]. This model trains providers to first ask questions in a nonjudgmental manner about the patient's views of the etiology of their disease and treatment plan, to share the biomedical model, to compare the patient's views with the provider's views, and to negotiate a treatment plan through collaboration. This approach has been shown to help providers avoid coming to a premature conclusion and instead incorporate the patient's views regarding the treatment plan.

Conclusions

Until very recently, it has been essentially unheard of for a high-profile athlete to speak openly about their mental health struggles. A new generation of athletes, with the support of their teammates, coaches, family, and mental health providers, is beginning to shift this trend. With building momentum, it is imperative for the provider to understand the stressors identified throughout this chapter as they can be critical to the understanding of an EA when facing mental health symptoms or disorders. Implementation of the BPSCS model can be one method that the provider can use to help understand cultural differences and close gaps related to health inequities and cultural incompetence. While it is not feasible for all providers to be experts in all cultures, we should strive to recognize our own biases and have the awareness to conduct research and ask questions that will help us understand cultures different from our own. The hope is that the provider will work toward fostering cultural humility in their practice. Without this, it can be impossible to build a strong therapeutic alliance with an EA. In Sir William Osler's words, "the good physician treats the disease; the great physician treats the patient who has the disease."

References

1. O'Toole JK, Alvarado-Little W, Ledford CJW. Communication with diverse patients: addressing culture and language. Pediatr Clin N Am. 2019;66(4):791–804.
2. Borrell-Carrio F, Suchman AL, RM E. The biopsychosocial model 25 years later: principles, practice and scientific inquiry. Ann Fam Med. 2004;2(6):576–82.
3. Benning TB. Limitations of the biopsychosocial model in psychiatry. Adv Med Educ Pract. 2015;6:347–52.
4. Wright CD, Tiani AG, Billingsley AL, Steinman SA, Larkin KT, McNeil DW. A framework for understanding the role of psychological processes in disease development, maintenance, and treatment: the 3P-disease model. Front Psychol. 2019;10:2498.
5. Rice SM, Purcell R, De Silva S, Mawren D, McGorry PD, Parker AG. The mental health of elite athletes: a narrative systematic review. Sports Med. 2016;46(9):1333–53.
6. Petruccelli K, Davis J, Berman T. Adverse childhood experiences and associated health outcomes: a systematic review and meta-analysis. Child Abuse Negl. 2019;97:104127.
7. Felitti VJ, Anda RF, Nordenberg D, Williamson DF, Spitz AM, Edwards V, et al. Relationship of childhood abuse and household dysfunction to many of the leading causes of death in adults. The Adverse Childhood Experiences (ACE) Study. Am J Prev Med. 1998;14(4):245–58.
8. Brown BJ, Jensen JF, Hodgson JL, Schoemann AM, Rappleyea DL. Beyond the lines: exploring the impact of adverse childhood experiences on NCAA student-athlete health. J Issues Intercoll Athl. 2020:8–38.
9. Zondi PC, AV A. A question of colour: systemic racism in sports and exercise medicine. Br J Sports Med. 2021;55(10):519–30.
10. DSM-5 handbook on the cultural formulation interview. American Psychiatric Publishing, Inc.; 2016.
11. Jeckell AS, Copenhaver EA, Diamond AB. The spectrum of hazing and peer sexual abuse in sports: a current perspective. Sports Health. 2018;10(6):558–64.
12. Jeckell AS, Copenhaver EA, Diamond AB. Hazing and bullying in athletic culture. In: Hong ERA, editor. Mental health in the athlete. Cham: Springer; 2020. p. 165–79.
13. Hoover NC, Pollard NJ. National survey: initiation rites and athletics for NCAA sports teams. New York: Alfred; 1999.
14. Sullivan T. Today's athletes must tread carefully in an increasingly hostile worl of social media. The Boston Globe; 2021.
15. Global Athlete Survey Results: athlete rights, welfare, and representation. Global Athlete; 2020.
16. Management RW. Professional athletes need a retirement game plan. Royal Bank of Canada Website; 2021.
17. Biggin IJ, Burns J, Uphill MA. An investigation of athletes' and coaches' perceptions of mental ill-health in elite athletes. J Clin Sport Psychol. 2017;11:126–47.
18. Gulliver A, Griffiths KM, Christensen H. Barriers and facilitators to mental health help-seeking for young elite athletes: a qualitative study. BMC Psychiatry. 2012;12:157.
19. Souter G, Lewis R, Serrant L. Men, mental health and elite sport: a narrative review. Sports Med Open. 2018;4(1):57.
20. Stambulova N, Alfermann D, Statler T, Côté J. ISSP position stand: career development and transitions of athletes. Int J Sport Exerc Psychol. 2009;7:395–412.
21. Park S-h, Lavallee D, Tod D. Athletes' career transition out of sport: a systematic review. Int Rev Sport Exerc Psychol. 2013;6:22–53.
22. Beable S, Fulcher M, Lee AC, Hamilton B. SHARPSports mental Health Awareness Research Project: prevalence and risk factors of depressive symptoms and life stress in elite athletes. J Sci Med Sport. 2017;20(12):1047–52.
23. Gouttebarge V, Frings-Dresen MH, Sluiter JK. Mental and psychosocial health among current and former professional footballers. Occup Med (Lond). 2015;65(3):190–6.
24. Leatherwood WE, Dragoo JL. Effect of airline travel on performance: a review of the literature. Br J Sports Med. 2013;47(9):561–7.
25. Steenland K, Deddens J. Effect of travel and rest on performance of professional basketball players. Sleep. 1997;20:366–9.
26. Reardon CL, Factor RM. Sport psychiatry: a systematic review of diagnosis and medical treatment of mental illness in athletes. Sports Med. 2010;40(11):961–80.

27. Junge A, Prinz B. Depression and anxiety symptoms in 17 teams of female football players including 10 German first league teams. Br J Sports Med. 2019;53(8):471–7.

28. Belz J, Heidari J, Levenig C, Hasenbring M, Kellmann M, Kleinert J. Stress and risk for depression in competitive athletes suffering from back pain—do age and gender matter? Eur J Sport Sci. 2018;18(7):1029–37.

29. Jones TV. Predictors of perceptions of mental illness and averseness to help: a survey of elite football players. J Ment Health. 2016;25(5):422–7.

30. Newman HJ, Howells KL, Fletcher D. The dark side of top level sport: an autobiographic study of depressive experiences in elite sport performers. Front Psychol. 2016;7:868.

31. Schuring N, Aoki H, Gray J, Kerkhoffs G, Lambert M, Gouttebarge V. Osteoarthritis is associated with symptoms of common mental disorders among former elite athletes. Knee Surg Sports Traumatol Arthrosc. 2017;25(10):3179–85.

32. Gouttebarge V, Jonkers R, Moen M, Verhagen E, Wylleman P, Kerkhoffs G. The prevalence and risk indicators of symptoms of common mental disorders among current and former Dutch elite athletes. J Sports Sci. 2017;35(21):2148–56.

33. Kilic Ö, Aoki H, Haagensen R, Jensen C, Johnson U, Kerkhoffs G, et al. Symptoms of common mental disorders and related stressors in Danish professional football and handball. Eur J Sport Sci. 2017;17(10):1328–34.

34. Biggins M, Cahalan R, Comyns T, Purtill H, O'Sullivan K. Poor sleep is related to lower general health, increased stress and increased confusion in elite Gaelic athletes. Phys Sportsmed. 2018;46(1):14–20.

35. Gerber M, Holsboer-Trachsler E, Pühse U, Brand S. Elite sport is not an additional source of distress for adolescents with high stress levels. Percept Mot Skills. 2011;112(2):581–99.

36. Gonzalez Hofmann C, Fontana R, Parker T, Deutschmann M, Dewey M, Reinsberger C, Claussen MC, Scherr J, Jeckell AS. Sports psychiatry and medical views on mild traumatic brain injury in competitive sport: a current review and recommendations. Dtsch Z Sportmed. 2021; 72: 293–9. https://doi.org/10.5960/dzsm.2021.501.

37. Houltberg BJ, Wang KT, Schnitker SA. Religiousness and perceived god perfectionism among elite athletes. J Christ Soc Kinesiol Leis Sport Stud. 2017;4(1):29–46.

38. Eime RM, Young JA, Harvey JT, Charity MJ, Payne WR. A systematic review of the psychological and social benefits of participation in sport for children and adolescents: informing development of a conceptual model of health through sport. Int J Behav Nutr Phys Act. 2013;10:98.

39. Dimech AS, Seiler R. Extra-curricular sport participation: a potential buffer against social anxiety symptoms in primary school children. Psychol Sport Exerc. 2011;12:347–54.

40. Easterlin MC, Chung PJ, Leng M, Dudovitz R. Association of team sports participation with long-term mental health outcomes among individuals exposed to adverse childhood experiences. JAMA Pediatr. 2019;173(7):681–8.

41. Pluhar E, McCracken C, Griffith KL, Christino MA, Sugimoto D, Meehan WP III. Team sport athletes may be less likely to suffer anxiety or depression than individual sport athletes. J Sports Sci Med. 2019;18(3):490–6.

42. Johnston SA, Roskowski C, He Z, Kong L, Chen W. Effects of team sports on anxiety, depression, perceived stress, and sleep quality in college students. J Am Coll Heal. 2021;69(7):791–7.

43. Allan V. The suprising role of chilldhood trauma in athletic success the conversation. The Canadian Press; 2018. https://nationalpost.com/pmn/news-pmn/the-surprising-role-of-childhood-trauma-in-athletic-success.

44. Lekas H-M, Pahl K, Fuller Lewis C. Rethinking cultural competence: shifting to cultural humility. Health Serv Insights. 2020;13:1178632920970580.

45. Kutob RM, Bormanis J, Crago M, Harris JM Jr, Senf J, Shisslak CM. Cultural competence education for practicing physicians: lessons in cultural humility, nonjudgmental behaviors, and health beliefs elicitation. J Contin Educ Heal Prof. 2013;33(3):164–73.

46. Brewer BW, Van Raalte JL, Linder DE. Athletic identity: Hercules' muscles or Achilles heel? Int J Sport Psychol. 1993;24(2):237–54.

47. Coyle M, Gorczynski P, Gibson K. "You have to be mental to jump off a board any way": elite divers' conceptualizations and perceptions of mental health. Psychol Sport Exerc. 2017;29:10–8.

48. Hammond T, Gialloreto C, Kubas H, Hap Davis H. The prevalence of failure-based depression among elite athletes. Clin J Sport Med. 2013;23(4):273–7.

49. Mousavi A, Mousavi MKV, Yaghubi H, editors. Defense mechanisms in psychological health and sport success of athletes; 2017.

50. Nixdorf I, Frank R, Beckmann J. Comparison of athletes' proneness to depressive symptoms in individual and team sports: research on psychological mediators in junior elite athletes. Front Psychol. 2016;7:893.

51. Nixdorf I, Frank R, Hautzinger M, Beckmann J. Prevalence of depressive symptoms and correlating variables among German elite athletes. J Clin Sport Psychol. 2013;7:313–26.

52. Doherty S, Hannigan B, Campbell MJ. The experience of depression during the careers of elite male athletes. Front Psychol. 2016;7:1069.

53. Jensen SN, Ivarsson A, Fallby J, Dankers S, Elbe A-M. Depression in Danish and Swedish elite football players and its relation to perfectionism and anxiety. Psychol Sport Exerc. 2018;36:147–55.

54. Lundqvist C, Raglin JS. The relationship of basic need satisfaction, motivational climate and personality to well-being and stress patterns among elite athletes: an explorative study. Motiv Emot. 2015;39(2):237–46.

55. Prinz B, Dvořák J, Junge A. Symptoms and risk factors of depression during and after the football career of elite female players. BMJ Open Sport Exerc Med. 2016;2(1):e000124.

Mental Health in Youth Elite Athletes

Courtney C. Walton, Simon M. Rice, and Rosemary Purcell

As documented throughout the various chapters of this book, elite athletes are exposed to a range of stressors and risk factors, which may predispose them to experiencing mental health symptoms and disorders [1, 2]. However, there are specific subgroups of athletes who experience elite sport differently (i.e., due to age, gender, culture), potentially contributing in varied ways to their mental health. In this chapter, we will discuss how elite youth athletes can face a range of distinct issues that are relevant to clinical care and the likelihood of experiencing mental health symptoms and disorders [3, 4]. Within this chapter, we consider youth athletes as those aged 12–18 years. While *youth* is increasingly considered to encompass a larger age group (typically 12–25 years of age) on the basis of accomplishment of social and economic milestones (e.g., leaving home, obtaining employment), we focus here on those under 18 who are faced with specific barriers prior to reaching young adulthood.

Common mental health disorders such as various types of mood and anxiety disorders are highly prevalent among young people [5]. Approximately half of all mental health disorders begin by middle adolescence [6]. It is estimated that approximately 20–25% of adolescents and young adults in the general community will experience a diagnosable disorder in any given year [5]. A number of factors are believed to contribute to this heightened prevalence, including aspects related to puberty, identity formation, changing interpersonal relationships, and a range of risk factors such as experiencing abuse, neglect, bullying, and social disadvantage [5, 7]. Therefore, prior to any environmental factors relating to sport, young athletes are already at an increased risk of men-

tal health symptoms and disorders owing directly to their age and developmental period. In the following section, we highlight how specific aspects of the youth sports environment can further contribute to youth athletes' experiences around mental health.

Mental Health and the Youth Sports Environment

It is important to consider that, typically, youth sport is a valuable and beneficial environment for child and adolescent development. This may be particularly relevant in nonelite settings, where psychosocial development can be prioritized over performance and competition-based outcomes. In addition to these environments intrinsically supporting mental health, they are also well-suited for delivering targeted education and early intervention programs [8, 9]. Physical exercise and sport are believed to provide benefits to the mental health of young people via numerous biological, psychological, and social effects such as the positive neurophysiological effects of physical activity, improved self-esteem, and increased social integration, respectively [4]. An influential review by Holt et al. [10] illustrated that sport can contribute to positive youth development in the form of enhanced self-perceptions, problem-solving skills, stress management, goal setting, responsibility, perseverance, and independence, in addition to developing friendships, communication skills, and leadership. Vella et al. [11] have demonstrated that the relationships between sports participation and adolescent mental health are bidirectional, with time involved in organized sport predicting better future mental health and vice versa. Meta-analysis has also generally supported these relationships, with adolescents engaged across various forms of sports participation showing *lower* levels of anxiety and depressive symptoms [12]. Predominantly, however, these findings relate to *recreational* or *community* sport, which is often more social and less-competitive or pressurized by nature. The positive effects of youth sport on mental health

C. C. Walton (✉) · S. M. Rice · R. Purcell
Elite Sport and Mental Health, Orygen, Melbourne, VIC, Australia

Centre for Youth Mental Health, The University of Melbourne, Melbourne, VIC, Australia
e-mail: courtney.walton@orygen.org.au;
rosie.purcell@orygen.org.au; simon.rice@orygen.org.au

are therefore not necessarily a given in elite environments, where other factors may come into play.

Despite increased interest in the mental health of elite athletes, surprisingly little research has examined those involved at the youth level. This represents an important and underexplored population, given the varying and potentially interacting factors that may be influential, including age, schooling, and biopsychosocial development. With regard to the general prevalence, only a small number of studies have examined this population. For example, Weber et al. [13] provided some insights into the experience of depression and anxiety in young athletes at an elite level. Among a large sample of student athletes from an elite sports school in Germany, 7.1% and 3.1% were classified as possible and probable cases of anxiety, respectively, whereas this was 9.5% and 3.7%, respectively, for depression, lower than many comparative samples. Brand et al. [14] also compared the rates of mental health symptoms among student athletes at elite sports schools in Germany. Generally, results pointed to more significant symptoms in female athletes and in those who had recently been deselected from progressing in their sport. In addition to gender and the current competition status, further evidence of contextual risk factors exists, with one study demonstrating youth athletes in individual sports to have more significant depressive symptoms than those in team sports [15].

Although there is no strong evidence to link elite sports participation in youth to either improved or worsened mental health in a general sense, there are a number of contextual factors and stressors that may influence the mental well-being in youth athletes. Not least is the fact that youth sports environments are increasingly specialized with higher rates of professionalism expected at younger ages. Potential negative psychosocial outcomes of young athletes engaging in early specialization include social isolation, poor academic performance, increased anxiety, greater stress, inadequate sleep, decreased family time, and burnout [16].

Stressors Encountered by Elite Youth Athletes

There are numerous stressors that can affect how a youth athlete may experience their sport [17] and, subsequently, their mental health. Here, we will loosely separate these based on (1) individual factors, relating to particular cognitive, emotional, and behavioral traits and (2) environmental or external factors, relating to the environment and those within it. However, although this distinction is helpful on a descriptive level, in reality, there is a significant overlap between this binary classification. We also emphasize that the stressors described below do not necessarily "predict" mental health symptoms and disorders, but can provide insights into the potential difficult experiences that an elite youth athlete may face, to be considered by practitioners working to maintain their mental well-being or to respond to mental health symptoms or disorders.

Individual Factors

Youth athletes competing within elite and competitive settings are exposed to pressure to perform from increasingly earlier ages. Such pressure likely contributes to the significant rates of perfectionistic attitudes seen in youth athletes [18]. Perfectionism is typically conceptualized as including at least two key factors: (1) 'perfectionistic concerns', which relate to the pursuit of exacting standards imposed by significant others and (2) 'perfectionistic strivings', which relate to the pursuit of self-imposed goals and standards accompanied by harsh self-criticism [19]. Meta-analytic evidence suggests that while perfectionistic strivings tend to be associated with more adaptive outcomes in both performance and well-being, perfectionistic concerns are associated with poorer well-being and a higher likelihood of experiencing anxiety, while providing no clear benefit to sporting performance [20]. Furthermore, perfectionistic concerns have regularly been associated with the experience of burnout in youth athletes [18, 21], which can be a problematic experience contributing to poor mental health.

Burnout in sport is typically characterized by both physical and emotional exhaustion, along with a reduced sense of accomplishment and sport devaluation [22]. Early sport specialization is becoming increasingly common in the context of the growing professionalization of youth sport [16]. Athletes, coaches, and parents may anticipate that this early focus will increase a young person's chances of future success; however, burnout is a possible outcome. A study by Granz et al. [23] employed complex classification analytic techniques to identify youth athletes at risk of burnout. They identified factors associated with burnout including involvement in technical, endurance, aesthetic, or weight-dependent sports, training under an autocratic or a laissez-faire coach, high subjective stress outside of sport, a low willingness to make psychological sacrifices, lack of sleep, and female sex. On the other hand, fewer hours of training, low social pressure, low subjective stress outside of sport, a high willingness to make psychological sacrifices, and high health satisfaction were protective [23].

As identified above [23], poor sleep can exert significant effects on burnout, and there is a well-established link between sleep quality and mental health generally [24]. While achieving adequate sleep can be an ongoing problem for athletes already (see Chap. 5 for a broader overview), this may be further accentuated in young people. This is owing to the facts that (1) adolescents generally demonstrate poorer sleep patterns than do adults and (2) competing sporting, academic, and social demands of elite youth athletes may affect sleep schedules. Evidence from one systematic review showed that child and adolescent athletes had impaired sleep when assessed via sleep time, sleep efficiency, and waking after sleep onset [25].

An additional significant risk factor for mental health symptoms and disorders in youth athletes is body image and weight concerns. Given the complex presentation and management of these concerns, readers are encouraged to refer to Chap. 9, which focuses entirely on eating disorders. Adolescents are at a risk of eating disorders [26]. In adolescent athletes specifically, a large study reported 8% *constantly* trying to lose weight, 12% using compensatory methods (e.g., fasting or purging), and 32.5% fulfilling the criteria for an eating disorder [27]. Unfortunately, little is known about the specific risk factors for youth athletes, given the frequent inconsistencies in the literature [28]. Furthermore, while eating disorders are more commonly associated with female athletes, male athletes have been relatively neglected in the literature [29].

Environmental Factors

In addition to the experiences described above, there are a range of external or environmental factors that can potentially contribute to mental health symptoms and disorders among elite youth athletes. Potentially exerting the most influence on youth athletes—both positive and negative—is the role of responsible adults, primarily parents and coaches, within these spaces. It is important to keep in mind that for the most part, parents have a protective impact on youth athletes' experiences in sport. This can be through providing emotional, behavioral, financial, and logistical support. However, parents of athletes can also be a key contributor to stress or discomfort by being sources of negative or critical feedback, anger, or inappropriate behavior during competition or training and by holding unrealistic expectations for the young athlete [30]. Similarly, coaches can have a supportive role for youth athletes and their mental health in particular [31]. However, there is an inherent power imbalance that exists between the athlete and the adults who are responsible for decisions critical to their sporting ambitions and desires (e.g., playing time, selection, medical treatment, training priority). Furthermore, there is potential for abuse to occur in youth sports environments [32, 33]. Experiences such as these can have significant and ongoing effects on the mental health of young people involved in sport [34].

In addition to interpersonal stressors, injuries, including concussions, are common occurrences for athletes at all levels, as covered in Chap. 17. However, youth athletes are at a particular risk due to the ongoing physical and physiological

changes being undertaken as well as underdeveloped coordination, skills, and perception [35]. Similarly, the role that concussion has in mental health is receiving increasing attention in the sports literature [36]. Of particular concern in this population is that adolescent athletes may underreport postconcussive symptoms, due to not wanting to leave the game, not wanting to *let their team down*, or misunderstanding the severity or consequences of concussive injuries [37]. Although research is currently limited, some studies have shown a range of worsened mental health outcomes following concussive injuries [38–40], and extreme care should be taken in supporting youth athletes following their occurrence [41].

Clinical Considerations for Working with Youth Athletes

Mental health-care professionals who work with elite youth athletes should be aware of a range of factors that are relevant throughout assessment and treatment. Youth athletes provide a particularly complex presentation, in which multiple relationships and environmental considerations must be considered. Central to this is understanding the key systems within which the individual operates. As discussed by Purcell et al. [42], an ecological systems approach is critical for supporting elite athletes' mental health. In youth sport settings, a range of key systems all have the potential to impact an athlete's behaviors, attitudes, and experiences. Specifically, these include (1) the family subsystem (the athlete, parents, and siblings), (2) the team subsystem (the athlete, peers, and coaches), and (3) the environmental subsystem (organizations, communities, and societies) [43]. It is recommended that clinicians obtain a full understanding of how the youth athlete relates to the relationships within these systems.

To understand how an athlete's mental health may relate to sport, practitioners can encourage athletes to describe *both* their positive and negative experiences in sport, with specific attention to key relationships with peers, coaches, and parents. It is advisable to refrain from automatically assuming and communicating the worst of these relationships or environments, as this is likely to reduce the rapport with the young person; allowing the athlete to describe the positive aspects of their sport can instead assist in trust formation. Despite this, clinicians should be active in listening and prompting for any potential abuse or maltreatment that may be occurring, given that unguided disclosure is often unlikely [33]. Understanding the youth athlete's interpretation of perceived pressures around body image and weight, performance, and playing through injury (particularly concussion) is important, as is an understanding of the extent to which the athlete is balancing sports participation with academic and social responsibilities and desires. Identifying the ways in which athletes view and relate to themselves, especially with regard to athletic identity and perfectionistic concerns, can inform clinical formulation.

Another key factor that can be overlooked among elite youth athletes due to age is substance misuse. In particular, this may be relevant to athletes experiencing adversity or transitions out of sport. For example, in the aforementioned study by Brand et al. [14], deselected male athletes were significantly more likely to report using alcohol, nicotine, or illicit substances than were currently active elite youth athletes or nonathletes. Female deselected athletes, on the other hand, were significantly more likely to report using prescription drugs. Such findings suggest that youth athletes may use substances in response to negative changes in their sport, and this should be carefully considered, especially where complex issues of confidentiality and risk are relevant [44].

A consideration when working with young athletes is that they may not openly disclose their mental health difficulties, owing to a range of fears and concerns about their reputation or playing consequences. Sport is a domain where mental toughness is encouraged, which may wrongly [45] be interpreted by young people as requiring them to downplay or minimize mental health symptoms and disorders. This may be especially significant in youth athletes, as they are still developing confidence and self-understanding. Demonstrating the potential barriers to help-seeking in youth athletes, one study reported how athletes believed that they should not show weaknesses and worried about what their teammates, coaches, and parents would think of their ability to perform to their best if they were struggling with their mental health [46]. Given these real and *perceived* ramifications (e.g., to playing time, selection, reduced trust), any practitioner working in these spaces needs to be conscious of language, should ensure confidentiality, and should maximize opportunities for psychoeducation. Indeed, relating to language, some individuals may respond more favorably to framing around performance optimization, rather than treatment of a 'disorder' [47].

Unfortunately, the evidence base is limited regarding the assessment and treatment of elite youth athletes experiencing a mental health disorder. Practitioners are encouraged to draw on evidence-based approaches from the broader literature. For example, a range of general mental health screening tools considered appropriate for this age group has been recommended by the Neurobiology in Youth Mental Health Partnership [48]. Although the Sport Mental Health Assessment Tool 1 (SMHAT-1) [49] represents the first measure specifically designed to assess mental health symptoms within the sporting context, this tool is only appropriate for athletes 16 years of age and older. It is hoped that subsequent versions of the SMHAT may address assessment of younger elite athletes. Treatment approaches also remain underexplored for this population, and readers are encouraged to adapt established therapies—both psychological (Chap. 2) and pharmacological (Chap. 3)—as appropriate.

Conclusions

Elite youth athletes are exposed to a range of stressors that may predispose them to experience difficulties with mental health. Although sport is generally considered to have a positive influence on young people, those at an elite level may struggle with the pressure to perform and perfectionism, burnout, coach or parental pressures, abuse or maltreatment, injury, concussion, body image and weight concerns, and disrupted sleep. Practitioners working with young athletes should develop a strong understanding of these experiences and how young people relate to their sport and the people within it. Given that clear youth-specific approaches to management are not yet well-established in sport, practitioners are encouraged to lean on the broader literature of sports psychology and youth mental health in order to appropriately manage presenting concerns.

References

1. Rice SM, Purcell R, De Silva S, Mawren D, McGorry PD, Parker AG. The mental health of elite athletes: a narrative systematic review. Sports Med. 2016;46(9):1333–53.
2. Reardon CL, Hainline B, Aron CM, Baron D, Baum AL, Bindra A, et al. Mental health in elite athletes: International Olympic Committee consensus statement (2019). Br J Sports Med. 2019;53(11):667–99.
3. Walton CC, Rice S, Hutter RI, Currie A, Reardon CL, Purcell R. Mental health in youth athletes: a clinical review. Adv Psychiatry Behav Health. 2021;1(1):119–33.
4. Vella SA. Mental health and organized youth sport. Kinesiol Rev. 2019;8(3):229.
5. Patel V, Flisher AJ, Hetrick S, McGorry P. Mental health of young people: a global public-health challenge. Lancet. 2007;369(9569):1302–13.
6. Kessler RC, Amminger GP, Aguilar-Gaxiola S, Alonso J, Lee S, Ustün TB. Age of onset of mental disorders: a review of recent literature. Curr Opin Psychiatry. 2007;20(4):359–64.
7. Rudolph KD, Lansford JE, Rodkin PC. Interpersonal theories of developmental psychopathology. In: Developmental psychopathology; 2016. p. 1–69.
8. Walton CC, Carberry S, Wilson M, Purcell R, Olive L, Vella S, et al. Supporting mental health in youth sport: introducing a toolkit for coaches, clubs, and organisations. Int Sport Coach J. 2021:1–8.
9. Vella SA, Swann C, Batterham M, Boydell KM, Eckermann S, Ferguson H, et al. An intervention for mental health literacy and resilience in organized sports. Med Sci Sports Exerc. 2021;53(1):139–49.
10. Holt NL, Neely KC, Slater LG, Camiré M, Côté J, Fraser-Thomas J, et al. A grounded theory of positive youth development through sport based on results from a qualitative meta-study. Int Rev Sport Exerc Psychol. 2017;10(1):1–49.
11. Vella SA, Swann C, Allen MS, Schweickle MJ, Magee CA. Bidirectional associations between sport involvement and mental health in adolescence. Med Sci Sports Exerc. 2017;49(4):687–94.
12. Panza MJ, Graupensperger S, Agans JP, Dore I, Vella SA, Evans MB. Adolescent sport participation and symptoms of anxiety and depression: a systematic review and meta-analysis. J Sport Exerc Psychol. 2020;42(3):1–18.

13. Weber S, Puta C, Lesinski M, Gabriel B, Steidten T, Bär K-J, et al. Symptoms of anxiety and depression in young athletes using the Hospital Anxiety and Depression scale. Front Physiol. 2018;9:182.

14. Brand R, Wolff W, Hoyer J. Psychological symptoms and chronic mood in representative samples of elite student-athletes, deselected student-athletes and comparison students. Sch Ment Heal. 2013;5(3):166–74.

15. Nixdorf I, Frank R, Beckmann J. Comparison of athletes' proneness to depressive symptoms in individual and team sports: research on psychological mediators in junior elite athletes. Front Psychol. 2016;7:893.

16. Brenner JS, LaBotz M, Sugimoto D, Stracciolini A. The psychosocial implications of sport specialization in pediatric athletes. J Athlet Train. 2019;54(10):1021–9.

17. Hayward FPI, Knight CJ, Mellalieu SD. A longitudinal examination of stressors, appraisals, and coping in youth swimming. Psychol Sport Exerc. 2017;29:56–68.

18. Esmie PS, Andrew PH, Howard KH. Perfectionism, burnout, and depression in youth soccer players: a longitudinal study. J Clin Sport Psychol. 2018;12(2):179–200.

19. Stoeber J. The dual nature of perfectionism in sports: relationships with emotion, motivation, and performance. Int Rev Sport Exerc Psychol. 2011;4(2):128–45.

20. Hill AP, Mallinson-Howard SH, Jowett GE. Multidimensional perfectionism in sport: a meta-analytical review. Sport Exerc Perform Psychol. 2018;7(3):235–70.

21. Madigan DJ, Stoeber J, Passfield L. Perfectionism and burnout in junior athletes: a three-month longitudinal study. J Sport Exerc Psychol. 2015;37(3):305.

22. Raedeke TD. Is athlete burnout more than just stress? A sport commitment perspective. J Sport Exerc Psychol. 1997;19(4):396.

23. Granz HL, Schnell A, Mayer J, Thiel A. Risk profiles for athlete burnout in adolescent elite athletes: a classification analysis. Psychol Sport Exerc. 2019;41:130–41.

24. Baglioni C, Nanovska S, Regen W, Spiegelhalder K, Feige B, Nissen C, et al. Sleep and mental disorders: a meta-analysis of polysomnographic research. Psychol Bull. 2016;142(9):969.

25. Vlahoyiannis A, Aphamis G, Bogdanis GC, Sakkas GK, Andreou E, Giannaki CD. Deconstructing athletes' sleep: a systematic review of the influence of age, sex, athletic expertise, sport type, and season on sleep characteristics. J Sport Health Sci. 2021;10(4):387–402.

26. Campbell K, Peebles R. Eating disorders in children and adolescents: state of the art review. Pediatrics. 2014;134(3):582–92.

27. Giel KE, Hermann-Werner A, Mayer J, Diehl K, Schneider S, Thiel A, et al. Eating disorder pathology in elite adolescent athletes. Int J Eat Disord. 2016;49(6):553–62.

28. Stoyel H, Slee A, Meyer C, Serpell L. Systematic review of risk factors for eating psychopathology in athletes: a critique of an etiological model. Eur Eat Disord Rev. 2020;28(1):3–25.

29. Karrer Y, Halioua R, Mötteli S, Iff S, Seifritz E, Jäger M, et al. Disordered eating and eating disorders in male elite athletes: a scoping review. BMJ Open Sport Exerc Med. 2020;6(1):e000801.

30. Elliott SK, Drummond MJN. During play, the break, and the drive home: the meaning of parental verbal behaviour in youth sport. Leis Stud. 2017;36(5):645–56.

31. Mazzer KR, Rickwood DJ. Mental health in sport: coaches' views of their role and efficacy in supporting young people's mental health. Int J Health Promot Educ. 2015;53(2):102–14.

32. Kerr G, Battaglia A, Stirling A. Maltreatment in youth sport: a systemic issue. Kinesiol Rev. 2019;8(3):237–43.

33. Mountjoy M, Rhind DJA, Tiivas A, Leglise M. Safeguarding the child athlete in sport: a review, a framework and recommendations for the IOC youth athlete development model. Br J Sports Med. 2015;49(13):883–6.

34. Vertommen T, Kampen J, Schipper-van Veldhoven N, Uzieblo K, Van Den Eede F. Severe interpersonal violence against children in sport: associated mental health problems and quality of life in adulthood. Child Abuse Negl. 2018;76:459–68.

35. Caine D, Purcell L, Maffulli N. The child and adolescent athlete: a review of three potentially serious injuries. BMC Sports Sci Med Rehabil. 2014;6:22.

36. Rice SM, Parker AG, Rosenbaum S, Bailey A, Mawren D, Purcell R. Sport-related concussion and mental health outcomes in elite athletes: a systematic review. Sports Med. 2018;48(2):447–65.

37. Ferdinand Pennock K, McKenzie B, McClemont Steacy L, Mainwaring L. Under-reporting of sport-related concussions by adolescent athletes: a systematic review. Int Rev Sport Exerc Psychol. 2020:1–27.

38. Grubenhoff JA, Currie D, Comstock RD, Juarez-Colunga E, Bajaj L, Kirkwood MW. Psychological factors associated with delayed symptom resolution in children with concussion. J Pediatr. 2016;174:27–32.e1.

39. Covassin T, Elbin RJ, Beidler E, LaFevor M, Kontos AP. A review of psychological issues that may be associated with a sport-related concussion in youth and collegiate athletes. Sport Exerc Perform Psychol. 2017;6:220–9.

40. Kontos AP, Covassin T, Elbin RJ, Parker T. Depression and neurocognitive performance after concussion among male and female high school and collegiate athletes. Arch Phys Med Rehabil. 2012;93(10):1751–6.

41. Rivara FP, Tennyson R, Mills B, Browd SR, Emery CA, Gioia G, et al. Consensus statement on sports-related concussions in youth sports using a modified Delphi approach. JAMA Pediatr. 2020;174(1):79–85.

42. Purcell R, Gwyther K, Rice SM. Mental health in elite athletes: increased awareness requires an early intervention framework to respond to athlete needs. Sports Med Open. 2019;5(1):46.

43. Dorsch TE, Smith AL, Blazo JA, Coakley J, Côté J, Wagstaff CRD, et al. Toward an integrated understanding of the youth sport system. Res Q Exerc Sport. 2020:1–15.

44. Duncan RE, Williams BJ, Knowles A. Adolescents, risk behaviour and confidentiality: when would Australian psychologists breach confidentiality to disclose information to parents? Aust Psychol. 2013;48(6):408–19.

45. Gucciardi DF, Hanton S, Fleming S. Are mental toughness and mental health contradictory concepts in elite sport? A narrative review of theory and evidence. J Sci Med Sport. 2017;20(3):307–11.

46. Gulliver A, Griffiths KM, Christensen H. Barriers and facilitators to mental health help-seeking for young elite athletes: a qualitative study. BMC Psychiatry. 2012;12(1):157.

47. Donohue B, Gavrilova Y, Galante M, Gavrilova E, Loughran T, Scott J, et al. Controlled evaluation of an optimization approach to mental health and sport performance. J Clin Sport Psychol. 2018;12(2):234–67.

48. Lavoie S, Allott K, Amminger P, Bartholomeusz C, Berger M, Breakspear M, et al. Harmonised collection of data in youth mental health: towards large datasets. Aust N Z J Psychiatry. 2019;54(1):46–56.

49. Gouttebarge V, Bindra A, Blauwet C, Campriani N, Currie A, Engebretsen L, et al. International Olympic Committee (IOC) Sport Mental Health Assessment Tool 1 (SMHAT-1) and Sport Mental Health Recognition Tool 1 (SMHRT-1): towards better support of athletes' mental health. Br J Sports Med. 2021;55(1):30–7. https://doi.org/10.1136/bjsports-2020-102411.

Mental Health in Paralympic Athletes

Leslie Swartz

Within the structure of this book, this chapter is the last in the final section, entitled "Diverse Populations." A facetious, but not altogether inaccurate, version of this chapter could be "all of the above." It is important to state at the outset that every issue that has been dealt with in this book pertains to Paralympic athletes as well. In the history of how society thinks about disability, there are traditions that position people with disabilities as different from other people, inhabiting the world differently, or even, implicitly, inhabiting another world. This view of people with disabilities as inherently different from other people is inaccurate and, mercifully, falling out of favor in mainstream thinking.

Disability, Sport, and the Question of Inclusion

So, if people with disabilities are essentially no different from other people, then why have a separate chapter in a book like this to explore questions of mental health in Paralympic athletes? In some ways, it has become more possible to envisage a future world within which people with disabilities are fully included in society and sport, making the need for this chapter disappear. However, we are not there yet, by any means, and part of the reason we are not there yet goes to the heart of what we understand by disability.

The United Nations Convention on the Rights of Persons with Disabilities (UNCRPD), the foundational document for contemporary understandings of, and policies around, disability, defines disability as follows:

> Persons with disabilities include those who have long-term physical, mental, intellectual or sensory impairments which in interaction with various barriers may hinder their full and effective participation in society on an equal basis with others [1].

L. Swartz (✉)
Department of Psychology, Stellenbosch University,
Stellenbosch, South Africa
e-mail: Lswartz@sun.ac.za

Behind this widely accepted definition is a long history of struggle around how we should understand disability. There is not enough space here to go into detail about the debates regarding disability models and definitions (for some discussions of this, see [2–4]), but some key issues in the development of thinking are important to note. Historically, in what has been termed the "medical model," a disability was essentially defined as a bodily defect. A disability could be defined as no more and no less than what was wrong with a person's body; the goal of improving the lives of people with disabilities was, commonly, to conduct treatments to fix or ameliorate bodily impairments [5]. A disability, it was believed, was a matter of the body.

If we look at the UNCRPD definition quoted above, then we can see how far definitions of disability have come. Crucial for the definition is the phrase "in interaction with various barriers." The UNCRPD does not deny the importance of the body and mentions "long-term physical, mental, intellectual or sensory impairments," but these impairments are not the whole story. In a tradition of thinking that goes back to what was termed the "social model" of disability, coined in the 1970s, disability is far more than a problem or what disability would call, an impairment of the body—disability is constituted through the "various barriers" that people with impairments experience in the world [6].

Many models of disability have been proposed since the establishment of the social model [7–13], and debates concerning disability definitions remain heated within disability studies [14–16]. For the purposes of this chapter, what all of these approaches share is a recognition of the key role that the environment (including the physical, social, and virtual aspects) plays in the constitution of disability.

The Paralympic Movement started in 1948 at Stoke Mandeville, with the original emphasis on rehabilitation. The person credited with founding the Paralympic Movement, Dr. Ludwig Guttman, was a Jewish refugee from Nazi Germany; theorists have suggested that from the beginning of the movement, Guttman brought his own experience of social exclusion, discrimination, and oppression to the work of disability sport [17–19]. Although there was clearly in Guttman's mission a focus on physical rehabilitation, he understood from the beginning the importance of social inclusion and acceptance. In this important respect, though it historically predates the social model of disability, since its inception, the Paralympic Movement has been intertwined with an appreciation of the centrality of social exclusion as key to the experience of disability and, indeed, to disablement itself. There is growing evidence that discrimination of various kinds may be associated with psychological distress and mental health symptoms or disorders [20–25]; a key feature of contemporary thinking about disability and its relationship with mental health concerns focuses not on disability itself but on disablism, a social process akin to racism, sexism, or homophobia, for example [26–29].

The central rehabilitative mission of the Paralympic Movement, then, can be viewed in this light as focusing not just on the body of the athlete but, possibly more centrally, on the social conditions that exclude such bodies. From a mental health theory and a practice point of view, improving mental health conditions, which includes alleviating symptoms and preventing mental health disorders from developing in the first place, becomes not just a question of therapeutics as conventionally understood but also of social justice and social inclusion [30–34]. The issue of social inclusion is, of course, an issue for all people and all athletes, but may be of particular relevance, given the reality of disablism, to Paralympic athletes. However, how is inclusion achieved?

The Complex Politics of Inclusion

The South African Human Rights Commission, following international practice, in 2002, promulgated a report on disability called *Towards a barrier-free society* [35]. This report concludes with the statement, "Prejudice remains the greatest disability". Regardless of whether this comparative statement can be empirically supported, if we accept that prejudice is a key factor affecting social inclusion, then what role does Paralympic sport play in reducing prejudice and in improving mental health? Elsewhere in this book, the authors have explored the burden borne by all elite athletes in terms of what is expected of them as performers and role models and the potential contribution of expectations to mental health symptoms and disorders [36–38]. In the absence of many studies comparing mental health symptoms and disorders in elite athletes with appropriate control groups, it is difficult to isolate the potential mental health impacts on athletes from the burden of expectations on them. This question becomes more complex when con-

sidering the case of Paralympic athletes. As I will show later in this chapter, the number of studies comparing mental health issues and their genesis in Paralympic versus other athletes, or even comparing Paralympic athletes to the general population, remains small. It is nevertheless important at this stage of the science to consider contextual factors that may have a bearing and that should be explored in future work.

Critical theorists of disability sport, notably P. David Howe [39–42], have pointed out how the Paralympics have evolved from having an essentially rehabilitative focus from Stoke Mandeville roots to being a global television and social media-mediated spectacle [43, 44]. Many claims have been made for the Paralympics, and the London 2012 Paralympics in particular, to effect social change, and there is considerable debate as to whether these games have changed perceptions in an enduring manner or improved the lives of people with disabilities [45–47].

At the level of the athletes themselves, and their mental health, concerns have been expressed in the literature about the possible impact of representation of sportspeople with disabilities as "inspirational" or "superhuman." Critiquing this phenomenon, which is known as the "supercrip" phenomenon, the late disability activist and comedienne Stella Young used (and is credited with having coined) the term "inspiration porn"; her TED talk on this topic has been viewed close to four million times [48].

Discussing this phenomenon and Young's contribution, Grue [49] defines inspiration porn in the following manner:

> Inspiration porn is the representation of disability as a desirable but undesired characteristic, usually by showing impairment as a visually or symbolically distinct biophysical deficit in one person, a deficit that can and must be overcome through the display of physical prowess ([49]: 838).

Debates about "supercripping" and "inspiration porn" are extensive and are part of broader discussions about disability and representation [50, 51]—discussions that cannot be fully summarized here. The key issue of this chapter, though, is that portraying people with disabilities as overcoming odds is not just a portrayal of reality but a reproduction of ideas about what disability is and should be [52]. It is certainly better for people with disabilities to be portrayed as overcoming odds and being inspirational than it is to have them portrayed as pathetic, weak, dangerous, or "freaks" [53], but these issues of representation are not simple, and as Nario-Redmond et al. [52] have suggested, there may be many forms of ableism that are not overtly hostile but which may be demeaning, including paternalistic views. In summary, few, if any, would argue that inclusion is a bad thing—far from it—but inclusion brings with it a complex representational politics of its own.

The Paralympic Paradox: Body, Society, and Mental Health

As we have seen, the social model of disability and the approaches stemming from it have been central in showing that disability is not only, or essentially, about the body but also about the interaction between impairment and social and other environmental issues. A second feature of the social model was its insistence that by virtue of impairment, there is no reason to assume that people with disabilities inevitably experience more mental health challenges, or mental health disorders, than do members of the general population [26, 28, 29], with contemporary theorists emphasizing the continuities rather than inherent the categorical differences between lives lived with and without a disability [49]. These two features, taken together, create related challenges for studying mental health symptoms and disorders in Paralympic athletes.

The first problem is that if researchers look for evidence of mental health symptoms and disorders in athletes with disabilities, then they may fear leaving themselves open to being accused of being old-fashioned medical modelists, conflating bodily differences with emotional problems [54–56]. In my own work with disability activists in Africa [57], I have very often had colleagues with impairments saying, "I may be disabled, but I am not mad or stupid." Quite apart from the fact that statements like this may be read as reproducing stereotypes of people with psychosocial or intellectual disabilities, this statement does indicate some of the struggles for equality experienced by people with disabilities. Over the course of the development of the Paralympic Movement, furthermore, the emphasis has been on other, supposedly more positive, qualities of athletes with disabilities, such as grit, determination, and resilience [58]. Just as there is stigma associated with physical impairment, there is stigma associated with mental health symptoms and disorders [59–61], and it would not be surprising if researchers were to avoid this field of research, which, however unfairly, could be seen as yoking two sets of stereotyping—that against disabilities and that against mental disorders—together.

A second issue potentially affecting research into mental health symptoms and disorders in Paralympic athletes is that with the emphasis on social and environmental factors as constitutive of disabilities, there may be, paradoxically, a lack of attention to issues of the body and how these may differentially affect athletes with disabilities. The differential attribution of suffering and pain to Paralympic as opposed to other athletes without evidence is an ideological problem [62]; the empirical question of whether athletes with impairments experience more pain or different types of injuries than do those without [63, 64] is another matter and is a question central to good health and, specifically mental health, care for athletes. The relationship between general physical pain and mental distress is well-researched [65, 66]. Bodily experiences of pain, and of issues related to the classification of bodies by impairment through the Paralympic classification system, are unlikely to be irrelevant to the questions of mental health for Paralympic athletes, but a reluctance to focus on and pathologize the disabled body may explain the relative lack of information on mental health symptoms and disorders in Paralympic athletes.

Mental Health Symptoms and Disorders in Paralympic Athletes: Data and Issues for the Future

In our narrative review on mental health symptoms and disorders in Paralympic athletes [23], we noted the paucity of information on the topic. This situation has not changed substantially [67–69]. Olive et al. [69] have demonstrated that the rates of mental health disorders between athletes with and without disabilities may not differ much (a point that underscores the "all of the above" comment at the outset of this chapter), and, in this regard, a recent chapter [70] has summarized a challenge relevant to thinking about mental health in Paralympians as opposed to other athletes, using the tagline "Same same but different"; specifically, the challenge remains of mainstreaming mental health symptoms and disorders in Paralympic athletes with mental health symptoms and disorders in all athletes, while not losing sight of the distinctive challenges. This is an example of more general questions around mainstreaming of disability issues and people with disabilities [71].

The key issues noted by Swartz et al. [23] and in related publications [67, 72] remain current. There is good evidence that participation in sport is helpful in a range of ways for the mental health of all people, including people with disabilities [73]; we need to know more, however, about the impact of trauma histories on the mental health of Paralympic athletes, a proportion of whom have become disabled through trauma, and about the impact of classification and reclassification of para-athletes as categories change and new patterns of exclusion may emerge [74]. We need to understand more about pain, medication, and assistive devices and their relationship with mental health symptoms and disorders in Paralympic athletes.

As in all contemporary studies on the genesis and development of mental health disorders, we need to take a lifespan approach, understanding the different trajectories to becoming a Paralympic athlete and also to life after this career. A central issue affecting all elite athletes is transition out of high-level sport participation; this issue takes on a particular meaning and significance for para-athletes [23, 75]. Given the high rates of social exclusion of people with disabilities, and lower employment rates, the path to life outside sport for former athletes may well be more trying for para-athletes, with the possibility of not only loss of employment but also loss of an elevated role. Supercrip status, as suggested earlier, may be a problem; the journey from this status to a marginalized category (persons with a disability) may be especially challenging.

As is the case with any understanding of mental health needs in elite athletes in general [76], it is essential to consider the global context of sport participation and mental health resources. As economic barriers to participation in parasport may, hopefully, be more recognized and dealt with [77], there may be more athletes from low- and middle-income countries participating in disability sport at the highest level. The challenges that these athletes may face in terms of infrastructure, support, access to appropriate assistive devices, transport, and more all need to be factored into any understanding of the mental health symptoms facing Paralympic athletes. The transition out of sport in low-income contexts, furthermore, may be especially challenging where resources are few and opportunities are scarce for the society as a whole.

Conclusions

In summary, the field of mental health for Paralympic athletes remains understudied and is not yet fully understood. A global approach is needed, allowing for inclusion of athletes from a wide range of countries and contexts, including contexts where formal mental health services are scant. Innovative, cost-effective, and culturally appropriate services are important, in line with contemporary thinking in global mental health [78, 79]. Culturally appropriate care is essential, and, in this regard, among the true experts on what is culturally relevant and acceptable to Paralympic athletes are the athletes themselves. Their voices need to be listened to in debates.

References

1. United Nations Department of Economic and Social Affairs: Disability. Article 1-Purpose. https://www.un.org/development/desa/disabilities/convention-on-the-rights-of-persons-with-disabilities/article-1-purpose.html. Accessed 15 Feb 2022.
2. Goodley D. Disability studies: an interdisciplinary introduction. London: Sage; 2016.
3. Shakespeare T. Disability rights and wrongs revisited. London: Routledge; 2013.
4. Shakespeare T. Disability: the basics. London: Routledge; 2017.
5. Smith B, Bundon A. Disability models: explaining and understanding disability sport in different ways. In: The Palgrave handbook of Paralympic studies. Springer; 2018. p. 15–34.
6. Oliver M. The social model of disability: thirty years on. Disabil Soc. 2013;28(7):1024–6.
7. Chisale SS. Politics of the body, fear and Ubuntu: proposing an African women's theology of disability. HTS Teol Stud/Theol Stud. 2020;76(3).
8. Dirth TP, Adams GA. Decolonial theory and disability studies: on the modernity/coloniality of ability. J Soc Polit Psychol. 2019;7(1):260–89.
9. Kavanagh C. What contemporary models of disability miss: the case for a phenomenological hermeneutic analysis. Int J Fem Approaches Bioeth. 2018;11(2):63–82.
10. Lawson A, Beckett AE. The social and human rights models of disability: towards a complementarity thesis. Int J Hum Rights. 2021;25(2):348–79.
11. Mitra S. The human development model of disability, health and wellbeing. In: Disability, health and human development. New York: Springer; 2018. p. 9–32.
12. Mji G, Gcaza S, Swartz L, MacLachlan M, Hutton B. An African way of networking around disability. Disabil Soc. 2011;26(3) https://doi.org/10.1080/09687599.2011.560419.
13. Ngubane-Mokiwa SA. Ubuntu considered in light of exclusion of people with disabilities. Afr J Disabil. 2018;7(1):1–7.
14. Cleary K. Disability studies. Fem Media Hist. 2018;4(2):61–6.
15. Garland-Thomson R. Misfits: a feminist materialist disability concept. Hypatia. 2011;26(3):591–609.
16. Salvador-Carulla L, Bertelli M, Martinez-Leal R. The road to 11th edition of the International Classification of Diseases: trajectories of scientific consensus and contested science in the classification of intellectual disability/intellectual developmental disorders. Curr Opin Psychiatry. 2018;31(2):79–87.
17. Akkermans R. Ludwig Guttmann. Lancet Neurol. 2016;15(12):1210.
18. Silver JR. Ludwig Guttmann (1899–1980), Stoke Mandeville Hospital and the Paralympic games. J Med Biogr. 2012;20(3):101–5.
19. Wedgwood N. Hahn versus Guttmann: revisiting 'sports and the political movement of disabled persons'. Disabil Soc. 2014;29(1):129–42.
20. Balakrishnan A, Kulkarni K, Moirangthem S, Kumar CN, Math SB, Murthy P. The Rights of Persons with Disabilities Act 2016: mental health implications. Indian J Psychol Med. 2019;41(2):119–25.
21. Comas-Díaz L, Hall GN, Neville HA. Racial trauma: theory, research, and healing: introduction to the special issue. Am Psychol. 2019;74(1):1–5). . American Psychological Association. https://doi.org/10.1037/amp0000442.
22. Nakkeeran N, Nakkeeran B. Disability, mental health, sexual orientation and gender identity: understanding health inequity through experience and difference. Health Res Policy Syst. 2018;16(1):9–19.
23. Swartz L, Hunt X, Bantjes J, Hainline B, Reardon CL. Mental health symptoms and disorders in Paralympic athletes: a narrative review. Br J Sports Med. 2019;53(12):737–40. https://doi.org/10.1136/bjsports-2019-100731.
24. Temple JB, Kelaher M. Is disability exclusion associated with psychological distress? Australian evidence from a national cross-sectional survey. BMJ Open. 2018;8(5):e020829.
25. Vargas SM, Huey SJ Jr, Miranda J. A critical review of current evidence on multiple types of discrimination and mental health. Am J Orthopsychiatry. 2020;90(3):374.
26. Marks D. Disability: controversial debates and psychosocial perspectives. London: Routledge; 2014.

27. Reeve D. Psycho-emotional disablism: the missing link? In: Routledge handbook of disability studies. London: Routledge; 2019. p. 102–16.

28. Watermeyer B, Swartz L. Disablism, identity and self: discrimination as a traumatic assault on subjectivity. J Community Appl Soc Psychol. 2016;26(3):268–76. https://doi.org/10.1002/casp.2266.

29. Watermeyer B. Towards a contextual psychology of disablism. Abingdon: Routledge; 2012.

30. Filia K, Menssink J, Gao CX, Rickwood D, Hamilton M, Hetrick SE, Parker AG, Herrman H, Hickie I, Sharmin S. Social inclusion, intersectionality, and profiles of vulnerable groups of young people seeking mental health support. Soc Psychiatry Psychiatr Epidemiol. 2021;57(2):245–54.

31. O'Donnell P, O'Donovan D, Elmusharaf K. Measuring social exclusion in healthcare settings: a scoping review. Int J Equity Health. 2018;17(1):1–16.

32. Scifo L, Chicau Borrego C, Monteiro D, Matosic D, Feka K, Bianco A, Alesi M. Sport intervention programs (SIPs) to improve health and social inclusion in people with intellectual disabilities: a systematic review. J Funct Morphol Kinesiol. 2019;4(3):57.

33. Tan RKJ. Social inclusion and social determinants of health. In: Liamputtong P, editor. Handbook of social inclusion: research and practices in health and social sciences. Springer; 2020. p. 1–21. https://doi.org/10.1007/978-3-030-48277-0_2-1.

34. Woodgate RL, Gonzalez M, Demczuk L, Snow WM, Barriage S, Kirk S. How do peers promote social inclusion of children with disabilities? A mixed-methods systematic review. Disabil Rehabil. 2020;42(18):2553–79.

35. SAHRC Report. Towards a barrier-free society; 2022. http://www.sahrc.org.za/home/21/files/Reports/towards_barrier_free_society.pdf2002.pdf. Accessed 15 Feb 2022.

36. Gouttebarge V, Bindra A, Blauwet C, Campriani N, Currie A, Engebretsen L, Hainline B, Kroshus E, McDuff D, Mountjoy M, Purcell R, Putukian M, Reardon CL, Rice SM, Budgett R. International Olympic Committee (IOC) Sport Mental Health Assessment Tool 1 (SMHAT-1) and Sport Mental Health Recognition Tool 1 (SMHRT-1): towards better support of athletes' mental health. Br J Sports Med. 2021;55(1):30–7. https://doi.org/10.1136/BJSPORTS-2020-102411.

37. Gouttebarge V, Castaldelli-Maia JM, Gorczynski P, Hainline B, Hitchcock ME, Kerkhoffs GM, Rice SM, Reardon CL. Occurrence of mental health symptoms and disorders in current and former elite athletes: a systematic review and meta-analysis. Br J Sports Med. 2019;53(11):700–6.

38. Rice SM, Gwyther K, Santesteban-Echarri O, Baron D, Gorczynski P, Gouttebarge V, Reardon CL, Hitchcock ME, Hainline B, Purcell R. Determinants of anxiety in elite athletes: a systematic review and meta-analysis. Br J Sports Med. 2019;53(11):722–30.

39. Howe D. The cultural politics of the Paralympic movement: through an anthropological lens. London: Routledge; 2008.

40. Howe PD. Cyborg and supercrip: the Paralympics technology and the (dis) empowerment of disabled athletes. Sociology. 2011;45(5):868–82.

41. Pullen E, Jackson D, Silk M. (Re-) presenting the Paralympics: affective nationalism and the "able-disabled". Commun Sport. 2020;8(6):715–37.

42. Silva CF, Howe PD. The (in) validity of supercrip representation of Paralympian athletes. J Sport Soc Issues. 2012;36(2):174–94.

43. Hodges CEM, Scullion R, Jackson D. From awww to awe factor: UK audience meaning-making of the 2012 Paralympics as mediated spectacle. J Pop Telev. 2015;3(2):195–212.

44. Pullen E, Jackson D, Silk M, Scullion R. Re-presenting the Paralympics: (contested) philosophies, production practices and the hypervisibility of disability. Media Cult Soc. 2019;41(4):465–81.

45. Ahmed N. Paralympics 2012 legacy: accessible housing and disability equality or inequality? Disabil Soc. 2013;28(1):129–33.

46. Postlethwaite V, Kohe GZ, Molnar G. Inspiring a generation: an examination of stakeholder relations in the context of London 2012 Olympics and Paralympics educational programmes. Manag Sport Leis. 2018;23(4–6):391–407.

47. Shakespeare T. The Paralympics—superhumans and mere mortals. Lancet. 2016;388(10050):1137–9.

48. Young S. TED: ideas worth spreading. I'm not your inspiration, thank you very much. https://www.ted.com/talks/stella_young_i_m_not_your_inspiration_thank_you_very_much?language=en. Accessed 15 Feb 2022.

49. Grue J. The problem with inspiration porn: a tentative definition and a provisional critique. Disabil Soc. 2016;31(6):838–49.

50. Garland-Thomson R. Staring: how we look. Oxford: Oxford University Press; 2009.

51. Sandell R, Dodd J, Garland-Thomson R. Re-presenting disability: activism and agency in the museum. London: Routledge; 2013.

52. Nario-Redmond MR, Kemerling AA, Silverman A. Hostile, benevolent, and ambivalent ableism: contemporary manifestations. J Soc Issues. 2019;75(3):726–56.

53. Tyrrell B. A world turned upside down: hop-frog, freak shows, and representations of dwarfism. J Lit Cult Disabil Stud. 2020;14(2):171–86.

54. Blacker CJ. What's wrong with you? JAMA Neurol. 2021;78(3):269–70.

55. Deacon L, Macdonald SJ, Donaghue J. "What's wrong with you, are you stupid?" Listening to the biographical narratives of adults with dyslexia in an age of 'inclusive' and 'anti-discriminatory' practice. Disabil Soc. 2020;37(3):406–26.

56. Kattari SK, Olzman M, Hanna MD. "You look fine!" Ableist experiences by people with invisible disabilities. Affilia. 2018;33(4):477–92.

57. Swartz L. Building capacity or enforcing normalcy? Engaging with disability scholarship in Africa. Qual Res Psychol. 2018;15(1):116–30. https://doi.org/10.1080/14780887.2017.1416801.

58. Cormier DL, Ferguson LJ, Gyurcsik NC, Briere JL, Dunn JGH, Kowalski KC. Grit in sport: a scoping review. Int Rev Sport Exerc Psychol. 2021:1–38.

59. Codjoe L, Barber S, Ahuja S, Thornicroft G, Henderson C, Lempp H, N'Danga-Koroma J. Evidence for interventions to promote mental health and reduce stigma in Black faith communities: systematic review. Soc Psychiatry Psychiatr Epidemiol. 2021;56(6):895–911.

60. Henderson C, Noblett J, Parke H, Clement S, Caffrey A, Gale-Grant O, Schulze B, Druss B, Thornicroft G. Mental health-related stigma in health care and mental health-care settings. Lancet Psychiatry. 2014;1(6):467–82. https://doi.org/10.1016/S2215-0366(14)00023-6.

61. Mascayano F, Toso-Salman J, Ho YCS, Dev S, Tapia T, Thornicroft G, Cabassa LJ, Khenti A, Sapag J, Bobbili SJ. Including culture in programs to reduce stigma toward people with mental disorders in low-and middle-income countries. Transcult Psychiatry. 2020;57(1):140–60.

62. Martínez-Bello VE, Bernabé-Villodre MM, Cabrera García-Ochoa Y, Torrent-Trilles L, Vega-Perona H. The representation of athletes during Paralympic and Olympic games: a Foucauldian analysis of the construction of difference in newspapers. Disabil Soc. 2021:1–23.

63. Grobler L, Derman W, Blauwet CA, Chetty S, Webborn N, Pluim B. Pain management in athletes with impairment: a narrative review of management strategies. Clin J Sport Med. 2018;28(5):457–72.

64. Willick SE, Webborn N, Emery C, Blauwet CA, Pit-Grosheide P, Stomphorst J, Van de Vliet P, Marques NAP, Martinez-Ferrer JO, Jordaan E. The epidemiology of injuries at the London 2012

Paralympic games. Br J Sports Med. 2013;47(7):426–32. https://doi.org/10.1136/bjsports-2013-092374.

65. IsHak WW, Wen RY, Naghdechi L, Vanle B, Dang J, Knosp M, Dascal J, Marcia L, Gohar Y, Eskander L. Pain and depression: a systematic review. Harv Rev Psychiatry. 2018;26(6):352–63.

66. Kirtley OJ, Rodham K, Crane C. Understanding suicidal ideation and behaviour in individuals with chronic pain: a review of the role of novel transdiagnostic psychological factors. Lancet Psychiatry. 2020;7(3):282–90.

67. Badenhorst M, Runciman P, Brown JC, Swartz L, Derman WE. Promotion of Para athlete well-being in South Africa (the PROPEL studies): profiles and prevalence of psychological distress. J Sci Med Sport. 2021;24(7):616–21. https://doi.org/10.1016/J.JSAMS.2020.12.013.

68. Currie A, Blauwet C, Bindra A, Budgett R, Campriani N, Hainline B, McDuff D, Mountjoy M, Purcell R, Putukian M. Athlete mental health: future directions. Br J Sports Med. 2021;55(22):1243–4. BMJ Publishing Group Ltd and British Association of Sport and Exercise Medicine.

69. Olive LS, Rice S, Butterworth M, Clements M, Purcell R. Do rates of mental health symptoms in currently competing elite athletes in Paralympic sports differ from non-para-athletes? Sports Med Open. 2021;7(1):1–9.

70. McKay CD, Callaghan L, Badenhorst M, Runciman P, Derman W. Injury psychology and para athletes: same same, but different. In: The mental impact of sports injury. London: Routledge; 2022. p. 208–22.

71. Makuwira J. Disability-inclusive development. In: Simms K, Banks N, Engel S, Hodge P, Makuwira J, Nakamura N, Rigg J, Salamanca A, Yeophantong P, editors. The Routledge handbook of global development. London: Routledge; 2022. p. 480–92.

72. Bantjes J, Swartz L. Social inclusion through parasport: a critical reflection on the current state of play. Phys Med Rehabil Clin N Am. 2018;29(2):409–16.

73. Aitchison B, Rushton AB, Martin P, Barr M, Soundy A, Heneghan NR. The experiences and perceived health benefits of individuals with a disability participating in sport: a systematic review and narrative synthesis. Disabil Health J. 2021;15:101164.

74. Patatas JM, De Bosscher V, Derom I, Winckler C. Stakeholders' perceptions of athletic career pathways in Paralympic sport: from participation to excellence. Sport Soc. 2022;25(2):299–320.

75. Bundon A, Ashfield A, Smith B, Goosey-Tolfrey VL. Struggling to stay and struggling to leave: the experiences of elite para-athletes at the end of their sport careers. Psychol Sport Exerc. 2018;37:296–305.

76. Reardon CL, Hainline B, Aron CM, Baron D, Baum AL, Bindra A, Budgett R, Campriani N, Castaldelli-Maia JM, Currie A, Derevensky JL, Glick ID, Gorczynski P, Gouttebarge V, Grandner MA, Han DH, McDuff D, Mountjoy M, Polat A, et al. Mental health in elite athletes: International Olympic Committee consensus statement (2019). Br J Sports Med. 2019;53(11):667–99. https://doi.org/10.1136/BJSPORTS-2019-100715.

77. Swartz L, Bantjes J, Rall D, Ferreira S, Blauwet C, Derman W. "A more equitable society": the politics of global fairness in Paralympic sport. PLoS One. 2016;11(12):e0167481. https://doi.org/10.1371/journal.pone.0167481.

78. Javadi D, Feldhaus I, Mancuso A, Ghaffar A. Applying systems thinking to task shifting for mental health using lay providers: a review of the evidence. Glob Ment Health. 2017;4:e14.

79. Patel V, Saxena S, Lund C, Thornicroft G, Baingana F, Bolton P, Chisholm D, Collins PY, Cooper JL, Eaton J. The Lancet Commission on global mental health and sustainable development. Lancet. 2018;392(10157):1553–98.

Index

A

Acceptance and commitment therapy (ACT), 10, 65
ACT's cognitive defusion techniques, 11
Adverse childhood experiences (ACEs), 198
Allostasis, 171
Amateur athletes (AAs), 119
Anabolic androgenic steroids (AAS), 186
Anti-doping organizations (ADOs), 18
Anti-nausea effects, 17
Anxiety, 7, 17, 18, 90
   clinical management, 64, 65
   competitive performance anxiety, 63, 64
   epidemiology, 61
   GAD, 62
   OCD, 63
   panic disorder, 63
   prevalence, 62
   risk factors, 62
   social anxiety disorder, 62, 63
   symptoms, 64
   systematic review and meta-analysis, 62
Assessment of sleep environment (ASE), 36
Athlete exposure (AE), 120, 121
Athlete Sleep Screening Questionnaire (ASSQ), 36
Attention-deficit/hyperactivity disorder (ADHD), 18, 19, 108
   characteristics, 91, 92
   comorbidities, 90, 91
   diagnosis, 89, 90
   differential diagnosis, 90, 91
   overview, 89
   prevalence, 90
   symptoms, 91
   treatment of
      neurofeedback, 92
      non-stimulants, 93
      psychosocial intervention, 92
      stimulants, 92, 93
Australian Institute of Sport (AIS), 5
Autism spectrum disorder (ASD), 90
Autonomic nervous system hypothesis, 174

B

Behavioral addictions
   components, 145
   factors, 145
   gambling problems/disorders
      accessibility and availability, 146
      diagnostic criteria, 147, 148
      growth, 146
      guidelines for helping athletes, 148

      impacts, 147
      online wagering, 146
      prevalence, 147
      susceptible to, 146
   gaming disorder
      e-sports, 149
      guidelines for helping athletes, 150
      measurement tools, 150
      overview, 148
      prevalence, 148, 149
      symptoms, 149
   mental health symptoms and disorders, 145, 146
   overview, 145
Berlin Questionnaire (BQ), 36
Binge eating disorder (BED), 19
Biopsychosocial cultural spiritual (BPSCS) model, 197, 198
Biopsychosocial models, 24
Bipolar disorder, 19, 20, 90
   assessment, 110–112
   diagnosis, 105
      depression, 106, 107
      hypomania, 106
      illness course, 107
      issues, 107
      manic episode, 106
      medical conditions, 106
      mixed states, 107
      psychosis, 108–109
      rapid cycling, 107
      subclassification, 105
   differential diagnosis
      ADHD, 108
      personality disorder, 107, 108
      substance use disorder, 107
   investigations, 112
   management
      acute mania/hypomania, 114
      depression, 114
      exercise, 113
      medication guidance, 113–115
      prophylaxis, 115
      psychosis, 115
      psychotherapy, 113
   physical examination, 112
   prevalence, 110
Bone stress injuries (BSIs), 81
Branched-chain amino acids (BCAAs), 174
Brief index of sleep control (BRISC), 36
Bruxism, 39
Burnout syndrome in athletes (BSA), 173
Buspirone, 17

PAN-ASIAN EXPRESS

Quick Fixes for Asian-Food Fans

Barbara Witt

BANTAM BOOKS
NEW YORK TORONTO LONDON SYDNEY AUCKLAND

PAN-ASIAN EXPRESS

A Bantam Book/February 1997

All rights reserved.
Copyright © 1997 by Barbara Witt.
Cover art copyright © 1997 by Renée Comet Photography, Inc.

BOOK DESIGN BY JAMES SINCLAIR.

Library of Congress Cataloging-in-Publication Data
Witt, Barbara, 1930–
Pan-Asian express : quick fixes for Asian-food fans / Barbara Witt.
p.   cm.
ISBN 0-553-37405-2
1. Cookery, Oriental.   I. Title.
TX724.5.a1W58   1997
641.595—dc20   96-31587
                                                                            CIP

Published simultaneously in the United States and Canada

Bantam Books are published by Bantam Books, a division of Bantam Doubleday Dell Publishing Group, Inc. Its trademark, consisting of the words "Bantam Books" and the portrayal of a rooster, is Registered in U.S. Patent and Trademark Office and in other countries. Marca Registrada. Bantam Books, 1540 Broadway, New York, New York 10036.

PRINTED IN THE UNITED STATES OF AMERICA

BVG   10   9   8   7   6   5   4   3   2   1

PAN-ASIAN EXPRESS

Contents

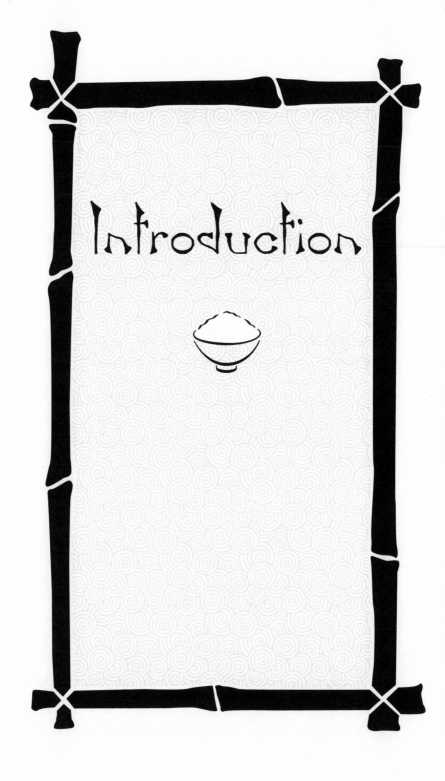

Introduction

*W*hen I was a kid growing up in Connecticut, dinner in Manhattan's Chinatown was my Dad's best, squeal-of-joy family treat. I loved everything about Mott Street but mostly its exotic little restaurants. Some were simply wondrous with lacquer red and gilt arches and pagoda roof lines, but most came in plain storefront wrappers. For me, stepping inside was a ride on a magic carpet; the dancing ceiling lanterns with silk tassels and square paper beads delighted me. So did the waiters with their braided licorice-stick ponytails as they wrote down our orders with dizzying speed— backwards. Their second-best trick was being able to harvest my chopsticks from midair when they inevitably flew away from me. Since they spoke little English, we smiled at each other a lot—inscrutably, of course.

I have an audible memory of those dented metal domes clanging on and off the food, and I can also conjure up the haunting steamed chicken and celery aroma of Cantonese-American chow mein. Surely those crispy little noodles we piled under and over everything paved the way for America's munch-a-bunch-of-crunch addiction. Although my adventurous Dad always wanted to try something different, Mom kept right on ordering the *egg foo yung*. My older brother was less interested in the culinary experience than in proving how much incendiary Chinese mustard he could slather on his egg roll without imploding. As for me, my favorite dish was the gooey, festive sweet-and-sour pork. Mom never fixed anything like *that* at home.

After we stuffed ourselves with two from Column A and three from Column B, I always had the same dessert: a scoop of vanilla ice cream sliding about in a stemmed metal compote still warm from the dishwasher. The final teapot heralded my favorite treats, the fortune cookies with real "Confucius say" quotations poking out like birthday snappers and those pale yellow cartwheel-size almond cookies with a whole toasted nut pressed into the center like a hub. The waiter would slip an extra one into my pocket when my Mother wasn't looking, and then we'd begin our after-dinner stroll down Mott Street.

Even after I grew up, I didn't grow out of the wonder and pleasures of Chinatown or my affinity for the exotic Far East. When I opened my own restaurant years later, specializing in international cheese dishes, I even rationalized a few Asian dishes into my constantly changing menu. Serving Korean *bulgogi*, Indian mulligatawny soup, curries, Vietnamese spring rolls, and Chinese stir-fries was pretty ludicrous considering the rarity of cheese in Asia, but the anomaly seemed to delight my customers as well as the chef, who shared my sense of the absurd and my fondness for Asian food.

Although many colorful inner-city ethnic communities have dispersed in the wake of urban neglect, sweet memories like mine are being formed daily by children being taken to authentic suburban restaurants. Not only did our national connection with Asian food start with the Chinese immigrants who fed the Gold Rush prospectors and built our first railroads back in the mid-nineteenth century, but our personal connection started when we were toddlers because Chinese restaurants were family owned and operated, as well as family priced. They welcomed and doted on children and their success with working Americans was easily earned by offering multiple, abundant dishes at a single low price—our first introduction to prix fixe.

There's scarcely a small town in America without a Chinese restaurant. Egg rolls are as much a national dish as hot dogs, so it's no surprise that when other Asian immigrants introduced their distinctive cuisines, we were ready for them. Today, ethnic restaurants of almost every nationality abound and Americans, who travel eagerly to these exotic countries, seem endlessly intrigued by them all.

But our craving for the variety of flavors this food can bring to our tables is often frustrated when the only way to satisfy it is by going to a restaurant. Of course there's always the take-out menu beckoning under the fridge magnet, but home delivery turns much of this food gloppy, and the low price doesn't justify the compromised quality.

If Asian food is such a natural and welcome part of our lives, why do we find cooking it ourselves so daunting? Is it the fear of mastering unfathomable new techniques, or do we think we'll have to buy a lot of baffling equipment and peculiar ingredients we dare not touch to the tips of our tongues? We never hesitate to order something in black bean sauce in a restaurant, but just the sight of those homely pellets imprisoned in their jars wrinkles up our noses like a whiff of shrimp paste.

Or perhaps we resist cooking Asian food because we're used to equating the length of a recipe's ingredient list with labor-intensive preparation, forgetting that its appeal is in the diversity of flavors. There may be more jars to pull out, but most are simply punctuation—a dot here, a dash there—and, with practice, they'll soon fly in and out of the cupboard with no measuring spoons in sight.

My intent is to prove these fears groundless by guiding you along the same easy path I took to enjoying some of those great tastes and textures at home, and to share my own experiments rustled up when nothing else would do but the taste of ginger, soy, cilantro, garlic, and chiles—easy on the seaweed. Because the dishes we crave are more memorable for their similarities than their differences, I've tried to demystify Asian cooking by relaxing the bonds of authenticity and blurring country boundaries so you can see how this approach works—the better to experiment yourself. You needn't learn the intricacies of all the cuisines of Asia to enjoy any one of them. One way I've tried to introduce you to the generalities of Asian cooking is by relating some recipes to American cooking and eating styles, revealing how naturally they blend in—see Coconut Hamburgers with Cucumber Salsa, Tokyo Guacamole, Asian Cole Slaw, and Shrimp Frittata. That's a pass at *fusion cooking,* the currently fashionable mingling of diverse ethnic cuisines. It's as inevitable as p.b. & j. on a croissant and as imminent as virtual reality. Indeed, the future is here in the youth-filled cafés of southern California with names like Hurry Curry of Tokyo, Mu Shu Mex, and Chez Izumi, where you can buy green tea popsicles and black bean shortcake. Clearly this isn't a slow and easy culinary melding of East and West—it's more like a high-speed wok-wreck.

The second way I've tried to welcome you to Asian cooking is to introduce a few of the simpler classic dishes and their techniques. Asian food is by character and necessity more improvisational than most and, in keeping with that spirit, these recipes are very forgiving. Quantities are merely guidelines to be fearlessly, but thoughtfully, adjusted. Ingredients that don't appeal to you, or you don't have on hand, can often be omitted or substituted in kind. You can't make grave errors; you can only risk a dull dish, and if it can't be rescued in mid-prep, you'll know how to make it sing the next time. What you're seeking is that characteristic yin and yang of texture and taste; the incomparable snap of perfectly cooked vegetables; the interplay of exotic and titillating seasonings over satiny fish or meat; and the familiar, comforting pleasure of rice or noodles weaving it all together.

After the equipment requirements in the first chapter, you'll notice that some of the recipes are arranged untraditionally by style of cooking, like Stir-Fry and Crisp-Fry. In Asian restaurants you're likely to sample several dishes at once, but at home you'll want to start out by cooking only one or two dishes. Besides, the cook-and-serve aspect of Asian food defies planning traditional courses. If you have my level of addiction, you can get your fix tonight by sprinkling a plain grilled fish fillet with spicy Coco-Peanut Crunch or marinating chicken thighs in Thais Like-It-Hot Barbecue Sauce. Or simply dip your french fries into Philippine Seasoned Vinegar, smear Cilantro and Mint Chutney on a broiled lamb chop, or toss your favorite pasta in Peanut Sauce and top it with a few garlicky shrimp. Make up a batch of Spicy Coco-Lime Macadamia Brittle to pop in your mouth when the urge strikes, or make a super-quick Saigon Pâté in the microwave for lunches at home or away. Make your next burger-on-a-bun a Wasabi Tuna Burger, or serve a small family supper of Singapore Noodles and a warm take-out roast chicken. Glazed Oyster and Jicama Kebabs don't have to preface an Asian meal, and Shrimp and Corn Fritters don't have to be a snack—they don't even need to be made with shrimp and corn.

When summer brings a plethora of farm-fresh vegetables to your kitchen, it's the perfect time to hone your stir-fry skills. The Stir-Fry chapter merely pricks the surface of what you can learn to create. More time is spent here telling you *how* to do it than what to cook. These beginner recipes range from Scallops with Pork and

Black Beans (adapted from a Chinese classic) to how to turn ground beef, a resident onion, and a handful of frozen green beans into a surprisingly tasty East-West dish. If you'll take a moment to read the introductory hints on general technique, each of the recipes should send you off into a different improv direction.

When winter's chill brings the drearies, or life is just being nasty, look through the Asian Comfort Food chapter for curries, rice, and noodles. How about a Quick Pad Thai or a steamy plate of Duck Fried Rice to make you feel whole again? On the way home from work, if there's only a bit of this and a snitch of that in the refrigerator, pick up some Asian wrappers at the market and turn to the Crisp-Fry chapter to see how to roll up nothing into something . . . and so it goes.

Above all, Asian food fills the eye and feeds the soul with its fanciful beauty and unrivaled contrasts. I hope you enjoy preparing these introductory recipes, which are merely suggestive of the venerable, centuries-old cuisines of the *majority* of people on this planet. Now, there's a sobering fact that should send us all to the nearest Asian market.

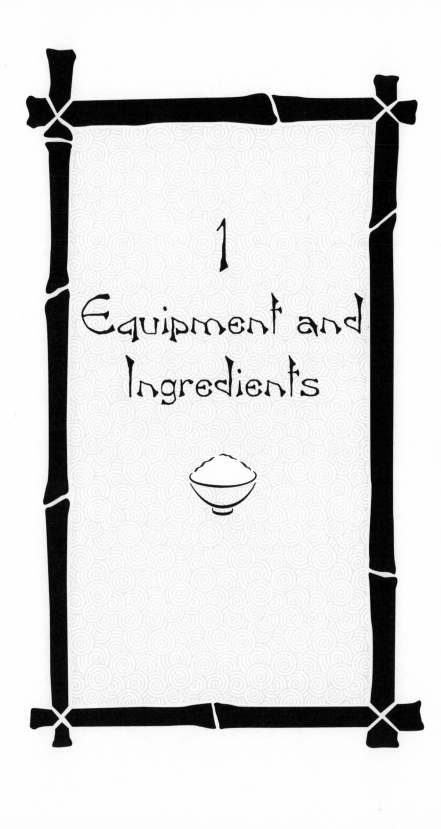

1
Equipment and Ingredients

EQUIPMENT

Good equipment saves time, builds confidence in the craft of cooking, and can make galley slaves hum. I assume you already have some of the everyday equipment like a sturdy cutting board at least 15 by 20 inches, a microwave oven, a toaster oven, a box grater, a little electric spice grinder, a mortar and pestle, and a food processor. The essentials for cooking from this book can be listed in one deep-breath sentence: a seasoned pan for stir-frying and shallow-frying, a heavy kettle for deep-frying, a fat thermometer, a slotted spoon or mesh strainer, a wide flat wooden spoon, a pair of metal tongs, a sharp chef's knife and paring knife, and a new vegetable peeler. That's all you really *need*, but at the risk of sounding frivolous, you won't have much fun—and having fun makes the food taste better. Here's what I urge you to acquire to get into the pace and rhythm of Asian cooking:

WOK: A good stove-top wok costs less than a meal at a Chinese restaurant. Its deep bowl shape makes it easy to keep the bite-size pieces of food moving, evenly cooked, and off the floor. My wok isn't a dusty stranger in the bottom cabinet since I often prefer my vegetables stir-fried and the pan's shape is equally great for tossing up skillet pasta, or even popping corn, using its dome lid.

Inexpensive woks can be purchased in Asian markets or restaurant supply houses. Look for a 12- to 14-inch spun steel pan with a long, cool handle and an opposing side bar or loop to make it easy to tip out the contents with both hands. There's no time for pot holders when you're stir-frying. I prefer a flat-bottom wok for the American range, whether gas or electric. Only a commercial range will produce a high enough flame to lick the sides of the pan. It's the shape and rapid heat conduction of the lightweight metal that makes the wok valuable. Test its weight by lifting it by the handle with one or both hands, moving it around in front of you at waist height. If your wrists can't support the weight empty, it won't work for you full.

Stainless or enameled steel, although handsome, are not intended for very high heat. Even a snow pea will stick if it isn't floating in oil. There are a lot of nonstick woks on the market; you can toss them in the sink when you're finished and fill them with water without fear of rust. But you pay a price for that convenience. You can't heat a nonstick wok without oil or you'll ruin the surface, and in stir-frying, the heat comes first.

To season an uncoated wok, scrub it well to remove any machine oil that may have been used as a protective coating. Dry it and thinly coat the surface with vegetable oil. Heat the wok very slowly over low heat for ten minutes, then wipe it out with paper towels. Repeat the entire process until the paper towels are no longer blackened. Once your wok is seasoned, just rinse it out with plain water to clean it, rubbing with paper towels to dry. Set it over the stove-top burner to dry thoroughly and store in a paper bag to avoid rusting. Don't use soap on it or you'll ruin the seasoning.

I don't recommend the countertop electric wok as the primary pan because it's immobile—you can't shake, toss, flip, or turn the food out quickly—so you have to rely on your dexterity with implements. And even though the thermostats are accurate, it's difficult to adjust the temperature quickly enough. However, if you have the storage room, the electric wok is not only a very efficient deep-fryer, because of its dependable thermostat and large surface capacity, it's also a wonderful back-up pan for company dinners, particularly for mounds of fried rice, or for keeping a pile of ribs warm without having to turn on the oven.

WOK ACCESSORIES AND UTENSILS: Be sure to buy a lid for the wok, so it can handle longer, moist cooking. It's also handy to have a hook-on side rack for holding cooked or raw food off the heat. If you ever want to try tea-smoking a chicken or duck, pick up a metal or bamboo trivet for the bottom of the wok.

I use my stacking basket steamers only for quantity cooking since I'm enamored of the way the microwave oven steams fish and vegetables; however, unless you're into zapping, basket steamers are the answer and of course they speak the Asian aesthetic. Two 10-inch trays ought to do it, but it's best to buy them when you pick out the wok to get the perfect fit. Don't forget the lid.

You'll need either a metal or wooden long-handled shovel for pushing and lifting and a wide, flat strainer for draining food out of its broth or oil. The Chinese make a simple brass woven wire mesh one with a wooden handle; there's an attractive and efficient

Thai version made of perforated coconut shell. There are many Western long-handled strainers that will work as well. I'm not quick enough with those long cooking chopsticks, so I prefer the shovel and a pair of 10- or 12-inch spring-loaded metal tongs used in restaurants and sold in most kitchen stores.

FRYER: A word about deep-fryers. Every experienced cook has his or her favorite pieces of equipment and this is one of mine: a feisty little electric fryer by Presto. Homely, inexpensive, and without bells and whistles, it comes in sizes from a little Fry Baby to a big Gran Pappy and has dependable fixed heat and a recovery range of 375 to 425 degrees. There's a hefty bucket handle and a plastic snap-on lid so you can leave the oil inside when you store it without fear of spills. A second wok, electric wok, or deep iron skillet can all do the job, but frying is messy when you have to empty out the oil with every use. I own the Fry Daddy, just the right size for two to four persons. Be sure to run a small sieve or handled strainer through the warm oil after each use. Straining the floating sediment will extend the oil's life.

KNIVES: My other favorite piece of equipment is my 7$^1/_2$ by 2$^1/_2$-inch Chinese vegetable cleaver, which I use for everything. Although it's smaller and lighter than the recommended all-purpose Chinese cleaver, I'm comfortable with it. If you keep it well sharpened, it will do everything for you except peel a grape. Mine is made in America by the Russell Company and engraved with Chinese characters. The blade is welded to a brass bevel fastened to a comfortable round wooden handle. The cleavers are inexpensive and available in most kitchen stores, as well as some Asian markets and restaurant supply houses. Try one in your hand to be sure it's a comfortable extension of your fingers. For good control, you must *feel* the action of the blade. Stainless carbon steel or chrome molybdenum are both rustproof and quick to sharpen. You'll also occasionally need a sharp paring knife.

GINGER GRATER: Not the beautiful Chinese wooden one that looks like a toy washboard but a whistle-clean white ceramic grater that mashes the fresh ginger perfectly. It has a grooved edge that pools the juice. It's a little tricky to push all the ginger out of the teeth, but the tip of a paring knife will do it and unclogging it is often just a matter of pouring whatever liquid you're working with over it. It cleans under running water in a flash and is one of those rare finds—a gadget that actually works. You can also mince ginger by pushing it through a garlic press.

BOWLS: You'll need a mess of little glass or china bowls to separate ingredients. Keep them on a tray next to the range where you can quickly reach for them and then stack them up when they're emptied. I like the inexpensive, small nesting glass bowls from Williams Sonoma.

GARLIC SLICER AND PEELER: These are fairly new, inexpensive little toys that you might want to play with. The slicer speeds up the job of making those ultra-thin fried garlic chips. The e-z-roll garlic peeler made by Omessi looks like a rubber cannoli. A few rolls on the counter top with the whole cloves inside and the husks fly off.

INGREDIENTS

Stocking an Asian pantry can be as uncomplicated as gathering the basic equipment, although even express cooking requires a well-edited shopping list. Be warned, once you put an Asian market on your regular shopping rounds, you'll be addicted. In the beginning, I felt like an interloper and the regular customers stared at me with kindly curiosity, as though E.T. were fingering the merchandise. Soon the excitement of such a dizzying array of goods gave me an acquisitive rush just walking through the door. I couldn't resist snatching up exotic trophies like stuffed rambutans, tree fungus, and Sri Lankan Maldive fish chips, though I had no inkling what to do with them.

You'll find, as I did, that ethnic food merchants delight in telling you about their national cuisine and often they, or their employee-relatives, are good cooks and can give you invaluable tips and advice.

The freezer cases are chock-full of convenience foods such as dumplings, wrappers, stuffed buns and other dim sum, Asian vegetables like Japanese edamame (the luscious pale green buttery soybean, better than limas), ready-to-cook scallion pancakes, flat bread doughs, and all manner of unusual goodies worth examining.

The fresh produce departments are a joy and they're so used to Western customers now that most things are marked in English. The scarce-elsewhere Japanese eggplant is common, cilantro rarely has its roots amputated, lemongrass isn't moldy, and the bean sprouts are blindingly white. The greatest stir-fry treasure is finding a bag of fluffy green snow pea vines *sans* peas, or a basket of fresh water chestnuts in among the baby bok choy, garlic chives, and Chinese broccoli.

I generally shy away from the meat and poultry department because the cuts of meat are unfamiliar and I'm not drawn to chicken feet, cockscombs, and other tips, tails, and entrails that appear bizarre to me. The barbecued pork and spareribs are a good buy, the Chinese sausage is a must, and often there are fantastic carry-out dishes like crispy duck, gingered chicken, and Thai curries. Expect a boggling array of fresh rice, wheat, and egg noodles and an equal variety of fresh homemade wrappers.

But that's just the beginning. How about the graphically stunning Japanese rice crackers, puckery Indian nibbles like *sev* and *chor,* bright green fried peas, cookies made in Hong Kong with ginger and mango cream fillings and peanut toppings—a tribute to British biscuit makers—and the sensibly large bottles of soy sauce, vinegar, cooking wines, and other essential seasonings costing a fraction of what you normally pay for multiple small bottles. Unsweetened Thai coconut milk is almost half the price, and it's better. There are all kinds of tropical fruits and juice, some very good; handsome raffia-tied jars of crystallized ginger; and rows of chutneys and pickled condiments. The baby corn is the proper immature sprout and not the sawed off, tough variety sold under some American labels, and the little Hümmel figure straw mushrooms are very appealing in stir-fries. My Indian store even has a whole back room devoted to bulk rice, including the prized aged basmati. You can leave these ethnic markets laden with groceries for far less than you regularly spend. That thought alone should make you an eager adventurer.

You do need to take the time to browse and read labels, and as soon as you realize the contents aren't so unfamiliar after all, you'll be hooked. You may even end up with your own can of Maldive fish chips.

What to do if you don't have an Asian market? Visit the international food section of your supermarket and your local specialty food store. Unless you check frequently, you'll be amazed at the growing selection of Asian ingredients on the shelves—probably everything you'll need for this book. Of course, you can also mail-order ingredients.

The checked items are those most frequently specified in the recipes, but everything listed is well worth having on hand.

Seasonings

✓ *CHILE PASTE:* Hot chiles ground into paste or jam with vinegar or tamarind, oil, salt, and garlic. There's Chinese (usually too salty for my taste), Thai (labeled *nam prik* and very hot), and Vietnamese (my first choice for its pleasant sweet-sour balance). Take your pick but use judiciously as the ones with visible seeds are scorchers. Chile paste is good for seasoning meat marinades, slow-cook dishes, and dips. A small jar goes a long way and keeps almost indefinitely in the refrigerator.

✓ *CHILE SAUCE, THAI (SRIRACHA):* My favorite all-around serrano hot pepper sauce is worth the shopping trip to an Asian market. It's made by Huy Fong Foods of Rosemead, California, and comes in a large, clear plastic squeeze bottle with a bright green top, which you've probably seen often on Thai restaurant tables. Look for the rooster on the label. It's specified repeatedly in this book, but is equally useful in Western cooking.

✓ *CHILES, DRIED:* The small dried red peppers so ubiquitous in Szechuan-Hunan and Thai cooking are available in cellophane bags in Asian markets and in tiny jars in gourmet stores. Use Italian crushed red pepper for a similar effect, but add this pepper with a light hand because you can't remove it while cooking and guests can't fish the little bits out at the table. Dried peppers eventually lose their power so replace them regularly.

✓ *CURRY POWDER AND PASTE:* There's lots of room for argument and personal preference here. You can make your own: see the curry powder recipe in the Condiments, Dips, and Sauces chapter. Or look for the Subahdar brand of curry paste imported from England. That whole line of Indian products is reliable. (Grab a box of Subahdar's coconut cream in a compressed block—very handy stuff; see listing for uses.) Curry paste keeps indefinitely, unlike powder, which conks out in three or four months. Ignore Chinese curry powder completely—it's nasty.

✓ *CURRY PASTE, THAI GREEN:* This pungently flavored seasoning base for green chile curries comes in tiny jars and keeps in the refrigerator two to three months before it starts losing strength. Handy for flavoring quick coconut milk curries.

✓ *FISH SAUCE, THAI NAM PLA OR VIETNAMESE NUOC MAM:* Take my advice: just buy it and use it as directed. Don't ask what's in it and, above all, don't smell it. It's thoroughly un-American, but wonderful. It's amazing what a huge extra dimension just a tiny bit of this sauce can add to a dish, so it's understandable why Asians dote on it. The best brand is the Thai King Lobster, which I suspect is a purely psychological opinion because there's no lobster in it. It doesn't need refrigeration, but my bulging cupboard has suffered a quart-size bottle for months, so look for a smaller size. Just be sure it's imported. Buy fish sauce in glass, not plastic bottles.

FIVE-SPICE POWDER: An appealing, fragrant, and balanced mixture of star anise, clove, cinnamon, fennel, and Szechuan peppercorns. It's finely ground like cinnamon, about the same color, and comes in small plastic bags or jars. Use sparingly. Store in tightly sealed jars, discarding it when the aroma wanes. There's also a five-spice oil on the market, which is convenient but doesn't seem to have the depth or balance of flavor.

GARAM MASALA: A subtle, vaguely sweet, cocoa-brown North Indian curry mixture made without the familiar yellow turmeric, it can be used as a sprinkling condiment over grilled or roasted meats or poultry and it seasons cold salads well. It contains cardamom, cloves, cinnamon, nutmeg, mace, cumin, coriander, and pepper and makes a mild, smooth-cooked curry sauce—a pleasant change from the more familiar South Indian seasonings.

✓ *GARLIC PUREE:* To make garlic puree, slice off just enough of the top of a head of garlic to expose the flesh in each clove. Set the head stem-side down on heavy-duty foil and drizzle the top with olive oil to moisten. Sprinkle salt and pepper on top. Seal the garlic tightly in the foil and bake at 350° for 1 hour. Squeeze the resulting paste from the husks and store it tightly sealed in the refrigerator for a mild, sweet garlic seasoning for dressings and sauces where freshly minced garlic may have too strong a bite. I usually roast three heads at a time since the puree keeps well and I often add some freshly grated ginger into the puree just for Asian cooking.

Asian markets carry already prepared garlic-ginger pastes and supermarkets and specialty stores stock all kinds of garlic in jars—whole, minced, preserved in oil, and even pureed.

✓ *HOISIN SAUCE:* A sweet pastelike condiment of fermented soybean, vinegar, garlic, sesame seed, star anise, and chile used primarily as a glaze for roasted or grilled pork and chicken. Add a little orange juice concentrate and a dash of dry red wine for a great basting sauce for duck. Thin it with soy and chile sauce to make a luscious barbecue sauce for spareribs or chicken. Hoisin's familiar flavor makes a good condiment for improvising. The Koon Chun Sauce Factory in Hong Kong makes a good one, as does Pearl River Bridge in China. Tightly lidded, it keeps indefinitely.

✓ *OYSTER SAUCE:* You don't have to eat oysters to love this ancient, thick and glossy, sea-salty, vaguely caramelized sauce. It's another one of those enigmatic Asian seasonings with a complexity of flavor contradicting its simple ingredients. It's delicious in vegetable or beef stir-fries, or just over noodles. A more expensive imported brand will be higher quality; the readily available Kame brand is weak in flavor so look for the smokier Lee Kum Kee with the garishly delightful label. You can definitely lick it from your fingertips.

PLUM SAUCE: The Koon Chun Sauce Factory also makes a well-balanced plum sauce to please anyone's palate; kids often embarrass their parents by smearing it over everything in a Chinese restaurant. This sauce is made with sugared plums, vinegar, ginger, spices, and garlic. It's a wonderful dip for chicken or lamb kebabs or grilled pork chops.

✓ *SAFFRON:* When you realize that about 500 crocuses must give up their bucolic lives every time you serve saffron rice, this pricey spice seems downright cheap. If you have a choice, buy the deeply colored threads in preference to saffron powder, which can be easily adulterated. The threads also keep their strength longer. Just crush them in a little hot water or milk to release their full flavor.

✓ *SESAME SEEDS:* Buy them in bulk at natural foods stores—taste them first to be sure they're fresh and sweet. They're also sold in large bags at Asian markets. Keep them tightly sealed in a cool, dry cupboard so they won't turn rancid. You can also freeze them. Toast some to keep handy for sprinkling over salads or steamed fish in need of a little crunch.

SHRIMP PASTE: You might be tempted to pick this up if you're shopping in an Asian market. It *sounds* delicious, but it's made from salted decomposed shrimp and smells like old tennis shoes. So will your whole refrigerator if you don't seal it like hazardous waste. Consider this just a friendly shopper's warning, although more advanced Asian cooks will have to succumb—literally. Thai and Malaysian shrimp pastes are milder, a good place to start if you must.

✓ *LIQUID SMOKE:* This seems a peculiar product for the Asian kitchen, but just a few drops can give dishes like Beef Chow Fun the appealing smoky taste you get in restaurants when the flames are high enough over the wok to lick the food with smoke. Wright's Liquid Smoke is available in most supermarkets.

✓ *SOY SAUCE:* A novella could be written about the subtle properties of fine soy sauce, but for everyday use the consistently best is the readily available Japanese-style Kikkoman soy sauce made right here in Wisconsin. They also make a low-sodium version for those who need it. Tamari is darker and has a stronger flavor. Soy sauce should be refrigerated after opening; it keeps six months.

✓ *SOY SAUCE, DARK:* Sometimes called black soy, this condiment is used when you don't want the extra liquid of thin soy sauce but do want the flavor and color. It's saltier than regular soy sauce, which is balanced a bit with a touch of intensifying molasses. Koon Chun is a good brand.

SOY SAUCE, MUSHROOM: This is a soy sauce flavored with straw mushrooms and is, as one might imagine, delightful sprinkled over any stir-fry. The only brand I've found is Pearl River Bridge, which is superb.

SOY SAUCE, SHRIMP: The Chinese equivalent of Thai and Vietnamese fish sauce. Look for the Pearl River Bridge brand. With the addition of soy sauce, the shrimp extract is darker and richer than its sister fish sauce, which makes it more suitable for stir-fries, marinades, and dipping sauces.

SOY SAUCE, INDONESIAN (KETJAP MANIS): This most important sauce in Indonesian cooking should not be confused with the less subtle Chinese sweet soy sauce. Although rarely called for in this book, it's nice to have on hand for satay dipping and improv cooking. Its familiar flavors (soy sauce, sugar, garlic, ginger, star anise, and bay leaf), if not the actual ingredients, work well in Western dishes based on shrimp and beef. It keeps forever.

✓ *SZECHUAN PEPPERCORNS:* These aromatic peppercorns are indigenous to China and are not peppercorns at all; they look like flower buds but actually they're berries. If you can't smell their camphorlike aroma they aren't fresh enough. They come in plastic bags and need to be picked over for debris before toasting for a few minutes in a skillet, then grinding. They are not hot, but can be used as an alternative to ground pepper; see Chinese Salt and Pepper (page 24). They keep for years in a well-sealed jar.

✓ *WASABI, PASTE OR POWDER:* Japanese green horseradish comes in powder form to be mixed with water or already reconstituted in a tube of paste. The paste is more convenient and keeps its snap well. This is the familiar horseradish dotted on sushi and its bite is not easily forgotten. Delicious mixed with mayonnaise as a cold shrimp dip.

OILS AND VINEGARS

✓ *COOKING OILS:* Peanut oil has a very high smoking point and is therefore particularly well suited to crisp-frying. It also imparts a slightly nutty flavor that you may perceive as an oilier taste. Peanut oil is relatively expensive; look for the excellent Lion and Globe brand from Hong Kong or the more readily available Akita brand from Canada. Flavorless corn oil also holds up well in high-heat cooking. Safflower or canola oil are good choices for the small quantities used in stir-frying.

CITRUS OILS: This American product comes from Boyajian in Massachusetts. It's useful in both Eastern and Western cooking. These are pure extracts of lime, orange, or lemon with no additives. It takes only a drop or two of these intense oils to add a citrus zing to stir-fries, sauces, marinades, and glazes—a convenient substitute for freshly grated zest. These oils are sold separately or in sets and keep indefinitely in the refrigerator.

SESAME OIL, AMERICAN: This is a good mild stir-fry and salad oil without the intense flavor of its toasted Asian counterpart. Refrigerate it.

✓ *SESAME OIL, ASIAN:* Pressed from toasted sesame seeds, this dark oil is purely for seasoning—not cooking. Use it sparingly. The first brand I ever bought was the Japanese Kadoya and since it's rich in flavor, color, and aroma, I've remained loyal. A dash of toasted sesame oil gives pizazz to marinades for grilled meat. It keeps well in the refrigerator but should be brought to room temperature before using.

✓ *RICE VINEGAR, JAPANESE:* The Marukan brand is excellent and less harsh than the Chinese. I use rice vinegar for salad dressings, chutneys, and salsas, always preferring a mild vinegar to a sharp one. (Look for the acid percentage on the label.)

PLUM VINEGAR (UME), JAPANESE: Small bottles of this salty, tart vinegar made from umeboshi are appearing in natural foods stores among the Eden line of products. Used in sparing amounts, it's interesting to experiment with in sauces and dressings. Add a dash of it to Chinese plum sauce to cut the sugar and use it for glazing roasts.

MANGO VIGNETTE: The California Consorzio Company's marketing moniker for a sophisticated blend of mango puree, champagne vinegar, sugar, and vanilla. It makes a delicious marinade for poultry, pork, lamb, or fish and a refreshing dressing for fruit or chicken salads. It keeps indefinitely in the refrigerator.

COOKING WINES

MIRIN, JAPANESE SWEET WINE: This isn't a drinking wine so don't be tempted to sip while you cook. It's a Japanese cooking ingredient, akin to sweet sherry, used in basting sauces for dishes like yakatori and teriyaki. The Marukan brand is reliable, but buy the smaller bottle since you probably won't use this too often.

✓ *SAKE, JAPANESE RICE WINE:* I'm very partial to the subtlety and smoothness of sake and use it wherever wine or sherry is specified. Its excellent glazing qualities make it wonderful for marinades if you boil off the alcohol first. All well-stocked liquor stores carry imported sake, but it doesn't keep indefinitely. Use it within a year for maximum flavor.

SHAOHSING, CHINESE YELLOW RICE WINE: This dry cooking wine can come in handy if you cook Chinese food often and have a back corner of the cupboard you want to fill. Since I use sake for every cooking wine need, mine props up a bag of tiger lily buds.

General Packaged Goods

✓ *BLACK BEANS, CHINESE SALTED:* The ancient and original soyfood that produced miso and soy sauce looks kind of pitiful. The fermented black soybeans add a certain *je ne sais quoi* to a steamed white fish, seafood, or chicken sauce. They come in thick plastic bags, but store them in a small screwtop jar in the cupboard or the refrigerator once opened. Finger the beans through the package to be sure they're plump and soft before you buy them. A popular brand is Mee Chun. Look at the ingredient label and avoid those flavored with five-spice powder; Pearl River Bridge is a good brand.

CHICKPEA FLOUR (BESAN): Used extensively in Indian cooking for batters and doughs, but this flour is pretty hard to find except in Indian markets and health food stores. It's called for here only in vegetable fritters.

CLAMS, THAILAND: Chopped clams just aren't what they used to be. I suspect they haul in one giant toughie to fill a whole case of cans these days. But check out the imported baby clams; Thai clams are sweet and tender, small enough for adding whole to fried rice and seafood salads.

CORN, CHINESE: Baby corn is as handy to have in the cupboard as straw mushrooms—always ready to join fresh vegetables in any stir-fry. These miniature ears of corn are sweet and appetizing. Taiwanese market brands change with every crossing, but they're all better than the European brands.

CRABMEAT, THAI: This canned crabmeat is quite satisfactory for adding to spur-of-the-moment spring rolls, rice paper rolls, soups, or Asian omelets.

✓ *COCONUT MILK, UNSWEETENED:* Coconut milk is used a great deal in Southeast Asia. It's sort of the Asian cream sauce, never to be confused with the sweetened variety used to make tropical drinks. I think the canned milk is as good as, if not better than, making your own from the fresh meat of the coconut, if you can buy a good imported brand like Chaokoh from Thailand. There are other acceptable brands on the market including the American label Taste of Thai, now found in most supermarkets. The distinction between good and best is the richness of flavor and the texture, which gives the necessary body to the sauce. If you need only a small amount, you can keep the rest in a clean screwtop jar in the refrigerator for several weeks. Happily, you can also buy little half-tins in Asian markets—I buy six at a time.

COCONUT CREAM: Subahdar, a line of Indian condiments imported from England, includes a small paper box containing a stick of condensed and solidified coconut cream. A curious product, not easy to come by, but very convenient as it keeps indefinitely in the refrigerator. Just chunk off a little piece to flavor any dish.

COCONUT, UNSWEETENED, GRATED: Natural foods stores stock grated and flaked dried coconut without added sugar. Refrigerate or freeze it for toasting or simply to add to condiments. Toasted flakes look wonderful sprinkled over salads, curries, or desserts. There's a big difference between this product and the processed canned one.

GHEE: Natural foods stores and Indian markets (much cheaper) are the best places to find this form of clarified butter in a jar. Clarified butter doesn't burn at the higher temperatures of Asian cooking and keeps a long time at room temperature. The one I buy comes from Deep Foods, a distributor of all manner of divine Indian food treasures.

✓ *GINGER, PICKLED:* You can't enjoy sushi without it. Thankfully, you can buy it almost everywhere, including your local sushi take-out. Paper-thin, pink, spicy, sweet, and vinegary, pickled ginger is a delight, even as a Western condiment or an addition to fresh fruit salsas. Asian markets also carry the Day-Glo red pickled ginger or the shredded Japanese Kizami Shoga, both of which make fanciful garnishes.

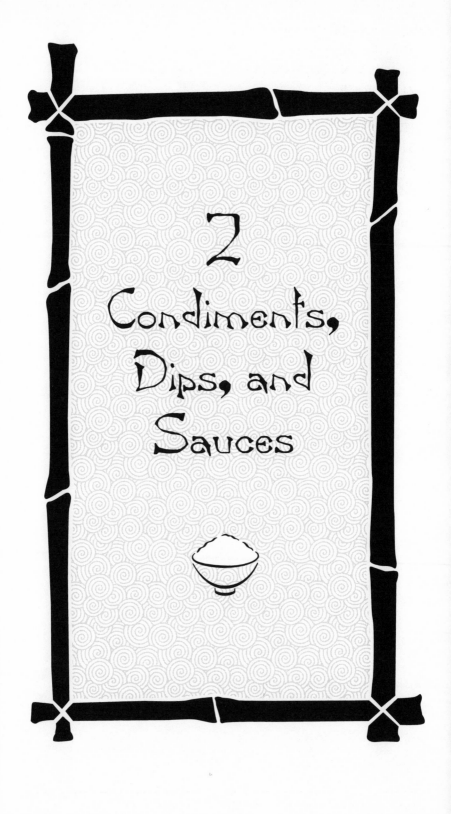

2
Condiments, Dips, and Sauces

Here are a few delightful Pan-Asian cooking seasonings, dipping sauces, and table condiments essential to—and instantly associated with—the food of that region. Many require no cooking at all, and those that can be made ahead and kept indefinitely should lure you into Asian cooking if you don't push them aside between ethnic cravings. Used regularly and imaginatively, they can spark up many a drab Western meal as well.

☯ Chinese Seasoning Oil ☯
Makes about 2 cups

*T*his infused oil can be used for practically any meat or fish sauté, as a quick oil rub for grilling or broiling, or even in salad dressings. Store it in a squeaky clean screwtop jar in a cool cupboard, where it keeps indefinitely and reach for it often. Soon you'll be spinning it out in your own variations. Barbara Tropp, chef-owner of San Francisco's revered China Moon restaurant, makes a more complex infusion called *ma-la* oil; see Mail-Order Sources.

1 cup peanut oil
6 large garlic cloves, smashed and peeled
4 bunches scallions, sliced, including 2 inches of green
8 quarter-size coins of peeled fresh ginger, smashed

Put the ingredients in a 1-quart measuring cup or pitcher, cover tightly with plastic wrap, and microwave on high for 5 minutes. Let the oil steep until cool, then strain and store in a clean half-pint screwtop jar or bottle.

◢ Since many of the recipes in this book call for hot peppers or chile sauce, there are none in this oil. If you want to boost the fire-power, add 3 or 4 tiny dried red chiles or a teaspoon or two of dried red pepper flakes to the infusion.

◢ Add a few drops of one of the citrus oils (see Ingredients) to vary this basic one.

✐ To make a seasoning oil and a condiment at once, see the recipe for Coco-Peanut Crunch (page 33).

☯ Chinese Salt and Pepper ☯

Makes ⅓ cup

This traditional toasted Szechuan salt and pepper is subtle and deliciously aromatic. Contrary to the food of that province, Szechuan pepper is not hot at all. It works well on all meats, fish, or poultry and is a welcome alternative to the universal salt and freshly ground black pepper. This mixture is balanced in favor of pepper because so many recipes call for salty soy sauce or fish sauce.

2 tablespoons coarse salt
3 tablespoons Szechuan peppercorns

Roast the salt and peppercorns in a dry heavy skillet over medium heat until the salt takes on a golden hue and the peppercorns start to smoke a bit, about 3 minutes. After the mixture cools, grind it in a spice mill or coffee grinder. Store in a clean screwtop spice jar. Keeps indefinitely.

☯ Toasted Sesame Salt ☯

Makes ½ cup

Toasted sesame-seed salt is a splendid shake for chicken and shrimp salad and for vegetables, particularly asparagus, green beans, and zucchini. If you were Korean, you could hardly live without it.

¼ cup sesame seeds, toasted
¼ cup coarse salt

✓ *MUSHROOMS, BLACK, DRIED:* I can remember when I thought *these* were weird—long before dried wild mushrooms started appearing in supermarkets and I discovered that the stinky Chinese dried mushroom is really our friend the shiitake. Fresh shiitakes are no substitute, however, because the flavor intensity is not the same. The good news is that dried shiitakes are now commonly available. They need to be soaked in hot water for about twenty minutes to soften before stemming and adding to any dish. If dry and cool, they keep indefinitely.

✓ *MUSHROOMS, STRAW:* The diminutive Chinese straw mushroom offers a winning glazed ceramic look to a stir-fry. They're used whole more for their looks and texture than for their rather bland flavor. Keep a can in the cupboard for spontaneous Chinese cooking.

PANKO: If you find cellophane bags of these Japanese bread crumbs in your Asian market, buy some. They make the crunchiest coating for fried shrimp, chicken, or eggplant. Simply dip the meat, fish, or vegetables in beaten egg (or cornstarch and then beaten egg white) and coat heavily with panko. Shallow or deep-fry until golden. You'll wonder where this product has been all your life.

✓ *RICE, JASMINE, BASMATI, AND SHORT-GRAIN:* Most gourmet stores and some supermarkets carry imported rice, all of which should be thoroughly rinsed before cooking. Soft, fragrant, medium-grain jasmine rice is lovely with almost any Asian meal. Medium-grain is best with Chinese food, and nutty basmati is the incomparable Indian rice ideal with spicy food. Creamy, short-grain Japanese rice is a must for sushi, but when the rice will be eaten plain, you can use arborio or Spanish paella rice.

RICE FLOUR: Not an essential but I keep it around to lighten fritter batters or dredge meat or fish for frying. It comes in plastic bags and keeps indefinitely.

SAUSAGE, CHINESE: These mild, sweet, air-dried pork sausage links are like no other and are sold in vacuum packs of six or eight in either the Chinese market deli case or in the store's freezer. They must be steam softened—easily done in the microwave—before slicing for dim sum, soup, stir-frys, or rice dishes. A few links always wait in my freezer.

TOFU: A bean curd made from dried soybeans, sold in blocks, and available nowadays in every supermarket. You can buy soft, firm, and variously flavored tofu. Soybeans are the only vegetable to qualify as a complete protein. The only descriptive adjective I can think of for tofu is innocuous, which is why you won't find more than a couple of recipes for it in this book. Aficionados like it deep-fried or sautéed with spicy ingredients, which kind of says it all.

Noodles and Wrappers

NOODLES: Noodles are detailed in the Asian Comfort Food chapter.
> **Dried:** Thai rice sticks *(banh pho)*, Japanese somen, Japanese buckwheat *(soba)*, Chinese rice vermicelli, Chinese cellophane noodles (mung bean)
> **Fresh:** Chinese rice sheets *(fun)*, Chinese egg noodles

WRAPPERS: Wrappers are detailed in the Crisp-Fry chapter.
> **Dried:** Vietnamese rice paper *(banh trang)*
> **Fresh:** Chinese egg roll and wonton, Philippine lumpia (often frozen)

Mail Order Sources

CHINA MOON CATALOGUE (food and equipment)
639 Post Street
San Francisco, CA 94639
415-771-Moon

DE WILDT IMPORTS, INC. (Asian food and specialties)
Fox Gap Road, R.D. #3
Bangor, PA 18013
1-800-338-3433

DEAN & DELUCA (international specialties and equipment)
560 Broadway
New York, NY 10012
212-431-1691

WILLIAMS SONOMA (international food and equipment)
P.O. Box 7456
San Francisco, CA 94120
1-800-541-2233

CINNABAR (Indian sauces, marinades, and chutneys)
1134 W. Haining Street
Prescott, AZ 86301
1-800-824-4563

ASIAN FOOD MARKET
217 Summit Avenue
Jersey City, NJ 07306
201-333-7254

SUPER ASIAN MARKET
2719 Wilson Boulevard
Arlington, VA 22201
703-527-0777

ADRIANA'S BAZAAR
317 West 107th Street
New York, NY 10025
212-877-5757

UWAJIMAYA
519 Sixth Avenue So.
Seattle, WA 98104
206-624-6248

DEEP FOODS (Indian food)
1090 Springfield Road
Union, NJ 07083
908-810-7500

Toast the seeds in a dry heavy skillet over low heat until golden and aromatic, or toast on a dinner plate in the microwave, stirring at 2-minute intervals. Mix the seeds with the salt and grind together in a spice mill or coffee grinder. Store in a clean screwtop jar. Keeps indefinitely in a cool, dry cupboard.

☯ Curry Powder ☯

Makes about ½ cup

I've been making this curry powder for many years and have never found one I like better. Be sure all your spices are super fresh. This makes about ½ cup, which should be enough to last the 3 to 4 months you can keep it. I buy bulk spices from a natural foods store and make a double recipe every year just before Christmas so I can share it with friends.

2 tablespoons coriander seeds
1½ tablespoons cumin seeds
¾ teaspoon mustard seeds
¾ teaspoon fenugreek seeds
1 tablespoon ground cinnamon
2 tablespoons black peppercorns, ground
¾ teaspoon grated nutmeg
¾ teaspoon ground cloves
1½ teaspoons ground cardamom
1½ teaspoons turmeric
1½ teaspoons ground ginger
2 teaspoons–1½ tablespoons cayenne pepper, for mild to
    very hot curry

Toast the seeds on a metal pie plate in a 325° oven until the mustard seeds begin to pop. Cool. Process or blend the seeds with the rest of the ingredients. Store in a cool dark place, preferably in a small tin. Keeps 3 to 4 months.

☯ Japanese Glazing Sauce ☯

Makes ³/₄ cup

*Y*ou can buy prepared teriyaki sauce, but now you have the quality components in your own pantry.

¹/₃ cup soy sauce
¹/₃ cup mirin or sake
2 teaspoons sugar, or 1¹/₂ tablespoons if using sake
2 quarter-size coins of fresh ginger, peeled and crushed
1 teaspoon Thai chile sauce, optional

In a 2-cup glass measure, mix the soy sauce, mirin or sake, and sugar. Add the ginger and optional chile sauce and bring to a boil in the microwave. Cook another minute or so until mixture thickens to a light glaze. Store in a clean half-pint screwtop jar. It will keep for months without refrigeration in a cool cupboard. It's best to baste this on the beef, chicken, or fish at the end of the grilling, so the sugar won't burn.

Philippine
☯ Seasoned Vinegar ☯

Makes 1¹/₄ cups

*V*inegar is an important ingredient in Philippine cooking, and dipping sauces like this one are used everywhere on grilled fish and meat, as well as on crispy fried foods.

1 cup rice vinegar
4 garlic cloves, peeled and lightly bruised
¹/₂ teaspoon coarse salt
1 teaspoon whole black peppercorns

Put all the ingredients in a half-pint screwtop jar or bottle and let the flavors develop for a week before using. This will keep indefinitely and can be used for hearty salad dressings.

≁ You can vary the effect of this condiment by adding a small amount of soy sauce or any Asian chile sauce to individual servings, thus preserving the keeping quality of the basic mixture. You can also use ¼ cup balsamic vinegar and ¾ cup rice vinegar, adding complementary complexity and sweetness. A couple of bruised quarter-coins of peeled fresh ginger are particularly good with this combination.

Vietnamese
☯ ## Table Seasoning ☯

Makes ⅔ cup

*N*uoc cham may never replace A-1 sauce on the Western table, but it's a snappy way to enliven grilled meats or chicken. Use it as a dip for spring rolls and chicken or lamb meatballs, or add it at the table to stir-fries or rice dishes.

2 fresh red chiles, seeded and minced
1 garlic clove, crushed and minced
1 teaspoon sugar
juice of 1 lime
1 tablespoon rice wine vinegar
¼ cup fish sauce *(nam pla* or *nuoc mam)*
¼ cup water

Mash the chiles and garlic together with the sugar in a mortar and pestle, rendering them as close to a paste as you can. Add the lime juice and mash some more. Add this mixture to the rest of the ingredients and store the sauce in a clean half-pint screwtop jar in the refrigerator. Shake before using.

≁ If you want to mix up this sauce in a flash and you have no fresh chiles, use any Asian chile paste (with or without garlic) or Thai chile sauce. A teaspoon will do it, and no mashing in a mortar is required. Add ½ teaspoon first, then taste.

☯ Thai Table Seasoning ☯

Makes about ½ cup

Like the Vietnamese *nuoc mam*, this Thai sauce called *nam prik* appears on every table to dip or drizzle at will. As you might suspect, this one is much hotter and a bit sweeter. Otherwise, the difference is minute.

- 2 tablespoons Thai fish sauce *(nam pla)*
- 2 tablespoons soy sauce
- 2 tablespoons fresh lemon or lime juice
- 2 tablespoons water
- 1 tablespoon light brown sugar
- 4 garlic cloves, pressed
- 2 fresh red chiles, minced, or more to taste

Combine all ingredients. This sauce isn't a keeper; make it the day you plan to serve it.

☯ Korean Table Seasoning ☯

Makes about ½ cup

This is a good communal dunking sauce for grilled meats.

- ¼ cup dark soy sauce
- 1 tablespoon toasted sesame oil
- 2 tablespoons plus 1 teaspoon rice vinegar
- 3 scallions, very thinly sliced, with 2 inches of green
- ¼ teaspoon or more cayenne pepper (optional)

Combine all ingredients. This sauce isn't a keeper; make it the day you plan to serve it.

Thais Like-It-Hot
Barbecue Sauce

☯   ☯

Makes 1 1/2 cups

This sauce is so versatile it isn't limited to slathering on grilled meat and chicken. Use it as a dip for wonton chips or cold shrimp. I've even used it to season gazpacho and stir-fried eggplant.

> 2 tablespoons safflower or light sesame oil
> 6 bottled jalapeño peppers, stemmed and chopped
> 1 tablespoon peeled and chopped fresh ginger
> 1/4 cup chopped shallots (about 3 large)
> 3 garlic cloves, chopped
> 1/4 cup chopped cilantro leaves and tender part of stems
> 3/4 cup tomato puree
> 2 tablespoons Thai fish sauce *(nam pla)*
> 1 tablespoon rice vinegar, or juice of 1/2 lime
> 1 1/2 tablespoons sugar
> 1 teaspoon salt

Put the oil and chopped ingredients into a food processor and process to a smooth paste. Add the liquid ingredients and blend well. Taste and adjust seasoning. Store in a clean pint-size screwtop jar. It will keep, refrigerated, for months.

✂ Oil-rub the chicken, beef, or shrimp and add the sauce toward the end of the grilling so it doesn't burn. Serve a separate bowl of it at the table.

✂ This sauce makes a wonderful topping for grilled burgers—beef, lamb, or chicken.

☯ Black Banana Sauce ☯

Makes about 1 1/2 cups

*O*ne day I got tired of pushing a bag of blackened Chiquitas around in my freezer. It wasn't frozen daiquiri weather and I hadn't made a loaf of banana bread in years. Reincarnating them into this sauce was a good move. It's excellent on barbecued ribs, chicken, or lamb and makes a spunky dip for Philippine lumpia, Madras chimichangas, or samosas.

3 overripe bananas
1 tablespoon Thai chile sauce or Tabasco sauce
2 garlic cloves, crushed and minced
2 tablespoons Mango Vignette (see Ingredients)
1 tablespoon fresh lime juice
brown sugar, to taste
1/4 cup unsweetened coconut milk

Mix all ingredients in a food processor or blender. Taste and adjust the tart-sweet balance and the heat to your preference. This sauce will keep in a screwtop jar for about a week.

✂ See notes (page 104) for Mango Vignette substitute.

✂ If you're going to use this on grilled meat or poultry, marinate the meat first in soy sauce, oil, crushed ginger, and garlic. Baste with the banana sauce toward the end of the grilling time so that it caramelizes nicely on the meat but doesn't burn. Save some sauce to add at the table.

✂ If you can shop at an Asian market, pick up a bottle of the spicy Philippine catsup called Jufran Hot Banana Sauce. It lasts indefinitely.

☯ Spicy Sesame Sauce ☯

Makes about ³/₄ cup

Less rich than peanut sauce, this deliciously creamy first cousin is excellent for dipping or dabbing on almost anything. It's great on fish, dumplings, or rice noodles topped with stir-fried asparagus or shrimp.

> **¹/₄ cup tahini (not Chinese sesame paste)**
> **1 teaspoon toasted sesame oil**
> **3 garlic cloves, pressed**
> **¹/₄ teaspoon peeled and grated fresh ginger, with juice**
> **2 tablespoons Indonesian soy sauce *(ketjap manis)* or**
>   **Chinese dark soy sauce**
> **6 scallions, minced, with some green**
> **¹/₂ teaspoon Thai chile sauce, or to taste**
> **1 tablespoon rice vinegar**
> **1 tablespoon water**

Combine all ingredients well. Store in the refrigerator in a clean half-pint screwtop jar. It should keep for a couple of weeks. Stir before using.

☯ Peanut Sauce ☯

Makes 2 cups

Peanuts are grown and eaten all over Asia—chopped, ground, whole, or pressed for cooking oil. They're sprinkled over salads, tossed into stir-frys, and mashed into spicy sauces metamorphosing our beloved childhood peanut butter into a socially acceptable grown-up treat. There are myriad versions of peanut sauce with or without coconut milk or fish sauce, mint or cilantro—not so hot or red hot, very simple or complex.

> **4 garlic cloves, crushed**
> **1 tablespoon chopped cilantro root, or 3 tablespoons**
>   **chopped leaves and stems**

2 fresh hot red or green chiles, seeded and chopped, or $\frac{1}{2}$
   teaspoon chile oil
$\frac{1}{4}$ cup Indonesian soy sauce *(ketjap manis)* or Chinese
   dark soy sauce
2 tablespoons Thai fish sauce *(nam pla)*
1 tablespoon fresh lime juice
1 cup smooth peanut butter
1 tablespoon toasted sesame oil
$\frac{1}{2}$ cup unsweetened coconut milk, preferably Thai
$\frac{1}{4}$ cup dry-roasted unsalted peanuts, chopped

Mince the garlic, cilantro, and chiles in a food processor with the soy sauce, then add the fish sauce, lime juice, peanut butter, and oil. Blend well. Pulse in the coconut milk in two parts so you can adjust the consistency for dipping. Fold in the chopped peanuts. Store the sauce in a clean pint-size screwtop jar in the refrigerator. It will keep for several weeks.

✄ In a thick version you can spread this delectable sauce on Japanese rice crackers, dip the top into black sesame seeds like jimmies, and roll the edge in finely minced cilantro.

✄ If you plan to serve this sauce with grilled satays, you can warm it in the microwave.

✄ You can replace the cilantro with chopped mint and add snipped chives.

✄ Add the fresh herbs on the day you plan to serve it.

Quick Vietnamese Peanut Sauce

☯   ☯

Makes about $\frac{3}{4}$ cup

$\frac{1}{4}$ cup smooth peanut butter
2 tablespoons hoisin sauce

1 teaspoon chile paste with garlic or Thai chile sauce

1 tablespoon dark soy sauce or fish sauce *(nam pla* or *nuoc mam)*

1 tablespoon catsup

$1/4$ cup chicken broth or water

Combine all ingredients until smooth. Store in a screwtop jar.

☯ Coco-Peanut Crunch ☯
Makes about 3 cups

*T*his wonderful topping adds an interesting fillip to rice, noodles, and curries, as well as chicken salad or grilled fish, lamb, or pork. Dip your grilled satay in a lime or vinegar dip and then in the coconut crunch as a switch from peanut sauce. Float it over red pepper, black bean, or lentil soup. It may seem complex, but the recipe makes almost a quart, which will last a very long time. Having made it once, you won't need to read the instructions a second time.

2 cups peanut oil

1 medium head garlic with firm fat cloves, peeled and thinly sliced

12 large, thinly sliced quarter-size coins of peeled fresh ginger

8 large shallots, thinly sliced

grated zest of 1 lime, or 4 drops pure lime oil

1 cup unsweetened coconut, toasted

1 cup honey-roasted peanuts, chopped

cayenne pepper, to taste (optional)

superfine or confectioners' sugar (optional)

Heat the oil in a wok or skillet over medium-high heat until it gathers a few bubbles around a chopstick. Spread out the garlic, ginger, and shallot slices separately on a layer of paper towels, cover with another layer, and press down with the heel of your hand to extract the surface moisture. This will allow quicker crisping. Add the shallot slices to the oil first, and when oil comes back to a gentle bubble, adjust the heat to keep it below a fast boil. Depending on the moisture content of the slices, it will take from 5 to 8 minutes for the shallots to turn walnut brown. Resist hastening the process at higher heat or they will darken before they dry.

As soon as they're brown, lift them from the oil with a fine strainer and fluff them out onto paper towels. You'll hear a papery rustle if they're crisp; if not, put them back for a minute or two. Blot the excess oil with another paper towel and fry the garlic slices, which will take only half as long to turn golden. The garlic doesn't need to reach as rich a brown as the shallots do to be crisp. Test one before you remove them all.

Cook the ginger slices the same way. Remove from the oil and blot in the same manner as the shallots. Mix all three together and let them cool.

In a food processor, process all but the peanuts and cayenne to a fine granular sprinkle, not a paste. Mix in the nuts and the cayenne. Taste the mix, and if it needs sweetening for balance, add a little superfine or confectioners' sugar to taste. Store in a clean 1-quart screwtop jar with a tight seal. Carefully protected, it will take weeks to lose its crunch and can be refreshed in the microwave when it does.

✒ Fried garlic, shallots (or onions), and ginger chips make a wonderful snack with cocktails. All they need is a little salt or Chinese Salt and Pepper.

✒ One of those little garlic slicers makes speedy work when you have this much to slice.

✒ If you can't find shallots, use a couple of finely chopped yellow onions and always fry them separately from the garlic because they have more moisture and it takes longer to crisp them. For the same reason, onion bits shrink when they're crisp-fried so don't mince them too finely.

✒ By all means save the remaining oil in a clean screwtop jar. You've just made a basic seasoning oil.

✂ Yes, you could use an electric deep-fryer for this project, but skimming such small bits from the depths of a deep kettle is tedious. The wok's larger surface allows the slices to float so you can capture them easily.

☯ ## Bog Berry Chutney ☯

Makes 2 quarts

Even though I'm a New Englander, I've always been content to eat cranberries only during the holidays. Working on this book at a friend's home on Nantucket inspired me to try them in a chutney. They're perfect for that necessary sweet-sour balance.

Since chutney makes such a welcome holiday hostess gift, I've made a note to myself to add some festive diced green pepper to this recipe for my gift batch. Pair it with a small jar of homemade curry powder for an impressive present. I'd rather have this chutney with my turkey than traditional cranberry sauce—put me in the stockade.

4 garlic cloves, crushed and minced
4 quarter-size coins of peeled fresh ginger, minced
¹/₂ large white onion, minced
zest from ¹/₂ tangerine or small orange, cut into thin strips
1 teaspoon sweet Indian curry powder (*garam masala*)
1 tablespoon Asian sesame oil
¹/₂ cup diced red and/or yellow sweet peppers
1 20-ounce can unsweetened chunk pineapple with juice,
    or ¹/₂ fresh pineapple, chopped
1 pound (1 bag) cranberries
1 semi-ripe papaya, peeled and chopped
¹/₂ cup light brown sugar
¹/₂ cup rice vinegar or distilled white vinegar
2 teaspoons Thai chile sauce
¹/₄ cup macadamia nuts, well toasted and chopped

Mix the garlic, ginger, onion, tangerine zest, and curry powder with the sesame oil. Soften the mixture in the microwave for a couple of minutes in a tightly covered dish large enough to hold the rest of the ingredients. Then add everything except the nuts, and microwave for 6 minutes. Stir and taste. Adjust the sugar and vinegar for a pleasant sweet-sour balance. If you prefer it spicier, add more chile sauce. Cook for another 5 minutes, uncovered. Taste again. If you want to further adjust the flavor or just reduce the quantity of juice, remove the fruit to a bowl with a slotted spoon and continue reducing the syrup. It will thicken slightly when cool and the flavors will permeate the fruit as the mixture mellows.

When the chutney is cool, fold in the toasted nuts and store in a couple of clean 1-quart screwtop jars. This has not been processed, so it must be refrigerated. It will keep perfectly at least a month.

✐ Commercial chutneys are fine, but often not memorable enough to turn us into devotees. I think you'll quickly appreciate chutney's merits if you prepare your own; it's so easy and satisfying to make. You can use almost any firm seasonal fruit. The microwave makes it super-quick and refrigerating it saves you the bother of processing.

Asian Pear and Mango Chutney with ☯ Crystallized Ginger ☯

Makes about 2 quarts

3 Asian pears, peeled and chopped
3 large semi-ripe mangoes, diced
¼ cup finely chopped crystallized ginger
¼ cup dried currants
2 garlic cloves, crushed and minced
1 tablespoon mustard seeds
1 tablespoon minced hot green chiles
½ cup rice vinegar
¼ cup balsamic vinegar
½ cup dark brown sugar
1 teaspoon salt

Put all the ingredients into a covered dish and cook in the micro-wave on high for 5 minutes. Stir and taste. Adjust the tart and sweet balance if necessary and cook another 5 to 8 minutes, uncovered. Store in clean 1-quart and half-pint screwtop jars in the refrigerator. It will keep for a couple of weeks.

To cube a mango: Stand the mango on its plump round bottom and slice down with a long sharp knife on each side of, and as close as possible to, the flat center pit. Now you have two mango cheeks. With the tip of the knife, score the flesh into cubes right down to the skin. Press the edges of each side downward with your thumbs while pressing the skin side up with your fingers. This will turn the mango half "inside out," forcing the cubes to pop up in relief. Cut them off right next to the skin. Peel the center slice containing the pit and, standing over the sink, rake off the sweet juicy flesh with your teeth—cook's treat.

Cilantro:

Fresh cilantro keeps several days, as fresh as the proverbial daisies, if you put it in a glass with its feet in shallow water and the leaves under a plastic bag.

Cilantro and Mint Chutney

Makes 1 cup

This fresh Indian chutney for herb lovers is a pungent dip for samosas, vegetable fritters, rice paper rolls, lumpia, kebabs, and satays either as is or mixed with yogurt. Leftovers can be used as a judicious seasoning for stews and soups, mixed with mayonnaise for chicken or shrimp salad, or spread on meat or cucumber sandwiches.

2 big bunches cilantro, leaves and tender part of stems
1/2–1 bunch mint, leaves only
2 canned pickled jalapeño peppers, stemmed, not seeded
2 shallots, chopped
4 garlic cloves, smashed
1 tablespoon fresh lime juice or rice vinegar
1/2 teaspoon sugar
1/4 teaspoon salt

Puree all the ingredients in a food processor or blender. Refrigerate in a half-pint screwtop jar.

⟋ Stir some of this chutney into well-drained yogurt, or half yogurt and half sour cream. Fold it into steamed rice. Top a baked sweet potato or soft scrambled eggs with it.

⟋ Add grated unsweetened coconut to the mixture for body and a pinch of cumin for more complexity. Spoon it onto grilled lamb or a pan-fried lamb burger, or spread it over grilled or broiled eggplant.

⟋ If you're not a cilantro lover, make the chutney with all mint or basil and mint.

⟋ Look for Nirav brand coriander and mint chutneys in your Asian market.

☯ Fresh Mango Chutney ☯
Makes almost 1 quart

*A*n unfussy and refreshing chutney that's perfect with poultry, duck, or grilled salmon or tuna.

2 semi-ripe mangoes, cubed
2 tablespoons unsweetened coconut
2 tablespoons minced cilantro
1 tablespoon minced peeled fresh ginger
1/2 teaspoon salt
1/8 teaspoon cayenne pepper
Fresh lime juice, to taste

Toss all the ingredients until well combined. Enhance the chutney lightly with a squeeze or two of lime. Cover and store in the refrigerator no more than 8 hours before serving.

Super Express

LAMB CHOPS: Smear chops with Cilantro and Mint Chutney 30 minutes before grilling them over white-hot charcoal. Serve them with grilled halves of Asian eggplant scored and brushed with garlic oil. Make a raita to serve on the side: seed and pulp 2 ripe tomatoes. Fold 3 minced shallots and the tomato pulp into drained yogurt and mix.

☯ Banana and Date Raita ☯

Makes about 2 cups

Indian raitas are relishes made of raw or cooked fruit or vegetables in a base of seasoned yogurt. Here are two quite different raitas that will perk up any simple meal, Indian or not.

2 bananas, sliced
4 fresh dates, pitted and chopped
1 heaping tablespoon minced red onion
2 teaspoons toasted sesame seeds
Grated zest of 1 small lime
pinch of salt
cayenne pepper, to taste
1 cup plain yogurt, drained

Fold all the ingredients into the yogurt and serve immediately, or refrigerate and store for up to 4 hours.

The jumbo, amber, soft unpitted dates sold in bulk in the produce departments in late fall and through the holidays are labeled "fresh," although they don't come right off the date palm in that form. Whether a misnomer or not, these dates, usually Medjools, are preferable to the drier, stickier ones that come in boxes.

Cucumber Raita with Mint

Makes approximately 3 cups

2 small cucumbers, seeded, blotted dry, and chopped
$1/2$ small onion, thinly sliced
1 jalapeño pepper, seeded and minced
$1/4$ teaspoon ground cumin
pinch of salt
1 tablespoon chopped fresh mint
1 cup plain yogurt, well drained in a sieve

Combine all the ingredients with the yogurt and serve immediately or refrigerate and store for not more than a day.

Seared Corn, Tomato, and Black Bean Relish

Makes about 2 1/2 cups

I'm so fond of corn relish that I couldn't resist trying my hand at an Asian version. If it doesn't disappear by the forkful from the refrigerator before you can serve it, try presenting this zesty relish with barbecued ribs, teriyaki chicken, or grilled swordfish or tuna.

1 tablespoon Chinese Seasoning Oil (page 23)
$1/2$ teaspoon chile oil

$^3/_4$ cup sweet onion, preferably Vidalia or Maui, diced into small pieces

$^1/_4$ cup diced sweet red pepper

2 large ears yellow corn, kernels cut from cob, or 1$^1/_2$ cups frozen corn, thawed

2 teaspoons light brown sugar

1 teaspoon yellow mustard seeds

$^1/_2$ teaspoon turmeric

pinch of ground cloves

$^1/_2$ teaspoon coarse salt

$^1/_4$ teaspoon ground Szechuan pepper

1 ripe tomato, seeded, pulped, and chopped

1 tablespoon chopped Chinese black beans

2 tablespoons rice vinegar

Heat the oils in a wok and add the diced onion. Toss and shake over high heat, searing the onion until it picks up small black flecks and softens slightly. Reduce the heat and add the red pepper. Toss and shake until the pepper softens slightly but retains some crunch. Remove the onion and pepper with a slotted spoon, leaving a film of oil in the wok. If you're using frozen corn, blot it very dry with paper towels. Add the corn to the hot wok and sear over high heat for about 30 seconds. Add the brown sugar. Adjust the heat to medium and let the corn caramelize slightly to a light golden brown, adding the mustard seeds, turmeric, cloves, salt, and pepper after 1 minute. Keep tossing the mixture until the mustard seeds start to pop. Add the tomato, tossing and stirring until it softens. Add the onion and pepper, along with the black beans and vinegar. Combine the ingredients well. Taste and adjust salt. Serve the relish at room temperature. You can make this a couple of days ahead. It will keep a week or so in the refrigerator.

✁ Chopped cilantro or fresh basil are both good additions to this relish. You can fold them in anytime after deciding which works best with the seasoning in your main dish.

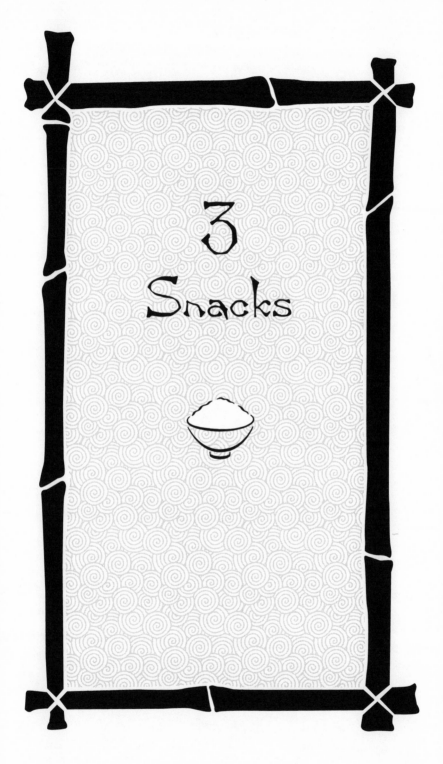

3
Snacks

☯ Curried Cashews ☯

Makes about 1 quart

This is a simplified version of the wonderful sweet-hot nuts a good friend and I used to produce for our little company called Certified Nuts.

1 jumbo egg white
1 tablespoon water
1 pound raw cashews
2 teaspoons salt
1 tablespoon curry powder
3 tablespoons superfine sugar
$^1/_2$ teaspoon cayenne pepper

Preheat the oven to 300°. Line a jelly-roll pan with aluminum foil and coat it lightly with vegetable oil spray. In a bowl large enough to hold the nuts, whisk the egg white with the water until it's frothy. Mix in the cashews, tossing them to coat. Turn them out onto the baking pan in a single layer. Mix the salt, curry powder, sugar, and cayenne, blending well. Sprinkle the mixture over the nuts, toss, and bake them for about 1 hour, stirring 2 or 3 times. When the nuts are completely cool, store them in an airtight tin or a couple of screwtop jars. They'll keep for weeks in low humidity.

☯ Fire Dust Peanuts ☯

Makes about 1 quart

These are too easy to be so good—perfect for the busy cook.

1 pound honey-roasted peanuts or mixed nuts
1 tablespoon five-spice powder
$^1/_4$ teaspoon cayenne pepper
salt, to taste

Pour the peanuts into a large bowl and mix the spices well in a small one. With a large spoon, scoop the nuts up and over, and sprinkle them with the seasoning mixture, coating and recoating the nuts thoroughly. Taste and add more seasoning and/or salt as needed. Store in an airtight tin or a couple of screwtop jars.

Garlic and Chile Almonds

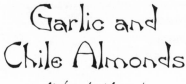

Makes about 1 pound

*S*tore the nuts and garlic for snacking or gifts, and use the spicy seasoned oil for cooking.

2 cups peanut oil
6–8 small dried red chiles
1 head of garlic, peeled and sliced
1 pound blanched almonds
1 teaspoon chile powder
salt

Pour the oil into a wok, add the chiles, and over medium-high heat, bring the oil up to 350°. Add the garlic slices and toast them to a light golden brown. Remove with a mesh skimmer or slotted spoon and turn out onto paper towels to crisp. Add the nuts to the hot oil and cook to a light golden brown, about 5 minutes. Turn out onto paper towels to drain. Sprinkle with chile powder and leave them to cool. Salt the nuts and taste for seasoning. Mix the almonds with the crispy garlic slices and store in an airtight container.

✎ Although the flavor won't be comparable, you can create the same effect more quickly by deleting the sliced garlic and tossing the nuts with a mixture of bottled garlic oil and chile oil to lightly coat them. Bake them at 350° for about 15 minutes, or until they start to take on color. Sprinkle with chile powder and salt when they're cool.

Spicy Coco-Lime
☯ # Macadamia Brittle ☯

Makes 1 cup

*H*ere's why I love my microwave: no muss, no fuss. You can have these luscious nuts ready to serve in a wink and no burnt-sugar skillet to clean up. I buy nuts in bulk and store them in the freezer just so I can turn out such treats any time. You can use 2 or 3 drops of lime oil instead of the zest; add it along with the coconut flavoring.

2 teaspoons grated lime zest
$^1/_2$ cup sugar
$^1/_4$ cup light corn syrup
1 cup roasted, lightly salted macadamia nuts
1 teaspoon natural coconut flavoring
$^1/_4$ cup shredded unsweetened coconut
$^1/_4$ teaspoon cayenne pepper
$^1/_2$ teaspoon baking soda

Grate the lime zest and spread it out on a small plate to dry. Meanwhile, stir the sugar and corn syrup together in a 1-quart glass or ceramic dish. Microwave on high for 3 minutes. Stir in the nuts and microwave on high for 3 minutes more, or until the mixture is light brown. Add the coconut flavoring, coconut, and cayenne pepper. Microwave on high for another 1$^1/_2$ minutes. Remove the nuts from the oven and gently stir in the baking soda until the mixture is light and foamy. Quickly turn the nuts out onto a sheet of aluminum foil lightly filmed with cooking spray and separate them with the tip of a knife, pushing the excess caramel to one side for a cook's treat. It will take a half-hour for the nuts to cool. If you like them super-spicy, sprinkle with additional cayenne, but taste them first—they kick back a little. Store the nuts in an airtight container or screwtop jars. Humidity will soften the glaze so they won't keep as well as roasted nuts.

✎ I recommend taking the extra time to sprinkle the nuts with the grated lime zest even if you use the oil, just because it *looks* so appetizing. Do it as quickly after they're spread out as you can. Sprinkle the dried zest directly over the nuts with a demitasse spoon. It will sink into the glaze and retain its bright green color.

☯   # ꟿadras Popcorn   ☯
Makes approximately 6 cups

Seasoning popcorn any which way is easy if you pop it on top of the stove; a hot-air popper or microwave won't work here. If you add the dry seasonings to the hot oil, as many recipes direct, you risk burning them. I learned a better way from Susan Feniger and Mary Sue Milliken at the Border Grill in Los Angeles, where they always offer giant bowls of the fluffy stuff at the bar.

$1/4$ **teaspoon cayenne pepper**
$1/4$ **teaspoon ground allspice**
$1/4$ **teaspoon ground coriander**
$1/4$ **teaspoon ground cumin**
$1/4$ **teaspoon turmeric**
$1/2$ **teaspoon salt**
2 tablespoons vegetable oil or ghee
$1/4$ **cup popcorn kernels**

Blend all the seasonings in a small dish and keep it near the stovetop. Heat the oil in a lightweight lidded saucepan or wok, or use a popcorn popper. The oil is ready when 1 kernel pops; when it does, add the rest of the corn and put on the lid. When the corn starts popping, lift the lid just enough to pitch the seasonings into the pan. Cook and shake until the corn is quiet.

Super Express

MAKE A TROPICAL ASIAN-STYLE SMOOTHIE: Blend yogurt, guava nectar, fresh pineapple chunks, mango slices, and lots of grated ginger and chopped mint leaves with a few ice cubes for a luscious liquid lunch.

Chickpea Puree with Ginger and Basil

☯ ☯

Makes approximately 3 1/2 cups

There's a hint of India in this creamy dip, which is great with pita, wonton, or chapati crisps and equally tasty with a mini-garden of fresh baby vegetables, or for dunking chunks of warm take-out rotisserie chicken.

- **1 1-pound can chickpeas (2 cups), rinsed and drained**
- **1 tablespoon roasted garlic puree, or 6 large garlic cloves, crushed and minced**
- **3 quarter-size coins of peeled fresh ginger, crushed and minced**
- **3 tablespoons safflower or canola oil**
- **1/2 teaspoon turmeric**
- **1 teaspoon salt**
- **1/4 teaspoon cayenne pepper**
- **2 tablespoons chopped fresh basil**
- **1 tablespoon fresh lemon juice**
- **3/4 cup yogurt**
- **1/4 cup sour cream**

Blend all the ingredients except the yogurt and sour cream in a food processor or blender until smooth. Quickly pulse in the yogurt and sour cream. Refrigerate for at least 1 hour to mellow the flavors. Bring to room temperature before serving.

↙ You can use fresh mint or cilantro instead of basil, if you prefer.

↙ To turn this into a delicious main-dish accompaniment, sauté the chickpeas in the oil with the minced garlic and ginger. Add the dry seasonings, and instead of basil or mint, toss in a couple fistfuls of stemmed flat-leaf spinach. Stir until the spinach is just limp, then add 1/4 cup each of yogurt and sour cream. Serve with chicken or lamb.

⤝ This puree makes an utterly delicious chilled soup, simply thinned with chicken broth and creamed out with a little more yogurt. Garnish with slivered seeded cherry tomatoes and snipped chives. It's not only great for a lunchbox thermos but it's elegant enough for company.

☯ Tokyo Guacamole ☯
Makes 1 cup

*H*ere's a tasty little discovery to offer guests, something surprisingly different. Serve the guacamole with deep-fried flour tortillas or wonton triangles (page 118).

1 tablespoon light mayonnaise or yogurt
$1/2$ teaspoon wasabi paste
1 ripe avocado
3 scallions, trimmed and minced, white part only
1 teaspoon minced pickled ginger
$1/2$ medium tomato, peeled, seeded, and minced
2 teaspoons chopped cilantro
salt and pepper

Mix the mayonnaise with the wasabi paste and mash it and the avocado with a fork, leaving some texture. Mix in the rest of the ingredients and serve slightly chilled.

☯ Silky Tofu Walnut Dip ☯
Makes 2 cups

I find crudités quite dull and experience has taught me they're often left untouched. But not when you serve this simple dip, which comes from a young food-smart grad student in Japan who served this with trimmed daikon, carrots, celery, bok choy, snow peas, and zucchini.

1 cup toasted walnut pieces
1 10.5-ounce package soft tofu
salt and pepper to taste
1 tablespoon minced dill or chives, for garnish

Toast the walnuts in a 325° oven for 12 minutes. Mince them in a food processor, almost to a paste. Add the tofu, salt and pepper, and pulse to mix well. Taste for salt, which brings this dip to life. Garnish with dill or chives.

Glazed Oysters and Jicama Kebabs

Serves 4–6

*A*ngels-on-Horseback has been my favorite hors d'oeuvre for years. It's an easy way to cook oysters if you don't like them raw and this version looks and tastes as if it should arrive on a red lacquer plate. I'm suggesting jicama because it's fresh and has no hint of the tinny taste associated with the traditional canned water chestnuts. If you can find fresh water chestnuts, by all means use them, or rinse canned ones well.

1 pint select oysters, well drained
$^1/_2$ cup Japanese Glazing Sauce (page 26)
$^1/_2$ pound lean smoked bacon, thinly sliced
1 small jicama, peeled, sliced $^1/_4$-inch thick, and cut into 1-inch squares; or sliced water chestnuts

Preheat the broiler. Soak short wooden skewers in water for at least 30 minutes so they don't burn. Marinate the oysters in the glazing sauce at least 15 minutes. One cut strip of bacon will wrap around 2 or 3 oysters. Blanch enough whole strips in the microwave to cover the number of oysters you want to broil—about 1 minute should do. The bacon will now crisp before the oysters overcook. When the bacon is cool enough to handle, blot it with a paper towel and cut the strips to fit around the oysters. Slide one slice of water chestnut, then one wrapped oyster on each skewer. Broil just until the bacon is crisp. Serve immediately.

⟋ A dab of wasabi is the perfect accent for these oysters. Or, if you prefer a less zippy one, try the Cilantro and Mint Chutney (page 37) made with all cilantro—or dilute the bite of wasabi with soy sauce and lemon juice.

Chilled Lime Scallops with
☯   Coconut Cream   ☯
Serves 4

*S*callops require no cooking at all to be safe to eat, so they're ideal for this simple seviche. The marinade can be made ahead and kept in the refrigerator for three or four days.

**3 small fresh red chiles, seeded and minced, or 1 teaspoon
    Thai chile sauce**
¹/₄ cup fresh lime juice, strained
3 tablespoons Thai fish sauce *(nam pla)*
2 teaspoons minced pickled ginger
6 scallions, including 2 inches of green, very thinly sliced
1 pint bay scallops
2 tablespoons minced cilantro
6 cherry tomatoes, seeded and slivered

DIP:
   **Whisk ¹/₂ cup unsweetened coconut milk with ¹/₄ cup sour
   cream and ¹/₂ teaspoon grated peeled ginger**

Mix the chiles, lime juice, fish sauce, ginger, and scallions in a glass bowl. Drain the scallops well and blot them dry if they're very juicy. Add the scallops to the marinade, cover, and refrigerate for at least 2 hours. When you're ready to serve, drain off the excess liquid and fold in the cilantro and tomatoes. Put the dip in the center of the bowl. Serve with picks.

⟋ Lime scallops make a lovely starter course for a dinner party. Peel an avocado half for each serving. Cut and reserve a round disk from the bottom of each half to steady it on the plate. Mound the scallops into the avocado, set it on a nest of cress, and cap with the reserved disk. Or just chop the scallops and avocado and make garden rolls.

Shrimp and Corn Fritters

⊙ ⊙

Makes about 30 2-inch fritters

*T*hese luscious fritters are closest to the Indonesian *perkedel;* they're crisp, lacy, and flat and make a terrific hors d'oeuvre or accompaniment to brunch or a light supper.

¹/₄ pound medium shrimp, in the shell
1 cup fresh (about 2 ears) or frozen white corn kernels
¹/₃ cup unsweetened coconut milk
3 tablespoons rice flour
3 tablespoons cornstarch
¹/₄ teaspoon baking soda
1 large egg, lightly beaten
2 garlic cloves, pressed, or 1 teaspoon roasted garlic puree
¹/₄ cup minced scallions, including 2 inches of green
pinch of ground cumin
pinch of cayenne pepper
¹/₄ teaspoon salt
peanut oil

Undercook the shrimp in the microwave in a covered dish in a splash of water for 1 minute or plunge them into boiling water to cover and set aside for 2 minutes. Drain, rinse in cool water to stop the cooking, shell the shrimp, and chop them roughly.

Put the corn and coconut milk into a food processor and pulse until the mixture is fairly smooth but not pureed. Add the flour, cornstarch, baking soda, and beaten egg and pulse a few times to combine. Pour the batter into a bowl and stir in the scallions and seasonings.

Heat about a ½ inch of oil in a large skillet, and when bubbles gather around an upright wooden chopstick held in the center of the pan, slide in 1 tablespoon of the fritter mixture. The batter will drop to the bottom and spread out. After about 3 minutes on each side, the fritters will be golden brown and crisp around the edges. Drain them on paper towels and serve warm or at room temperature. For larger fritters, increase the batter drop to 2 table-spoons.

✐ This recipe can be doubled with equally good results.

✐ You can use crab meat instead of the shrimp, or leave out the seafood altogether.

✐ You can add minced cilantro to the batter plus a dash of chile sauce for a spicier version. A simple mix of Indonesian soy sauce and rice vinegar is a good dip for these fritters.

✐ Since this batter contains an egg, you can cook the fritters in a nonstick skillet instead of floating them in oil and you'll have tender little pancakes.

Hot Peanut Banana Coins

Serves 4

*H*ere's a lighter way to handle an egg fritter batter. Cook the fritters in a nonstick skillet in a half-dollar size for canapés or in a silver-dollar size for an unusual accompaniment. This combination may have a Far Eastern personality, but it's reminiscent of the grilled peanut butter and banana sandwiches of my youth.

1 teaspoon peeled and minced fresh ginger
2 garlic cloves, minced
2 heaping tablespoons chopped sweet onion
$^3/_4$ teaspoon Thai chile sauce
$^1/_4$ cup chopped loosely packed cilantro—leaves and top
   part of stems
$^1/_4$ cup plus 1$^1/_2$ tablespoons extra-chunky peanut butter
2 strips crisp bacon, finely chopped
3 tablespoons rice flour
3 tablespoons cornstarch
$^1/_4$ teaspoon baking soda
$^1/_4$ teaspoon salt
1 large egg, beaten with $^1/_4$ cup water
1 semi-ripe banana

Put the ginger, garlic, onion, chile sauce, and cilantro in a food processor and blend until you have a thick paste. Add the peanut butter and bacon and pulse to combine. Add the flour, cornstarch, baking soda, and salt. Process briefly. Pour in the egg and water, and mix just until the batter sits up loosely on the tip of a spoon. Scrape the mixture into a bowl. Peel and slice the banana into $^1/_4$-inch rounds.

Heat a nonstick skillet and drop the batter in by the teaspoonful. The consistency of the batter is such that it will hold a perfect shape as it hits the heat so you can size them any way you like. This time, make them half-dollar size. As soon as they set up slightly, place a banana round in the middle and cover the banana with a little more batter. When tiny bubbles appear on the surface, flip the coins over. They cook quickly and should be golden brown when finished.

⤚ If you want to make these ahead, you can reheat them in a slow oven.

⤚ Serve these fritters with spareribs grilled or broiled with Thais Like-It-Hot Barbecue Sauce (page 29).

Free-Form Sushi

Serves 4

*N*igiri, the hand-formed Japanese sushi resembling oval Ping-Pong balls, with the sushi fillings draped over them, are a popular Japanese snack. Maneuvering these mounds on chopsticks in and out of the soy sauce without dumping the whole shebang makes a hilarious parlor game. Jennifer Brennan, who lives and writes cookbooks in Yokohama, says to do what busy Japanese sushi lovers do—arrange everything free-form in a rice bowl. Brilliant.

RICE
2 cups Japanese short-grain rice *(uruchi)*, sold in supermarkets as sushi rice
1¾ cups water mixed with ¼ cup rice vinegar, 1 teaspoon salt, and 2 teaspoons sugar

Wash the rice under running water in a sieve and soak it in cool water for 30 minutes. Bring the rice to a boil in the seasoned water over moderate heat, stirring frequently. Cover the pot tightly, reduce the heat to low, and cook for 15 minutes or until the water has evaporated. Let the rice stand, covered with a towel, for another 10 minutes.

Portion the rice into four individual bowls and give everyone a tiny vessel of soy sauce and a saucer with pickled ginger slices and wasabi paste. Arrange the toppings on a service platter or around the edge of the rice.

SUGGESTED TOPPINGS: Cooked salmon or salmon roe, smoked trout chevrons, grilled or raw tuna, cooked shrimp, lump crab, bay scallops, or slivers of teriyaki steak, pork tenderloin, or roast chicken. Also avocado cubes, asparagus tips, cooked kidney beans, shredded carrot and daikon, slivered tomato, diced cucumber and sweet red pepper, shredded raw or stir-fried flat-leaf spinach, and crumbled nori (crisp the sheets first on a hot, dry skillet).

SUGGESTED RICE GARNISHES: Dill or cilantro sprigs, chives, toasted sesame seeds, or a sprinkle of grated lime zest.

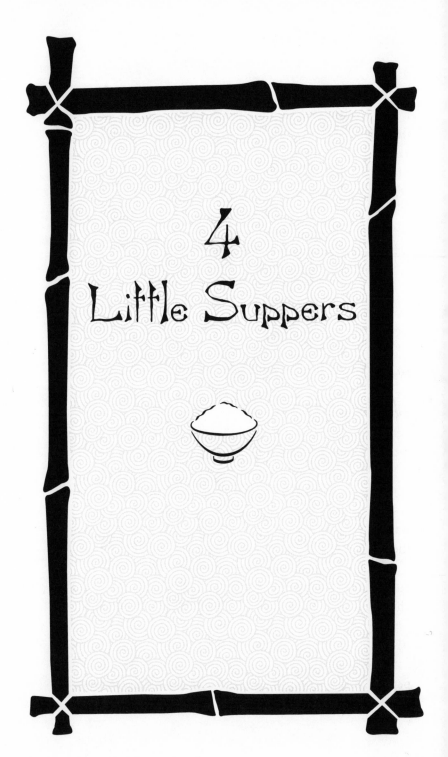

4
Little Suppers

Delhi Quesadillas

☯   ☯

Serves 1

*O*nce you taste one of these, you won't think it's such a hokey idea. You can use fresh whole-wheat chapatis instead of flour tortillas if you want to soften the cultural clash. However you make these exotic grilled cheese sandwiches, they're a great solution for spur-of-the-moment lunches, soup and salad suppers, and company starters. Serve them for Sunday brunch with Aidell's grilled Burmese or smoked lemon chicken sausages and a bowl of coconut fried rice garnished with mango and papaya.

1 tablespoon Chinese Seasoning Oil (page 23)
2 8–9-inch flour tortillas or Indian chapatis per serving
1 tablespoon Cilantro and Mint Chutney (page 37) or
    bottled coriander chutney
$1/2$ cup freshly grated Sonoma or Monterey Jack cheese
3 small slices tomato, blotted between paper towels

Heat the seasoned oil in a nonstick skillet. For each serving, spread 1 tortilla with chutney and top with the grated cheese. Arrange the tomato slices over the cheese without overlapping. Cover the filling with the second tortilla, making a sandwich, and place the quesadilla on the hot skillet. Let it cook over medium heat until the bottom is golden and crisp, then flip the quesadilla over. When it's done on both sides, slide it out on a cutting board and cut into wedges with a sharp knife.

⟍ Instead of the herb chutney, try a quality fruit chutney, such as homemade apple or pear. Omit the tomato, of course.

Southeast Burritos ☯

☯ ☯

Serves 4

Spicy Asian ingredients can rival those of a great Southwestern burrito. Marinate the meat the night before, and the next night you'll have a light, tasty supper in minutes.

MARINATED MEAT

1 flank steak, about 1¼ pounds
4 garlic cloves, crushed
2 quarter-size coins of peeled fresh ginger, crushed
¼ cup mushroom or dark soy sauce
3 tablespoons hoisin sauce
2 tablespoons oyster sauce
2 tablespoons sake or Chinese rice wine
1 teaspoon chile paste, or to taste
2 teaspoons sugar
1 tablespoon peanut oil
1 tablespoon toasted sesame oil, reserved for seasoning
   cooked meat
4 large flour tortillas

VEGETABLE FILLING

1 cup thin ribbons of romaine lettuce
8 scallions, slivered, with some green
⅓ cup cooked corn kernels (frozen is fine)
¾ cup roughly chopped bean sprouts

Flatten the steak, trim it of any fat, and slide it in the freezer for about 45 minutes. Meanwhile, combine the rest of the marinade ingredients except for the sesame oil. Slice the partially frozen meat very thin against the grain. Put in a covered dish to marinate for a couple of hours or overnight in the refrigerator.

Drain the meat from the marinade. Heat the wok until it's almost smoking. Quickly sear the meat over high heat in two 20-second batches. Season with the sesame oil, cover the wok, and remove it from the heat. Moisten the tortillas with wet hands and soften them on each side by holding them with tongs over an open flame or low electric burner for a second.

Make a nest of romaine, scallions, corn, and sprouts just front of center on each warm tortilla. Pile the meat on top and roll the burrito tightly, folding in the sides like an egg roll.

✂ Try leftover barbecued pork or chicken with shredded napa cabbage and the onions from Lamb Burgers with Seared Five-Spice Onions.

✂ The seared meat alone makes a tasty filling for steamed or baked buns made with frozen dinner-roll dough. Pull the thawed dough into 2-inch discs, leaving it slightly thicker at the center. Put a small amount of chopped cooked meat in the center and pull up the edges of the circle, twisting and pinching it closed. Let the buns rise for an hour on a sheet of wax paper. Either steam them in your wok for 15 minutes or egg wash and bake at 350° for 25 minutes. Serve hot or at room temperature.

☯ Pacific Rim Sandwich ☯

*W*e tend to think sandwiches are purely Western, if not all-American. Not true—it seems Lord Sandwich's influence was as far reaching as Marco Polo's. The whole world has a version of a satisfying sandwich.

BREAD
French demi-baguette (for a Vietnamese sub), hollowed-out crusty hard roll, or good bakery white bread, thickly sliced and lightly toasted

FILLINGS
• Thin slices of Saigon Pâté (page 65), onions seared in a hot wok with peanut oil and a dash of liquid smoke, sweet and/or hot roasted pepper strips, and a few sprigs of cilantro, or minced cilantro mixed into mayonnaise

- Cold roast lamb with thinly sliced sweet onion, red-ripe tomato, and Cilantro and Mint Chutney (page 37) mixed with drained yogurt
- Sliced grilled teriyaki chicken (or turkey) breast with a good fruit chutney and lots of chopped watercress
- Barbecued pork tenderloin (Thais Like-it-Hot Barbecue Sauce, page 29) with strips of grilled eggplant or Seared Corn, Tomato, and Black Bean Relish (page 40)
- Beef tenderloin tips stir-fried with garlic, thinly sliced onion, minced chiles, oyster sauce, and chopped basil. Line the roll or bread with sliced tomato and pile the savory meat on top.

Open-Face Chicken Sandwich ☯ on Asian Garlic Toast ☯

Serves 4

*A*lmost any leftover roasted or barbecued meat will produce a tasty mini-meal. However, what to do with a skinless chicken breast seems a national obsession. You won't be disappointed with this zesty alternative.

2 tablespoons peanut oil
4 boneless and skinless chicken breast halves
¼ cup chicken broth
4 ½-inch slices day-old Italian bread cut on the diagonal
1½ tablespoons softened butter
2 garlic cloves, pressed
1 tablespoon mixed minced mint, cilantro, and chives
1 large sweet onion, such as Vidalia, very coarsely chopped
3 red or green jalapeño peppers, seeded and sliced in thin strips
2 quarter coins of peeled fresh ginger, minced
pinch of sugar
salt and pepper

Heat the oil in a wok over high heat and sear the chicken on both sides. Pour in the broth, reduce the heat to medium low, and cover the wok. Cook the chicken for 20 minutes, checking once to make sure the pan doesn't dry out.

Preheat the oven to 350° or poach it, covered, in the microwave for about 6 minutes and spread the bread generously on the top side and lightly on the bottom with the butter seasoned with the garlic and herbs. Place it on a baking sheet in the center of the oven. The toast will take only about 15 minutes to reach a crisp golden brown. Remove the chicken from the wok and pour off any remaining liquid. Add a little more oil if needed and toss in the onion and remaining ingredients, sautéing over high heat until the onion wilts. Return the chicken to the wok, reduce heat to low, and cover while waiting for the toast. Serve 1 chicken breast half and some onion on each garlic and herb toast. Either a simple green salad or a mixed fruit salad would be perfect with this sandwich.

☯ Garden Rolls with Crab ☯

Serves 4

*T*he Vietnamese garden roll ought to become an American classic—it really matches our fondness for fast food. The rolls are easy to fix and their see-through wrappers tantalize, exposing a tangle of vegetables, seafood noodles, and herbs. If the filling is made ahead, there's nothing at all to cook, and the finished rolls will keep in the refrigerator all day. They make a wonderful warm-weather accompaniment to a grilled dinner and an ideal picnic dish. Either the round or triangular rice papers can be used, but the triangles make a prettier roll.

2 ounces cellophane noodles
$^{1}/_{2}$ cup bean sprouts
1 6$^{1}/_{2}$-ounce tin lump crab, or $^{1}/_{2}$ pound fresh backfin or
    claw crab meat
2 teaspoons fish sauce *(nuoc mam or nam pla)*
6 Boston lettuce leaves
1 carrot, grated

8 scallions, minced, white part only
1 tablespoon minced cilantro
1 tablespoon chopped mint
1 1/2 tablespoons finely chopped dry-roasted peanuts
1/2 teaspoon sugar
1/2 teaspoon salt
2 teaspoons fresh lime juice
8 Vietnamese rice paper wrappers
16 chives
8 cilantro sprigs

Soak the cellophane noodles in boiling water until they're transparent and soft, about 20 minutes. Drain and cool. Blanch the bean sprouts in a sieve by slowly pouring boiling water through them. Rinse with cool water and set aside to drain. In a large bowl, toss the crab meat with the fish sauce. Stack the lettuce leaves, 4 at a time, and roll the stack tightly. Cut across the roll into very thin strips and add to the crab, noodles, carrot, scallions, cilantro, mint, and peanuts. Add the sugar and salt to the lime juice and stir to dissolve. Toss the crab salad with the seasoned lime juice.

Hold 4 wrappers, one at a time, under a tepid water faucet stream and lay them out, side by side, on your work surface with the point away from you. Keep a water mister nearby to add more, or use your fingers. The wrappers will absorb the moisture and start puckering. They are sturdier than they look, so don't be afraid to mist enough to make them pliable and easy to handle.

Use 2 whole chives with a sprig of cilantro to mark the midline of each wrapper. The herbs will show through the finished roll. Lay one-eighth of the salad on top and fold in the sides. Holding the filling in place, roll the package up tight. The moistened point of the wrapper will adhere to the wrapper and automatically seal it. Repeat for remaining wrappers. Don't despair if the first couple you make are sloppy; it takes a few tries to achieve a tightly packed, plump cylinder that can be picked up without falling apart. They're really fun to do. If you want to store them at room temperature for a while, cover them well with plastic wrap and a dampened towel.

✑ Serve with Vietnamese Table Seasoning (page 27) or Peanut Sauce (page 31).

✑ You can also steam these filled rolls, either 15 minutes in a basket steamer or 3 minutes in the microwave.

✑ You can use shrimp instead of crab, or delete the seafood altogether for a vegetable garden roll. Add blanched and slivered snow peas to the mix for crunch and color. Or mix in chopped cucumber and slivers of seeded cherry tomato.

☯ # Saigon Pâté ☯

Serves 4

*T*his Vietnamese-style meatloaf is simple, quick, delicious, and economical. It's a subtly seasoned, easily sliced, dense loaf with many hot and cold uses, from canapés to main dish to sandwiches to salads. Traditionally this type of loaf is steamed in a wok for an hour, making it the perfect candidate for the microwave, which does the job in a mere 6 minutes. (Be sure your microwave is full power, or cook it a little longer.) What more could you ask?

6 dried Chinese black mushrooms
1 pound lean ground pork
3 large garlic cloves, minced
3 tablespoons minced shallot, or ¼ cup minced onion
3 tablespoons fish sauce *(nam pla* or *nuoc mam),* or 1
    tablespoon anchovy paste
2 rounded teaspoons chile paste, preferably Tommy Tang's
    Thai Roasted Chile Paste
¼ teaspoon ground cinnamon
¼ teaspoon powdered galangal or ground ginger
2–3 tablespoons white wine, chicken broth, sake, or water

Soak the mushrooms in boiling water to cover for at least 15 minutes, or until soft and pliable. Meanwhile, put the rest of the ingredients except wine in a large bowl and blend with a fork. Drain and stem the mushrooms, squeezing them dry between your fingers. Top side down, sliver them across, quarter-turn the slivers, and mince. Add the mushrooms to the meat mixture and get serious about blending the flavors. I like to turn the meat out onto a cutting board, wrapped with a sheet of wax paper to escape scraping and scrubbing the board, and knead it together with my hands. It's messy, but an effective way to work out any air bubbles.

Turn the mixture into a 2-cup microwave-safe dish—either round or rectangular, it doesn't matter. Drizzle the wine over the loaf and cover tightly with plastic wrap. Cook on high for 6 to 8 minutes. Let it stand for another 5 or 10 minutes before draining and serving, or wrapping and storing in the refrigerator or freezer.

➤ If you prefer to steam the loaf, put the uncovered dish in your steamer basket, cover the steamer, and cook for about 1 hour.

➤ Resist the temptation to salt the meat. The fish sauce provides enough.

➤ Since this loaf is meant to be dense, finely mince the garlic, shallots or onion, and mushrooms so you don't create pockets of moisture, which can cause the loaf to crumble when sliced.

➤ The reason for the somewhat subtle seasoning of this loaf is because no matter how you choose to serve it, the meat should be accompanied, in the Asian manner, by a pungent sambal or dip. Make your own choice from those in the Condiments chapter.

➤ Slice the loaf thinly and serve it with Japanese rice crackers and an herb sambal or fruit chutney as an hors d'oeuvre. Or cut it into chunks, pierce them with short wooden skewers, and provide a spicy dip like Black Banana Sauce (page 30). Use the loaf like any good cold sandwich meat, as in the Pacific Rim Sandwich suggestions (page 61). Serve the loaf hot for a main dish with generous sprigs of cilantro and/or mint or basil and soft noodles, or vegetable fried rice.

Cilantro and Ginger Omelet

☯ ☯

Serves 4

*T*his is a variation of the Indian Parsi *akoori*, which is a pungent soft-scrambled egg dish. It makes a refreshingly different omelet and the perfect little supper. Crusty hash brown potatoes and sautéed cherry tomatoes are just the right accompaniments.

THE FILLING
  2 tablespoons butter
  $1/4$ cup minced sweet onion, such as Vidalia
  1 teaspoon peeled and minced fresh ginger
  2 teaspoons minced fresh chile
  $1/4$ teaspoon turmeric
  $1/2$ teaspoon ground cumin
  $1/4$ cup chopped cilantro leaves
  salt

  knobs of butter for the pan
  8 large eggs, lightly beaten with 1 tablespoon water
  salt and freshly ground black pepper

Melt the butter in a skillet and sauté the onion, ginger, and chile over medium heat until the onion and chile are soft. Stir in the rest of the filling ingredients, salt lightly, and set aside. Melt a small knob of butter in a nonstick omelet pan and swirl it around. Over medium to low heat, pour in about one-fourth of the egg mixture, and as soon as it begins to set around the edges, gently pull a wooden spoon or heatproof rubber spatula through it to let most of the uncooked egg run to the bottom. While the omelet is still soft in the middle, spoon in one-fourth of the filling, front of center, and flick the front edge of the omelet up and over it. Gripping the handle of the pan with your left (or right) thumb on top, let the omelet roll out over itself onto the plate, using the pan to guide it. Keep the omelet warm in a low oven while you make the rest.

Shrimp Frittata

☯   ☯

Serves 4

I'm teasing—it's an *egg foo yung*. I'll bet there are as many Chinese Americans who secretly love this dish as there are American devotees who think it's Chinese. No matter—now that even supermarkets are carrying gorgeous fresh bean sprouts regularly, this flat omelet is a wonderful light fast meal. I've included shrimp in this one, although it's equally good with bits of roast pork. Serve with sautéed sugar snap peas or snow peas.

1 tablespoon peanut oil
1/2 pound raw shrimp, shelled and diced, or 1/2 cup diced
   roast pork
4 extra-large eggs, lightly beaten
1 cup fresh bean sprouts
1 tablespoon cornstarch
6 shiitake mushrooms, stemmed and slivered
4 large scallions, minced

THE SAUCE
1 cup chicken broth, homemade or low-sodium canned
1 teaspoon rice wine, sake, or dry sherry
1/2 teaspoon Chinese Salt and Pepper (page 24)
1 tablespoon oyster sauce
1 tablespoon cornstarch, dissolved in 2 tablespoons broth

Heat the oil in a nonstick omelet pan over medium-high heat and sauté the shrimp very quickly until they barely turn pink and are still springy to the touch. Turn them out onto a paper towel–lined plate. Whisk the eggs in a medium bowl. Pick over the sprouts, pulling off any loose bits. Break them into bite-size lengths. Put the cornstarch into a small sieve and sift just enough of it over the sprouts to coat them very lightly. Shake away the excess. Stir the sprouts, shrimp, mushrooms, and scallions into the eggs.

Bring the broth to a boil. Add the rest of the sauce ingredients, reduce the heat to medium, and cook 2 to 3 minutes until the sauce is thickened and clear. Set aside on the range to keep warm.

Swirl a little oil around in the omelet pan and heat it over medium heat. Ladle the mixture onto the skillet as you do pancakes. Lightly brown them on one side and turn to cook on the other. Keep them warm in a low oven until they're all finished. Spoon the warm sauce over them.

☯ ## Philippine Tortilla ☯

Serves 4

*W*hen the Spaniards left the Philippines, many of their culinary traditions remained—especially using tomatoes with garlic and olive oil. The flat omelet, or tortilla, is just one reminder of that Spanish influence. This tortilla is a meal in itself and needs only a dollop of Black Banana Sauce (page 30).

1 tablespoon olive oil
3 garlic cloves, minced
$^1/_2$ cup diced onion
1 pound ground round or chuck
salt and pepper
$^1/_2$ teaspoon dried oregano, or 1 tablespoon minced fresh
1 tablespoon minced flat-leaf parsley
1 large tomato, seeded, pulped, and chopped
1 medium waxy potato, cooked and chopped
4 large eggs, lightly beaten with 1 teaspoon water

Heat the olive oil in a 10-inch nonstick skillet and sauté the garlic and onion until soft. Add the ground beef and sauté over medium-high heat, pressing down with the back of a wooden spoon to separate the clumps. Add the seasonings and blend well. Fold in the tomato and potato, and pour the beaten eggs over all. When the tortilla has set, cut it into wedges to serve.

⤙ A romaine salad with onion rings and hearts of palm dressed with Philippine Seasoned Vinegar (page 26) and olive oil would be just the right accompaniment.

Savory Corn Custard with
☯ Scallops and Spinach ☯
Serves 4

*B*oth the Chinese and the Japanese enjoy savory custards. Here's an Asian-style corn custard that teams well with sautéed scallops and fresh spinach.

**1 cup Asian Chicken Broth or Quickly Seasoned Canned
   Broth (pages 81 and 82)**
³/₄ cup white corn kernels (about 2 ears) or thawed frozen
1 tablespoon milk
¹/₄ teaspoon sugar
¹/₈ teaspoon salt
2 large eggs
2 teaspoons oyster sauce
1 tablespoon minced chives
2 teaspoons peanut oil
2 garlic cloves smashed and minced
2 pounds flat leaf or baby spinach
1 pint bay scallops, drained
2 tablespoons sake
salt and pepper

Preheat the oven to 350°. In a food processor or blender, puree the corn kernels with the milk, sugar, and salt, leaving some texture. Pulse in the eggs, oyster sauce, and chives. Pour one-third of the hot broth into the corn mixture and pulse once to mix. Now slowly pour the custard into the rest of the hot broth and then distribute the custard into four ¹/₂-cup ramekins spritzed with a touch of vegetable oil spray. Put the ramekins in a roasting pan with enough hot water to come halfway up the sides of the dishes. Bake for 20 minutes or until the custard is just set; you can use a cake tester to check the centers.

Ten minutes before the custards are ready, heat a wok, add the oil, then the garlic, stirring until softened. Add the spinach in batches, cooking it down over medium-high heat. Simmer for 5 minutes and remove to a sieve. Press out the excess water and keep the spinach warm.

Wipe out the wok and sauté the scallops over high heat, tossing and flipping them in the hot wok to heat through and pick up golden flecks. Add the sake and let it sizzle and reduce, glazing the scallops.

Divide the spinach among 4 plates, turn the custards out on top and surround with the scallops.

✑ These savory custards are also delicious with ¼ cup slivered, sautéed shiitake mushrooms instead of corn. Increase the eggs to 3 and the broth to 1½ cups, and delete the milk and sugar. Serve with hoisin-glazed pork chops or a roasted lemon chicken.

✑ Substitute a can of whole baby clams for the scallops and use ½ cup bottled clam juice and ½ cup chicken broth.

Jakarta Tart

Serves 4

*E*ggs may be prohibitively expensive in Indonesia but they are occasionally eaten in omelets and other forms. This is an abundant vegetable quiche hauntingly accented with coconut.

1 8-inch frozen deep-dish pie shell, Oronoque Orchards preferred
1 tablespoon peanut oil
½ cup chopped onion
2 garlic cloves, crushed and minced
3 quarter-size coins of peeled ginger, crushed and minced
1 cup thinly sliced green cabbage
1 young carrot, thinly sliced
½ cup cut green beans (frozen are fine)
½ sweet red or yellow pepper, seeded and sliced
2 plum tomatoes, thinly sliced
3 large eggs, lightly beaten
½ cup unsweetened coconut milk

1 tablespoon Indonesian soy sauce *(ketjap manis)*
¹/₄ teaspoon salt
¹/₂ teaspoon Thai chile sauce or to taste
Coco-Peanut Crunch (page 33)

Preheat the oven to 425°. Thaw the pie shell for 15 minutes, then bake the pie shell for 10 minutes; reduce oven to 350°. Heat the peanut oil in a wok or skillet and stir-fry the onion, garlic, and ginger until soft but not brown. Blanch the cabbage, carrot, and green beans in the microwave for a couple of minutes, drain, and pat dry. (If the green beans are frozen, you need only thaw them.) Toss the cooked vegetables together and strew them into the pie shell. Add the sliced tomatoes, tucking them in randomly. Whisk the eggs with the coconut milk, soy sauce, salt, and chile sauce. Pour the mixture into the shell. Bake for 50 minutes or until a knife inserted in the center comes out clean. Sprinkle the top with Coco-Peanut Crunch.

☯ Pacific Steak and Fries ☯

Serves 4

*E*ven a juicy pan-sautéed steak and crispy french fries can be steered eastward. A dash of this and that exotica can transform a familiar Western supper into an Asian one. Accompany the steaks with french-fried sweet potatoes or frozen shoestrings and a mixed green salad with an Asian vinaigrette.

1 tablespoon Chinese Seasoning Oil (page 23)
4 beef filet or ribeye steaks
1¹/₂ tablespoons oyster sauce
2 teaspoons Thai fish sauce *(nam pla)*
1 tablespoon low-sodium soy sauce
¹/₂ teaspoon Thai chile sauce, or to taste
¹/₄ teaspoon sugar
¹/₄ cup shredded or grated daikon, blotted dry

Heat the oil in a skillet large enough to hold 4 steaks. Sear them well on both sides over high heat. Reduce the heat to medium high and cook the steaks until done to your taste. Mix the liquid ingredients and the sugar. Remove the steaks to a warm plate. Deglaze the hot skillet with the seasonings and drizzle the syrupy sauce over the hot steaks. Pile the shredded daikon on top of each serving.

Burmese Sesame Chicken Wings

Serves 4

*T*his recipe comes from Michael Min Khin, a former Burmese restaurateur turned med student. The wings are glossy, bright, beautiful—and thoroughly messy. A big platter of these wings with a bowl of Curried Coconut Rice (page 162), Asian Cole Slaw (page 96), and a raft of paper napkins is a must for close friends and family.

12 whole chicken wings
1 tablespoon Chinese fermented black beans
1 tablespoon cold water
1 tablespoon peanut or light sesame oil
2 garlic cloves, crushed
2 quarter-size coins of peeled fresh ginger, crushed and minced
3 tablespoons soy sauce
2 tablespoons rice wine, sake, or dry sherry
1/4 teaspoon ground white pepper
1 tablespoon toasted sesame oil
1 tablespoon sesame seeds, toasted
8 scallions
sprigs of mint and/or basil, for garnish

Chop off the wing tips and discard or freeze for stock. Cut the wings in two at the joint. Crush the beans with the flat of your cleaver and let them stand in the cold water. Heat the oil over high heat in a wok and stir-fry the garlic and ginger for 2 to 3 seconds. Reduce the heat to medium high and add the chicken wings. Toss them around until they're golden brown all over, about 3 minutes. Add the soy sauce, wine, black beans, and pepper. Cover the wok and simmer for 10 minutes.

Remove the wok cover, turn the heat back to high, and reduce the liquid in the pan until it's almost entirely evaporated. Stir in the sesame oil and cook briefly until the wings are beautifully glazed. Pile the wings on a platter and sprinkle with the toasted sesame seeds. Garnish the platter with the scallions and herbs.

Asian Burgers

*W*e can all use a few suggestions for sparking up ground beef and lamb, as well as chicken and turkey. Tuna and salmon burgers are extravagant newcomers that also lend themselves well to Asian seasonings and Western presentations.

Lamb Burgers with Seared ☯ Five-Spice Onions ☯

Serves 4

*S*erve these with crisp green beans stir-fried in the wok, tossed with thin jicama sticks or sliced water chestnuts.

2 tablespoons peanut oil
2 large sweet white onions, such as Vidalia, roughly
   chopped
1¹/₂ teaspoons sugar
salt and freshly ground black pepper
¹/₄ teaspoon dried red pepper flakes (optional)
1 teaspoon minced pickled ginger
¹/₄ teaspoon five-spice powder
4 lean ground lamb patties

Heat the oil in a wok or skillet until very hot. Add the chopped onions and stir and toss over high heat until they begin to char. Reduce the heat and add the rest of the ingredients except the patties. Stir-fry until the onions are cooked through but not soft. Set the pan to the side of the range to keep warm. In a skillet, sauté the lamb patties until done to taste. After you have turned them to the second side, salt and pepper them and cover them with the charred onions.

Coconut Hamburgers with Cucumber Raita

Serves 4

Serve these with a basmati rice pilaf with currants, or on toasted buns spread with chile or ginger butter.

1½ pounds lean ground chuck
Chinese Salt and Pepper (page 24)
3 garlic cloves, pressed
1½ teaspoons ground cumin
1½ teaspoons peeled and grated fresh ginger
1 teaspoon ground coriander
¼ cup minced onion
1 large egg, beaten with 1 tablespoon yogurt
½ cup unsweetened grated coconut
1 medium cucumber, peeled and seeded
2 tablespoons yogurt
1 tablespoon minced fresh mint leaves
2 tablespoons peanut oil

Combine the beef with all the ingredients except the cucumber, yogurt, mint, and oil. Form into 8 patties or meatballs. Blot the cucumber very dry and grate on the largest holes of a box grater. Spread them out on paper towels to drain some more. Lightly salt them and then mix with just enough of the yogurt to lightly coat the cucumber. Stir in the fresh mint and set aside.

Heat ¼ inch of oil in a wok or skillet until very hot. Add the meatballs or patties and fry until golden brown. Drain and serve with the cucumber raita.

☯ Wasabi Tuna Burgers ☯

Serves 4

Serve these with Asian Cole Slaw, thin fingers of crispy jicama and carrot, or a basket of root chips, such as Terra Chips.

¹/₃ cup mayonnaise, Hellmann's or Best Foods
1¹/₂ teaspoons wasabi paste
1¹/₄ pounds fresh albacore tuna
1 tablespoon minced chives
1¹/₂ tablespoons finely minced scallions, white part only
2 teaspoons sake
1 teaspoon avocado or light sesame oil
¹/₂ teaspoon Toasted Sesame Salt (page 24)
cornstarch, for coating
4 soft hamburger buns, lightly toasted
8 to 12 thin slices pickled ginger
4 thin slices ripe tomato
¹/₂ avocado, thinly sliced
4 lettuce leaves

Whisk together the mayonnaise and wasabi paste and set aside. Slice the tuna thinly across the grain, then mince the slices. Albacore tuna cuts into rings like an onion, so it's easy to mince without mashing the flesh. Mix in the rest of the seasonings. Gently form the tuna into 4 plump patties and dust them with the cornstarch. Sauté them in a nonstick skillet over medium-high heat about 2¹/₂ minutes on each side, leaving the center to continue cooking after leaving the heat. Spread the toasted buns with wasabi mayonnaise, add a few thin slices of pickled ginger, a tomato slice, and a few avocado slices. Put the lettuce on the bottom and turn out the tuna burgers on top.

Sesame Orange Salmon Burgers

☯ ☯

Serves 4

1¼ pounds thick salmon fillet, or 4 small steaks with
   bones removed
1 teaspoon grated orange zest or 2 drops of pure orange oil
2 tablespoons minced scallion, with some green
1 teaspoon grated peeled ginger, with juice
2 teaspoons Indonesian soy sauce *(ketjap manis)*
½ teaspoon Asian sesame oil
2 tablespoons cornstarch
1 tablespoon sesame seeds
1 tablespoon light sesame oil or peanut oil
4 toasted onion rolls
1 bunch watercress, stemmed

Mince the salmon with a very sharp knife to simulate coarsely
ground beef or pulse briefly in a food processor. Mix in the orange
zest, scallions, ginger, soy sauce, and Asian sesame oil. Loosely form
the salmon into 4 balls. Sift the cornstarch onto a plate. Sprinkle
the sesame seeds over it. Turn each ball around in the coating,
lightly pressing it in. Gently flatten the balls into patties. Put the oil
in a nonstick skillet over medium-high heat, and when the pan is
hot, sear the salmon burgers on both sides. Lower the heat slightly
and cook the patties about 3 minutes on each side. Make a nest of
watercress on each bun half and set the burger on top. Either butter the other half or spread it with mayonnaise spiked with wasabi
to taste. Serve with strips of fresh tropical fruit. Papaya and mango
are wonderful complements.

☯ Ginger Chicken Burgers ☯

Serves 4

6 dried Chinese black mushrooms
1½ pounds ground chicken; or half chicken, half turkey
¼ cup minced scallions, with some green
1 teaspoon grated peeled ginger, with juice
3 tablespoons minced water chestnuts or jicama
½ teaspoon grated lemon zest or 3 drops pure lemon oil
1 tablespoon oyster sauce
1 teaspoon mushroom soy sauce
Chinese Salt and Pepper (page 24)
1 teaspoon safflower or peanut oil
½ teaspoon toasted sesame oil
hoisin sauce
4 or 5 soft hamburger buns, warmed
shredded Boston lettuce

Soak the mushrooms in boiling water until they're soft and flexible. Drain, rinse, and pat dry. Cut the stems off at the base and discard. Mince and mix the mushrooms with the chicken, scallions, ginger, water chestnuts, and seasonings, combining them well. Form the mixture into 4 or 5 patties and sauté them in the two oils in a nonstick skillet over medium heat for 3 to 4 minutes on each side. In the last minute, glaze both sides of the patties by brushing them with hoisin sauce and turning them over in the hot pan. Serve on warmed buns with shredded lettuce.

Super Express

CORNISH HEN: Mix tandoori powder (available in specialty stores or Indian markets) with drained yogurt and pressed garlic, and rub the mixture over and under the skin of a Cornish hen. Let it marinate overnight before roasting or grilling. This treatment is also good for a butterflied leg of lamb on the grill, served with steamed baby carrots drizzled with ginger-lime butter.

5
Soups

☯ Asian Chicken Broth ☯

Makes 3—4 quarts

I always keep quarts, pints, and cubes of this essential broth in my freezer as a ready base for main-dish soups and an enrichment for sauces, noodles, rice, and stir-fries. When the broth called for in a finished recipe remains clear, as in soups, do try to use home-made; it makes all the difference. There is, however, a hurry-up version at the end of the recipe.

There are two easy ways to collect the chicken bones necessary to make a good rich broth. One is to harvest them from various chicken dinners, stashing them in the freezer until you have enough. This won't work if you eat only chicken breasts. The second way is to make stock from scratch and enjoy poached chicken several ways in the coming week. Here's how to make both a rich and flavorful broth and juicy, tender chicken.

1 roasting chicken or 2 fryers, about 5 pounds total
6 extra wings with tips, or extra bones from freezer
2 leeks, trimmed, cleaned, and split, or 1 white onion,
   quartered
2 large celery ribs, broken in half
1 carrot, scraped and split
4 large garlic cloves, crushed
6 quarter-size coins of fresh ginger, unpeeled; or 3 crushed
   knobs from the sides of the root
1 teaspoon mixed black and Szechuan peppercorns
1 teaspoon salt

Remove the wrapped entrails from the chicken cavity, saving only the neck for the stock, and wash the chicken inside and out under cool water, pulling out any debris. Cut off the legs at the thigh joint. Cut off the wings at the base. Remove the whole breast from the carcass with poultry shears or a sharp knife, and store in the re-frigerator in a plastic bag. Split the back into 2 or 3 pieces with a cleaver. Remove all excess skin and flaps or any visible pockets of fat.

In a large 6- or 8-quart soup pot, lay the back, neck, and wings, vegetables, and seasonings, and finally the whole legs. Fill the pot with water to barely cover the contents. Set the lid and turn the heat to medium. When the water comes to a low boil, reduce the heat to the lowest setting, using a flame tamer on a gas range. The liquid should not boil but remain at a barely visible simmer for 45 minutes. Remove the legs and put the whole chicken breast in their place. Cover the pot and continue simmering for 30 minutes. Remove the breast. Pull the meat from the legs and breast and return the bones to the pot. Cover and simmer for another 30 to 45 minutes. Let the leg and breast cool before storing.

When the broth is finished, uncover the pot and lift out the solids into a colander set over a bowl. Return the collected drippings to the pot. Taste the broth. If it isn't rich and intense, bring it back to a simmer and reduce it, uncovered, by one-third. Let the broth cool a bit and pour it through a fine sieve into freezer storage containers, leaving room for expansion. Store them in the refrigerator, without their lids, overnight or all day. The broth will gel when cold so you can easily scrape off any fat.

✐ Quickly Seasoned Canned Broth: When you run out of homemade chicken broth, season a can of low-sodium broth with a crushed garlic clove, a bruised quarter-coin of ginger, a few peppercorns, and a split scallion. Bring the broth to a boil in the microwave and let it steep for 30 minutes, or simmer it on your stove-top for about 10 minutes and let it steep until cool. Strain and store. Makes about 1¹/₂ cups.

✐ If you prefer storing homemade broth without Asian seasoning so it can serve other uses, delete the garlic, ginger, and Szechuan pepper. Season the thawed broth with these ingredients as suggested for canned broth.

✐ Be sure to store the broth in containers of varying sizes, from ice-cube portions for small add-ins to quarts for soup. When you use up the cubes, thaw another quart and refreeze it in ice cube trays. They're just too handy to be without. Remember to measure the amount of liquid your ice tray holds so you can mark the cube quantity on the freezer bag.

Hurry-Up Soups Using Asian Chicken Broth

➤ Add thinly sliced onion, strips of chicken breast, a dash of fish sauce, and a bunch of stemmed, flat-leaf spinach

➤ Add pre-soaked rice stick noodles, minced cilantro, scallions, a little chile sauce, and Florida rock shrimp

➤ Add diced cooked potato, minced shallots, slivered seeded tomato, some frozen peas, chicken sausage slices, a little heavy cream, and green curry paste to taste. Top with slivered toasted almonds.

Chinese Vegetable Soup with Shaomai

☯ ☯

Serves 4

*P*ure and satisfying, vegetable soup in any language speaks to all the senses. Since you already have a stash of Asian broth, you have only to add the vegetables and the dumplings. If you really want to speed things up, you can prepare the vegetables the night before and keep them covered in the refrigerator, ready to pop into the simmering stock.

6 cups Asian Chicken Broth (page 81)
1 stalk lemongrass
1 carrot, peeled and cut into thin half-rounds
2 dried Chinese black mushrooms, soaked, stemmed, and slivered
3 stalks bok choy, trimmed and chopped crosswise
8 snow peas, stringed and slivered, or whole sugar snap peas
¼ large red sweet pepper, stemmed, seeded, and diced
8 ears canned baby corn
4 scallions, trimmed and slivered

8 canned straw mushrooms

2 fistfuls flat-leaf spinach, stemmed

12 frozen shaomai, preferably Royal Dragon, microwaved
per package instructions

Pour the broth into a soup pot. Trim off the dry top of the lemon-grass stalk, remove the tough outer layer from the bulb, and split it in half. Drop the lemongrass into the broth and bring the liquid to a boil over moderate heat. Reduce the heat to medium low and simmer for 5 minutes. Remove the lemongrass and discard. Add the carrot and black mushrooms and simmer for a minute. Then add the rest of the vegetables and simmer until the carrot and bok choy are tender but still crunchy, 3 to 4 minutes. Drop in the shao-mai to reheat.

Egg Drop Soup with Chinese ☯ Sausage and Basil ☯

Serves 4

The Italian classic *uovo in brodo* is my idea of the ultimate com-fort food, and I think many would put egg drop soup in the same league. I've added sweet Chinese sausage for substance and herbs for contrast, but it could just as easily be slivers of poached chicken breast or bits of smoky ham and some lump crab meat.

1 Chinese sweet sausage

1½ quarts Asian Chicken Broth or Quickly Seasoned
Canned Broth (pages 81, 82)

3 scallions, white part only, trimmed and slivered

6 basil leaves, cut into ribbons, or 2 tablespoons minced
cilantro

Chinese Salt and Pepper (page 24)

1 tablespoon cornstarch, mixed with 1 tablespoon soy
sauce

1 large egg, beaten

toasted sesame oil

Duck Broth

The next time you have dinner at your favorite Chinese restaurant and order Peking Duck, ask to take home the carcass—and any others in the kitchen they can spare. Duck bones make the most delicious broth for soups.

In a covered microwave dish, steam the sausage in a couple of tablespoons of water for 3 minutes. Slice into thin rounds. Bring the broth to a simmer and add the scallions, basil, salt, and pepper to taste. Stir the cornstarch and soy sauce and add it to the broth. Increase the heat and stir until the soup is slightly thickened. Remove the pan from the heat and slowly drizzle in the beaten egg, stirring gently. Add the sausage to reheat. The final touch of a few drops of sesame oil gives the soup a heady aroma.

☯ Saffron Squash Bisque ☯

Serves 6–8 as a starter

*T*he inspiration for this unusual velvety soup came from a buttercup squash in the farmer's market that had my name written on it. I had no idea what I was going to do with it, but this luscious soup turned out to be one of those memorable creations called cook's luck. You can use butter*nut* squash, which is more readily available, but not so sweet and unctuous as buttercup—so look for it.

4-pound buttercup squash, split and seeded
1 foil package (.0045 ounce) powdered Spanish saffron, or
    pinch of threads, crumbled
1 quart Asian Chicken Broth or Quickly Seasoned Canned
    Broth (pages 81, 82)
1 2¹/₂–inch strip lemon zest

¹/₈ teaspoon cayenne pepper
1 teaspoon fruit vinegar, preferably Japanese ume plum
¹/₂ cup unsweetened coconut milk
1 tablespoon chopped dry-roasted peanuts
4 cilantro sprigs

Remove any fibrous membrane from the squash. Steam the split halves in a microwave oven for about 12 minutes, cut side down, covered with wax paper. The flesh should be tender when pierced with a toothpick. Or place squash on a steamer rack over water and cook for 20 minutes. Steep the saffron in ¹/₄ cup of the broth by heating it in the microwave and letting it sit for a couple of minutes.

Bring half the broth to a boil in a large saucepan with the lemon zest. When the squash is cool enough to handle, scoop squash out of shell and puree in the processor or blender with the remaining cool chicken broth. Remove the lemon peel from the warm broth and add the puree. Stir in the saffron, cayenne, vinegar, and coconut milk. Serve with a garnish of chopped peanuts and a sprig or two of cilantro.

Hot and Sour Vegetable Noodle Soup

Serves 4

*W*ith rich homemade broth tucked away in your larder, this version of a familiar favorite can be made in minutes. It would be a lively beginning to a meal of grilled chicken or fish or a main course with the chicken or fish added to it.

SOUP
2 quarts Asian Chicken Broth, or Quickly Seasoned
   Canned Broth (pages 81, 82)
3 lemongrass stalks
2 small dried red chiles, or ¹/₂ teaspoon red pepper flakes
¹/₄ cup rice vinegar
2 teaspoons sugar

 ¹/₂ **cup very finely shredded cabbage**
 1 carrot, peeled and thinly sliced
 ¹/₂ **cup cut frozen green beans**
 2 tablespoons frozen petite peas
 6 dried black mushrooms, stemmed, soaked to soften, and
    slivered
 3 ounces rice vermicelli, soaked to soften
 lime wedges

Put the broth in a 4-quart saucepan. Trim off the dry tops of the lemongrass stalks, remove the tough outer layer from the bulbs, and split in half. Drop the lemongrass into the broth along with the chives, vinegar, and sugar. Bring the liquid to a simmer and cook for 5 minutes over moderate heat. Fish out the lemongrass and chiles. Taste for seasoning. Add the cabbage and carrot and simmer for 3 minutes. Add the beans and peas and simmer for 2 minutes more. Add the noodles and mushrooms and serve the soup in heated bowls with lime wedges.

⟨ If you'd like to thicken this soup slightly, stir in 3 table-spoons of cornstarch dissolved in 3 tablespoons of the broth.

Curried Roasted Eggplant
☯ and Carrot Soup ☯

Serves 4–6

If you share my taste for eggplant, you'll be pleased with this sur-prisingly delicious soup. It's silky and only seemingly rich, and it's tempting either hot or cold. The eggplant puree is self-thickening and the sweet carrots cancel out any bitter edge.

 1 medium eggplant (about 1 pound)
 6 young carrots, scraped and chopped
 2 tablespoons safflower oil
 2 garlic cloves, crushed and minced

1 teaspoon coarse salt
2 teaspoons curry powder
1 quart chicken broth, homemade or canned
$1/2$ cup plain yogurt
chives, for garnish

Preheat the oven to 375°. Pierce the eggplant with a fork several times, place it on a piece of foil, and bake until it collapses and the flesh is soft, about 40 minutes, or roast it on a stove-top grill.

Steam the carrots (or microwave them) until very tender. In a small skillet, heat the oil and gently sauté the garlic, salt, and curry powder over low heat until it's fragrant and the garlic is soft. Scrape the cooled eggplant from its skin and drain the carrots. Puree the vegetables with the broth in batches in a food processor or blender. Pour the mixture into a storage container or a saucepan, and whisk in the seasoned oil and the yogurt, blending well. Chill or heat and sprinkle with snipped chives.

Five-Spice Onion Soup with Beef Tenderloin

Serves 4

This is a quick adaptation of the more complex Vietnamese *pho* and is particularly wonderful made with Vidalia, Maui, or Texas sweet onions. Look for their tiny glued-on labels in season. Traditionally, bean sprouts are passed at the table with this soup.

2 quarts beef broth, homemade or canned
4 quarter-size coins of peeled ginger, bruised
3 garlic cloves, crushed
$1/4$ teaspoon five-spice powder
2 large sweet white onions, halved and thinly sliced
1 fresh red chile, stemmed and slivered
$1/2$ teaspoons Vietnamese fish sauce (*nuoc mam*)
1 teaspoon fresh lime juice

salt and white pepper
4–5 ounces rice noodles or vermicelli
2 1-inch-thick beef fillets, very thinly sliced
6 scallions, minced
1 tablespoon chopped cilantro

Simmer the broth with the ginger, garlic, five-spice powder, and onions until the onions are soft. Add the chile, fish sauce, and lime juice. Salt and pepper to taste. Boil the noodles in about 3 quarts of salted water until tender. Drain and divide among the soup bowls. Drop the beef slices into the gently simmering onion soup and cook for 30 seconds. Serve the soup and beef over the noodles and garnish with scallions and cilantro.

Roast Chicken Mulligatawny

Serves 4

*R*ather than strain to figure out what to serve with it, turn a take-out roast chicken into an instant dinner soup. Serve it with a warm flat bread and a big spinach salad with lemon vinaigrette and a few chickpeas for garnish.

3 tablespoons clarified butter *(ghee)*
1 medium onion, chopped
2 garlic cloves, minced
3 quarter-size coins of peeled ginger, minced
2 teaspoons ground coriander
1 teaspoon turmeric
1 teaspoon ground cumin
1/4 teaspoon cayenne, or to taste
1 teaspoon salt
instant flour, as needed
1 tablespoon rice vinegar
5 cups chicken broth, homemade or canned
1 cup unsweetened coconut milk

3 cups pulled meat from roast chicken
1 cup cooked basmati rice
cilantro sprigs

Melt the butter in a heavy-bottomed 3-quart saucepan. Soften the onion, garlic, and ginger over medium heat without browning it. Add all of the seasonings, stirring constantly. When the butter and spices start to bubble, shake in just enough of the instant flour to absorb the fat and make a medium-thick, but loose, paste. Add the liquids slowly at first to allow the roux to thicken the broth slightly. Heat the chicken and rice in the seasoned broth and serve piping hot. Garnish with cilantro sprigs.

Gingered Spinach Soup with Sea Bass and Pine Nuts

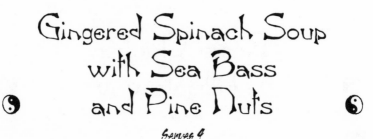

Serves 4

*I*f you like fish but hate to cook it, this sweet, mild fish in well-seasoned broth will please you. Many Asian soups are more like light versions of our stews—a meal in a bowl, delicious and spontaneous.

$^1/_2$ package (7$^3/_4$-ounce) cellophane noodles
1 lemongrass stalk
$^1/_2$ cup sake
5 cups Asian Chicken Broth, or Quickly Seasoned Canned
    Broth (pages 81, 82)
4 shallots, minced
4 quarter-size coins of peeled ginger, minced
$^1/_2$ teaspoon white pepper
1$^1/_2$ pounds sea bass fillets, preferably Chilean, or cod
1 pound spinach, washed and stemmed, or two 6-ounce
    bags baby spinach
2 tablespoons fish sauce *(nuoc mam or nam pla)*

salt, to taste
2 tablespoons pine nuts, toasted

Soak the cellophane noodles in boiling water, or hot tap water, until they're soft and pliant, about 5–10 minutes. Drain and set aside. Trim the lemongrass—remove the dried top, root end, and tough outer stalk; split and quarter the remaining white bulb. Put the sake and 1/2 cup of chicken broth in a 2-cup glass measure with the lemongrass, shallots, ginger, and pepper. Bring to a simmer in the microwave, then let steep until almost room temperature. Trim the fish into 4 servings and place the fillets in a microwave-safe dish with the seasoned sake. Cover tightly with plastic wrap and steam the fish in the microwave for 4 minutes. Bring the rest of the chicken broth to a simmer in a 3-quart saucepan. Add the spinach and then the fish sauce. Cook over medium-low heat until the spinach wilts. Carefully place the fillets and sake into the broth and simmer for 3 or 4 minutes. Add the noodles. Taste for salt. Ladle the soup into shallow bowls and garnish with the toasted pine nuts.

☯   # Bean Paste Soup   ☯
Serves 4–6

I think miso soup *(miso shiru)*, like olives, is an acquired taste for most of us, but it's such a quick soup to prepare that you might want to see if you're a member of its very large fan club.

1 1/2 quarts dashi*
1/4 cup red bean paste (miso)
4 scallions, diagonally sliced with some green
8 1 1/2-inch squares soft tofu
6 shiitake mushrooms, stemmed

Bring the dashi to a boil. Stir a ladle of it into the bean paste to smooth it out, then add to the broth and stir. Add the rest of the ingredients and serve when the mushrooms are soft.

---

*Dashi, an instant Japanese dried fish and seaweed broth, can be made by adding boiling water to a powder or liquid available in Asian markets or specialty food stores. The quantity of water to the instant dashi varies so follow the package instructions to reconstitute enough for the miso soup.

⚊ Instead of the dashi and water, you can use 2 cups clam broth and 2 cups chicken stock.

6
Salads

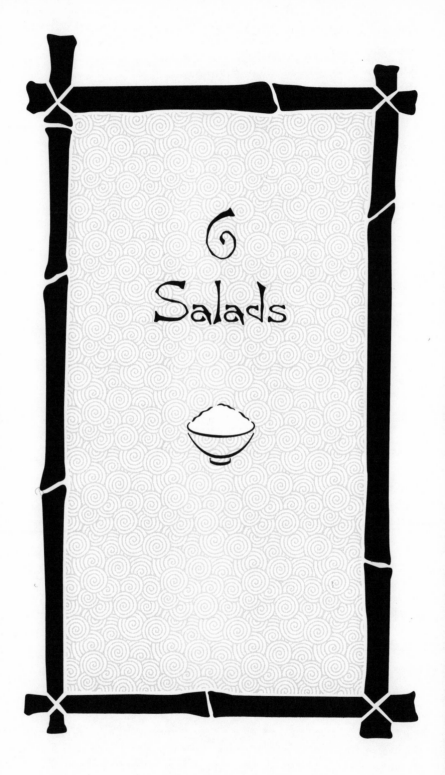

SIDE SALADS

Romaine Salad with
☯ Lemon Soy Dressing ☯
Serves 4

*V*ariations on Asian dipping sauces and seasonings make interesting dressings for American salads, including the perennial
tossed green salad, which we pair so often with simple grilled or
roasted meat or fish. This is kind of an Asian Caesar salad.

HERB TOAST
  4 slices day-old French bread, ¹/₂ inch thick
  **1¹/₂ tablespoons Chinese Seasoning Oil (page 23) or garlic
    oil**
  2 teaspoons minced fresh mint or basil
  1 teaspoon minced chives

SALAD
  **1 small head romaine lettuce, washed, trimmed, and torn
    into bite-size pieces**
  6 scallions, white part only, trimmed and slivered

DRESSING
  ¹/₄ cup avocado or safflower oil
  1 garlic clove, pressed
  1 teaspoon soy sauce
  2 drops pure lemon oil, or ¹/₄ teaspoon grated lemon zest
  **¹/₄ teaspoon fish sauce *(nam pla* or *nuoc mam)*, or 2
    minced anchovies**
  1 tablespoon rice vinegar
  pinch of sugar

Preheat the oven to 350°. Make the herb toast: Put the bread slices
on a baking sheet. Mix oil with herbs and brush bread slices lightly

on both sides with the oil. Bake until golden and crisp, 10 to 12 minutes. Make the salad: Put the lettuce and scallions in a large salad bowl and whisk the dressing ingredients. Taste for balance. Toss the greens with the dressing and tear the herb toast into croutons to scatter on top.

⟋ Avocado wedges and seeded slivered cherry tomatoes are particularly good on this salad.

⟋ A quarter-size coin of peeled ginger can be minced into the dressing.

⟋ Don't hesitate to adjust the proportions and ingredients to suit your taste. If you make this dressing your own, you'll use it often, whether or not you're preparing an Asian meal.

How to Shred Vegetables

For firm vegetables like carrots, daikon, turnips, jicama, squash, broccoli stems, etc., use a vegetable peeler to cut thin strips, stack the strips, and cut the vegetables into threads with a sharp cleaver or chef's knife. Or, for a small pile of vegetable threads, use a citrus zester to shred them.

☯ Asian Cole Slaw ☯

Serves 4

This is a *really* tasty cole slaw—a refreshing alternative to the beloved American picnic slaw and definitely veering toward Korean *kimchi*. In fact, if you change the cabbage to napa, let it wilt a few hours under a sprinkling of salt before dressing it, and put in garlic and enough chile powder to launch a rocket, you'll have a good approximation of *kimchi*. Try this first. Almost every country in Southeast Asia has its version of pickled cabbage slaw.

---

3 cups very thinly sliced green cabbage

3 tablespoons grated onion, squeezed dry in a kitchen
 towel

2 teaspoons minced pickled ginger

$^1/_2$ teaspoon Chinese Salt and Pepper (page 24)

cayenne pepper, to taste

$2^1/_2$ teaspoons sugar

$1^1/_2$ tablespoons Chinese Seasoning Oil (page 23) or garlic
 oil

2 teaspoons Asian sesame oil

1 tablespoon soy sauce

$1^1/_2$ tablespoons rice vinegar

Cut the cabbage into quarters. Cut out the hard white core and discard. Pull off 4 or 5 leaves at a time and fold them over on the center rib. With a Chinese cleaver or chef's knife, cut the leaves into
the finest possible strips. This method gives you far better control
and thinner shreds than you can get wrestling with the compact
head. Put the cabbage in a large bowl and add the remaining ingredients as listed, tossing after each addition. Taste and adjust the
seasoning, if necessary.

✐ I like to add minced cilantro and/or mint to this slaw, depending on the seasonings in the rest of the meal.

✐ Toasted sesame seeds are a good textural garnish.

Vegetable and Rice Noodle Salad

☯ ☯

Serves 4

*T*his is the kind of salad I love because a refrigerator search
usually turns up enough variety to make it a good one. You
do need to be thoughtful in choosing complementary ingredients,
however, or you'll end up with a mere tangle of leftovers.

1 8-ounce package of rice stick noodles *(banh pho)*

DRESSING

3 tablespoons mirin, or sake and a pinch of sugar
3 tablespoons soy sauce
2 tablespoons fish sauce *(nam pla or nuoc mam)*
juice of 1 small lime

VEGETABLES

¼ cup corn kernels, fresh or frozen
1 teaspoon peanut oil
8 shiitake mushrooms, stemmed and slivered
½ sweet red pepper, seeded and diced
3 tablespoons diced jicama, or slivered water chestnuts
1 small ripe tomato, seeded, pulped, and slivered
1 small cucumber, peeled, seeded, and cut into half rounds
Chinese Salt and Pepper (page 24)

GARNISH

red-leaf lettuce
Coco-Peanut Crunch (page 33) or just the fried shallots or
    garlic chips from the same recipe
crumbled fried noodles (see Sesame Orange Chicken, page
    105)

Soak the rice stick noodles in boiling water for 3 to 4 minutes until pliable. Drain and cool to lukewarm. Mix the dressing ingredients, pour it over the noodles, and combine well. Taste for seasoning. Set aside for 1 hour. If you're using frozen corn, let it thaw and blot dry with paper towels. Pan-roast the corn in the peanut oil in a hot wok until it caramelizes slightly, taking on some charred flecks. Turn it out onto a plate to cool.

In the same hot wok, sauté the slivered mushrooms over medium-high heat until they wilt. Turn them out onto a separate plate to cool. Now toss in the red pepper and stir-fry for 15 seconds. Toss the pepper dice into the corn and remaining salad ingredients and dressed noodles, adding any mushroom juice. Taste for salt and pepper. Heap the noodle salad over red leaf lettuce arranged on a platter. Garnish the edge of the salad with Coco-Peanut Crunch or fried chips and the crumbled noodles.

↙ The crunchy garnish is important to the textural contrast of the dish—one of the delights of Asian cooking. As an alternative to the Coco-Peanut Crunch, plug in a deep-fryer, explode some rice vermicelli in hot oil, and use it around the edge. You could also use packaged shrimp chips, root chips, or sweet-potato chips.

Lemon Rice Salad with Minted Peas and Carrots

☯ ☯

Serves 4

*R*ice salad often gets a bad rap, which is a pity because it can be very good, indeed. The rice itself is often the problem. If it's an absorbent, overcooked, processed rice, the salad will be just a gummy porridge. This very refreshing recipe is a perfect foil for seafood or lamb and makes a particularly nice buffet dish.

1 cup basmati rice, picked over and rinsed
1¹/₂ cups water
1 teaspoon salt
1 small carrot, scraped and grated
¹/₂ cup frozen petite peas, thawed and blotted dry
2 tablespoons minced chives or scallions, with some green
2 tablespoons minced fresh mint leaves
¹/₄ cup safflower or avocado oil
1 teaspoon finely grated lemon zest
1 tablespoon fresh lemon juice
salt and pepper

Bring the rice, water, and salt to a boil in a heavy, tightly lidded saucepan. Reduce the heat to its lowest point, using a flame tamer over a gas burner. Check the rice in 15 minutes by lifting the lid to see if all the water has evaporated and a couple of craters have appeared in the surface. Taste a kernel of rice; it should be soft on the outside, with a slightly chewy center. If the rice is old, it might take a bit longer. In that case, drizzle in a couple tablespoons of water, re-cover, and cook another 5 minutes. Test again, as above.

Turn the rice out into a mixing bowl. When it's cool, fold in the vegetables and herbs. Don't cook either the grated carrot or the frozen peas. Mix the oil, lemon zest and juice and dress the salad, tasting for salt and pepper. Serve immediately or the peas will darken.

Sweet Potato Salad with Pickled Okra and Coconut Cream

Serves 4

*S*weet potatoes lend themselves well to East-West cooking. They are popular in Asia, often in desserts, but my research confirms that, in any country, an interesting sweet potato recipe is hard to find. Here's a quirky combination.

2 large sweet potatoes, peeled and cubed (4 cups or more)
$^1/_2$ cup minced red onion
6 Talk o' Texas hot pickled okra, stemmed and thinly sliced
2 teaspoons light brown sugar
$^1/_4$ cup unsweetened coconut milk
$^1/_4$ cup sour cream or drained yogurt
salt and pepper
$^1/_4$ cup minced fresh mint
chopped unsalted roasted peanuts for garnish

In a shallow microwave-safe dish, steam the potatoes with about $^1/_4$ cup of water for 5 minutes. Remove and stir. Steam for another 3 minutes. They should be cooked through but not mushy. Drain the potatoes and toss them, warm, with the onion, okra, and brown sugar. Cool. Fold in the coconut milk and sour cream. Salt and pepper to taste. Do not refrigerate. Scatter the mint and peanuts on top when serving the dish.

➤ If you refrigerate leftovers, the potatoes may absorb most of the coconut-cream dressing. Add more sour cream when the salad has come back to room temperature.

➤ Jars of both hot and mild pickled okra can be found in supermarkets with the Talk o' Texas label, usually hiding in the exotic condiments section.

➤ If you're not fond of okra, use cut green beans and add hot chile sauce to the blend.

➤ You might want to experiment with a curried sweet potato salad by mixing drained yogurt with mayonnaise, curry paste, and ground cumin. Fold in minced onion or scallions and cooked petite peas. This variation can also be made with half white and half sweet potatoes.

Main-Dish Salads

Many Splendored Chicken Salads

Whether we hanker for Eastern or Western renditions, leftover roast or poached chicken begs to be tossed up into one of our all-time favorites, chicken salad. Now that we have spit-roasted chickens twisting and turning on every corner, we can make salad on a whim and on the run—all the more reason for trying something new.

I prefer the flavor balance of both light and dark meat, but of course you can use breast meat only in any of these recipes. Each salad is presented differently: one is wrapped in lettuce, one stuffed into a pineapple shell, another mounded high over both soft and crisp noodles, and the fourth is a pristine Japanese-style presentation. Any one of these salads can be served Western-style on a bed of mixed greens.

☯ Peanut Chicken Salad ☯

Serves 4

*L*ettuce wrappers are a great way to present chicken salad on a multiple-dish buffet, for a casual family supper, or even as a lunch-on-the-run. Accompany the salad with individual bowls of steamed rice.

3 cups take-out chicken, skinned, boned, and pulled into bite-size pieces
¹/₂ cup grated raw carrot
¹/₂ cup finely diced celeriac or celery heart
8 scallions, finely sliced, with some green
salt
1 head soft lettuce

DRESSING
¹/₂ cup Peanut Sauce (page 31) at room temperature
1 tablespoon fresh lime juice
2 tablespoons light mayonnaise, Hellmann's or Best Foods

Mix the salad ingredients in a large bowl. Whisk the dressing and toss the salad together with half the dressing at a time, stopping when mixture is just moist and flavorful. Taste and adjust the seasonings if necessary. If you want to boost the heat level, add a squirt or two of Thai chile sauce.

Serve this salad at room temperature with a stack of soft lettuce leaves on each plate for rolling up the chicken.

✒ This salad pairs perfectly with ripe mango and looks stunning with red leaf lettuce.

✒ Refrigerated leftovers can become unappetizingly dry because the chicken tends to absorb its dressing in storage. Stir in a little more mayonnaise to revive the creamy glaze. Resist adding more Peanut Sauce or the flavor will overwhelm the chicken.

✒ Leftover Peanut Sauce tastes great on roast pork, grilled chops, or jumbo shrimp.

Pineapple Stuffed with Mango
☯ Curry Chicken Salad ☯

Serves 4

This version is reminiscent of the Indian Raj—and the sumptuous presentation would have made a Bombay bearer proud.

2 ripe medium pineapples
3 cups bite-size chunks roasted or poached chicken
1 tablespoon currants
$^1/_2$ cup slivered water chestnuts or jicama
$^1/_3$ cup (about 12) scallions, finely sliced, with some green
$^1/_4$ cup minced fresh cilantro, optional
salt, to taste

DRESSING
2 teaspoons curry powder
1 tablespoon Conzorsio's Mango Vignette (see
   Ingredients)
$^1/_2$ teaspoon grated peeled ginger, with the juice
1 tablespoon nut or safflower oil
$^1/_3$ cup mayonnaise, Hellmann's or Best Foods
$^1/_3$ cup sour cream
$^1/_3$ cup plain yogurt

GARNISH
$^1/_4$ cup slivered almonds
$^1/_2$ cup unsweetened coconut flakes (or shreds)

Cut the pineapples lengthwise from the base to the top where the leaves are attached. Pull the base apart and the leaves will separate from each half perfectly without cutting. If the leaves are lush and green, don't trim them; otherwise, clip off any blemishes or remove any brown outer leaves. Carefully remove the fruit from the shell in chunks, leaving 4 smooth $^3/_4$-inch-thick shells. Take a very thin slice off the rounded side of each shell to make it sit evenly on the plate. All of this can be done ahead and the shells stored in the refrigerator in plastic bags. Sliver the pineapple along the grain, and reserve 1$^1/_3$ cups.

Stir the curry powder, the Mango Vignette, and the ginger into the oil and heat it in the microwave for 30 seconds to release its flavor. When it's cool, whisk it with the mayonnaise and yogurt. Toss the salad ingredients with the dressing.

Toast the almonds and coconut on separate pieces of foil, in a 325° oven for about 8 and 5 minutes, respectively. The natural sugar in coconut burns quickly, so keep a keen eye on it, fluffing it up once or twice while toasting. The nuts are done when they're golden and there's a noticeable nutty aroma.

Divide the slivered pineapple between the shells and mound the chicken salad on top. Sprinkle the almonds and coconut generously over all.

⤙ Instead of the toasted almonds and coconut, use Coco-Peanut Crunch (page 33).

⤙ Saffron garlic toast—just add a pinch of saffron to the garlic butter—is delicious with this salad.

⤙ If the salad doesn't fill the shells adequately, you can dummy-up the bottom with some shredded lettuce or fill in around the edge of the shells with garden sprouts or sprigs of mint.

⤙ If the Mango Vignette isn't available, puree the flesh of $^1/_2$ mango with 2–3 tablespoons of fruited vinegar. It won't be as intense as the commercial brand. Store the rest in the refrigerator to use for marinades or fruit-salad dressings.

⤙ If you're serving this salad for a company brunch or summer supper, you can add a bit of high drama by cutting a couple of fuchsia and white *Dendrobium* orchid sprays in half and inserting them into the shells at the leaf end. These orchids are inexpensive and can often be found in supermarket floral departments.

✒ Diced jicama provides a moist crunch similar to water chestnuts. Fresh water chestnuts are glorious but scarce morsels—well-rinsed canned ones will do.

Sesame Orange Chicken with Asparagus and
☯ Two Kinds of Noodles ☯

Serves 4

*O*nly Washington's cherry blossoms herald spring more sweetly than fresh asparagus. This is a lovely, refreshing salad for asparagus season that looks every bit as good as it tastes.

4 whole boneless and skinless chicken breasts, cut into fingers or 6 chicken tenders
1 tablespoon Chinese Seasoning Oil (page 23)
1 garlic clove, minced
1/4 teaspoon Thai chile sauce or chile paste
Chinese Salt and Pepper (page 24)
16 fresh asparagus spears, trimmed
1 teaspoon toasted sesame oil
4–6 skeins from 1 package (10 ounces) somen noodles
1/2 cup diced daikon

DRESSING
1 tablespoon frozen orange juice concentrate
1 tablespoon rice vinegar
1 tablespoon balsamic vinegar
1 tablespoon soy sauce
2 teaspoons honey Dijon mustard
2 shallots, minced
2 teaspoons grated peeled ginger with juice, or pickled ginger
1 1/2 tablespoons avocado or safflower oil

GARNISH
2 tablespoons sesame seeds, toasted
$1/2$ sweet red pepper, seeded and cut into tiny dice
2 navel oranges, sectioned

Stir-fry the chicken fingers in the seasoning oil, garlic, and chile sauce over medium-high heat until they turn opaque. Turn the heat down to medium and cook for another 2 to 3 minutes or until the chicken is just firm to the touch. Sprinkle lightly with salt and pepper. Set the chicken aside to cool. This can be done a day ahead or the night before. Let the chicken come to room temperature before assembling the salad.

If you haven't time to peel the asparagus spears after snapping off their bottoms, at least peel the heavy ends—both color and texture will benefit. Roll them around in the sesame oil and spread them out singly on the broiler rack of your toaster oven or regular oven. It takes less than 5 minutes to broil them. They're done when they begin to wrinkle and the tips look a little toasty. (Broiling the asparagus approximates the Chinese technique of double frying; the natural flavor not only intensifies but it develops a nutty taste.) Set the asparagus aside to cool. (You can also cook the asparagus in the microwave with a minimum of water, covered, for about 3 minutes, retaining some crisp texture. Plunge them into ice water to cool and hold their bright green color. Drain on paper towels.)

Put 4 skeins of somen noodles into a large pot of boiling water and cook 2 to 3 minutes or until al dente, testing strands as they boil. Drain in a colander and run under cool water to stop the cooking. For a delicious crunchy addition to this salad, crisp-fry the other two noodle skeins for a minute or so. They will crisp very fast. Lift the skeins out of the oil and drain on paper towels. Lay another sheet of paper towel on top and crush the noodles with the heel of your hand.

Put a serving of the cooked noodles on each plate with the chicken fingers and daikon on top. Rest 4 asparagus spears around the salad, tips at the top. Mix the dressing ingredients and dress the salad, reserving any excess for another use. Garnish the salad with the sesame seeds, diced red pepper, and the orange sections.

Sake-to-Me Chicken Salad

Serves 4

*T*his is the ultimate chicken salad for those dog days of summer. It's clean, crisp, and spare.

8 boneless chicken breast halves
$^1/_2$ cup Asian Chicken Broth or Quickly Seasoned Canned Broth (pages 81, 82)
$1^1/_4$ cups sake, boiled for 1 minute
1 tablespoon sugar
1 teaspoon salt
$^1/_2$ cup light mayonnaise, Hellmann's or Best Foods
2 teaspoons wasabi paste
$^1/_2$ seedless European cucumber
2 bunches watercress
avocado or safflower oil
12 cherry tomatoes, halved and seeded

Skin the chicken breasts and remove the tenderloin strip underneath. Freeze the tenders for other uses. Trim the breasts of any extraneous bits of flesh or fat, leaving each piece in a near-perfect smooth oval. Place the breasts in a shallow microwave-safe dish with the chicken broth and $^1/_4$ cup of the sake. Cover with plastic wrap and microwave on high for about 8 minutes. Add the remaining sake, sugar, and salt. Let the chicken cool to room temperature and then refrigerate overnight, or at least 4 hours.

Mix the mayonnaise with the wasabi paste. Without peeling the cucumber, slice it tissue thin and spread the slices out on paper towels. Blot them dry. Drain the chicken and place 1 piece on either side of a nest of watercress. Glaze the tops of the chicken breasts very lightly with a brush dipped in the avocado or safflower oil. Arrange overlapping cucumber slices and cherry tomato halves in a pristine Japanese manner. Serve the wasabi mayonnaise in individual ramekins for dipping the chicken.

⊂ Accompany the salad with icy cold, lightly dressed soba noodles.

Spinach Salad with Chinese
☯ Sausage and Chicken ☯
Serves 4

*O*ne habit you'll adopt when you start easing into Asian cooking is saving chicken tenders, the loose strip of flesh that cozies up under each half of the breast. I pull them off into a small zippered freezer bag until I have enough for a stir-fry or spinach salad. These full-meal hot and cold salads are very appealing any time of the year. They're a snap to put together, and they look and taste so special you could serve them to company.

2 large bunches flat-leaf spinach, washed and stemmed

DRESSING
2 garlic cloves, crushed
2 quarter-size coins of peeled ginger, crushed and minced
2 teaspoons honey Dijon mustard
pinch of cayenne pepper
1 tablespoon rice vinegar
2 teaspoons Thai fish sauce *(nam pla)*
2 tablespoons safflower or American sesame oil

2 Chinese sausages, lightly steamed and sliced into thin rounds
2 teaspoons Chinese Seasoning Oil (page 23) or peanut oil
1 large egg, beaten with a splash of water
4–6 chicken tenders or 2 skinless breast halves, boned
1 red onion, sliced into very thin rings

Put the spinach into a large salad bowl. Whisk together the dressing ingredients and set aside.

Steam the sausages in the microwave in a little water until they soften, about 3 minutes. Heat an 8-inch nonstick skillet over medium heat with 1 teaspoon of the oil. Pour in the beaten egg and immediately swirl it around to thinly film the bottom of the skillet, running it a little bit up the sides if necessary. The egg will set instantly. Slide it out of the pan and roll it up. Cut the tenders on the diagonal into thin strips and stir-fry them in the seasoned oil for a minute. Add the steamed sausage rounds and continue stir-frying until the sausage browns a bit and the chicken is opaque. Cut the rolled egg crosswise into thin ribbons. Toss the spinach with the dressing and the onion rings, and divide among the dinner plates. Arrange the sausage rounds and chicken strips around the edge. Fluff out the egg ribbons and drape them over the top.

Fried Dumplings on Napa Cabbage

Serves 4

*A*sian markets often sell large bags of frozen uncooked pork, shrimp, or vegetable dumplings and they're quite inexpensive. Sometimes you can order them uncooked from your favorite Chinese restaurant. It's worth seeking out a source because they're marvelous to have on hand for dropping into broth, steaming or frying for a quick supper, or for turning out onto this highly flavored, crispy salad.

2 dozen frozen Chinese dumplings
2 teaspoons peanut oil
$^1/_2$ cup water or chicken broth

DRESSING
2 teaspoons roasted garlic puree
1 tablespoon Dijon horseradish mustard
1 tablespoon dark soy sauce
2 teaspoons balsamic vinegar
2 teaspoons fresh lemon juice
$^1/_4$ cup mayonnaise, Hellmann's or Best Foods

1 head napa cabbage, thinly sliced
salt and freshly ground black or Szechuan pepper
whole chives and thin slivers of sweet red pepper, for
   garnish

Divide the dumplings, side by side, flat edge down, between two nonstick skillets with 1 teaspoon of oil in each. (Or cook them in relays.) Over medium-high heat, sauté the dumplings until the bottoms are lightly brown. Add half the chicken broth to each skillet, put lids on the skillets, and simmer the dumplings until the dough is transparent and most of the broth is absorbed or evaporated. Remove the lids and continue cooking until all the liquid is gone and the dumpling bottoms are richly browned. Slide the dumplings onto a platter and set aside.

Put all the dressing ingredients except the mayonnaise in one of the skillets, simmering and whisking for a minute to blend and thicken slightly. Remove from the heat and whisk in the mayonnaise.

Put a bed of cabbage on each plate and salt it lightly. Arrange 6 warmed dumplings on each salad and drizzle the dressing equally over each serving. Scatter whole chives and red pepper slivers over the top of each salad.

Tropical Fruit, Avocado, and Tofu Salad

☯ ☯

Serves 4

*E*ven when mangoes, papaya, and avocados are plentiful they're not exactly inexpensive, unless you live in the tropics. Using these luscious fruits for a main dish helps to move them out of the extravagant class. Combining tofu with the fruit adds protein, and its silkiness is a match for the ripe fruit. Crunchy contrast comes in the piquant greens, jicama, and topping. In less lavish proportions, this salad is also a colorful and tempting side dish.

DRESSING
   1 garlic clove, mashed and minced
   2 quarter-size coins peeled ginger, crushed and minced

2 tablespoons Mango Vignette or raspberry vinegar

1 teaspoon fish sauce *(nuoc mam* or *nam pla)*

6 tablespoons avocado or American sesame oil

SALAD

1 10.5-ounce package firm tofu, drained, blotted dry, and
cut into fingers

7 cups mesclun (mixed baby greens)

1 bunch watercress, stemmed, or 1 cup baby spinach leaves

salt and freshly ground pepper

2 mangoes

1 papaya

1 avocado

$1/4$ cup diced jicama

8 scallions, trimmed and slivered

2 tablespoons Coco-Peanut Crunch (page 33) or chopped
dry-roasted peanuts

Whisk together the dressing ingredients and marinate the tofu strips in it. Toss together the mesclun and watercress or spinach, and divide among the plates. Salt and pepper the greens lightly.

Standing them on their round bottoms, cut each mango in half lengthwise against the flat pit. Score the flesh diagonally down to the skin in both directions, forming cubes. Press each half firmly from the skin side, forcing the sections to pop up. With a paring knife, cut the cubes from the skin and divide them among the servings. Cut the papaya in half and spoon out the seeds. Peel the fruit and slice the flesh lengthwise, dividing the slices among the servings. Quarter and peel the avocado and make 4 fans by cutting narrow lengthwise strips, leaving the flesh intact 1 inch from one end. Fan out the strips slightly between your fingers, and place on salads. Scatter the scallion slivers over the salads. Lift the tofu strips from the dressing and place them on the greens, then drizzle on the balance of the dressing. Sprinkle with Coco-Peanut Crunch.

This salad makes an ideal base for grilled duck breast or strips of Peking duck ordered from your favorite Chinese take-out.

Thai Barbecued Shrimp Salad

Serves 4

*A*sian barbecued shrimp parked on top of a good base salad with chopped herbs make an adventurous supper. You should be able to find excellent shrimp in your seafood market—seek them out. But watch out for the tasteless, pop-art striped tiger shrimp.

1 pound jumbo shrimp, peeled, tails on
¹/₂ cup Thais Like-It-Hot Barbecue Sauce (page 29)
1 tablespoon safflower or American sesame oil
1 small head red-leaf lettuce, trimmed and torn
2 hearts romaine lettuce, trimmed and shredded
1 cucumber, peeled, seeded, and chopped
2 carrots, grated
1 medium tomato, seeded, pulped, and slivered
¹/₄ red onion, very thinly sliced
1 dozen basil leaves, shredded
toasted pine nuts (optional)

DRESSING
¹/₄ cup safflower or avocado oil
2 garlic cloves, pressed
1 tablespoon rice vinegar
salt and pepper, to taste

Marinate the shrimp in ¹/₄ cup of the barbecue sauce for 1 hour.

Heat the oil in a wok or skillet. Sauté the shrimp over medium-high heat, adding more barbecue sauce as it darkens and caramelizes; the shrimp will be done in 3 to 4 minutes.

Toss the salad greens, vegetables, and basil very lightly with the dressing and pile it high in the center of individual serving plates. Place the shrimp around the salad, drizzling on some of the barbecue sauce and sprinkle the salad with the pine nuts.

≺ You could also make this salad with swordfish, tuna, or sea scallops.

Teriyaki Steak and
⚊ Soba Noodle Salad ⚊

Serves 4

This is a great way to enjoy the taste of a good steak and avoid that feeling of having eaten too much of a good thing. In such judicious portions, you can select the most handsome, well-marbled prime meat you can find, and if you don't mind firing up the grill for two steaks, the flavor will be memorable. Use the dying embers to roast some peppers.

2 thick strip steaks, 1 inch or more, totaling 1 pound
1 recipe Japanese Glazing Sauce (page 26) with the
    optional Thai chile sauce
2 teaspoons safflower oil
1 8.8-ounce package Japanese buckwheat noodles (soba)
16 fresh shiitake mushrooms, stemmed and sliced
$1/2$ cup chopped fresh bean sprouts
$1/4$ cup sliced scallions, including some green
$1/4$ sweet green pepper, seeded and diced
6 cherry tomatoes, seeded and slivered

DRESSING
3 tablespoons Japanese Glazing Sauce
2 tablespoons rice vinegar
1 tablespoon Asian sesame oil
2 tablespoons safflower oil
2 pressed garlic cloves
2 teaspoons hoisin sauce
dash of Thai chile sauce, optional

Marinate the steaks in glazing sauce and oil for at least 3 hours.

Put the noodles into a pasta pot of rapidly boiling water. Cook for 1 to 2 minutes, until the noodles are al dente. Test a strand before turning them into a colander. Run cold water over the noodles to stop the cooking.

Grill the steaks over white-ash coals until rare, about 4 minutes each side, 5 for medium. Or sauté them over medium-high heat for 3 to 4 minutes on each side. Let the steaks cool slightly before cutting them on the diagonal into ¼-inch slices. While the steaks are cooling, sauté the mushrooms briefly until they are just limp.

Toss the noodles with the vegetables. Whisk the dressing and coat the noodle salad lightly. Taste for seasoning. Divide the salad among the dinner plates and top with slices of steak.

⤜ A delicious alternative is to simply dress the soba noodles with Peanut Sauce thinned with a little teriyaki sauce.

⤜ You can use bottled Teriyaki sauce—just add Thai chile sauce to taste.

Super Express

EGGPLANT: Broil peeled slices brushed lightly with oil until just tender. Salt and pepper and fill a gratin dish. Cover the top with a mixture of half drained yogurt, half sour cream, and lots of chopped fresh mint. Just before serving, run the dish under the broiler for a few minutes to heat the eggplant and set the topping.

SWEET POTATOES: bake—or reheat leftover sweet potatoes— and mash the flesh with unsweetened coconut milk, salt, five-spice powder, and cayenne pepper to taste.

OKRA: Steam a package of frozen okra with 2 smashed coins of ginger and 2 smashed garlic cloves. Drain and fish out the ginger and garlic. Add them to 2 tablespoons of peanut oil in a hot wok and stir-fry cherry tomatoes until the skins start to pop. Toss in a handful of slivered scallions, then add the okra and a dash of hot sauce.

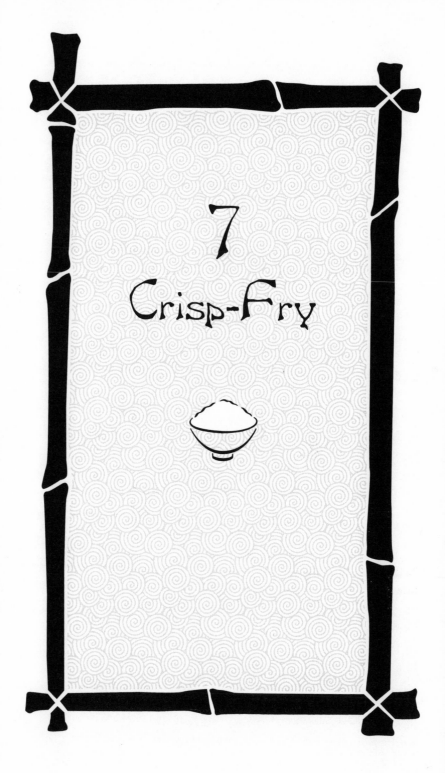

7
Crisp-Fry

*L*et's fess up, we're all fried food freaks and Asians are among the planet's best fry cooks. In that part of the world, these little surprise packages are snack food, part of the offering at dim sum teahouses, or the crisp accent to an abundant feast. What versatile small bites all these mysterious crackly wrappers make and what fun they are to dip in those tongue-tickling sauces and sambals. Along with noodles, kids love them best, and I've discovered there's no cajoling required to enlist little fingers to roll and seal. Hard to make? Not at all. Even if you're klutzy, these will taste just fine as long as you seal them well. All the wrappers are terrific for experimenting with leftovers.

Frying in deep oil at the right temperature actually results in less fat absorption than sautéing in less fat at lower temperatures. Controlling the *amount* of fat is important in sautéing, whereas in deep-frying it's the *temperature* and *quality* of the oil that are key. Of course, there are other factors too, such as how porous the coating is, the freshness of the oil, and the skill of the cook. Japanese tempura, in the hands of a master chef, is the epitome of light deep-frying.

Do give yourself permission to enjoy the Asian crisp foods. They're so important to the balance and joy of these cuisines. Before getting started with the recipes, here's some essential information about the wrappers, the fillings, and the oil.

The Wrappers

EGG ROLL AND WONTON WRAPPERS: Think fresh pasta. These doughs are made from wheat flour, eggs, and water. If you can't find Frieda's Finest in your supermarket, and you haven't time for an Asian market run, fresh lasagna sheets can be cut into 3$^1/_2$- or 5$^1/_2$-inch wonton and egg roll squares. Conversely, you can use quality egg roll wrappers for ravioli, cannelloni, or even lasagna. Either dough can be boiled, steamed, or fried. The only difference between them is that pasta sheets are thicker and won't produce the ethereal results of the traditional Chinese wrapper.

To experiment with this dough, buy a package of wonton wrappers, heat up the fryer, and cut half the stack in two on the diagonal. Drop the triangles into the hot oil where they'll puff and brown almost instantly. Turn them over with tongs and then quickly out onto paper towels to drain. When cool, dust them lightly with seasoned salt and serve them with stir-fries or salads or store them in a tight tin for dipping or snacking.

SPRING ROLL WRAPPERS: There's no substitute for the formidably peculiar *banh trang*—Vietnamese dried rice paper wrappers—which come in either 8-inch rounds or triangles. These starched organza playing cards with a shadowy bamboo pattern are straight out of *Alice in Wonderland,* but they become obediently pliable when spritzed with water. When softened and/or steamed, they're called garden rolls, enclosing light fillings that can be eaten out of hand like a Western sandwich.

Using sugar or beer in the softening water encourages browning. Use a spray bottle for spritzing or a shallow bowl wide enough to dip the wrappers without bending them. Spread a clean towel over your work surface so the wrappers don't sit in puddles of water.

You can expect the stiff wrappers to occasionally crack or tear in handling, but they're blessedly cheap so just pitch the rejects. Deep-fried, they make the especially delicious Vietnamese spring roll—one of the great joys of Asian food.

The Chinese spring roll wrapper is a flour and water crepe available frozen in Asian markets. It's very similar in end result to the

Vietnamese wrapper, but the rice paper version is more versatile because it doesn't require refrigeration and can be enjoyed with no cooking at all.

LUMPIA WRAPPERS: These Philippine wrappers are available in the frozen food section of Asian markets, and they make the most crackly wrapper of all. They're not a rolled dough like egg roll, wonton wrappers, or pasta. They're actually a paper-thin batter crepe made with cornstarch and egg; when they're homemade, they're eaten fresh with a lettuce leaf lining and room-temperature fillings. When frozen, they're best for crisp-fry snacks. They make a superior spring roll and excellent Indian samosas. They're easier to handle than the rice paper wrapper and thinner and/or crunchier than egg roll or spring roll wrappers.

The Fillings

There are three important rules for making fillings:

1. The ingredients must be cut finely enough to prevent pulling out a clothesline full of food with your teeth. Not only is that startling and embarrassing, but you risk a nasty burn. The imprisoned steam in wrapped, fried foods is extremely hot.

2. If the vegetables you choose have a naturally high water content (such as celery, bean sprouts, or onions), blanch, drain, and blot them to keep the wrapper from getting soggy.

3. Mixed-ingredient fillings require a little thickening agent to keep the parcel together for dipping. You don't want the filling to tumble out all over the plate to be hopelessly chased by chopsticks. A slurry of cornstarch and water is the preferred binder.

The Oil

My preference is 100 percent peanut oil, which can reach a higher temperature before "breaking" than other edible oils and can be reused more often. Yes, it's relatively expensive. Look for economical jumbo sizes in Asian markets, food warehouses, and discount clubs. Corn or canola oil is a good alternative.

The proper oil temperature for most crisp-fry recipes is 375° and the quantity you'll need in a wok is about 1 quart. When adding raw food, always pause a few seconds between each round for the thermometer or thermostat to recover.

How often the oil needs to be replaced depends a lot on what and how much you cook in it and how clean you keep it between uses. Always skim and/or sieve the oil of floating debris after each use while the oil is still warm and before the cooked particles have a chance to drop to the bottom and turn into sludge. The most reliable gauge for when to discard and replace the oil is to watch how quickly it recovers temperature or take notice when the food no longer seems crispy when it's done. Three or four uses is about the maximum before the oil begins to break down. When you have to replace it, be sure to scrub out the deep fryer with soapy water and rinse well before pouring in fresh oil.

Cantonese Egg Rolls and Wontons

Makes approximately 1 dozen

These treats, both large and small, make great appetizers as well as welcome additions to one-dish suppers. When you cook Asian food regularly, there are always little leftovers—extra filling from the last spring roll orgy, snips of cooked meats or fish too choice for the cat, or assorted stir-fry veggies that don't quite add up to a second round. These are the things you can reinvent and twist up into egg roll or wonton wrappers. Freeze them individually, then bag them. The fillings don't have to match and, remember, they don't have to be crisp-fried, either. You can drop them into boiling stock or steam a bowlful.

The folding and shaping of traditional wontons *is* a fussy task, but you don't have to follow tradition. Make a simple triangular fold, sealing both edges well, or roll them up and twist the ends. Any which way, as long as they stay sealed so the filling doesn't leak out or the oil soak in. Always dampen the edges to be sealed with a "glue" of egg or cornstarch beaten with a little water.

Pan-Asian Express

Here's the egg roll filling recipe I've used for many years. If you're into nostalgia, this is as good as an egg roll gets. I've updated the procedure to make quick use of the microwave, but the taste is classic. Serve these with good old-fashioned Chinese mustard and plum sauce.

FILLING
2 tablespoons grated raw carrot
2 tablespoons grated celery
2 tablespoons minced scallions, with a little green
2 teaspoons light sesame or peanut oil
1/4 pound minced pork
1/4 pound medium shrimp, peeled, deveined, and minced
2 garlic cloves, pressed
1 teaspoon cornstarch, mixed with 1 teaspoon soy sauce
1/2 teaspoon salt
freshly ground black pepper

1 package egg roll wrappers
1 large egg, beaten with 1 teaspoon water
oil, for frying

Put the carrot and celery in a small dish with a teaspoon of water. Cover and cook in the microwave for 30 seconds. Drain and squeeze dry in a paper towel when cool. Mix with the scallions.

Heat the oil in a wok. Toss the pork and shrimp with the garlic, cornstarch-soy sauce mixture, salt, and pepper. Stir-fry over medium-high heat until the shrimp and pork look barely cooked. Cool and toss all the ingredients together. You may refrigerate the filling for a day or two, or freeze it for later use.

Place 4 wrappers at a time in a diagonal position on a work surface lightly dusted with cornstarch. Put 2 tablespoons of filling in the center of each wrapper. Fold the point nearest you completely over the filling, tucking the tip under it. Fold both side points to meet at the center. Moisten the remaining flap with the beaten egg. Shallow-fry in about 2 inches of oil or in deep oil in a kettle fryer. Turn them over as the underside turns deep golden brown. They'll be cooked through when both sides are equally brown, about 6 minutes. Drain them on paper towels and serve.

⌇ This same filling can be used in wonton, spring roll, or lumpia wrappers.

⌇ HAM AND SCALLOP SNAPPERS: Marinate tiny bay scallops in dark soy sauce, oyster sauce, and a drop of lemon oil for 1 hour. Drain and reserve the marinade. Lay out the wrappers straight. Use a narrow strip of Black Forest ham or prosciutto as a center line marker. Put one or two scallops on top like Tootsie Roll segments. Egg-wash the top edge and the two sides. Roll up the dough like a party snapper, seal the ends together, twist them, and press to keep the shape. Crisp-fry and add minced ginger and garlic to the marinade for a dip. Float a thin lemon slice on top.

☯ Vegetable Spring Rolls ☯
Makes approximately 1 dozen

T he delicate, even elegant, nature of the Vietnamese spring roll is most pronounced when the filling is composed entirely of vegetables. Like garden rolls, cellophane noodles are often used to knit everything together. There are no rules about vegetable choices. Just select complementary flavors and contrasting textures. All of this may look complex, but spring rolls go together quite quickly. The third time you'll need no recipe. Serve these with Vietnamese Table Seasoning, Peanut Sauce, or soy sauce.

FILLING
   4 ounces (¹/₂ package) cellophane (mung bean) noodles or cooked Japanese somen noodles
   6–8 dried Chinese black mushrooms
   1 teaspoon light sesame or safflower oil
   1 large egg, whisked with 1 teaspoon water
   ²/₃ cup roughly chopped bean sprouts
   ¹/₂ cup slivered dark greens (flat-leaf spinach, chard, kale, romaine)

$^1/_2$ cup shredded carrots
$^1/_2$ cup finely shredded napa or green cabbage
$^1/_4$ cup minced scallions, with some green
$^1/_4$ cup finely diced water chestnuts or jicama
salt and freshly ground black pepper

18 round rice paper wrappers
1 cup water, mixed with 1 tablespoon sugar, or $^3/_4$ water
    and $^1/_2$ cup beer
oil, for frying

Soak the cellophane noodles in warm water for 15 to 20 minutes, or until they're soft. Drain and dry on paper towels. Cut the noodles with scissors into approximately 2-inch lengths and drop them into a mixing bowl. Soak the mushrooms in hot water for 30 to 60 minutes, or until they're soft. Squeeze them dry, then stem and mince them. Toss with the noodles.

Heat the oil in a wok or nonstick skillet and swirl the beaten egg around to thinly coat the bottom. As soon as the egg sets, slide it out into a tight roll onto a plate. Cut the cooled omelet crosswise into thin ribbons. Add to the filling. Put the bean sprouts in a sieve over a small bowl and blanch them by pouring boiling water over them and letting them sit there for a second or two. Lift the sieve out and run cool tap water over them to stop the cooking. Drain on paper towels and chop into short segments. Add to the filling. Wilt the greens in the microwave in a splash of water. Blot dry and chop. Add to the rest of the filling ingredients and salt lightly as you mix.

Spritz or dip 4 wrappers in the sugar or beer water in sequence and lay them out on the counter. Wait a couple of seconds and you'll notice the wrappers begin to pucker and soften. If they're ornery, spritz again. Fold up the side nearest you, round edge to center line. This gives you a sturdier base for the filling. Place 1 or 2 tablespoons of filling between the fold line and the center and shape it lightly into a log, tucking in the loose shreds. Turn the wrapper and filling a half-roll and, keeping it all together with firm fingers, fold over the two sides. Now, remembering how an egg roll looks, finish a tight roll and lightly press down the moist flap. Turn the roll over, with the flap down to keep it sealed. Your fingers will get the feel of it very soon—don't despair. You can also unwrap a messy one and start over; the wrappers aren't as fragile as they look. Now, you're ready for another round of 4 wrappers. By the time you get to the end, your second career is assured. You can cover and store the filled spring rolls in the refrigerator all day or freeze them to fry another day.

Shallow-fry the spring rolls in about 2 inches of oil or in deeper oil in a kettle fryer. Turn the rolls over as the underside turns deep golden brown. They'll be cooked through when both sides are brown—in 5 or 6 minutes. Drain them on paper towels and serve.

⚞ THAI CRAB ROLLS: Omit the cabbage and water chestnuts. Add 2 pressed garlic cloves, 1 teaspoon Thai chile sauce, and ¼ cup of chopped cilantro.

⚞ If you freeze the spring rolls, partially thaw them and blot them before cooking.

☯ Madras Chimichangas ☯
Serves 4

*F*lour tortillas are hardly Asian, but they're great for experimenting with whimsical, nontraditional fillings. To get you started, here's one with an Indian twist. If your natural foods store carries them, of course you can make these with chapatis.

FILLING
2 tablespoons safflower or peanut oil
1 cup chopped onion
1 pound ground lamb or beef
3 garlic cloves, minced
4 quarter-size coins peeled ginger, minced
1 teaspoon curry powder
½ teaspoon ground cumin
salt, pepper, and cayenne pepper, to taste
1 cup canned black beans, well drained

4 8-inch flour tortillas or chapatis
oil, for frying
$1/2$ cup well-drained plain yogurt
1 ripe tomato, seeded, pulped, and minced
$1/4$ cup chopped cilantro

Heat the oil in a wok or skillet and stir-fry the onion over high heat until brown flecks appear. Remove from the pan when tender but still crisp. Sauté the meat in the same well-oiled pan, pressing down on it with the back of your spoon to separate the clumps. Cook until no raw bits remain. Scrape the meat into a bowl with the onion. In the same pan, sauté the garlic, ginger, curry powder, cumin, salt, pepper, and cayenne. When the garlic is soft, add the beans. Cook and stir for a couple of minutes; mash the beans with a fork just enough so they cling together, mixing in the seasonings well. Add a little water if the beans seem dry.

To assemble the rolls, dampen the tortillas slightly by rubbing them with wet hands. Soften them for rolling by flipping them over the gas or electric burner for a second on each side. Spread the beans first, leaving a 2-inch margin all around. Pile on the meat and onion in the center. Fold the edge nearest you up over the meat, tucking it under, then fold in the sides and roll in the same manner as an egg roll. Fasten the final flap with a toothpick, or hold it together with tongs for a second or two when it hits the hot oil.

Shallow-fry the rolls until the tortilla is golden and crisp on all sides, about 6 minutes. Remove the toothpick. Mix the yogurt with the tomato and cilantro. Serve.

⟋ Leftover fried rice makes a good base for tortilla rolls. Add strips of cooked chicken or shrimp and vegetables like bamboo shoots, diced cooked carrot, and slivered snow peas.

Philippine Lumpia

ॐ   ॐ

Makes 6 rolls

T he lumpia is a gutsy Philippine version of the Asian spring roll, often served in the form of a cornucopia with a ruffled lettuce liner and fresh hearts of palm poking out. But those taste best when the crepes are fresh off the griddle, so this variation on the theme will be fried—an equally popular Philippine snack. The cornstarch in the lumpia batter makes the wrappers delightfully crisp, almost shattering, when fried. I've also used this wrapper for the beloved Indian snack, samosas.

FILLING

- 1 tablespoon peanut oil
- 1 sweet medium onion, such as Vidalia, finely chopped
- 2 garlic cloves, crushed and minced
- ³/₄ pound ground pork loin or boneless country ribs
- 2 tablespoons fish sauce (*nam pla* or *nuoc mam*)
- 1 large sweet potato, cooked and diced (about 1 cup)
- ¹/₄ cup chopped cooked green beans
- ¹/₂ cup blanched finely sliced cabbage
- 1 large ripe tomato, seeded, pulped, and diced
- ¹/₄ cup finely chopped celery
- ¹/₄ cup chopped roasted peanuts
- salt and freshly ground pepper

- 6 lumpia wrappers
- a squeeze or two of fresh lime
- 1 large egg, lightly beaten with 1 teaspoon water
- oil, for frying

Heat the oil in a wok or skillet and, over medium-high heat, sauté the onion and garlic until soft and translucent. Add the meat and stir-fry until there's no sign of red. Cook 1 minute longer, then stir in the fish sauce. Toss the vegetables with the seasoned meat and onion. Salt and pepper to taste, heavy on the pepper, and add the lime.

Peel the wrappers from the stack and don't fret if they come off as unwillingly as Band-Aids. Mound a couple tablespoons of filling, front of center, adjusting the quantity by eye. Roll the crepe in the same manner as a round spring roll wrapper. Seal the flap with the egg wash and fry as Egg Rolls (page 120).

For a dip: Blend ¼ cup soy sauce with 3 tablespoons Philippine Seasoned Vinegar (page 26), 2 teaspoons sugar, and hot sauce of choice. Taste and adjust. In the Philippines, they fancy the sour tastes.

Fresh Fish Lumpia Rolls: Use any firm flesh fish like tuna, mahimahi, swordfish, sea bass, or grouper. Make a bed of Seared Corn, Tomato, and Black Bean Salsa (page 40) in the center of the wrapper. Put a raw, thumb-size piece of fish on top. Roll up and crisp-fry. Serve with a dip of half mayonnaise, half drained yogurt spiced with Thai chile sauce.

☯ Samosas ☯

Makes 6 dozen

These delectable Indian snacks are great pleasers and, like wontons, deserve some room in the freezer for impromptu company or family snacks while you finish flipping the stir-fry or firing the grill. Lumpia and wonton wrappers both work well for samosas, but I prefer the lighter quality of the lumpia crepe, even though it has to be cut to make the smaller size turnover. Cut a few when you buy them, and keep the smaller rounds in the freezer for later use.

FILLING

1 tablespoon safflower oil
2 garlic cloves, crushed and minced
1 teaspoon minced peeled ginger
1 cup minced onion
salt and pepper, to taste
½ pound ground beef, lamb, or chicken

2 teaspoons curry powder
$^1/_2$ teaspoon ground cumin
$^1/_4$ teaspoon ground cinnamon
pinch of cloves
2 tablespoons chopped mint

8 lumpia wrappers
1 large egg lightly beaten with 1 teaspoon water
oil, for frying

Heat the oil in a wok or large skillet and, over medium-high heat, cook the garlic, ginger, and onion until limp and translucent. Add salt and pepper. Add the meat or poultry along with the dry herbs and stir-fry, pressing down on the meat with the back of your spoon to break up the clumps. Cook until there is no sign of raw bits of meat. Add the fresh mint.

Cut five or six 3-inch circles out of each lumpia wrapper with a cookie or biscuit cutter and then cut each circle in half. Laying out 6 semicircles at a time on your work surface, moisten the edges with the egg wash—fingertips are a fast way. Put a small mound of filling in the center of each piece and make a simple foldover, pressing the moistened edges together well. The samosas are ready to crisp-fry or pack in heavy zippered plastic bags and freeze. To fry the samosas, drop 8 to 10 at a time into deep 375° oil and cook until the wrappers are deep golden brown, about 4 minutes. Drain on paper towels and keep hot in a warm oven until the rest are ready.

Cilantro and Mint Chutney is the perfect dip, made easier to scoop by mixing it with a little plain yogurt.

One of the classic samosa fillings combines diced cooked potato and peas with the above onion, garlic, ginger, and curry seasonings. Omit the meat.

main-dish garnish. If you want to serve a whole tempura meal with vegetables, fish, and spicy soba noodles, *and* you have an electric wok or a portable butane burner, cook the tempura right at the dining table. Use attractive bowls for the ice and batter, and attentively arrange the vegetables and seafood on a handsome tray. Use long cooking chopsticks for dropping in the food and drain the finished pieces on a basket tray lined with paper napkins. Everyone will enjoy watching the dinner crisp-fry and, once set up, it's super simple for the cook. This is a great patio meal.

Crispy Fish with Spicy Ginger-Lime Sauce

4 servings

*C*risping fish fillets for an ordinary supper shouldn't faze you a bit. This is the kind of Asian treat I favor with a serving of brilliantly colorful stir-fried veggies and a small bowl of steamed rice or noodles to catch the last drops of sauce.

BATTER
Tempura batter (page 132), or stir enough beer or tonic into ¹/₂ cup all-purpose flour to make a velvety coating

FISH
1¹/₂ pounds of any firm, thick, white fish fillets (Chilean sea bass, grouper, mahimahi, cod)

GINGER-LIME SAUCE
¹/₄ cup ginger preserves
juice of 2 limes
2 tablespoons soy sauce
1 small red chile, partially seeded and minced
2 teaspoons minced chives

Prepare batter according to Tempura recipe. Rinse and dry the fillets and make a few slashes in the flesh with a razor-sharp knife to allow the batter to run over a greater surface. Dip and fry the fish in the same manner as for Tempura.

Bring all sauce ingredients, except chives, to a simmer in a 2-cup glass measure in a microwave. Let it steep for a while. Taste and adjust the spiciness or sweet-sour balance to your taste. Warm the sauce and stir in the chives just before serving.

☯ Vegetable Fritters ☯

Makes enough batter for 4 servings

You can call them *pakoras or bhajjias,* or you can call them *perkedel,* or *philouries*—but I just call them delicious. They differ slightly from North and South India to Indonesia, but the batter is a snap to mix and it keeps in the refrigerator for a day or so. These tasty treats can début for company cocktails and the leftover batter can reappear the following day for lunch or supper with totally different ingredients. There are options for the batter as well as the vegetables, but the combination of half chickpea and half rice flour, thinned with soda, gives optimum results. As an alternative you could use all rice flour or all chickpea flour.

BATTER
- $1/2$ cup chickpea or all-purpose flour
- $1/2$ cup rice flour or cornstarch
- $1/4$ teaspoon baking soda
- $1/2$ teaspoon salt
- 1 teaspoon turmeric, $1/2$ teaspoon ground cumin, and $1/2$ teaspoon cayenne pepper; or $1 1/2$ teaspoons Curry Powder (page 25) and $1/4$ teaspoon cayenne pepper
- 1 cup club soda, tonic, or beer
- Optional: 1 tablespoon very finely minced scallion and garlic combined and/or 1 teaspoon peeled, grated ginger
- 1 quart peanut oil
- vegetables for frying (see below)

Combine the flours, baking soda, salt, and seasoning. Add the soda or tonic slowly, beating continuously, until the mixture flows like a medium cream sauce. Of course you can do this in the food processor, but it's so easy to mix by hand it seems pointless. Stir in the minced seasonings, if using, and blend thoroughly. Cover and let the batter stand at room temperature for at least 30 minutes, until you're ready to make the fritters.

Heat peanut oil in your wok to a temperature of 375° or use an electric fryer.

Blot the vegetables very dry and stir in just enough batter to hold them together. Scoop up a rounded tablespoon of the fritter mixture and slide it off into the hot oil with the tip of a teaspoon. Fry slowly until they're golden and crisp. Drain on paper towels and serve immediately, or hold in a slow 200° oven. You may also pre-fry the fritters like french-fried potatoes. Fry them halfway, leaving them aside at room temperature, and finish in hot oil just before serving.

• MIXED VEGETABLE FRITTERS: Whole chickpeas and chopped fresh spinach leaves; diced cooked peas, carrots, and turnip; cooked cut green beans; minced onion; and chopped red pepper.

• SINGLE VEGETABLE FRITTERS: Slices of cooked sweet or white potato; 1/4-inch slices of sweet onion separated into rings (these are the *best* onion rings ever and take a well-seasoned batter); lightly cooked cauliflower or broccoli florets; slices of plantain or underripe banana; slices of cooked beets; thinly sliced eggplant; hot pickled okra (blot okra dry and season batter cautiously—I like curry powder, minced garlic, and a pinch of cayenne).

✎ Serve these fritters with Cilantro and Mint Chutney, a sweet-sour dip of Indonesian soy sauce and rice vinegar, or well-drained yogurt whipped with lots of minced fresh mint and snipped chives.

✎ Fritters are wonderful supper accompaniments to grilled fish or sautéed lamb burgers.

✎ If you really want to please your dinner guests, make a teaser batch of fried okra, onion rings, and sticks of fontina cheese early in the day and finish them off while drinks are being prepared. The fritters are satisfying enough to keep tummies from rumbling while you get the dinner together, and they preclude any thought of a first course.

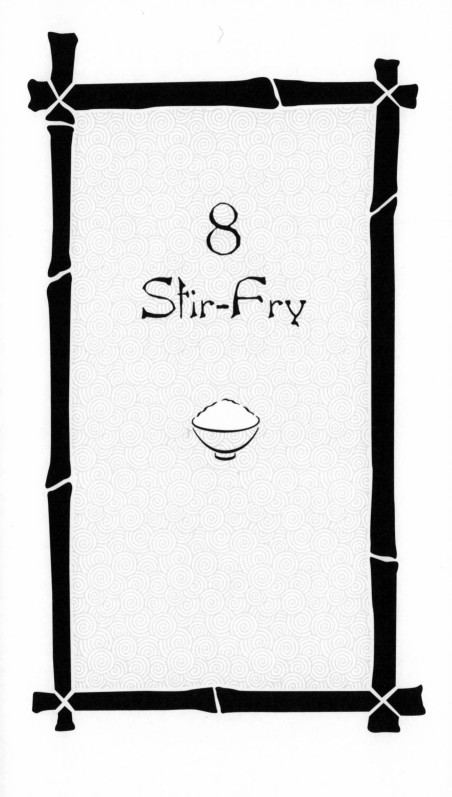

8
Stir-Fry

*T*he centuries-old Chinese method of express cooking, called stir-frying, produced the world's first fast food, a sensible technique for an agrarian diet and a solution to the basic dilemma of a scarce fuel supply. All people really needed was a market bouquet of ingredients; a light, hammered-steel wok; and a high-licking flame.

What is stir-fry cooking anyway? It's the constant flipping and tossing of bite-size pieces of food, in a small amount of oil, over very high heat. The reason for that forward slide and backward flip the professional chefs do so effortlessly is to minimize the time the food *feels* the intense heat of the wok. Quick and even cooking is the whole point of stir-frying. It sounds pretty simple, but producing a properly textured, perfectly cooked, glistening stir-fry can be a humbling experience—not because the wrist action is hard to master but because you have to be a highly organized, intensely focused, hyperactive control freak to pull it off. *But,* it's only for a couple of minutes. As soon as the wok is empty, you can revert to your usual cool demeanor.

THE PREPARATION
Cutting

If you master the simple slant-cut and perfect the familiar dice and slice, your stir-fries will cook properly and look acceptably authentic. You must, however, work with a sharp knife. Practice the slant-cut on a celery rib. Make a sharply diagonal slice at either end of the rib and, resting the tip of the cleaver on the cutting board, shift the handle so the blade lines up with the first cut. Now, tilt the blade backwards slightly, which will effect an even deeper slant. Keeping your fingertips curled under, slide the celery along under the rocking blade. You'll end up with uniform diagonal pieces of celery intended to expose more surface for even and fast cooking. This is the most important form-follows-function dictum in Chinese cooking. For express cooking, the decorative embellishments are best left to the pros.

A properly diced vegetable should be a small, meticulous chop no more than $1/2$-inch square. Cubes should be about $3/4$ inch and chunks 1 inch. A minced ingredient, like garlic or ginger, is worked through by the cleaver so often the pieces are miniscule. Shredding, or repetitive slicing, produces julienne strips, matchsticks, or slivers. Thin slices of meat should be $1/8$-inch thick, medium-thin slices $1/4$-inch thick. Meat should be sliced *against* the grain and fish *with* the grain. It's easier to slice meat thinly if it's partially frozen first.

Blanching

You'll need to blanch fibrous vegetables like carrots, broccoli or asparagus stems, turnips, celery, or green beans that might not cook through when they're briefly stir-fried. *Blanching* just means undercooking as a preface to finished cooking. You can microwave them for a few seconds in a splash of broth or water—sequentially according to the length of time each vegetable requires—or you can steam or parboil them for the brief time it takes to soften the raw edge but retain crispness. For example, carrots should be blanched for 1 minute, snow peas for 30 seconds. Run the veggies immediately under cold water and drain. Repetition will teach you the best timing. You can blanch ahead of time—even the night before. Once the prep is done, stir-fries take mere minutes to complete.

The Cooking

Unless you're using a nonstick pan, heat the wok until it's about to smoke *before* you add the oil. This forces the oil to "float" over the hot metal and prevents sticking. Remember to swirl the oil around the inside of the wok, as the entire surface of the pan is used in proper stir-frying. If you need more oil during the cooking, drizzle it down the side of the wok so it's hot when it reaches the food. Never overload the wok or the ingredients will sear unevenly and the vegetables will have a dull, steamed look instead of that appetizing bright glaze. It's better to work in relays, turning ingredients out into a large bowl as they're done and combining them all in the wok briefly at the end. If you stir-fry at the right pace, nothing has time to cool off. And, remember, over such high temperatures the food will continue cooking even after it has left the wok.

That's about all you need to *know*—now here's what you need to *do*.

BE ORGANIZED

✓ Read through the recipe and pull out all the ingredients along with a stack of small ingredient dishes. Clear off a space alongside the stove-top.

✓ Cut and marinate the meat, poultry, or seafood. Trim and cut the vegetables. Blanch the fibrous ones.

✓ Mince and combine the fresh seasonings, like garlic, ginger, and chile.

✓ Combine any dry seasonings, such as dried red pepper flakes, curry powder, or five-spice powder.

✓ If the recipe calls for it, combine the cornstarch and liquid.

✓ If broth is needed, have it ready in a measuring cup or pitcher.

✓ Stir-frying should be the last thing you do before diners sprint to the table.

✓ Don't answer the telephone—or the smoke alarm.

Eight Easy Steps to a Perfect Stir-Fry

1. Heat the wok to searing, add and swirl the oil.
2. Add combined fresh or dry seasonings.
3. Stir-fry the meat/poultry/seafood. Remove to a bowl.
4. Stir-fry the vegetables.

5. Add the combined liquid seasonings.
6. Return meat/poultry/seafood to wok.
7. Thicken the sauce, if required.
8. Serve immediately!

Stir-Fry Troubleshooting

✎ *Too Watery* means vegetables were not dry when they went into the wok or not enough cornstarch was added to bind the liquid

✎ *Too Sticky* means too much cornstarch—try thinning out with more broth

✎ *Vegetables Not Brightly Colored* means the wok and the oil weren't hot enough

✎ *Some Vegetables Not Crisp* means some should have been blanched before stir-frying, or there was too much food in the wok at once.

Once you've mastered it, I urge you to delve inventively into stir-frying. It's the most exuberant and dazzling technique in the art of Chinese cooking. Here are some start-up samples of basic dishes from which you can extrapolate endlessly.

Ground Beef with Sweet Onions and Green Beans

Serves 4

This recipe brings the flexibility of the stir-fry about as close to home as you can get. It was my solution one night to the frustration of having little in the house except a partially thawed hamburger and a bag of frozen baby green beans. Sound familiar? Try this after you've stocked your kitchen with a few of the Asian essentials but you're not up to facing a whole new ritual. Serve with plain rice or wheat vermicelli.

1 tablespoon Chinese Seasoning Oil (page 23)

The Fresh Seasonings
3 garlic cloves, crushed and minced

The Meat
1 1/2 pounds ground chuck
Chinese Salt and Pepper (page 24)

The Vegetables
1 large sweet onion, rings separated and cut in 1-inch
squares
2 cups frozen baby green beans, thawed and blotted dry

The Liquid Seasonings
2 tablespoons oyster sauce
2 tablespoons soy sauce
2 teaspoons cornstarch, dissolved in 1/4 cup beef broth

Heat the wok. Add the oil and heat. Add the garlic and stir-fry for about 15 seconds. Add the meat and stir-fry, pressing out large clumps, until there's no raw meat showing. Remove the beef to a bowl. Pour off any drippings, leaving just enough oil for frying the onion.

Add the onion and stir-fry over high heat until it wilts slightly, retaining some crispness. It should pick up a few charred patches. Reduce the heat slightly and add the green beans. Shake and toss briefly. Return the meat to the wok, then add the oyster and soy sauces. Push the wok contents aside and drizzle in the cornstarch mixture one-half at a time, which will allow you to control the quantity of sauce as well as its consistency. If sauce is too thick, add more broth. Serve immediately.

✐ If you're buying the chuck specifically for this recipe, select the meat in a single piece and ask the butcher to grind it only once.

☯ Korean Bulgogi ☯

Serves 4

*T*raditionally, the marinated beef is grilled on a tabletop griddle. With a quick hand and a hot wok, you can successfully stir-fry it. Serve it with a piping hot bowl of rice and the spicy dipping sauce.

$1^1/_2$ **pounds beef tenderloin or flank steak, partially frozen for easy slicing**

The Marinade
6 scallions, slant-cut at $^1/_8$-inch intervals, including 2 inches of green
3 garlic cloves, crushed
2 quarter-size coins of peeled ginger, crushed
3 tablespoons dark soy sauce
2 tablespoons rice wine or sake
$1^1/_2$ teaspoons sugar
2 teaspoons cracked or freshly ground black pepper
1 tablespoon sesame seeds, toasted and crushed
2 teaspoons toasted sesame oil

The Cooking Oil
$1^1/_2$ tablespoons peanut oil or Chinese Seasoning Oil (page 23)

The Dipping Sauce
slivered scallions, for garnish
Korean Table Seasoning (page 28)

Cut the tenderloin against the grain into very thin slices or strips. If you're using flank steak, cut the meat with the grain into 3 lengthwise strips before slicing it against the grain. Combine the marinade ingredients, add the beef strips, cover, and refrigerate for at least 3 hours.

Heat the wok and add the peanut oil. Stir-fry the meat over high heat, searing it quickly for no more than 1 minute. Do not overcook. Serve immediately with slivered scallions scattered on top and individual dishes of table seasoning.

Super Express

MUSSELS: Let scrubbed mussels open in a piping-hot dry wok or skillet for 1 to 2 minutes. Tap the stubborn ones to nudge them along. Discard any unopened mussels. Remove the mussels to a serving dish lined with a layer of hot steamed rice and set them up on their hinges. Whisk about 2 teaspoons of oyster sauce per serving into the pan juices along with some grated ginger, minced garlic, and snipped chives. Drizzle the sauce over the mussels.

SEA SCALLOPS: Blot sea scallops dry with a paper towel, then dip them in a beaten egg (or just the white) and then in Japanese bread crumbs *(panko)*, pressing the crumbs in well. Shallow-fry in 375° oil until they're golden. Drain on paper towels and serve with mayonnaise spiked with finely grated lime zest and a squirt of Thai chile sauce.

FISH FILLETS: Steam firm white fish fillets (mahimahi, sea bass) in the microwave with 2 tablespoons per serving of unsweetened coconut milk seasoned with mild or hot curry powder. Serve with baby new potatoes and petite peas.

GOAN FISH SAUCE: Sauté thinly sliced onion with 1 minced garlic clove, 1/4 teaspoon ground ginger, 1 teaspoon turmeric, and cayenne pepper to taste. Serve over steamed or grilled fish fillets.

Scallops with Pork and Black Beans

☯ ☯

Serves 4

*S*callops and shrimp are, for me, the quintessential stir-fry elements. Nature made them just the right size, they're well behaved in the heat of the wok, and they're perfect with Asian seasonings. This is a livelier adaptation of a Cantonese classic enriched with a little ground pork. Serve with plain rice.

The Cooking Oil
2 tablespoons peanut oil

The Fresh and Dried Seasonings
1 teaspoon crushed and minced garlic
1 teaspoon minced fresh ginger
^{1}/$_2$ teaspoon freshly ground Szechuan pepper or white
   pepper
pinch of sugar

The Meat and Seafood
^{1}/$_4$ pound ground pork loin
1^1/$_2$ pounds bay scallops, drained and blotted dry

The Vegetables
5 scallions, slivered, including some green
1 tablespoon Chinese fermented black beans

The Liquid Seasoning
2 tablespoons oyster sauce
^{1}/$_2$ cup Asian Chicken Broth (page 81), or low-sodium
   canned

The Thickening
1 tablespoon cornstarch dissolved in 3 tablespoons
   chicken broth

Heat the wok, then add the oil. Add the garlic and ginger and stir-fry briefly to soften. Add the pepper and sugar. Add the pork and stir and toss, pressing out any clumps. As soon as the meat is cooked through and granular in appearance, remove it to a bowl. Add the scallops and stir-fry in the hot wok, adding a drizzle of oil if needed. Toss and stir until the scallops are opaque and firm. Add the scallions, black beans, oyster sauce, and broth; stir to combine. When the mixture is simmering, add the cornstarch mixture and stir until thickened. Taste and adjust the seasoning.

Bronzed Shrimp with Jasmine Rice

☯   ☯

Serves 4

This is a very easy and unusual Vietnamese stir-fry that can also be prepared with chicken or pork. The caramel syrup can be made ahead and stored in the cupboard for several weeks, so it's a versatile recipe to add to your repertoire.

The Caramel Syrup
1/2 cup sugar
1/2 cup plus 2 tablespoons water

The Rice
1 1/2 cups jasmine rice
2 1/4 cups water
1 1/4 teaspoons salt

The Cooking Oil
2 tablespoons peanut oil

The Fresh and Dried Seasonings
6 large garlic cloves, crushed and minced
3 large shallots, sliced
2–4 dried hot chiles, or 1/4 teaspoon dried red pepper flakes
1/2 teaspoon freshly ground black pepper

The Seafood
1 1/2 pounds medium shrimp, peeled

The Liquid Seasoning
2 teaspoons fish sauce (*nuoc mam* or *nam pla*)

The Garnish
2 scallions, trimmed and finely sliced, including 2 inches
  of green
1 tablespoon chopped cilantro

Prepare the caramel syrup. Put the sugar and 1/2 cup of water in a 2-cup glass measuring cup and boil it, uncovered, in the microwave on high for 12 minutes. The syrup will be deep gold but will turn to a rich brown after it leaves the oven. If not, return it for another minute. After you remove it from the heat, wait a couple of minutes; when it stops foaming, *slowly* dribble in the 2 tablespoons water, pausing between dribbles and stirring vigorously all the while. Let the syrup cool, and reserve 2 teaspoons for recipe. Store remainder in a screwtop jar. (You can also make this in a heavy saucepan or skillet on the top of the stove, which takes just as long and you'll have a sticky pan to wash.) Makes 1/2 cup syrup.

Put the rice, water, and 1 teaspoon salt in a heavy pan with a tight-fitting lid. Bring the rice quickly to a boil, reduce the heat to its lowest point, cover, and cook for 15 minutes. Turn off the heat and let the rice rest for another 5 minutes.

Heat the wok. Heat the oil over medium-high heat. Stir-fry the garlic, shallots, chiles, pepper, and remaining 1/4 teaspoon salt for about 30 seconds. Add the shrimp and fish sauce and stir-fry until the shrimp are tender-cooked and the fish sauce is absorbed. Add the reserved caramel syrup. Garnish with the scallions and cilantro, and serve immediately with the hot rice.

If you're *only* going to use the caramel syrup for Asian cooking, substitute fish sauce for the 2 tablespoons of water and hold your nose. A few drops of pure lime oil or 1/4 teaspoon grated lime zest would also be a smart addition. This way you save a couple of steps when you whip up some caramel chicken or pork. The trade-off for the shortcut is that the caramel will be cloudy and won't provide the lovely gloss to the dish.

Salmon with Seared Celery ☯ and Sugar Snap Peas ☯

Serves 4

*N*ow that sugar snap peas are widely available, I often use them in lieu of snow peas, not only because they have more flavor but also because their greater bulk gives the stir-fry a pleasing dimension. As for lackluster celery, it really snaps to attention seared in a hot wok and teamed with spicy salmon.

1½ **pounds salmon, boned steaks or thick fillets**

The Marinade
2 tablespoons mushroom soy sauce
1 teaspoon peeled and grated ginger with the juice

The Cooking Oil
1 tablespoon Chinese Seasoning Oil (page 23)

The Fresh Seasonings
1 teaspoon minced garlic
½ **teaspoon minced fresh hot green chile**

The Vegetables
4 celery ribs, strings peeled and slant-cut
5 ounces sugar snap peas, blanched
¼ **sweet yellow pepper, diced**
4 scallions, slant-cut, including 2 inches of green

The Liquid Seasonings
2 teaspoons soy sauce
2 teaspoons hoisin sauce
2 teaspoons Chinese yellow rice wine or sake

¹/₄ cup Asian Chicken Broth or Quickly Seasoned Canned
    Broth (pages 81, 82)
1¹/₂ teaspoons cornstarch, dissolved in 1 tablespoon water

Remove any skin from the salmon and cut into 1-inch chunks.
Combine the mushroom soy sauce and ginger and marinate the
salmon for at least 1 hour.

Heat the wok and add the oil. When it's hot, add the garlic and
chile and stir-fry for a couple of seconds. Add the salmon chunks,
tossing and flipping until the flesh turns opaque. Remove to a bowl.
Add more oil if necessary, and sear the celery until it's crisp-tender.
Add the rest of the vegetables and stir-fry until hot. Return the
salmon to the wok and add the soy sauce, hoisin sauce, wine, and
broth. Push the wok ingredients to one side; stir the cornstarch mixture, then drizzle into the wok and cook until the sauce is thickened.

Confetti Vegetables with Chicken

☯   ☯

Serves 4

With the popularity of Hunan and Szechuan provincial cooking, we've almost forgotten how delicious an abundant,
colorful Cantonese vegetable stir-fry can be. I've added chicken to
this recipe, which could just as easily be golden strips of fried tofu.
Without the chicken, these vegetables would be a sparkling accompaniment to a simple grilled fish or a thick and juicy lamb chop.
Any compatible selection of vegetables can be used—all garden
fresh would be wonderful, but I've included a couple traditional
Chinese canned ones for sentiment's sake.

**4 whole boneless and skinless chicken breasts, cut into
    strips**

The Marinade
2 tablespoons soy sauce
1 tablespoon Chinese yellow rice wine or sake
1 teaspoon Asian sesame oil

The Cooking Oil
1 tablespoon peanut oil or Chinese Seasoning Oil (page 23)

The Fresh Seasonings
2 garlic cloves, crushed and minced
3 quarter-size coins of peeled ginger, crushed and minced

The Vegetables
2 young carrots, slant-cut and blanched
1 cup baby bok choy stalks, slant-cut and blanched
1 cup broccoli florets, separated into walnut-size pieces and blanched
16 snow pea pods, ends cut and strings removed, blanched
1 sweet red pepper, diced into $1/2$-inch pieces, blanched
1 medium yellow squash, sliced into half rounds, blanched
12 whole canned Chinese baby corn
6 scallions, slant-cut, white part only
16 canned Chinese straw mushrooms
$1/4$ cup sliced water chestnuts, fresh or canned

The Liquid Seasonings
$1/2$ cup Asian Chicken Broth (page 81) or canned vegetable broth
1 tablespoon Chinese yellow rice wine or sake
1 teaspoon Asian sesame oil

The Dry Seasonings
$1/2$ teaspoon sugar
$1/4$ teaspoon white pepper
$1^1/2$ teaspoons cornstarch, dissolved in 1 tablespoon broth

Combine the marinade ingredients and marinate the chicken for at least 30 minutes.

Heat the wok. Heat and swirl the oil. When it's hot, stir-fry the garlic and ginger for 1 minute. Add the chicken and cook until the meat is opaque. Remove it to a bowl.

Stir-fry the vegetables in 2 batches, if necessary, so the wok is never overloaded. Stir in the broth, wine, sesame oil, sugar, and pepper. Combine all the vegetables and the chicken. Stir the cornstarch mixture, then add to wok. Cook briefly until thickened and serve.

Hunan Steak with Watercress

Serves 4

*U*nlike the French, the Chinese *cook* watercress, which is just assertive enough to balance the intensely flavored beef in this dish. You can also prepare this dish with spinach, chard, kale, or mustard greens.

I'm slipping a new technique into the stir-fry equation, called *slippery-coating*, which is a tenderizing method particularly effective for the more fibrous cuts of beef like flank steak. It shouldn't throw you off your stride, but if you're brand new to the stir-fry process, you might want to save making this recipe for when you have the basics down to a routine.

The Meat and Coating
1 pound flank steak
1 large egg white
2 teaspoons cornstarch, dissolved in 2 tablespoons rice wine or sake
$^1/_2$ teaspoon sugar
$^1/_2$ teaspoon Chinese Salt and Pepper (page 24)
2 teaspoons peanut oil

The Vegetable
2 bunches watercress

The Seasonings
1 teaspoon minced ginger
1 tablespoon minced garlic
1 tablespoon minced scallions, white part only
2 teaspoons chopped dried red chile, with the seeds

The Thickening
$4^1/_2$ tablespoons rice wine or sake
1 tablespoon dark soy sauce
2 teaspoons cornstarch
2 teaspoons Asian sesame oil

The Cooking Oil
2 cups peanut oil
Chinese Salt and Pepper

Cut the flank steak *against* the grain into segments 3 to 4 inches in length. Seal each segment in plastic wrap and partially freeze for about 30 minutes to make the meat easier to cut. Slice each segment *with* the grain into $^1/_4$-inch slices, then cut the slices like carrot sticks. Put the beef strips into a bowl and add the coating ingredients in the order listed. Work the coating into the meat with your fingers. Refrigerate the beef, which helps to set the coating, for 30 minutes or longer.

Trim the heavy stems from the watercress and cut it into 3-inch lengths. Combine the seasonings in one small dish and the thickening mixture in another.

Heat the wok. Heat the peanut oil to 300°. Add the beef and stir it in the oil for about 15 seconds. The beef will be gray, not brown. Strain it from the oil and set aside. Pour off all but a couple of tablespoons of oil.

Reheat the oil left in the wok. Add the watercress and stir and toss quickly. Add the remaining $^1/_2$ tablespoon wine and the salt and pepper. Stir and toss for 5 or 6 seconds, then turn out onto a warmed serving dish large enough to hold the meat on one side and the watercress on the other.

Add another tablespoon of oil to the wok and heat it, but not too hot this time. Add the ginger-garlic mixture and stir-fry for a few seconds to soften. Add the beef and toss and stir; don't sear the meat. It should be rare inside and barely brown on the outside. Sprinkle it with the salt and pepper. Stir the thickening mixture, turn up the heat, and add to the wok. Bring the mixture quickly to a simmer, until the sauce thickens a little. Turn the meat out next to the cress and serve immediately.

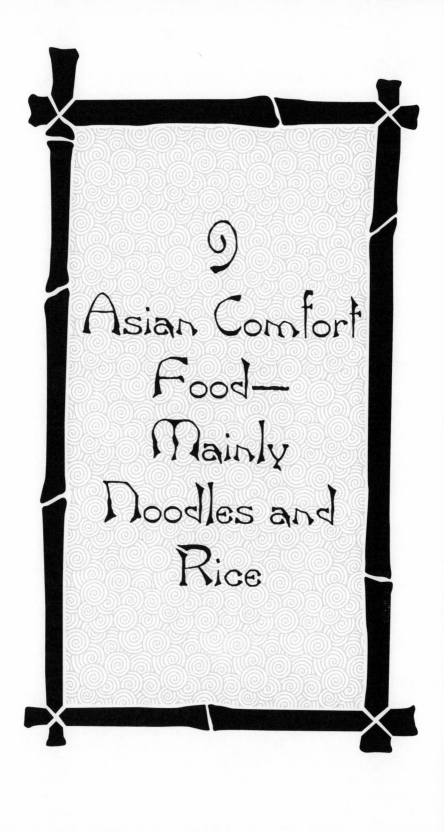

9

Asian Comfort
Food—
Mainly
Noodles and
Rice

*R*ice and noodles, oodles of rice and noodles. Rice or noodles for breakfast, lunch, dinner, and in-between. Rice and noodles are the fast food and staff of life of Asia, hawked by street vendors and magically, dexterously, slurped and shoveled in cafés and noodle shops everywhere. Rice is divine, a gift from the gods; and noodles—well, they were a gift from China.

It's hard to comprehend that Asians consume *eighteen times* as much rice per capita each year as do Americans. We can't even manage to eat what rice we grow and have to ship most of our excellent Carolina, Texas, and Mississippi Delta rice abroad. Although there was a brilliant rice cuisine in our past, we are just beginning to catch on to the interesting nuances of flavors and textures. American growers are doing their best to fire our interest by introducing hybrids combining the best qualities of American long-grain rice with the unique flavors and aromas of Asian rice, like jasmine and basmati. The sweet and nutty aroma of steaming jasmine or basmati rice can bring you to the table when you didn't know you were hungry. I encourage you to get beyond the box of standard processed rice that falls into your shopping cart and experiment with some of the more exotic varieties.

As for Asian noodles, the noodle section of an Asian market can send you into a tailspin of confusion and indecision. What *are* all those unfamiliar sticks and bundles? Some look and snap like shipping box straps and others are gathered and tied so artistically they should hang around your neck. The best advice I can offer is, take it slow and learn to handle the milky white dried rice noodle first, which you've probably enjoyed often in Thai and Vietnamese restaurants. All rice noodles have an appealing nondoughy chewiness that keeps the robust seasonings from being muffled. The rice stick noodle, resembling a thinner fettuccine, and rice vermicelli, just as thin as its namesake, are the noodles to use for most saucy Asian dishes.

When it comes to comfort food, the hands-down winner is the weirdly unattractive, but pristinely white, fresh rice noodle sheet. It's stocked in Asian markets in a sealed plastic bag, folded over like lasagna dough, sort of slimy and unyielding until it's cut into strips and quickly steamed. Like magic, the strips metamorphose into the most unctuous, slithery, yummy noodle ever. They can become a serious addiction.

The Japanese have elevated noodle making to an art form, and the eggless buckwheat soba is particularly worth your attention. The nutty taste and smooth texture makes it especially good for cold dipping and Asian salads. To my taste, the starchy udon so popular in those unpleasant little instant noodle cups tastes like extruded library paste. Perhaps the homemade udon has more to redeem it.

As for dried wheat noodles, I see no superiority in packaged Asian noodles over Italian.

DRIED NOODLES

RICE STICK OR RIBBON NOODLES: Most commonly imported from Vietnam under the Vietnamese name *banh pho.* These noodles aren't boiled—in fact, if they're overcooked, they will disintegrate. Just soak the rice sticks in boiling water until they're pliable. Lay the noodles out flat in a rectangular baking dish and pour boiling water over them. You have to test them frequently for the right texture because the timing will vary depending upon the age and dryness of the noodle. It won't take long—never more than 30 minutes. If you plan to stir-fry them, be sure to keep them chewy or they'll turn to mush in the wok. If you're using them cold, drain them as soon as they're soft enough to slurp.

RICE VERMICELLI: These noodles can be hot-water soaked and drained in the same manner as the rice sticks. They are so thin that you don't need to heat water at all if your tap water is very hot. They will soften in less than 10 minutes. When dry rice vermicelli is dunked in hot oil, it instantly puffs and fluffs into pure white curly fleece—the familiar "wool" in Chinese wooly lamb, the crispy *mee* in Thai *mee krob,* and a delightful crumble atop Asian salads.

To fry rice vermicelli, do it in small batches. If you try to put a large amount of vermicelli in the fryer or wok at one time it will swell up over the top and startle you. If you want a large bed of this wooly wonder, use the wok and a thermometer. If the oil isn't on the upside of 375°, the noodles won't puff; and if the oil is too hot, they'll brown before they puff. Test a few strands before you drop in the rest. These are so good it's worth playing around with them. They make a wonderful bed for grilled kebabs or an attractive nest for first courses. You do need to crumble the fried noodle with your fingers to get a workable volume, but don't try breaking them before they're cooked or you'll cut yourself. Use scissors.

CELLOPHANE OR GLASS NOODLES: The cellophane or glass noodle isn't made from rice. It is extruded from mung bean paste and the package is often marked "mung bean noodles" or "bean threads." They're transparent when cooked and have a viscous quality that I'm not fond of, but they're useful for bulking out the fillings for garden rolls or spring rolls and for adding substance to clear broth soups. I don't recommend them for stir-fries, where their bland elasticity and tendency to clump over high heat adds nothing special to the dish. Soak and drain them like rice noodles. They'll soften in less time.

DRIED SOBA NOODLES: I've read a lot of hocus-pocus about cooking Japanese soba noodles, but I just cook them in 3 or 4 quarts of boiling salted water for a couple of minutes and that works just fine.

Fresh Noodles

RICE SHEET NOODLES: Rinse off the folded bundle, but don't try to open it flat or the noodle will break on the fold. Cut wide ribbons straight through the wad and then pull them apart into single thicknesses. You don't need to soak these noodles if you're using them in a stir-fry, because the minute they feel steam from the broth they soften dramatically and *fast*. You definitely want to preserve the chewy quality in all rice noodles, but these fresh ones especially require TLC.

CHINESE EGG NOODLES: The fresh egg and flour noodles are certainly worth experimenting with if you're shopping in an Asian market, but like all fresh pasta, they're only as good as the maker. If you have a favorite Italian pasta shop, stick with their fettuccine or vermicelli. If you're fortunate enough to live near an Asian shop where they're homemade, that's a noodle of a different color.

If the egg noodles are very thin, cook as soba noodles; otherwise, add a minute or two to the cooking time. In other words, cook like Italian pasta.

Rice

Just because there are whole books written about rice doesn't mean you need an encyclopedic knowledge of this super grain to cook a proper Asian meal. It's a much less complex subject than the care and feeding of noodles because we have far fewer choices of grain here than in Asia. Just remember that cooked short grains are the most glutinous and sticky; medium grains are gently cohesive; and long grains are separate and fluffy.

FOR CHINESE AND JAPANESE DISHES: Short or medium white rice is the rule. The rice will stick to the chopsticks, and the food morsels to the rice. Either imported or American rice will do but for Japanese sushi it's best to look for the short grain specifically intended for that dish.

FOR INDIAN DISHES: The nutty imported basmati rice is available not only in ten-pound burlap sacks in Indian and Asian markets but, for a lot more money, boxed in some supermarkets and specialty food stores. Natural foods stores often carry it in bulk—it may be imported or just an admirable American imposter.

FOR THAI DISHES: The slender aromatic jasmine rice is preferred in Thailand. Although it's a long-grain rice, it's soft and the grains adhere to each other. The sweetly feminine quality of jasmine rice complements the macho seasoning of the Thai cuisine.

Medium-grain white rice is the best all-purpose choice for Pan-Asian cooking, whereas glutinous short-grain rice is primarily a specialty rice used for stuffings, sushi, and desserts. Brown rice is seldom used in Asia.

☯ Just Plain Rice ☯

Makes 3 cups cooked rice

To rinse and soak, or not to rinse and soak? If you're using American rice, there's nothing to rinse off except, possibly, some of the nutrients. If it's imported Asian rice, you can assume it's been coated with talc or cornstarch so rinsing *is* recommended. Put the rice in a fine-mesh, long-handled sieve and rest it in a bowl of water for a minute—or longer if you're busy. When you're ready to cook the rice, let cool tap water run through it for about 30 seconds while rubbing the rice lightly between your fingers. I see no reason for the long soaking of rice, but if you're a dedicated soaker, I guess there's no harm in it, either.

1 cup long-grain white rice
1¹/₂ cups water
¹/₂ teaspoon salt

Bring the rice, water, and salt to a rapid boil. Reduce the heat to the lowest point—using a flame tamer if possible—place the lid on the pot, and cook the rice for 15 minutes. Lift the lid and if the water is absorbed, replace it and let the rice rest, off the flame, for another 5 minutes. If the water has not yet been absorbed, cook for another couple of minutes before letting it rest.

✐ Although this is the water-to-rice ratio that has always worked best for me, rice is no more equal than the personal preferences for chewy or soft grains. I have a basmati rice in my pantry right now that cooks up so fast, and perfectly, I can hardly believe it. If you were to cook medium-grain jasmine rice for the same length of time as Carolina long-grain, you'd have rice pudding. Adjust the amount of water and cooking time to the particular rice you're using and to your own texture preference.

✐ COCONUT RICE: Simply use unsweetened coconut milk in lieu of water. Interesting variations come instantly to mind, depending upon how you plan to use the rice. Grated lime zest is a good foil for the natural sweetness of coconut, or add sautéed shallots and chopped toasted macadamia nuts. A judicious touch of allspice or ground cardamom would be nice, and so would thin ribbons of fresh basil or mint.

✐ CURRIED COCONUT RICE: Melt a tablespoon of butter in the rice pot and add $1/2$ teaspoon curry powder. Add the rice and stir until all the grains are coated. Add the coconut milk—or chicken broth, if you prefer—and cook as above.

Fried Rice

The best fried rice I ever put in my mouth was merely a casual side dish at Mr. Chow's in London, a trendsetting restaurant back in the late 1960s and 1970s and still flourishing today. That's the moment I discovered that fried rice wasn't a brown, oil-slicked excuse for unloading leftovers but a country bouquet in a rice bowl—a discovery made indelible by the amusement of having splendid Chinese food served by cheeky Italian waiters. There isn't a cook in Asia who doesn't have a personal fried rice recipe, so if it isn't a regular choice in your home, perhaps I can help you make it one.

☯ Duck Fried Rice ☯

Serves 4

This is a wonderful way to use doggy-bag duck from a Chinese restaurant—and you get the leftover rice, too.

2 tablespoons American sesame or safflower oil

3 garlic cloves, crushed and minced

3 quarter-size coins of peeled ginger, crushed and minced

6 fresh shiitake mushrooms, stemmed and diced

$^{1}/_{2}$ cup slivered snow peas, ends and strings removed

1 young carrot, cut into quarters lengthwise, diced, and
blanched

$^{1}/_{4}$ cup diced sweet red pepper

$^{1}/_{2}$ cup diced baby pattypan or yellow crookneck squash
(optional)

$^{1}/_{4}$ cup water chestnuts or jicama in $^{1}/_{4}$-inch dices

6 scallions, trimmed and thinly sliced

$^{1}/_{2}$ teaspoon Chinese Salt and Pepper (page 24)

2 cups shredded cooked duck, with some crispy skin

3 cups day-old cooked rice

1 tablespoon Asian sesame oil

$^{1}/_{4}$ cup hot chicken broth, if required

Heat the wok. Add the oil and swirl it. When it is hot, add the garlic and ginger and stir-fry until soft. Add the mushrooms and snow
peas and stir-fry a few seconds. Reduce the heat. Add the rest of the
ingredients except the rice, two-by-two, in the order listed.
(Adding the ingredients slowly will prevent the wok from cooling
down. Add the vegetables requiring longest cooking time first.) Stir
in the rice and sesame oil and combine well. If the dish seems too
dry or sticks to the pan, drizzle in a little hot broth to create
enough steam to moisten it. Fried rice should be fluffy, not wet or
clumped together.

✎ Mix 3 tablespoons soy sauce and either a few drops of chile
oil, a minced fresh chile, or a squeeze of Thai chile sauce. Serve this
sauce on the side for those who prefer spicy food, or who want to
eat some of their rice pure, and some sullied with soy sauce.

✎ This same recipe can be used for other fried rice. Substitute
shrimp and chicken, or chicken and Chinese barbecued pork for
the duck, and use asparagus tips, baby spinach, or slivered chard
for the snow peas and minced bok choy for the water chestnuts—
or keep it vegetarian and add diced tofu.

✂ THAI FRIED RICE: Lump crab meat and slivered Black Forest ham or crispy bacon bits would be a typical substitute for the duck. Add minced shallots along with the garlic and ginger, and for the vegetables, use bean sprouts, sweet red pepper, and slivered red and green chiles. Add a tablespoon of fish sauce while stir-frying the vegetables and add in thin egg ribbons made with 2 eggs just before serving: see Quick Pad Thai procedure on page 167.

✂ MALAYSIAN FRIED RICE: Use leftover coconut rice and shrimp instead of duck. For the veggies, use blanched carrots, thawed frozen peas, and slivered napa cabbage. Add 1 teaspoon of Thai chile sauce or 1/2 teaspoon chile paste to fire it up, and instead of the egg ribbons, top each serving of rice with a fried egg, sunny-side up. Don't forget the fish sauce.

Fiery Garlic Shrimp with Cilantro

☯   ☯

Serves 4

If you have rice stick noodles and chile sauce in your cupboard, all you need to pick up is the shrimp, a bag of mixed salad greens, and plenty of paper napkins. Some well-iced Asian beer would be ideal.

12 ounces rice stick noodles, soaked in boiling water until pliable, about 15 minutes
2 tablespoons Chinese Seasoning Oil (page 23)
6 garlic cloves, crushed and minced
1 1/2 pounds large fresh shrimp in their shells, legs removed
1 tablespoon Thai chile sauce or other Asian hot sauce, to taste
2 tablespoons catsup
1 tablespoon light or dark brown sugar
1 tablespoon Thai fish sauce *(nam pla)*
1 tablespoon fresh lime juice
1/4 cup chopped cilantro
2 tablespoons minced chives or scallions

While the noodles soak, heat the wok. Add the oil, then the garlic and cook and stir until the garlic softens. Add the shrimp and flip and toss over medium-high heat until they turn pink. Add the chile sauce, catsup, brown sugar, fish sauce, and lime juice. Stir to coat the shrimp. Turn up the heat and flip and toss the shrimp again until the sauce forms a caramelized glaze over the shells and charred spots appear. Slide the shrimp onto a warm pie plate and sprinkle with the cilantro. Sprinkle the chives over the noodles and heat them in the unwashed wok, scraping any remaining shrimp sauce into the noodles. Serve the shrimp over the noodles.

Marco's Cathay Noodles and ☯ Spicy Meatballs ☯

Serves 4

*F*ew dishes are better than fresh tomato sauce on pasta, with plump and zesty meatballs, but this Asian rice noodle variation comes close.

2 boneless and skinless chicken breast halves
¹/₂ pound boneless pork, with some fat
4 garlic cloves, crushed and minced
1¹/₂ tablespoons Indonesian soy sauce (*ketjap manis*)
2 teaspoons ground white pepper
cornstarch, sifted
2 tablespoons peanut oil
1 tablespoon sake
2 teaspoons minced, peeled ginger
4 large shallots, minced
3 large ripe tomatoes, peeled, seeded, and chopped
2 teaspoons sugar
2 tablespoons fish sauce (*nam pla* or *nuoc mam*)
3 tablespoons sake or Chinese yellow rice wine
1 teaspoon Asian sesame oil
12 ounces rice stick noodles, soaked and drained, or fresh egg noodles, cooked
¹/₄ cup thin ribbons of basil or mint leaves

Process the chicken and meat with the garlic, soy sauce, and pepper until it clumps together under the blade. Do not process to a mousse-like paste. Alternatively, buy the chicken and pork already ground and combine well with your fingers. Lightly oil your hands and form the meat into about 24 walnut-size balls and roll them directly onto a plate of cornstarch.

Heat the wok. Add the peanut oil. When it's hot, sauté the meatballs over medium-high heat for 3 minutes, or until they're brown and crusty. Add the sake, cover the wok, and braise the meatballs for another 2 to 3 minutes. Remove them with a slotted spoon.

Add the ginger and shallots to the remaining oil and pan juices and stir-fry briefly. Add the tomatoes, sugar, fish sauce, sake or rice wine, and salt and pepper. Stir and cook over high heat until the sauce has reduced but is still chunky. Add the sesame oil. Toss the noodles in the sauce and heat through. Serve with the warm meatballs and garnish with the basil or mint ribbons.

✂ You'll have a few meatballs left over. Freeze them to serve as canapés with a sweet-and-sour dip.

Baby Clams with Bacon and Oyster Sauce

Serves 4

Thailand exports so many baby clams that they're even distributed in the United States under popular Italian labels. Whether you're making spaghetti *alle vongole* or rice vermicelli with *hoy lai*, fresh Manila clams from a reliable seafood market are the most succulent choice, but the canned baby clams are surprisingly sweet and tender. Asian markets carry the direct imports at a better price. It's a handy specialty item to have on your shelf.

3 tablespoons finely diced slab bacon
2 garlic cloves, crushed and minced
3 shallots, minced
$^1/_4$ teaspoon dried red pepper flakes (optional)

1 tablespoon fish sauce (*nam pla* or *nuoc mam*)
2 tablespoons oyster sauce
2 teaspoons fresh lemon juice
2 10-ounce cans baby clams, with broth and enough water
   to make ¹/₂ cup
2 teaspoons cornstarch, dissolved in 1 tablespoon water
4 ounces rice vermicelli, soaked and drained
2 tablespoons diced sweet red pepper, for garnish

Heat the wok and crisp-fry the bacon bits. Pour off all but a couple teaspoons of the bacon fat. Add a teaspoon of seasoning oil and heat it. When hot, stir-fry the garlic, shallots, and pepper flakes until the shallots are soft. Add the fish sauce, oyster sauce, and lemon juice. Bring quickly to a simmer.

Add the clams and their broth. When the clams are hot, push them aside and drizzle in the cornstarch mixture. As soon as it's thickened and clear, toss the vermicelli with the sauce and garnish with the red pepper.

✒ This would be an equally delicious dish if you substituted diced Chinese sausage for the bacon. Steam-soften it in the microwave for a couple of minutes before stir-frying. Since the sausage is somewhat sweet, I recommend using at least some of the optional red pepper flakes.

☯ # Quick Pad Thai ☯

Serves 4

*T*he trouble with this delectable noodle dish is that I can't resist ordering it every time I go to a Thai restaurant, denying myself the opportunity to try new things. The solution? Learn to make a quick *pad thai* at home.

2 large eggs, whisked with 1 teaspoon water
3 tablespoons peanut oil
6 garlic cloves, crushed and minced
4 shallots, minced

1 teaspoon shrimp paste

¼ teaspoon chile powder or cayenne pepper

1 tablespoon light brown sugar

2 teaspoons grated lime zest

2 tablespoons fresh lime juice

3 tablespoons fish sauce (*nam pla* or *nuoc mam*)

¾ pound cooked shrimp, coarsely chopped

1⅓ cups bean sprouts

6 scallions, trimmed and thinly sliced, including 2 inches
   of green

12 ounces rice stick noodles, soaked

¼ cup finely chopped dry-roasted, unsalted peanuts

3 tablespoons chopped cilantro

dried red pepper flakes

Pour the whisked egg, one-half at a time, into a hot nonstick skillet and swirl it around so that it forms a tissue-thin coating. As soon as the omelet is dry on the top, slide it out and roll it up. When both omelets have cooled, slice the rolls into thin ribbons, fluff them out, and set aside for garnish.

Heat the wok. Add the oil and heat. When hot, add the garlic, shallots, and shrimp paste and cook until the shallots are softened. Add the chile powder, brown sugar, and lime zest and combine.

When the sugar starts to melt, add the lime juice and fish sauce. Add the shrimp and heat them through. Add the bean sprouts and scallions, cook for 1 minute, and then toss in the noodles, peanuts, and cilantro. Serve immediately, with the omelet ribbons on top and a dish of red pepper flakes to add to taste.

✄ Here's how you can turn this recipe into a good approximation of another favorite, Singapore noodles. Delete the shrimp paste and chile powder, and add a rounded ½ teaspoon curry powder. Use half-cooked chicken or pork, and add 1 tablespoon rinsed and chopped Chinese black beans and ⅓ cup frozen petite peas.

Beef Chow Fun

☯   ☯

*W*hen I grow too old to make it to the kitchen, this is the supper I want brought to my room on a tray.

1 pound flank steak, partially frozen

The Marinade
2 teaspoons cornstarch
1 tablespoon Chinese yellow rice wine or sake
2 tablespoons mushroom soy sauce

The Cooking Oil
2 tablespoons peanut oil

The Vegetables
1 sweet onion, rings separated and cut into 1-inch squares
1 cup fresh green beans, blanched, or frozen baby green beans, thawed

The Fresh Seasonings
3 garlic cloves, crushed and minced
3 quarter-size coins of peeled fresh ginger, crushed and minced

The Liquid Seasonings
3 tablespoons oyster sauce
3 tablespoons canned beef broth
1 teaspoon toasted sesame oil

The Noodles
1 12-ounce package fresh rice noodle sheets, cut into $1/2$-inch ribbons and separated
$1/4$ teaspoon liquid smoke

Slice the flank steak against the grain into $1/8$-inch strips. Rub the marinade into the meat and set aside for at least 30 minutes.

Heat the wok. Add the oil and heat. When hot, stir-fry the onion over high heat until it picks up flecks of char and is softened but not limp. Remove to a bowl with a slotted spoon. In the remaining oil, stir-fry the beans, garlic, and ginger briefly and remove to the bowl of onion. Stir-fry the beef for only a couple of minutes, tossing constantly while adding the oyster sauce, beef broth, and sesame oil. Lift the meat on top of the hot vegetables with tongs and quickly add the noodles to the pan juices. Stir and toss the noodles, keeping the heat high. Add the liquid smoke and a splash of broth or water, creating a little puff of steam to soften the noodles. As soon as the noodles wilt down, stir the vegetables and meat back into the wok. Stir and toss until everything is piping hot and serve immediately.

✄ What makes this dish so tantalizing in a Chinese restaurant is the mysteriously smoky flavor that results from wok *hei*—the licking of the flame over the sides of the wok. Adding the Liquid Smoke is the best I can do, but it really does heighten the appeal of *chow fun*.

Cold Soba Noodles

Icy cold noodles are very popular in the noodle shops of Japan, where they're served nested in baskets over bowls of ice. The nutty flavor of the buckwheat soba noodle seems just right for cool slurping and they're a refreshing side dish for skewers of meat or fish hot from the grill.

Cook the noodles according to the directions on page 159. Drain them well, cover, and chill thoroughly. Serve these noodles in a loose tangle with individual dipping bowls of sesame oil, mushroom soy sauce mixed with wasabi paste and a squeeze of lime, or dark soy sauce, rice vinegar, and judicious drops of toasted sesame oil. Pass a dish of chopped cilantro and another of slivered scallions.

When you see big, billowy bunches of flat-leaf spinach in the market, think of this dish. Broccoli is also good, and when you can find it, baby bok choy with slivered shiitakes is terrific. What *doesn't* work is a mélange of veggies of varying textures. It's the slithery quality of this dish that makes it pure comfort food.

Curried Tofu, Mushrooms, Peas, and Potatoes

Serves 4

Curried peas and potatoes are a familiar filling for Indian samosas—an ideal marriage. Adding meaty, sliced portobello mushrooms and golden-fried tofu cubes to this curry makes this a very satisfying vegetarian main dish.

2 cups peanut oil
1 10.5-ounce package firm tofu, cut into 1-inch cubes
3 tablespoons butter, or half butter, half safflower oil
3 garlic cloves, minced
3 quarter-size coins of peeled fresh ginger, minced
4 shallots, thinly sliced
1 large or 2 small portobello mushrooms, sliced
salt and pepper
2 teaspoons curry powder
1 cup unsweetened coconut milk
1/4 teaspoon grated lemon zest
8 baby new potatoes, steamed
1/2 cup frozen petite peas, thawed

Heat the oil in a wok to a temperature of 375° or use an electric fryer. Deep-fry the cubed tofu until crisp and golden. Set aside and reserve the oil for another use.

Heat the butter and sauté the garlic, ginger, and shallots until the shallots are soft. Add the sliced mushrooms, salt and pepper, and curry powder and stir-fry over medium-high heat until the mushrooms are soft. Pour in the coconut milk and bring it to a simmer.

Add the potatoes and the peas, and cook for 2 or 3 minutes until the sauce thickens. Taste and adjust the seasoning if required.

Curried Lamb with
☯ Mango and Kumquats ☯
Serves 4

*D*on't skip this recipe because you can't find kumquats. They're an interesting fillip but not a necessity—grated orange zest offers a similar flavor and aroma boost. It's just that I always look longingly at kumquats when I see a little basket of them in my market, sometimes even in summer. *Kumquat* means "golden orange" in Cantonese—where the kumquat is revered and given to friends to bring good fortune in the new year. The round ones are sweeter than the oval ones, but both can benefit from a half-minute of blanching in boiling water to soften the bitter edge. Plain rice is the best accompaniment here.

2 tablespoons butter
3 tablespoons minced shallots or onion
$^1/_2$ teaspoon peeled and grated ginger, with juice
$^3/_4$ teaspoon curry powder
$^3/_4$ cup chicken broth, homemade or canned
$^1/_4$ cup unsweetened coconut milk or heavy cream
2 tablespoons cornstarch
2 tablespoons rice flour or all-purpose flour
salt and pepper
8 loin lamb chops, 1$^1/_4$ inches thick, trimmed of all fat
1 tablespoon clarified butter *(ghee)*, or half oil, half butter
1 tablespoon fresh lime juice
1 ripe mango, cubed
2 kumquats, blanched and minced, or $^1/_2$ teaspoon grated
   orange zest
$^1/_4$ cup Coco-Peanut Crunch (page 33)

Heat the butter in a small nonstick skillet. Sauté the shallot and ginger until soft. Add the curry powder and cook for 1 minute. Increase the heat and drizzle in the broth, stirring continuously. Let the sauce reduce a bit. Add the coconut milk or cream and simmer to thicken slightly. The coating on the chops will thicken the curry sauce further.

Mix the cornstarch, flour, and salt and pepper. Dredge the chops in the seasoned mixture. Heat the butter in a large nonstick skillet and fry the chops about 4 minutes on each side. Test for doneness with the tip of a sharp knife; the lamb should be pink in the center. Add the curry sauce, lime juice, mango cubes, and kumquats or orange zest. Turn the lamb in the sauce several times, then serve topped with the Coco-Peanut Crunch.

Country Pork with Caramelized
☯ Shallots and Garlic   ☯

Serves 4

*M*y favorite cut of pork is country ribs because it tastes the closest to the wonderful Sunday pork roasts of my youth, when pork didn't shamelessly try to pass as "the other white meat." If you've tried Bronzed Shrimp with Jasmine Rice and have some leftover caramel sauce, you might like to try this adaptation of a Vietnamese classic, in which the garlic and shallots become buttery and glazed. These succulent caramel stews are tantalizing. Serve with plain crispy-bottom rice and a vinegary side salad of sliced cucumber and shredded carrot with a little pickled ginger.

salt and a generous amount of freshly ground black pepper
1¼ pounds boneless country ribs, trimmed and cut into chunks
⅓ cup Caramel Syrup (page 147)
¼ cup fish sauce (*nam pla* or *nuoc mam*)
juice of 1 lime
12 whole garlic cloves, peeled

12 whole shallots, peeled
2 fresh hot chiles, minced but not seeded, or ¹/₄ teaspoon
    dried red pepper flakes

Salt and pepper the meat and add all the other ingredients to a heavy, lidded casserole. Cover the pot and cook over low heat, stirring occasionally, until the pork is fork-tender, 45 minutes to 1 hour. Remove the meat and vegetables, increase the heat, and reduce the sauce to a shiny, syrupy glaze. Taste and add more caramel syrup or lime juice to balance the sweet and sour taste. Return the stew to the hot glaze and stir to coat.

✍ This recipe can also be made with half shrimp in their shells and half pork, in which case the shrimp are added at the end of the cooking time. Try it with chicken thighs, shallots, and whole baby carrots. Garnish with lots of chopped mint.

Green Chicken Curry with Grilled Eggplant
☯ ☯

Serves 4

*A*s you've heard before, there are as many curries as there are cooks, but we don't curry our food often enough to get beyond the familiar versions. Now it's even easier and faster to produce a decent Thai or Indian curry because the marketplace abounds with specialty products that take all the work out of it. Serve this curry with basmati or jasmine rice.

3 long, pale purple Asian eggplants, or 4 small Italian
    eggplants
2 tablespoons Chinese Seasoning Oil (page 23)
4 chicken thighs and 4 single breasts, boned and skinned
1 cup Thai unsweetened coconut milk
¹/₄ teaspoon grated lime zest, or a couple drops pure lime
    oil
2 tablespoons fish sauce (*nam pla* or *nuoc mam*)

2 tablespoons Thai green chile paste
2 teaspoons light brown sugar
16 large basil leaves
2 or more hot chiles, seeded and slivered (optional)

If grilling the eggplant, prepare the grill and wait for white-ash coals. If you have Asian eggplants, there's no need to peel them. Slice in half lengthwise and then again crosswise. If you're using the little Italian eggplants, peel them and cut them in lengthwise quarters. Brush the strips lightly with the oil and grill or broil them until they're fork-tender, about 5 minutes.

Cut the chicken into attractive chunks and put it in a wok. Add the coconut milk and bring the chicken and milk to a simmer, cooking it until the oil rises to the surface. Remove the cooked chicken to a bowl. Add the lime zest, fish sauce, chile paste, and brown sugar. Stir and mix until everything is well combined and continue simmering until the sauce is smooth. Taste for seasoning. Add the cooked chicken and simmer for another 10 minutes. Stir in the basil and chiles, and serve as soon as the curry is piping hot.

Coconut Salmon with
☯ Sesame Citrus Chips ☯

Serves 4

*S*ince I stumbled on these surprisingly delectable little citrus chips while working on the Crisp-Fry chapter, I've been trying to figure out how to share them with you without adding more work to the dish. This steamed salmon is the answer. There's nothing to fix *but* the citrus chips. Stir-fried sugar snap peas and rice vermicelli would be lovely accompaniments.

8 paper-thin slices of lime
4 paper-thin slices of lemon, seeds removed
4 paper-thin slices of navel orange
2 tablespoons cornstarch, sifted with 2 tablespoons rice
flour or all-purpose flour

1 tablespoon toasted sesame seeds
1–2 cups peanut oil
1½ pounds thick salmon fillets, skin removed
chile powder or cayenne pepper

As you slice the citrus, carefully lay the slices out on a paper towel to blot the surface. Mix the cornstarch and flour with the sesame seeds and spread it out on a saucer. Dip the citrus slices into the sesame mix on both sides, coating completely. Place them on a sheet of wax paper to dry a little.

Heat the oil in a wok or kettle fryer to 375°. Pick up the citrus pieces with tongs, redusting them a little, if needed. Lower them into the hot fat until they are golden and then remove them with a wire-mesh scoop. Lay them on a paper towel to drain. They need to be only warm to serve.

Cut the salmon into 4 serving pieces and place them in a glass or ceramic gratin or pie plate. Pour just enough coconut milk over the salmon to bring the level up to about ¼ inch. Cover the dish with plastic wrap and microwave on high for 5 minutes. Remove one side of the plastic wrap and spoon the milk up and over the fish once again. Test for doneness and return the fish to the microwave for another 2 to 3 minutes, if necessary. Do not overcook.

Sprinkle the salmon lightly with chile powder or cayenne, drizzle each serving with some of the coconut milk, and top with overlapping citrus chips.

10
Desserts

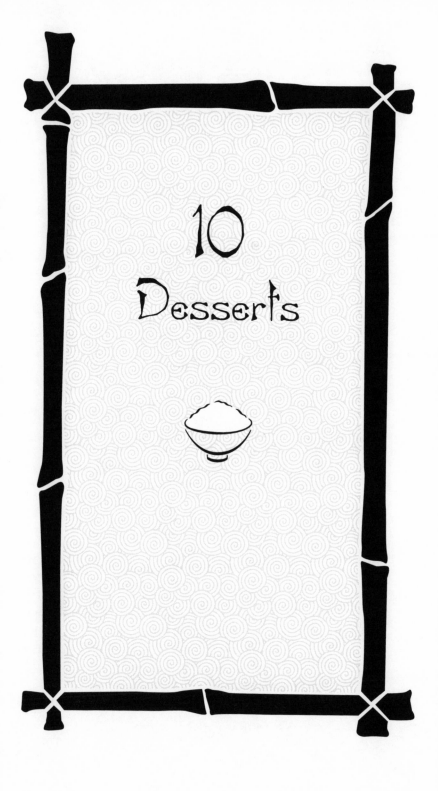

*H*ave you ever noticed what a poor dessert showing there is on Asian restaurant menus? That isn't because they don't *like* sweets. They simply don't eat them after dinner, preferring a bowl of chilled fruit, some crystallized ginger and honeyed nuts, or a few fennel or cardamom seeds to refresh the breath. Sweets are reserved for tea time or snacks.

However, should this book fulfill its purpose and make you comfortable with cooking Asian food, you might decide to share your talent at the wok and invite a friend or two over for dinner. What should you do about dessert? My own preference after spicy food is something very cold, light, and refreshing, which spells ice cream or sorbet, and perhaps a plate of the wonderful Asian cookies described in the Ingredients section. So here are a few simple dessert ideas for which you don't need recipes. They might set you to even more creative thinking.

Tempura Baby Bananas

Baby bananas from Central America are about 3 inches long and are very sweet and dry. Dip them in tempura batter and crisp-fry for about 1½ minutes or until golden. Pour a pool of caramel syrup on each dessert plate. Set the tempura bananas on top and garnish with mint sprigs. If you have some raspberry or mango puree in the freezer, either one would be as delicious as the caramel syrup.

☯ Green Tea Granita ☯

You'll find green tea ice cream and sorbet in Asian markets, where you'll also find a selection of tropical fruit sorbets that never reach regular stores. If you want to serve something interesting, select a boutique green tea at your specialty store, brew it properly, and sweeten it slightly. Let it cool and then freeze it in your ice cream maker or in a tray in your freezer until it's just slushy. Scoop it out into stemmed flutes and serve with lemon cookies. Republic of Tea, a specialty store brand, has tempting flavor choices such as Moroccan mint, cinnamon plum, and ginger ginseng.

Melon Balls with
☯ Ginger Cream ☯

No mystery here. Make whipped cream sweetened with confectioners' sugar, and beat in grated peeled ginger with the resulting juice to taste. If you don't want to scoop melon balls, just serve wedges and put a puff of the ginger cream into the melon cavity. If you prefer, finely mince some crystallized ginger and sprinkle it over the cream instead.

☯ Chow Mein Cookies ☯

This recipe is too silly for words, but pretty good. Buy a bag of Chun King chow mein noodles—the skinny curly ones—and a bag of real chocolate chips. Put the noodles in a bowl and melt the chips in the microwave. Pour the chocolate over the noodles and, with a pair of tongs, drop little mounds of them on a sheet of wax paper. If you want to get fancy, sprinkle the top with toasted coconut before the chocolate sets or add chopped macadamia nuts and chopped crystallized ginger to the mix.

Coco-Pineapple Frozen Yogurt

Buy vanilla frozen yogurt. Make a chunky pineapple puree with unsweetened canned crushed or fresh pineapple processed with a couple of tablespoons of frozen piña colada mix, and add a healthy splash of rum or not. If not, the pineapple might freeze. Put the yogurt in a bowl and let it soften just until you can make "roads" in it with a spoon. Swirl in the pineapple salsa and refreeze the yogurt. Serve with toasted coconut on top or just a sprig of mint.

Let's Hear It for Ben & Jerry

Caramelize slices of fresh pineapple in a nonstick skillet with brown sugar and dark rum—they won't get really sticky because there's too much liquid in the fruit, but the flavor will be terrific. Do them ahead and let them cool, reserving all the pan juices. Serve with a small scoop of Rainforest Crunch ice cream in the center and drizzle the pan juices over the top.

Ginger Pepper Jelly Sundae

Melt ginger pepper jelly in the microwave and pour it warm over honey ice cream. Stick a couple of waffle cookies in the top. Have you got any paper umbrellas?

Javanese Oranges ☯

Peel and thickly slice navel oranges and arrange them in an overlapping circle on each plate. Pour some caramel sauce over them and garnish with Coco-Peanut Crunch (page 33).

Cardamom Custard ☯

Make your favorite microwave custard or flan, flavored with a pinch of ground cardamom or almond extract. Serve with drained and chilled canned litchies and a couple of slices of kiwi fruit.

Almost Plain Mango ☯

Slice a mango on either side of the pit. Score each side to the skin diagonally with a sharp paring knife, then again in the opposite direction. Turn the halves inside out so the scored chunks pop up on top. Keeping the cupped shape, place them on plates and sprinkle with a tablespoon of coconut liqueur. Garnish with thin lime slices or chopped pistachios.

Malaysian Tropical Fruit ☯

Arrange a colorful and abundant centerpiece platter of colorful fruit such as pineapple, banana, papaya, mango, star fruit, and kiwi. Cover it with finely minced fresh mint and drizzle it with Malaysian ginger juice with honey, available in Asian markets, or minced preserved ginger with some of the syrup.

. . . and don't forget the fortune cookies.

Index